Syndrome of Nonverbal
Learning Disabilities

Syndrome of Nonverbal Learning Disabilities

Neurodevelopmental Manifestations

Edited by
BYRON P. ROURKE

THE GUILFORD PRESS / **New York London**

Last digit is print number: 9 8 7 6

Library of Congress Cataloging-in-Publication Data

Syndrome of nonverbal learning disabilities: neurodevelopmental
  manifestations / edited by Byron P. Rourke.
      p.   cm.
  Includes bibliographical references and index.
  ISBN 0-89862-155-0
  1. Learning disabilities—Physiological aspects. 2. Pediatric
neurology. 3. Learning disabilities—Pathophysiology. I. Rourke,
Byron P. (Byron Patrick), 1939–
  [DNLM: 1. Learning Disorders—etiology. 2. Nervous System
Diseases—in infancy & childhood. 3. Nervous System Diseases—
complications. 4. Abnormalities. 5. Neurologic Manifestations.
WS 110 1995]
RJ496.L4S96 1995
618.92'8588—dc20
DNLM/DLC   95-3981
for Library of Congress   CIP

Contributors

Peter E. Anderson, Department of Psychology, University of Windsor, Windsor, Ontario, Canada

Timothy P. Bohan, Departments of Neurology and Pediatrics, University of Texas Medical School at Houston, Houston, Texas

Michael E. Brandt, Departments of Psychiatry and Behavioral Sciences and Pediatrics, University of Texas Medical School at Houston, Houston, Texas

Bonnie L. Brookshire, Department of Pediatrics, University of Texas Medical School at Houston, Houston, Texas

Domenic V. Cicchetti, Department of Psychiatry and Yale Child Study Center, Yale University School of Medicine, New Haven, Connecticut

Kevin C. Davidson, Department of Psychology, University of Houston, Houston, Texas

Audrey Don, Department of Psychology, University of Windsor, Windsor, Ontario, Canada

Catherine B. Dool, Department of Psychology, University of Windsor, Windsor, Ontario, Canada

Linda Ewing-Cobbs, Department of Pediatrics, University of Texas Medical School at Houston, Houston, Texas

Jack M. Fletcher, Departments of Pediatrics and Neurosurgery, University of Texas Medical School at Houston, Houston, Texas

Katy B. Fuerst, Department of Psychology, University of Windsor, Windsor, Ontario, Canada

Ami Klin, Yale Child Study Center, Yale University School of Medicine, New Haven, Connecticut

Maxine Krengel, Department of Psychology, Boston Department of Veterans Affairs Medical Center, Boston, Massachusetts

Harvey S. Levin, Division of Neurosurgery, University of Maryland Medical System, Baltimore, Maryland

Erin M. Picard, Department of Psychology, University of Windsor, Windsor, Ontario, Canada

Byron P. Rourke, Department of Psychology, University of Windsor, Windsor, Ontario, Canada; Yale Child Study Center, Yale University School of Medicine, New Haven, Connecticut

Joanne Rovet, Psychology Department, Hospital for Sick Children, Toronto, Ontario, Canada

Lisa A. Smith, Department of Psychology, University of Windsor, Windsor, Ontario, Canada; Department of Psychology, Ottawa General Hospital, Ottawa, Ontario, Canada

Sara S. Sparrow, Yale Child Study Center, Yale University School of Medicine, New Haven, Connecticut

Katherine D. Tsatsanis, Department of Psychology, University of Windsor, Windsor, Ontario, Canada

Fred R. Volkmar, Yale Child Study Center, Yale University School of Medicine, New Haven, Connecticut

Roberta F. White, Department of Neurology and Environmental Health, Boston University School of Medicine and Public Health, Boston, Massachusetts; Department of Psychology and Boston Environmental Hazards Center, Boston Department of Veterans Affairs Medical Center, Boston, Massachusetts

Preface

This book was designed to address many important types of neurological disease, disorder, and dysfunction in children from a specific clinical/developmental and theoretical perspective. It is composed of chapters on a particular subset of pediatric neurological diseases and forms of dysfunction in which, to a greater or lesser extent, the syndrome of Nonverbal Learning Disabilities (NLD) is manifested. Throughout the work, emphasis is placed upon the relationships between the disease or disorder in question on the one hand, and the syndrome of NLD and the "white matter model" designed to account for its complex manifestations (Rourke, 1989) on the other.

To introduce these topics, the first chapter is devoted to an explication of the NLD syndrome and the white matter model; the second, to a discussion of white matter physiology and pathology. The third chapter details a specific form of neurological disorder, with particular attention paid to its white matter dimensions. These three chapters serve to introduce the reader to the discussions of pediatric neurological disease and disorder that follow. Two chapters toward the end of the work constitute attempts to extend the implications of the NLD syndrome and the white matter model to neurological disease in adults. An appendix contains the outline of an intervention program that we have found to be effective in the treatment of children and adolescents who exhibit NLD.

Throughout the book, our aim was to couch the best available research on the topics in question within the framework of the NLD syndrome and the white matter model, and to determine whether, to what extent, and under which sets of circumstances the syndrome and the model "fit" the disease or disorder in question. The results of this exercise are mirrored somewhat in the order of the table of contents—beginning with those diseases and forms of dysfunction in which the phenotypic manifestations of the NLD syndrome are seen most clearly, and moving to those in which these manifestations are less well defined and/or clouded by other types of neuropsychological dysfunction. The fruits of this pursuit are summarized in Chapter 18, which contains a more precise view of the developmental manifestations of the NLD syndrome and their relationships to the white matter model. (Indeed, the reader may wish to peruse Table 18.1 so that the context of this exercise may be more clearly appreciated.)

The contributions to this book could not have been written without the painstaking and insightful efforts of the researchers and theorists whose work is cited herein. For this, the authors are abundantly grateful. In addition, I wish to acknowledge, with considerable gratitude, the efforts of Marilyn F. Chedour, Katy B. Fuerst, and Katherine D. Tsatsanis, without whose expertise and tireless efforts this book would never have come to fruition.

BYRON P. ROURKE

REFERENCE

Rourke, B. P. (1989). *Nonverbal learning disabilities: The syndrome and the model.* New York: Guilford Press.

Contents

Introduction: The NLD Syndrome and the White Matter Model

Byron P. Rourke

This chapter contains a description of the characteristics and dynamics of the syndrome of Nonverbal Learning Disabilities (NLD) and the elements of the white matter model. These explications are presented in virtually the same manner as they were in Rourke (1989), because the 1989 version constituted the starting point and the standard used by the authors of this work for the comparisons effected in their chapters.

THE NLD SYNDROME: CHARACTERISTICS AND DYNAMICS

I begin with a description of the characteristics of the NLD syndrome, and then move to a brief explication of the dynamic interactions among and between the various levels of this syndrome's basic and derived manifestations. I turn then to a more specific discussion of these dynamics.

Summary of Characteristics

In this outline of the characteristics of the NLD syndrome, a clear, although minimally articulated, description of each of the dimensions (assets and deficits) in question is provided. To these are added statements regarding the developmental course of each. Within each major category,

The bulk of this chapter is reprinted, with minor modifications, from Rourke (1989, pp. 80–100, 111–118). Copyright 1989 by The Guilford Press. Reprinted by permission.

some notions regarding hypothesized interactional dynamics within and between categories are mentioned.

Two features of this description of NLD syndrome characteristics should be borne in mind:

1. Because of our focus on children and adolescents, manifestations of NLD in persons within these developmental stages are emphasized.

2. This description is couched in terms of the "developmental" manifestation of the NLD syndrome—that is, in terms of its characteristics in a child who has been so afflicted since his or her earliest developmental stages. Some modifications in the manifestations of the syndrome are necessary when we turn to considerations of the onset of the syndrome in an older child, adolescent, or adult who has enjoyed a normal early developmental course.

Note on Dynamics. The following summary of the assets and deficits of the NLD syndrome should be viewed within a specific context of cause-and-effect relationships; that is, the basic neuropsychological assets and deficits are thought to lead to the secondary neuropsychological assets and deficits, and so on, within the four categories of neuropsychological dimensions. Moreover, these assets and deficits are seen as causative vis-à-vis the academic and socioemotional/adaptive aspects of the syndrome. In this sense, the latter dimensions are, essentially, dependent variables (i.e., effects rather than causes) in the NLD syndrome. Figure 1.1, provided later, may be of some assistance in understanding the dynamics that are proposed to obtain in the NLD model.

Neuropsychological Assets

Primary Assets

Simple motor. Simple, repetitive motoric skills are generally intact, especially at older age levels (middle childhood and beyond).

Auditory perception. After a very early developmental period when such skills appear to be lagging, auditory-perceptual capacities become very well developed.

Rote material. Repetition and/or constancy of stimulus input—especially through the auditory modality, but not confined to it—is well appreciated. Repetitious motoric acts, including some aspects of speech and well-practiced skills such as handwriting, eventually develop to average or above-average levels.

Secondary Assets

Attention. Deployment of selective and sustained attention for simple, repetitive verbal material (especially that delivered through the auditory modality) becomes very well developed.

Tertiary Assets

Memory. Rote verbal memory and memory for material that is readily coded in a rote verbal fashion becomes extremely well developed.

Verbal Assets

Speech and language. Following an early developmental period when linguistic skills appear to be lagging, a number of such skills emerge and develop in a rapid fashion. Excellent phonemic hearing, segmentation, blending, and repetition and very well-developed receptive language skills and rote verbal capacities are evident, as are a large store of rote verbal material and verbal associations, and a very high volume of speech output. All of these characteristics tend to become more prominent with advancing years.

Academic Assets

Following initial problems with the visual–motor aspects of writing and much practice with a writing instrument, graphomotor skills (for words) reach good to excellent levels. Following initial problems with the development of the visual–spatial feature analysis skills necessary for reading, good to excellent single-word reading (decoding) skills are in evidence. Single-word spelling-to-dictation skills also develop to above-average levels. Misspellings are almost exclusively of the phonetically accurate variety. Verbatim memory for oral and written verbal material can be outstanding in the middle to late elementary school years and thereafter.

Neuropsychological Deficits

Primary Deficits

Tactile perception. Bilateral tactile-perceptual deficits are evident, usually more marked on the left side of the body. These deficits tend to become less prominent with advancing years.

Visual perception. There is impaired discrimination and recognition of visual detail and visual relationships, as well as outstanding deficiencies in visual–spatial–organizational abilities. Deficits in this area tend to increase with advancing years.

Complex psychomotor. Bilateral psychomotor coordination deficiencies are prominent; these are often more marked on the left side of the body. These deficits, except for well-practiced skills such as handwritting, tend to increase in severity with age.

Novel material. As long as stimulus configurations remain novel, they are dealt with very poorly and inappropriately. Difficulties in age-appropriate accommodation to, and a marked tendency toward overassimilation of, novel events increase with advancing years.

Secondary Deficits

Attention. Attention to tactile and visual input is poor. Deficiencies in visual attention tend to increase over the course of development, except for material that is programmatic and overlearned (e.g., printed text). Deployment of selective and sustained attention is much better for simple, repetitive verbal material (especially that delivered through the auditory modality) than for complex, novel nonverbal material (especially that delivered through the visual or haptic modalities). The disparity between attentional deployment capacities for these two sets of materials tends to increase with age.

Exploratory behavior. There is little physical exploration of any kind. This is the case even for objects that are immediately within reach and could be explored through visual or tactile means. A tendency toward sedentary and physically limited modes of functioning increases with age.

Tertiary Deficits

Memory. Memory for tactile and visual input is poor. Deficiencies in these areas tend to increase over the course of development, except for material that is programmatic and overlearned (e.g., spoken natural language). Memory for nonverbal material, whether presented through the auditory, visual, or tactile modalities, is poor if such material is not readily coded in a verbal fashion. Relatively poor memory for complex, meaningful, and/or novel verbal and nonverbal material is typical. Differences between good to excellent memory for rote material and impaired memory for complex material and/or that which is not readily coded in a verbal fashion tend to increase with age.

Concept formation, problem solving, strategy generation, and hypothesis testing; appreciation of informational feedback. Marked deficits in all of these areas are apparent, especially when the concept to be formed, the problem to be solved, and/or the problem-solving milieu are novel or complex. Also evident are significant difficulties in dealing with cause-and-effect relationships and marked deficiencies in the appreciation of incongruities (e.g., age-appropriate sensitivity to humor). Most noticeable as formal operational thought becomes a developmental demand (i.e., in late childhood and early adolescence), deficits in these areas tend to increase markedly with advancing years, as does the gap between performance on rote (overlearned) and novel tasks.

Verbal Deficits

Speech and language. Mildly deficient oral–motor praxis, little or no speech prosody, and much verbosity of a repetitive, straightforward, rote nature are characteristic. When paraphasic errors are in evidence, these are much more likely to be of the phonological than of the semantic variety. Also typical are content disorders of language, characterized by very poor psycholinguistic pragmatics (e.g., "cocktail party" speech) and reliance upon language as a principal means for social relating, information gathering, and relief from anxiety. All of these characteristics, except for oral–motor praxis difficulties, tend to become more prominent with advancing years.

Academic Deficits

Graphomotor. In the early school years, there is much difficulty with printing and cursive script; with much practice, handwriting most often becomes quite good.

Reading comprehension. Reading comprehension is much poorer than is single-word reading (decoding). Deficits in reading comprehension, especially for novel material, tend to increase with advancing years.

Mechanical arithmetic and mathematics. There are outstanding relative deficiencies in mechanical arithmetic as compared to proficiencies in reading (word recognition) and spelling. With advancing years, the gap between good to excellent single-word reading and spelling and deficient mechanical arithmetic performance widens. Absolute level of mechanical arithmetic performance only rarely exceeds the Grade 5 level; mathematical reasoning, as opposed to programmatic arithmetic calculation, remains poorly developed.

Science. Persistent difficulties in academic subjects involving problem solving and complex concept formation (e.g., physics) are prominent. The gap between deficiencies in this type of complex academic endeavor and other, more rote, programmatic academic pursuits widens with age.

Socioemotional/Adaptational Deficits

Adaptation in novel situations. There is extreme difficulty in adapting to (i.e., countenancing, organizing, analyzing, and synthesizing) novel and otherwise complex situations. An overreliance on prosaic, rote (and, in consequence, inappropriate) behaviors in such situations is common. These characteristics tend to become more prominent with advancing years.

Social competence. Significant deficits are apparent in social perception, social judgment, and social interaction skills; these deficits become more prominent as age increases. There is a marked tendency toward social withdrawal and even social isolation with advancing years.

Emotional disturbance. Often characterized during early childhood as afflicted with some type of acting-out or conduct disorder, such children are very much at risk for the development of "internalized" forms of psychopathology. Indications of excessive anxiety, depression, and associated internalized forms of socioemotional disturbance tend to increase with advancing years.

Activity level. Children who exhibit the syndrome are frequently perceived as hyperactive during early childhood. With advancing years, they tend to become normoactive and eventually hypoactive.

Summary of Dynamics

The principles relating to the dynamics that are inferred to be operative between the various levels and dimensions of the NLD model are presented schematically in Figure 1.1. More specific explications of these principles are given below.

Details of Characteristics and Dynamics

This section is designed to provide a fuller description of the characteristics of the NLD syndrome and to place them within the context of their developmental dynamics. It is structured in a manner that assumes that the reader will make reference to Figure 1.1 whenever necessary to follow the discussion.

Note on Terminology. In all of what follows in this section, I refer to the "developmental presentation" of the NLD syndrome, by which I mean the presentation that appears to have been evident at birth or shortly thereafter, and that is not complicated by subsequent neurological disease, disorder, or dysfunction. Although the same general principles—and especially the dynamics of the syndrome—hold for other children and adolescents who have experienced a normal course of development before suffering an untoward event (e.g., significant craniocerebral trauma) that eventuates in the NLD syndrome, there are important differences between the "developmental" and "other" presentations of the syndrome, the latter being due to neurological disease superimposed upon a normally developing brain. These differences are especially evident when we compare the neuropsychological presentations of children whose early months and years of cognitive development have been "normal" with those of children who have been affected adversely by the elements and dynamics of the NLD syndrome since a very early developmental stage.

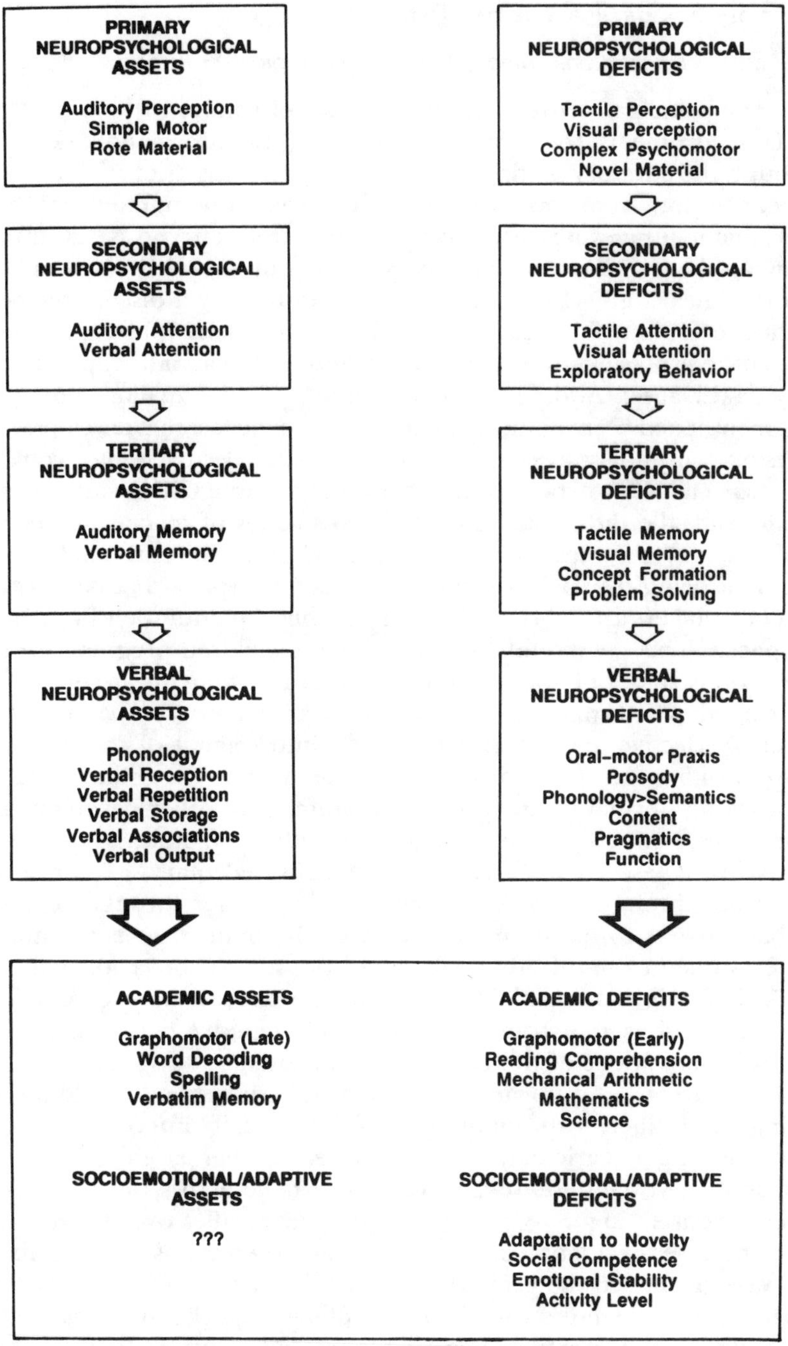

PRIMARY
NEUROPSYCHOLOGICAL
ASSETS

Auditory Perception
Simple Motor
Rote Material

SECONDARY
NEUROPSYCHOLOGICAL
ASSETS

Auditory Attention
Verbal Attention

TERTIARY
NEUROPSYCHOLOGICAL
ASSETS

Auditory Memory
Verbal Memory

VERBAL
NEUROPSYCHOLOGICAL
ASSETS

Phonology
Verbal Reception
Verbal Repetition
Verbal Storage
Verbal Associations
Verbal Output

PRIMARY
NEUROPSYCHOLOGICAL
DEFICITS

Tactile Perception
Visual Perception
Complex Psychomotor
Novel Material

SECONDARY
NEUROPSYCHOLOGICAL
DEFICITS

Tactile Attention
Visual Attention
Exploratory Behavior

TERTIARY
NEUROPSYCHOLOGICAL
DEFICITS

Tactile Memory
Visual Memory
Concept Formation
Problem Solving

VERBAL
NEUROPSYCHOLOGICAL
DEFICITS

Oral–motor Praxis
Prosody
Phonology>Semantics
Content
Pragmatics
Function

ACADEMIC ASSETS

Graphomotor (Late)
Word Decoding
Spelling
Verbatim Memory

ACADEMIC DEFICITS

Graphomotor (Early)
Reading Comprehension
Mechanical Arithmetic
Mathematics
Science

SOCIOEMOTIONAL/ADAPTIVE
ASSETS

???

SOCIOEMOTIONAL/ADAPTIVE
DEFICITS

Adaptation to Novelty
Social Competence
Emotional Stability
Activity Level

FIGURE 1.1. Elements and dynamics of the NLD syndrome.

Neuropsychological Assets and Deficits

Early Presentation: Primary Neuropsychological Skills and Abilities

The principal neuropsychological asset of children who exhibit the NLD syndrome is their capacity to deal with information delivered through the auditory modality. Virtually all other assets of such children appear to flow from this basic strength. It should be pointed out, however, that in infancy it is often suspected that children who are eventually shown to have a developmental presentation of the NLD syndrome are "hard of hearing." This impression is reinforced by a discernible delay in the acquisition of speech. (Fortunately, advances in evoked audiometry now make it possible to discern the integrity of the auditory apparatus at very tender ages). Adding to the seriousness of this situation during the first months and years of these children's lives is the fact that developmental milestones, including speech, are clearly delayed. Indeed, it is fairly common for such children to be scrutinized carefully during their early months of life, with the differential diagnostic possibilities of mental retardation, deafness, and/or severe (pervasive) emotional disturbance in mind.

This being the case, it should come as no surprise that parents and other caretakers are overjoyed when such children utter their first sounds of speech. This joy mounts thereafter as the children progress through the various stages of speech and language development at what seems to be an above-normal rate of speed. This is usually accompanied by the parents' selective and effusive positive reinforcement of this linguistic output, with a correlative disregard for the fact that the children are still not making normal progress in the attainment of other developmental milestones, especially those having to do with locomotor and manipulative skills. These children remain essentially sedentary, exploring the world not through vision or locomotion, but rather through receiving verbal answers to questions posed about the immediate environment. An example of the differences between the style of behavior exhibited by normally developing children and those with NLD may serve to illustrate the serious shortcomings in terms of cognitive development that the early limitations of the NLD syndrome entail.

Consider what a normal child entering toddlerhood would do in a sitting room filled with antiques and other visually interesting objects. The following scenario may very well ensue, once her parent is distracted: She spots a visually interesting vase on a table across the room from where she is sitting. She gets to her feet and toddles over to the table, feels the vase for a moment, picks it up, and then tosses it in the air. As the vase crashes to the ground, she hears her parent shriek, "My God! That's Aunt Gertrude's vase!" This is followed quickly by a swat across the child's nether portions and subsequent admonitions to avoid Aunt Gertrude's vase (and all others like it) in the future. Contrast this scenario with that which is likely to ensue when a child with NLD is involved in the same situation: Lounging with his parent in the sitting room, he sees the vase but makes no move to wend his way over to it. Rather, he asks his parent what it is. The reply comes immediately: "That's Aunt Gertrude's vase." He pays no further heed to the vase. Instead, he proceeds to ask more questions about objects in the room, and his parent responds with verbal information about them.

Let us consider what each of these children learns in this process. The "normal" child spots the interesting object, then mobilizes her locomotor resources to reach it. While so doing, she maintains her path to the object by periodically sighting it, and, when first encountering the object, she touches it. This is followed by lifting it and tossing it in the air and by the sounds of the object crashing to the floor, the rattle of its scattered bits to the four corners of the room, and her parent's plaintive cry. This is followed quickly by a feeling of pain and further verbal utterances by the parent. It is quite possible that this sequence of events has occasioned the following: elementary, though crucial, notions regarding means–ends relationships, and the sense of efficacy and confidence that mobilizing one's resources successfully to accomplish the end (examine the target object) can promote; the notion that the object remains constant in the face of perturbations of the retinal size of the light reflecting from it; the realization that the object has a smooth surface and that it has a mass that allows the child to lift it; some elementary notions of the interactions between aerodynamics and gravity as the object flies through the air; the realization that an object that is smooth and of this weight disintegrates when it encounters a relatively immovable object such as a wooden floor; the name of the object; the consequences of engaging in this type of activity; and further verbal labels and qualifiers for this activity and for the object involved therein.

In all of this, it should be noted that, for the normal child, the object was assigned a label (name) only *after* many of its physical features had been encountered, if not explored, in some detail. I would submit that for the child in late infancy and early toddlerhood, this is not only the most *common* manner in which many labels are assigned to objects, but also the *preferred* manner for this naming activity to transpire at this time. The prerequisities for this sequence of events, of course, are the neuropsychological dimensions of tactile and visual perception, complex psychomotor skills, and the capacity to deal with novelty. Deficits in all of these are thought to constitute the basis of the NLD syndrome.

Thus, when we turn to a consideration of the learning that has transpired for the NLD child regarding Aunt Gertrude's vase, we are presented with a very simple answer to our query—namely, that he has probably learned that the object is a "vase" and that it bears some relationship to "Aunt Gertrude." Nothing else.

Even within the context of this simple example at a relatively tender age, we can see the beginnings of the complex interactions that tend to transpire between and among the neuropsychological abilities and deficits of children with NLD. For example, it would appear quite likely that such children will become progressively less likely to engage in physical exploration of their environment, precisely because the patent auditory channel and its rapidly emerging receptive linguistic correlates provide information without the difficulties and large expenditures of energy attendant upon the engaging of deficient psychomotor skills for such purposes. Indeed, the more often and the more elaborate the parents' and other caretakers' verbal answers to these children's questions, the more likely it becomes that they will engage in sedentary rather than exploratory behaviors. This in turn reduces the opportunities for encountering truly novel stimuli, with consequent negative repercussions for an already diminished capacity to deal with such stimuli. In all of this, of course, it is clear that the reinforcement histories of such children would be expected to exacerbate or partially mollify some of these effects.

As a final consideration with respect to early presentations of basic neuropsychological skills and abilities, some note should be made regarding simple motor skills. It is a basic principle of the NLD syndrome and model that the reduction of novelty to familiarity and the invocation of the stereotypy that comes from sustained practice of simple motoric acts should lead to proficiency in them. Thus, it should come as no surprise that throughout this developmental process, particular skills such as graphomotor activities, although extremely difficult for the child initially, tend to be mastered to a considerable extent as a result of extensive practice. This mastery is a function of the repetitive nature of the task and the familiar nature of the surroundings within which it is to be executed.

Attention, Exploratory Behavior, and Memory

The patent auditory channel of the child with NLD, in concert with difficulties in dealing with visual and tactile signals, would be expected to increase the likelihood of good auditory attentional deployment and poor tactile and visual attentional deployment. In addition, it would be expected that, for the distance senses (audition and vision), the gap between "attention" within these modalities would tend to widen with advancing years.

Tactile perception is a special case. Little effort is required to engage this sensory modality; it can be developed within the proximate space of even a virtually immobile child; it can be "practiced" extensively by a child who is prone to engage in repetitive rote behavior. For all of these reasons, it is expected that children with NLD will eventually show few or no marked, "hard" signs of deficiencies in the tactile modality, including the capacity to deploy attention within this modality. Hence, although visual attention (and other skills and abilities that are dependent upon this rather basic processing level) would be expected to decline relative to age-appropriate norms, such would not be expected in the case of the "contact" sense of touch.

Exploratory behavior is expected to be quite deficient in terms of frequency and quality because of (1) the child's penchant for rote material, (2) a correlative avoidance of novelty (because of an inability to "handle" its information-processing demands), (3) problems in deploying complex psychomotor skills (e.g., climbing), and (4) a tendency to prefer the auditory over the visual modality for the processing of information. All of these features should conspire early in the child's life to limit exploration of the environment; thus, for example, it is expected that the child will come to prefer to *hear* about the environment rather than to *see* or to *touch* it.

It is a small step from the latter developmental point to expectations regarding relative proficiency in auditory (especially auditory–verbal) memory over visual memory. It should come as no surprise that several investigators have found that the auditory–verbal memory skills of children with NLD characteristics are superior to their visual memory skills (e.g., Fletcher, 1985). Similar results have been obtained recently in our own laboratory (Brandys & Rourke, 1991). The chain of events in the case of the child exhibiting NLD would seem to suggest very strongly that well-developed attention and memory for auditory stimuli, and poorly developed attention and memory for visual stimuli, follow a cause-and-effect sequence as follows: good or poor sensory-perceptual capacity → good or poor attentional deployment skills → good or poor memory. Furthermore, the interactions along this sequence are important; that is, it would be expected that, just as all biological organisms have a strong tendency to practice what they do well and to avoid what they do poorly, the very existence of a "strength" (auditory analysis) would be expected to interfere with the practice of a "weakness." In other words, within the perception → attention → memory sequence, it would appear quite probable that the rich will get richer and the poor poorer. It is only with a balance between and among these capacities that one would expect "normal" information-processing development to occur.

Concept Formation, Problem Solving, Strategy Generation, Hypothesis Testing, and Appreciation of Informational Feedback

The analysis, organization, and synthesis of information constitute the cognitive building blocks that lie at the basis of the ability to form and modify concepts, generate reasonable solutions to complex problems, apply these solutions in a testable fashion, and deal systematically with feedback regarding the acceptability of solutions to the problems. Another important basis for such activity is the capacity to tolerate and even relish novelty.

It should be remembered that classic studies of creative thinking (e.g., Hutchinson, 1949a, 1949b) have, without exception, pointed to the necessity of knowing (i.e., studying, examining, exploring, and remembering) all feasible aspects of the problem to be solved, if a creative solution is to be the outcome. Although Edison may have been off the mark somewhat in his estimates of the relative contributions of perspiration (99%) and inspiration (1%) to creativity, there is no doubt that the former is a prerequisite for the latter. And it is in the former activities that children with NLD are not prone to engage. Such engagement would require systematic, careful visual (and sometimes) tactile exploration of the evidence; perhaps complex psychomotor manipulation of the elements of the problem; a capacity for dealing with novel material; and memory for what one has seen during the exploration of the problem. These capacities are deficient in children with NLD and, in the developmental presentation of this syndrome, would be expected to have been deficient since their earliest days.

Previous references to Piaget's notions regarding the genesis of intelligent behavior are certainly relevant here. The "contributions" of the sensorimotor phase of development for the eventual attainment of formal operational thought are necessary to the series of events just proposed. The disabilities in concept formation and other forms of higher cognitive processes that are exhibited by children with NLD are seen as a fairly direct consequence of a failure to acquire these cognitive building blocks.

Speech and Language

In this formulation of the NLD syndrome, it is hypothesized that these children's speech and language assets are fairly direct reflections of their more basic neuropsychological assets, and that deficits in this area are similarly a reflection of more basic neuropsychological deficits.

Well-developed capacities for auditory perception, attention, and memory would seem to be excellent (and virtually sufficient) for the development of natural language in nonretarded persons who attain some even rather elementary enunciatory and word-finding skills. Thus, good phonemic hearing, segmentation, and blending capacities should lead to good to excellent verbal reception, verbal repetition, verbal storage, and verbal associative skills. These are characteristics of children with NLD that tend to develop to above-average, even extreme, degrees; such developments are accompanied by increasingly larger volumes of verbal output.

In these children's early years, oral–motor praxis problems are in evidence, though rarely severe or even moderate in degree. But, mild difficulties in the enunciation of complex, multisyllabic words tend to persist throughout development. These are inferred to be one reflection of a more general problem in praxis that persists over time.

More telling deficits evident in the linguistic performance of children with NLD include their problems in appropriate prosody and, more important, the sometimes grossly deficient content and pragmatics of their linguistic productions. The deficiencies in content and pragmatics are viewed as direct results of difficulties in concept formation and other higher-order cognitive skills. These in turn are inferred to be reflections of more basic neuropsychological deficiencies, as is the marked tendency to favor the phonological aspects of oral communication over its semantic content.

The end result of this pattern of linguistic deficits is poor "functional" language, a concept that is conveyed somewhat by the aforementioned deficiencies in linguistic pragmatics. It is included here because the means–ends relationships that language promotes in normal persons are notably absent from the spoken and written language of persons with NLD. This shortcoming is usually evident as a general and pervasive deficit touching virtually every aspect of their communicative behavior. It almost always appears to reflect a much more basic problem in appreciating the functional role that language can play in achieving one's goals.

Academic Assets and Deficits

After a rather slow start in kindergarten, Grade 1, and perhaps into Grade 2, children with NLD exhibit remarkable gains in single-word reading (decoding). It is not uncommon for such children to be rated on word decoding at the Grade 6 level when they are in Grade 3, at the Grade 9 level when they are in Grade 4, and at the Grade 11 level when they are in Grade 5. Indeed, beyond Grade 3, their word recognition skills are usually well in excess of their age-expected grade level.

An obvious question to pose here is this: Why are children who exhibit the NLD syndrome often thought to be "at risk" for reading disability when they are in kindergarten and Grade 1? The answer is quite straightforward. Although this is something of an oversimplification, there are two prerequisities for beginning reading: (1) the natural language capacity (language age) of a $5\frac{1}{2}$- to 6-year-old, and (2) the visual–spatial feature analysis skills of the average child of this age. In the case of children with NLD, the first prerequisite is usually attained by the chronological age of 4 years; however, the latter may not occur until they are almost 7. Once this is attained, the rapid development of their word-decoding skills becomes quite apparent and begins to match or even exceed their apparent language age.

It is quite common to find that even very experienced kindergarten teachers and school psychologists are convinced that their students with NLD are at risk for reading failure upon entry to kindergarten. This "diagnosis" is usually confirmed after several months of experience with the child. Most often, remedial techniques are applied to such children, in an effort to enhance their reading readiness skills. When they do, in fact, begin to read single words and then virtually skyrocket in this skill, there is the sense among their caretakers that this good to excellent performance in reading is a result of their interventions. Unfortunately for their egos, the same result would have occurred if they had virtually ignored the children—or tried yoga, or megavitamin therapy, or any other currently "hot" intervention technique that enjoys little or no empirical support for its efficacy. The fact of the matter is that children with NLD will read at least well, and probably at a superior level, regardless of what is done to help them. All they need to accomplish this is access to print and a marginally supportive educational milieu.

The spelling ability of these children follows a course similar to that exhibited in single-word reading; however, there is an added complication. In written spelling, rather than oral spelling, it is necessary to engage in graphomotor activity. Of course, this involves basic neuropsychological deficits exhibited by children with NLD in the areas of tactile-perceptual, visual-perceptual, and complex psychomotor skills. As already noted, these children's graphomotor skills are usually very poor during the primary grades of school. Often, such poor script—which is produced quite slowly and laboriously—is difficult for teachers and even for the children themselves to decipher. This situation would be expected to lead to an underestimate of the children's capacities in spelling during the early elementary school years. Once again, however, with the advent of the visual–spatial prerequisites noted earlier in connection with single-word reading, spelling performance begins to pick up. Smooth, coordinated handwriting may be seen as early as Grade 5 or 6, but in any case it will develop at some point.

It should be emphasized that graphomotor script becomes smooth and effortless even though it involves the most basic neuropsychological deficits included within this syndrome. This would appear to attest to the capacity of children with NLD to routinize this activity completely. As noted in the Rourke (1982) model, the capacity for such routinization and stereotypic application is thought to be a process for which left-hemisphere systems are particularly geared.

Another important dimension of these children's spelling performance is its fidelity to the phonetic composition of the words to be spelled. This is certainly a predictable attribute, in view of their basic neuropsychological assets in phonemic hearing, segmentation, and blending. Misspellings are almost exclusively of the phonetically accurate variety (e.g., "nacher" for nature; "okupie" for occupy). In fact, it is common to find that better than 95% of their misspelled syllables are rendered in a phonetically accurate manner. (See Sweeney & Rourke, 1978, for an explanation of our syllable-by-syllable system for assessing phonetic accuracy.) This rather high percentage becomes more than an idle curiosity when we see it in light of the fact that English is approximately 75% "regular" with respect to phoneme–grapheme correspondences. (This should be compared with virtually 100% phoneme–grapheme correspondences in Finnish.) It is also the case that normal adolescent and adult misspellings tend to be approximately 75% phonetically accurate. Taking these facts together, it becomes clear that English-speaking children and adolescents with NLD are "hyperphonetic" in the analysis of words to be spelled.

Other aspects of this tendency to accentuate the phonetic qualities of words (often to the detriment of their semantic content) can be seen in these children's tendency to make far more phonological than semantic paraphasic errors during sentence repetition tasks. It is as though, when given the opportunity to "choose" between the way words sound and what they mean, the former triumphs over the latter.

Mechanical arithmetic poses considerable difficulty for these children. The problems in evidence appear to reflect basic neuropsychological deficits in visual–spatial–organizational and psychomotor skills, appreciation for novel data, and the interrelated dimensions of concept formation, strategy generation, and hypothesis testing. Limitations in judgment and reasoning tend to predominate in the productions of older children with NLD; these would include their apparent failure to realize the inappropriateness of answers to arithmetic problems. Perseveration and failure to shift set in serial arithmetic problem solving would appear to reflect such difficulties, as do the related penchants for stereotyped, routinized, programmatic unfolding of behavior in any number of situations.

Rarely does the mechanical arithmetic prowess of these adolescents or adults exceed the Grade 5 to 6 level. Up until the Grade 2, 3, or even 4 level, it is sometimes not possible to see the emerging discrepancy between word recognition and spelling (high) and arithmetic (low), because of the nature of the arithmetic problems that are considered to be within the ken of the 7- to 8-year-old child. After this point and beyond, however, this discrepancy is easily discernible.

One particular proclivity of children and adolescents with NLD in mechanical arithmetic deserves further comment, because it bears upon subsequent discussions regarding frankly brain-damaged individuals. This is their marked tendency to "forget to remember." This phrase applies to individuals who have stored memories that would be applicable to a given situation, but who fail to realize that a particular time and place call for the particular stored material in question. Thus, it can usually be shown that 10-year-old children with NLD "know" how to "carry" and "borrow," but do not access these stored arithmetic rules when it would be appropriate to do so. This problem is easy to understand when we consider that normal people do not ordinarily commit to memory the *occasions* when particular memories need to be employed, but rather "trust" that their judgment at any particular time will be such that a decision to scan memory for the appropriate rule will be forthcoming. Note that this "trust" is probably a long-term consequence of the repeated assurances that ensue from efficacious problem solving in novel situations.

This interaction between memory/remembering and good and poor higher-order reasoning skills is analogous to the difference between skilled and unskilled mathematicians. The skilled mathematician would never dream of committing, say, the Pythagorean theorem to memory, but would instead "reason it through" when required to do so. Those who must commit the theorem to memory so as to regurgitate it when asked to do so are to be applauded for their verbal memory and the capacity to respond appropriately to the cue that calls forth this remembered material. What they may very well lack is the capacity to engage in elementary mathematical thinking. In this connection, it is often found that adolescents with NLD perform much better in secondary school mathematics courses than they did in elementary school arithmetic. This is so to the extent that the secondary school mathematics courses require verbatim memory for theorems, corollaries, and the like, as opposed to adaptive problem solving. When these adolescents turn to subjects such as physics, their difficulties in concept formation, problem solving, and hypothesis testing become very apparent. These deficiencies are compounded by their failure to benefit from informational feedback in such problem-solving situations.

Socioemotional/Adaptational Deficits

Like the academic deficits just described, the socioemotional difficulties of children with NLD appear to result from interactions among and between their neuropsychological assets and deficits. The following are some examples of such interactions:

1. Deficits in social judgment would appear to result from more basic problems in reasoning, concept formation, and the like, which also lie at the root of difficulties in mechanical arithmetic and scientific reasoning.

2. Difficulties in visual–spatial–organizational skills are reflected in problems in identifying and recognizing faces, expressions of emotion,

and other subtle nonverbal identifiers of important dimensions of human communication.

3. Lack of prosody, in conjunction with a high volume of verbal output, tends to encourage negative feedback from those who find themselves forced to listen to the seemingly endless recitation of dull, drab, colorless statements that these youngsters seem impelled to deliver. In a word, the type of speech and the language characteristics exhibited by such children tend to alienate them from others, thus increasing the probability that they will experience socioemotional/adaptational difficulties.

4. The tactile-perceptual and psychomotor prowess required for smooth affectional encounters, in conjunction with these children's typically inappropriate judgments regarding nonverbal cues, renders intimate encounters all but impossible.

5. Adaptability to novel interpersonal situations is the hallmark of socially appropriate individuals. The combination of aversion to novelty, failure sometimes even to appreciate that an event is in fact novel, and poor problem-solving and hypothesis-testing skills conspires to render spontaneous, smooth adaptation to the constantly changing milieux of social groups and the interactions nascent therein all but impossible for individuals with NLD.

The dynamics of the changes in activity level that are quite commonly seen in the developmental presentation of the NLD syndrome are relevant within this context. Typically, children with NLD are seen as hyperactive when they are 4 or 5 years of age. They are constantly getting in the way of others; they seem to be disinhibited; they bump into other persons and objects; and they persist in such behavior over protracted periods of time. These manifestations of the sensorimotor and other deficiencies of the NLD syndrome are often taken as indicators of the presence of hyperactivity and, presumably, an underlying attention deficit disorder as well. For this reason, methylphenidate is often prescribed for such youngsters. After a time in school, their behavior tends to "normalize" in terms of activity level, and they may no longer be medicated. Thereafter (usually during the middle of the elementary school years), it is noticed that they appear to be somewhat hypoactive.

This is, of course, another example of a situation wherein it would be easy to infer that the pharmacological agent and/or any other form of intervention employed (e.g., behavioral shaping) has been effective in the reduction of hyperactivity. The fact that the child reads and spells well after a course of such therapy also suggests that any underlying attentional deficit has also been "cured."

It must be pointed out, however, that the natural history of these children involves moving from apparent hyperactivity through normoactive behavior and then on to a hypoactive response style. This occurs largely, if not exclusively, as a result of the rebuffs and outright physical punishments that these children experience as a result of their failure to anticipate the consequences of their actions. Age-mates and adult caretakers tend to react very negatively to such shenanigans. And, since there is no reason to think that children with NLD are anhedonic, there is good reason to infer that the negative consequences of their behavior will eventuate in the reduction of activity level. Of course, a very unfortunate by-product of this reduction in activity level is an even further reduction in exploratory behavior, with the negative consequences that this can entail for the children's cognitive development.

These few examples should suffice to illustrate the main point of this discussion—namely, that socioemotional/adaptational deficiencies are, essentially, dependent variables in the NLD matrix. Like academic deficits, they arise out of a common mix of neuropsychological assets and deficits that all but insures that they will occur and grow in intensity with the passing of years. Unfortunately, the eventual social and personal outcome for those with NLD is almost never a pleasant one. Withdrawal, isolation, and loneliness are common.

THE WHITE MATTER MODEL

In order to expand the generalizability and explanatory potential of the Rourke (1982) right → left model, it was felt necessary to formulate an extension of this model that would focus on differences and interactions between white and grey matter in the brain. In so doing, an attempt was made to incorporate the down ↔ up and back ↔ front neurodevelopmental dimensions that were not considered in the Rourke (1982) model. The resulting expansion of the model, which I have titled the Rourke right ↔ left, down ↔ up, back ↔ front model (Rourke, 1987, 1988), would appear to be particularly helpful in the explication of the development of assets and deficits in at least one well-defined subtype of learning disability, NLD. At the same time, this extension was designed to encompass a relatively broad range of the neuropsychological dimensions of human development and their ramifications in aspects of personal, academic, and social functioning. A brief review of some of the salient features of the Goldberg and Costa (1981) and Rourke (1982) models would be helpful as an introduction to this new model.

Background

The Goldberg and Costa (1981) model is based primarily upon data gathered and speculations derived from investigations of human adults.

Its principal developmental dimension is its emphasis upon the progressive left-hemisphere lateralization of functions throughout the lifespan. The Rourke (1982) model was an attempt to expand the elements of this model to encompass early developmental phenomena, especially as these relate to the etiology, course, and persistence of central processing deficiencies in children.

In the Rourke (1982) model, special emphasis was afforded to formulations regarding children who exhibit outstandingly deficient mechanical arithmetic performance relative to word recognition and spelling performance (group A). Of particular importance in the present context is the fact that these children show virtually all of the characteristics of children with NLD. In the Rourke (1982) model it was emphasized that group A children exhibit deficiencies in intermodal integration, problem solving, and concept formation (especially in novel situations), and that they have profound difficulty in benefiting from experiences that do not mesh well with their only existing well-developed, overlearned descriptive system (i.e., natural language). In terms of the formulations of the Goldberg and Costa (1981) model, it was hypothesized that these children exhibit deficient right-hemisphere capacities within a context of well-developed, modality-specific, intramodal, routinized, and stereotyped left-hemisphere skills.

It was emphasized that the deficiencies shown by these children in tactile-perceptual, visual–spatial, visual-perceptual, and psychomotor capacities (deficits that are assumed to have been present from their earliest years) within a context of adequate auditory-perceptual and (eventually) verbal expressive capacities, would be expected to alter substantially the normal course of their development of sensorimotor skills. In turn, it was thought probable that this state of affairs would contribute to considerable developmental deviation in their acquisition of cognitive skills. Specifically, it was thought that their problems in establishing cause-and-effect relationships on a physical, concrete basis during infancy and early childhood would be expected to limit their capacity to develop more abstract levels of thought. Furthermore, this constellation of deficiencies was viewed as causative vis-à-vis the academic and social learning disabilities that these children eventually develop. The dynamics of the NLD syndrome outlined above constitute, essentially, a systematic expansion of the interplay of these features first proposed in the 1982 model.

As an explanation for this state of affairs, it was hypothesized that such children could have deficient right-hemisphere systems and/or insufficient access to initially intact right-hemisphere systems. This level of model development was felt to be sufficient to account for the differences that were evident in the neurodevelopmental course and neuropsychological profiles of the group A youngster (i.e., one manifestation of the NLD syndrome), as compared to those who exhibited other patterns of central processing abilities and deficits.

What follows is an extension of the Goldberg and Costa (1981) and Rourke (1982) models to account for the specific aspects of early and subsequent neuropsychological development within those domains that are thought to characterize *all* children who exhibit the NLD syndrome.

Main Theoretical Principles and Deductions

The primary theoretical principles upon which an explanation of the phenomena of NLD in children appear to rest are as follows, couched in terms of three principal dimensions of the NLD model: amount of destruction/dysfunction; developmental stage of destruction/dysfunction; development and maintenance of learned behavior.

1. *Amount of white matter destroyed or dysfunctional.* In general, the more white matter (relative to total brain mass) that is lesioned, removed, or dysfunctional, the more likely it is that the NLD syndrome will be in evidence. (This is reminiscent of the "mass action" hypothesis of Lashley, 1938.)

2. *Type and developmental stage of destruction or dysfunction.* Which white matter is lesioned, removed, or dysfunctional and at which stage of development this occurs have an important bearing on the manifestations of the NLD syndrome. (This formulation is in clear contradistinction to Lashley's [1938] notion of strict equipotentiality.)

3. *Development and maintenance of learned behavior.* Right-hemisphere white matter is crucial for the *development* and *maintenance* of its specific functions, such as intermodal integration, especially when novel information-processing situations are encountered. For example, significant destruction or permanent disruption of right-hemisphere white matter would be expected to pose a permanent handicap to the acquisition of new descriptive systems at any developmental stage.

Left-hemisphere white matter is essential for the *development* but not necessarily the *maintenance* of its specific penchants. For example, isolable linguistic skills are often found to remain intact after significant damage to the left cerebral hemisphere in adults. In terms of the model under consideration, once natural language is acquired and automatized, specific functions presumably subserved by the prominent opercula of the left hemisphere would be expected to be relatively impervious to destruction or permanent disruption of white matter not immediately adjacent to and/or forming an integral part of the functioning of these opercula.

However, it would be expected that significant disruption of white matter within the left hemisphere during early ontogenetic stages would hamper or even prevent the development of language in the child.

These theoretical principles lead to the following deductions:

1. *Sufficiency.* A significant lesion confined to the right cerebral hemisphere may constitute a *sufficient* condition for the production of the NLD syndrome.

2. *Necessity.* The *necessary* (and "dose-sensitive") condition for the production of the NLD syndrome is the destruction or dysfunction of white matter that is required for intermodal integration. For example, a significant reduction of callosal fibers or any other neuropathological state that interferes substantially with "access" to right-hemisphere systems—and thus to those systems that are necessary for intermodal integration—would be expected to eventuate in the NLD syndrome.

White Matter

At this point it would be well to describe briefly the three principal types of white matter fibers in the brain. In the following, a designation regarding the three principal axes of neurodevelopment is employed for each type of white matter:

1. *Commissural fibers (right ↔ left).* These nerve fibers cross the midline and interconnect similar regions in the two cerebral hemispheres. There are three sets of such fibers: the corpus callosum, made up of fibers that radiate to interconnect the left and right homologous regions of the frontal, parietal, temporal, and occipital lobes; the anterior, posterior, and habenular commissures; and the hippocampal commissural fibers, of which there are very few in humans. By far the largest set of these fibers is that which constitutes the corpus callosum.

2. *Association fibers (back ↔ front).* These are fibers that interconnect cortical regions of the same cerebral hemisphere. They are classified as short association or arcuate fibers, connecting adjacent convolutions within the hemisphere, and long association fibers, connecting cortical regions of the different lobes within the same hemisphere.

3. *Projection fibers (up ↔ down).* These fibers project from the diencephalon to the cerebral hemispheres and from the hemispheres to the diencephalon, the brain stem, and the spinal cord. The internal capsule, which handles the "input–output" of the hemispheres, contains projection fibers.

All of these fibers, of course, can be destroyed or rendered dysfunctional by various sorts of neurological disease; however, there are some observations that should be made at this point regarding the *probability* of destruction or disorder within these various types of white matter. First, it is clear that general white matter disease would be expected, by definition, to affect all three types of white matter, with consequent negative impact on all three of the principal axes of neural development.

Second, conditions such as hydrocephalus would be expected to have their principal effects upon commissural (right ↔ left) and projection (down ↔ up) fibers, leaving associational (back ↔ front) fibers relatively intact.

Third, a disease that affects the callosal fibers would be expected to interfere with right-hemisphere ↔ left-hemisphere "communication." Such a disease would be expected to have a more profound effect upon the functioning of the right hemisphere than the left, because of the right hemisphere's greater "dependence" upon white matter functioning, especially with regard to its apparent "specialization" for the intermodal integration of novel stimuli. On the other hand, left-hemisphere systems, many of which are relatively "encapsulated" within the three major opercular (grey matter and short association fibers), may maintain enough stimulation within and between each other that some fairly sophisticated intramodal integrations can proceed with little or no input from the right cerebral hemisphere. The upshot of all of this is that left-hemisphere systems are probably able to function reasonably well in the face of callosal and projection fiber damage, so long as association fibers are intact. Even in the latter instance, however, intact associational fibers would appear to be necessary for the *development* but not for the *maintenance* of left-hemisphere functioning.

One deduction that can be made from this state of affairs is that one would expect to see the principal (primary, secondary, and tertiary) neuropsychological features of the NLD syndrome *plus* global linguistic deficiencies (as in autism) only if there is early associational fiber disease within the left cerebral hemisphere *plus* white matter disease that affects intermodal integration. Associational fiber destruction, disorder, or dysfunction in the left hemisphere *after* natural language has been acquired should lead to aphasia (of the conduction or similar varieties) but not to autism.

It was my expectation that close clinical neuropsychological monitoring of children and adolescents with the various types of neurological disease, disorder, and dysfunction referred to here would eventuate in profiles characterized as being typical of the child with NLD. Investigation of children and adolescents with neuropsychiatric disorders, the published accounts of which bear a striking resemblance to the manifestations of the NLD syndrome (e.g., those who exhibit Asperger syndrome, alexithymia, and/or inadequate/immature types of delinquency), were expected to yield similar findings. In addition, it was my expectation that, in the future, studies employing sophisticated neural imaging techniques that are capable of assessing metabolic changes during central processing tasks would eventually demonstrate that the white matter versus grey matter relationships suggested in this model were causative with respect to the NLD syndrome.

General Developmental Implications

Integrity of function in white matter (long myelinated fibers) would appear to be necessary for the *development* of systems within both hemi-spheres, and crucial for both the *development* and the *maintenance* of those functions subserved primarily by systems within the right-hemispheral systems, but not necessary for the *maintenance* of some functions sub-served primarily by systems within the left hemisphere.

The NLD syndrome would be expected to develop under any set of circumstances that interferes significantly with the functioning of right-hemisphere systems, as in the case of any general deterioration of white matter or with substantial destruction of white matter within the right hemisphere, and/or access to neuronal intercommunication with these systems, as in the case of callosal agenesis.

Furthermore, the likelihood that the NLD syndrome will be mani-fested is increased by any neurological disease that has the effect of "isolating"—from each other and/or from right-hemisphere systems—one or more of the three prominent opercula of the left hemisphere that play a crucial role in its essentially intramodal functions of routinization and stereotypic application of previously acquired descriptive systems (e.g., natural language). Such a scenario would effectively handicap the affected individuals in the acquisition of new descriptive systems, and would increase the likelihood that they would apply previously acquired descriptive systems in a rigid, stereotyped, perseverative fashion within situations where such application is not necessarily adaptive. The set of phenomena associated with normal aging may be one example of such a state of affairs; symptoms associated with advanced stages of any num-ber of demyelinating diseases may be another. It should be noted that, for both of these examples, a *general* deterioration in white matter, rather than a *specific* deterioration of left-hemisphere white matter, would be expected to be the rule rather than the exception.

In any case, the loss of the capacity to generate new descriptive systems helps to explain the essentially downward course over successive developmental epochs that is observed in individuals who manifest the NLD syndrome. Considering the entire developmental course of this syndrome, it would seem that it is less apparent at the age of 7 to 8 years (Ozols & Rourke, 1988, 1991) than at 10 to 14 years (Rourke & Finlayson, 1978; Rourke & Strang, 1978; Strang & Rourke, 1983), and that it becomes progressively more apparent (and more debilitating) as adulthood approaches (Rourke, Bakker, Fisk, & Strang, 1983, pp. 247–253; Rourke, Young, Strang, & Russell, 1986).

In connection with this last observation, it should be noted that formal operational thought (a feature of higher-order cognitive functioning that is notably deficient in older children and adolescents who manifest the NLD syndrome) is not within the developmental capacities of the 7- to 8-year-old child. Since it becomes a developmental task/demand as the child approaches puberty—and, of course, increases in adaptive importance as the individual progresses through adolescence and into adulthood—it should come as no surprise that progressive deterioration in skills associated with such capacities (e.g., socioemotional adaptation) is the rule rather than the exception. Evidence of such deterioration is apparent in the cross-sectional and longitudinal studies of such individuals cited earlier in Rourke (1989).

FINAL COMMENTS

The descriptions of the NLD syndrome and the white matter model presented above are those that the authors in this work were asked to employ in their presentations. In addition to considerations regarding such issues as etiology, course, and prognosis, each author was asked to present the set of neuropsychological assets and deficits that constitutes the phenotype for the disorder in question. Of course, because of limitations regarding available literature and less than comprehensive neuropsychological analyses of some of these disorders, a phenotype complete enough to make comprehensive comparisons with the NLD syndrome was not always possible. Furthermore, the neurological disease, disorder, or dysfunction in question often involves a developmental course wherein the phenotypic manifestations change in a substantive fashion. Of course, this is to be expected, and was anticipated in the tenets of the NLD syndrome and the white matter model (see above).

Finally, it should be emphasized that the syndrome and the model employed by the authors in this work appeared first in 1987 and was last revised in 1989. In the interim, it has become apparent that some dimensions of the model can be expanded upon and refined; this is especially the case with respect to the anterior–posterior gradient. These refinements are contained in Chapter 18. Other publications emanating from our own laboratory and that of others have also been important in model development (e.g., Casey & Rourke, 1992; Casey, Rourke, &

Picard, 1991; Fletcher et al., 1992; Harnadek & Rourke, 1994; Rourke, 1993; Rourke & Fisk, 1988, 1992; Rourke & Fuerst, 1991; Sparrow, 1993).

Chapter 2 presents a more detailed examination of white matter physiology and pathology.

REFERENCES

Brandys, C. F., & Rourke, B. P. (1991). Differential memory capacities in reading- and arithmetic-disabled children. In B. P. Rourke (Ed.), *Neuropsychological validation of learning disability subtypes* (pp. 73–96). New York: Guilford Press.

Casey, J. E., & Rourke, B. P. (1992). Disorders of somatosensory perception in children. In I. Rapin & S. J. Segalowitz (Eds.), *Handbook of neuropsychology: Vol. 6. Child neuropsychology* (pp. 477–494). Amsterdam: Elsevier.

Casey, J. E., Rourke, B. P., & Picard, E. M. (1991). Syndrome of nonverbal learning disabilities: Age differences in neuropsychological, academic, and socioemotional functioning. *Development and Psychopathology, 3*, 329–345.

Fletcher, J. M. (1985). External validation of learning disability typologies. In B. P. Rourke (Ed.), *Neuropsychology of learning disabilities: Essentials of subtype analysis* (pp. 187–211). New York: Guilford Press.

Fletcher, J. M., Bohan, T. P., Brandt, M. E., Brookshire, B. L., Beaver, S. R., Francis, D. J., Davidson, K. C., Thompson, N. M., & Miner, M. E. (1992). Cerebral white matter and cognition in hydrocephalic children. *Archives of Neurology, 49*, 818–825.

Goldberg, E., & Costa, L. D. (1981). Hemisphere differences in the acquisition and use of asymmetries in the brain. *Brain and Language, 14*, 144–173.

Harnadek, M. C. S., & Rourke, B. P. (1994). Principal identifying features of the syndrome of nonverbal learning disabilities in children. *Journal of Learning Disabilities, 27*, 144–154.

Hutchinson, E. D. (1949a). The nature of insight. In P. Mullahy (Ed.), *A study of interpersonal relations: New contributions to psychiatry* (pp. 421–445). New York: Grove Press.

Hutchinson, E. D. (1949b). The period of frustration in creative endeavor. In P. Mullahy (Ed.), *A study of interpersonal relations: New contributions to psychiatry* (pp. 404–420). New York: Grove Press.

Lashley, K. S. (1938). Factors limiting recovery after central nervous system lesions. *Journal of Nervous and Mental Disease, 88*, 733–755.

Ozols, E. J., & Rourke, B. P. (1988). Characteristics of young learning-disabled children classified according to patterns of academic achievement: Auditory-perceptual and visual-perceptual abilities. *Journal of Clinical Child Psychology, 17*, 44–52.

Ozols, E. J., & Rourke, B. P. (1991). Classification of young learning-disabled children according to patterns of academic achievement: Validity studies. In B. P. Rourke (Ed.), *Neuropsychological validation of learning disability subtypes* (pp. 97–123). New York: Guilford Press.

Rourke, B. P. (1982). Central processing deficiencies in children: Toward a developmental neuropsychological model. *Journal of Clinical Neuropsychology, 4*, 1–18.

Rourke, B. P. (1987). Syndrome of nonverbal learning disabilities: The final common pathway of white-matter disease/dysfunction? *The Clinical Neuropsychologist, 1*, 209–234.

Rourke, B. P. (1988). The syndrome of nonverbal learning disabilities: Developmental manifestations in neurological disease, disorder, and dysfunction. *The Clinical Neuropsychologist, 2*, 293–330.

Rourke, B. P. (1989). *Nonverbal learning disabilities: The syndrome and the model.* New York: Guilford Press.

Rourke, B. P. (1993). Arithmetic disabilities, specific and otherwise. *Journal of Learning Disabilities, 26*, 214–226.

Rourke, B. P., Bakker, D. J., Fisk, J. L., & Strang, J. D. (1983). *Child neuropsychology: An introduction to theory, research, and clinical practice.* New York: Guilford Press.

Rourke, B. P., & Finlayson, M. A. J. (1978). Neuropsychological significance of variations in patterns of academic performance: Verbal and visual–spatial abilities. *Journal of Abnormal Child Psychology, 6*, 121–133.

Rourke, B. P., & Fisk, J. L. (1988). Subtypes of learning-disabled children: Implications for a neurodevelopmental model of differential hemispheric processing. In D. L. Molfese & S. J. Segalowitz (Eds.), *Brain lateralization in children: Developmental implications* (pp. 547–565). New York: Guilford Press.

Rourke, B. P., & Fisk, J. L. (1992). Adult presentations of learning disabilities. In R. F. White (Ed.), *Clinical syndromes in adult neuropsychology: The practitioner's handbook* (pp. 451–473). Amsterdam: Elsevier.

Rourke, B. P., & Fuerst, D. R. (1991). *Learning disabilities and psychosocial functioning: A neuropsychological perspective.* New York: Guilford Press.

Rourke, B. P., & Strang, J. D. (1978). Neuropsychological significance of variations in patterns of academic performance: Motor, psychomotor, and tactile-perceptual abilities. *Journal of Pediatric Psychology, 3*, 62–66.

Rourke, B. P., Young, G. C., Strang, J. D., & Russell, D. L. (1986). Adult outcomes of childhood central processing deficiencies. In I. Grant & K. M. Adams (Eds.), *Neuropsychological assessment of neuropsychiatric disorders* (pp. 244–267). New York: Oxford University Press

Sparrow, S. S. (1993). Asperger's syndrome and Nonverbal Learning Disabilities syndrome: Developmental and clinical aspects. *Journal of Clinical and Experimental Neuropsychology, 15*, 41.

Strang, J. D., & Rourke, B. P. (1983). Concept-formation/non-verbal reasoning abilities of children who exhibit specific academic problems with arithmetic. *Journal of Clinical Child Psychology, 12*, 33–39.

Sweeney, J. E., & Rourke, B. P. (1978). Neuropsychological significance of phonetically accurate and phonetically inaccurate spelling errors in younger and older retarded spellers. *Brain and Language, 6*, 212–225.

2

White Matter Physiology and Pathology

Katy B. Fuerst
Byron P. Rourke

The purpose of this chapter is to familiarize the reader with the basic composition and arrangement of the major white matter fiber tracts in the brain. The progression of myelination in the developing brain is also presented, followed by a general discussion of the structure and function of myelin. The global effects of major classes of white matter pathogens during embryogenesis are illustrated through a discussion of hormonal and teratogenic influences. A brief presentation of the classification of white matter diseases provides a context for the following chapters, which discuss many of these diseases and syndromes in detail. To complete this lifespan perspective, the effects of aging on white matter, both in the healthy elderly and in dementia patients, are touched on.

TYPES OF WHITE MATTER FIBERS

The two cerebral hemispheres of the human brain are made up of the convoluted grey cortex, the underlying white matter, and the deep nuclei known collectively as the basal ganglia. The large mass of white matter in the cerebral hemispheres extends from the cortex to the subcortical nuclei and the ventricular system. The most central region is often referred to as the centrum semiovale, because of its oval appearance in horizontal slices of the brain. Cerebral white matter consists of three major types of fibers: (1) commissural or "right–left" fibers, (2) association or "back–front" fibers, and (3) projection or "up–down" fibers.

Commissural Fibers

Commissural fibers connect corresponding cortical regions of the two hemispheres in a reciprocal fashion. In humans, these fibers are arranged into two principal bundles—namely, the corpus callosum and the anterior commissure (Carpenter, 1985). The corpus callosum is a large band of myelinated fibers that forms both the floor of the hemispheric fissure and much of the roof of the lateral ventricles. As the fibers exit the dense medial region, they fan out in a large callosal radiation to interconnect gross regions of the cortex in all lobes with homologous contralateral regions. Beginning anteriorly, the corpus callosum is subdivided into four parts: the rostrum, genu, body, and splenium. Fibers connecting anterior regions of the frontal lobes course through the genu, while fibers from the posterior parts of the frontal lobes and the parietal lobes form the body of the corpus callosum. The splenium contains fibers that interconnect regions of the temporal and occipital lobes.

The anterior commissure is a small but dense bundle of myelinated fibers that crosses the midline rostral to the columns of the fornix. Although not discernible on gross inspection, this structure comprises two parts. A small anterior portion of the commissure connects the two olfactory bulbs, while the larger posterior part interconnects regions of the middle and inferior temporal gyri. The two cerebral hemispheres are also interconnected by two smaller fiber bundles, the posterior and habenular commissures, and occasionally through hippocampal commissural fibers.

Association Fibers

Association fibers interconnect various cortical regions of the same hemisphere and can be divided into short and long types. Short association fibers traverse the floor of each sulcus, forming arches that connect cells in adjacent gyri. These fibers are aligned perpendicular to the long axis of the sulci. Long association fibers connect intrahemispheric cortical regions in different lobes, forming three main fiber bundles: the cingulum, the uncinate fasciculus, and the arcuate fasciculus. The primary bundle of association fibers, the cingulum, is located in the white matter of the cingulate gyrus on the medial aspect of the hemisphere. Its fibers interconnect regions of the frontal and parietal lobes with parahippocampal and temporal areas. The uncinate fasciculus, located beneath the insular cortex, connects the orbital frontal gyri with anterior portions of the temporal lobe. One deeply situated portion of this fasciculus, the inferior occipitofrontal fasciculus, is thought to connect the frontal and occipital lobes. The arcuate fasciculus courses around the insula to connect the superior and middle frontal gyri with regions of the temporal lobe. A superior portion of this bundle, the superior longitudinal fasciculus, extends caudally into parietal and occipital regions.

Projection Fibers

Projection fibers carry signals in both directions between the cortex and distant loci. Afferent and efferent cortical fibers enter the cerebral hemisphere in a radial fashion, forming the corona radiata, and converge toward the brain stem into a compact bundle known as the internal capsule. Horizontal sections reveal anterior and posterior limbs of the internal capsule. The anterior limb partially separates the caudate nucleus and the putamen of the corpus striatum. The posterior limb traverses between the thalamus and the lentiform nucleus of the corpus striatum. Fibers in the caudal portion of the posterior limb form the optic radiation. Afferent fibers in the internal capsule are primarily thalamo-cortical radiations, originating in the thalamus and projecting to diverse cortical regions. Efferent (corticofugal) fibers emanate from deep layers of various cortical regions and project to nuclei in the brain stem and spinal cord.

MYELINATION

The myelination of white matter in the developing brain is significant because it facilitates the transmission of neural impulses (Ritchie, 1984). The maturation of particular regions of the brain can be used to establish normal anatomical and functional developmental milestones. Myelination of the human brain begins during the fifth fetal month and proceeds rapidly during the first 2 years of postnatal life. Thereafter the process slows but continues well into adulthood, particularly in association areas of the brain. Histological studies have demonstrated that various fiber systems of the central nervous system (CNS) begin to myelinate at different points in development, and continue to do so at various speeds. Thus, rather than existing as a unitary process, myelination consists of series of temporally ordered sequences resulting in a hybrid of unmyelinated, partly myelinated, or completely myelinated tracts during early development. These cycles of myelination reflect the functional hierarchy of the developing nervous system (Yakovlev & Lecours, 1967).

Magnetic Resonance Imaging of Myelination

Until recently, it remained unclear how the progression of myelination determined through pathological studies was related to this process in normal and delayed development (Barkovich, Kjos, Jackson, & Norman, 1988). Recent advances in magnetic resonance imaging (MRI) have provided a means of studying the process of myelination *in vivo*; MRI now surpasses both computed tomography (CT) and ultrasound in contrast sensitivity. Changes in signal intensity on MRI of the developing brain correlate well anatomically and sequentially with Yakovlev and Lecours's (1967) classic histological demonstration of myelination (Barkovich et al., 1988; Martin et al., 1988). This suggests that myelin is a causal factor in the contrast observed between the grey matter, immature white matter, and myelinated white matter on MRI of the developing brain. There is also biochemical evidence favoring this supposition (Barkovitch, 1991).

Milestones of normal white matter maturation as demonstrated on MRI have been established for both T1 and T2 weighted images. At birth, the relative intensities of cerebral grey and white matter are reversed from the normal adult pattern. In the adult brain, white matter is hypointense relative to grey matter on T2 (long TR/TE [repetition time/echo time]) images, and hyperintense compared to grey matter on T1 (short TR/TE) images. Conversely, infant white matter is of high signal intensity with respect to grey matter on T2 images and of low signal intensity in comparison to grey matter on T1 images. Thus, white matter maturation, or myelination, appears as decreasing signal intensity on T2 weighted images and as increasing signal intensity on T1 images (Barkovitch, 1991). Changes in signal intensity caused by myelination are detected earlier on T1 weighted images than on T2 weighted images. Therefore, T1 weighted images are more sensitive to brain maturation during the first 6 months of life, whereas T2 weighted images are more accurate from 6 months of age onward.

Barkovich et al. (1988) have endeavored to explain this difference in the emergence of white matter maturation milestones between T1 and T2 weighted images. They have proposed that the earlier changes on the T1 images correspond to the accumulation of the precursors of myelin, such as cholesterol and glycolipids. As these compounds accumulate, there is an increase in bound water, and the resultant decrease in the amount of free water probably produces the changes seen on T1 images. On the other hand, the changes seen on T2 images correspond temporally to the actual formation of myelin and are probably related to the altered water distribution in mature myelin. The later emergence of white matter changes on the T2 weighted images also correlates more highly with the progression of myelination as demonstrated through histochemical studies (Yakovlev & Lecours, 1967; Barkovich et al., 1988). Therefore, in order to avoid duplication, only the sequence of myelination as detailed on T2 images is described here in detail.

The Progression of Myelination in the Developing Brain

In general, CNS myelination proceeds in an orderly fashion, beginning in the brain stem and progressing in a caudocranial temporal sequence, recapitulating phylogeny. Generally speaking, paleontologically older structures are myelinated prior to more recent structures. In addition, nervous system tracts typically become myelinated as they become functional (Valk & van der Knaap, 1989). Fiber systems mediating sensory input to the thalamus and cerebral cortex, located primarily in the brain stem, myelinate prior to systems that relate the sensory data to movement (Barkovich et al., 1988). Thus, the median longitudinal fasciculus, lateral and medial lemnisci, and inferior and superior cerebellar peduncles, which transmit vestibular, acoustic, tactile, and proprioceptive stimuli, are partially myelinated at birth. The ventral lateral region of the thalamus also begins to myelinate prenatally. Conversely, the middle cerebellar peduncles, which relay cerebral activities to the cerebellum, do not begin to myelinate until the second or third postnatal month and continue to do so more slowly. The same pattern holds true as myelination progresses in the cerebrum. During the first month of life, the somesthetic and propriokinesthetic sensory areas of the postcentral and precentral gyri begin to myelinate, whereas the posterior parietal and frontal areas, which integrate this information, acquire myelin later.

By approximately 2 months postnatally, myelination begins in the optic tracts and radiations, continuing posteriorly into the calcarine cortex by approximately 4 months. Myelination of the corpus callosum appears to progress in a posterior-to-anterior fashion, with white matter first evident in the splenium by 6 months and in the genu by 8 months. The corpus callosum appears uniformly myelinated by approximately 10 months of age. The internal capsule also acquires myelin from posterior to anterior, beginning with sensory tracts, followed by motor and then association tracts. The anterior portion of the posterior limb is partially myelinated by approximately 7 months and continues to acquire myelin through the ninth month. The anterior limb of the internal capsule is usually myelinated by the end of the 11th postnatal month. The majority of the deep white matter tracts are myelinated between 6 and 12 months of age.

The basal ganglia begin to myelinate at approximately 6 months and can be differentiated from the adjacent subcortical white matter of the centrum semiovale until approximately 10 months, when this area also acquires myelin. Other than the calcarine and pre- and postcentral areas, the subcortical white matter matures last. Here myelination begins during the 9th to 12th month in the occipital lobe and proceeds anteriorly to the frontal lobes. The majority of the deep frontal white matter is myelinated by approximately 14 months. Arborization of the white matter generally begins at 8 months of age, and continues until the extensive fine arborization is complete by approximately 8 to 24 months.

MYELIN

CNS white matter is made up of axons coursing to and from the grey matter of the cortex and other centers in the brain and spinal cord. White matter also contains two types of neuroglial cells, astrocytes and oligodendrocytes. Glial cells are thought to serve many structural, organizational, and nutritive functions, and may also be involved in neuronal repair and regeneration. However, they are best known for the role of oligodendrocytes in the production and maintenance of the myelin sheath surrounding CNS axons. Myelin, which constitutes the bulk of white matter in the CNS and imparts the characteristic white color, surrounds each axon.

Myelin plays a critical role in the insulation of axons and facilitation of impulse propagation by saltatory conduction. The speed of action potential propagation is functionally important to the efficiency of the nervous system. The conduction velocity of an axon can be increased either by an increase in its diameter or by myelination. Myelination is the better option, because it causes a much larger decrease in the axial resistance and capacitance of the axon than can be achieved through increases in diameter. Thus, conduction in myelinated axons is faster than conduction in unmyelinated axons of the same diameter. Demyelinating diseases result in the slowing or even blockage of action potential conduction, leading to a profound deterioration in the ability to control behavior. Unmyelinated sections of axon membrane, called nodes of Ranvier, are essential in the periodic boosts to the amplitude of the action potential, assuring its continuation along the entire length of the axon. The action potential seems to jump from node to node, because transmission is very fast through the myelinated internodes and slows considerably at the high-capacitance nodal regions; hence, the term "saltatory conduction" (Koester, 1985).

In the formation of the myelin sheath, a flat paddle-like extension from the oligodendrocyte wraps around a portion of a CNS axon in a spiral fashion. In mature myelin, there is cytoplasm remaining in these processes only in the paranodal region. The remainder of the sheath becomes a condensed mass of concentric layers of modified oligodendrocyte cell membrane. One oligodendrocyte is capable of forming up to 50 of these extensions simultaneously, each one insulating an internodal axon segment of as many different neurons. Thus, the destruction of even a single oligodendrocyte can result in significant demyelination (Valk & van der Knaap, 1989).

Myelin is a fatty substance with alternating protein–lipid–protein lamellae as the repeating subunit. The morphology of myelin is unique in comparison to other molecular bilayers, in that it has a very high lipid content and contains primarily very-long-chain saturated fatty acids. Whereas unsaturated fatty acid chains have a loose, unstable configuration, saturated lipids bind together very closely, creating a dense and steadfast structure. In addition, longer-chain fatty acids create a stronger membrane than short-chain fatty acids, because the longer hydrocarbon chain affords a better bond between the lipid molecules. It is also possible that the long-chain fatty acids of the lipid bimolecular leaflet somehow intertwine their hydrocarbon tails, increasing the integrity of the bond. In order to impinge on the inherent stability of the myelin membrane, many of the diseases affecting white matter do so by altering the composition of the lipids in the bilayer (Valk & van der Knaap, 1989).

Although the process of myelination unfolds with regularity, the nature of the stimulus initiating myelination remains unclear. It appears that the neuronal axons exert some influence over the proliferation, differentiation, and migration of oligodendrocytes, as well as the subsequent formation of the myelin sheath. For example, the diameter of the axon seems to play a role in the initiation of myelination, as well in the resultant thickness of the myelin sheath and the internodal length. An axon in the CNS destined to be myelinated begins to do so when it reaches a diameter of approximately 1 μm. With increasing fiber diameter, the internodal length is increased. In the peripheral nervous system (PNS), larger-diameter fibers have thicker myelin sheaths. Although this relationship has also been observed in the CNS, it is not entirely consistent (Raine, 1984). Impulse conduction is also believed to play an important role in the onset of myelination, as blocking nerve conduction results in decreased myelination. Thus, there seems to be a relationship between the neuron and the oligodendrocyte in initiating myelination, but it is unclear which structure exerts the control and by what means this control is effected. However, given that oligodendrocytes have been shown to produce myelin sheaths in the absence of neurons, other factors are clearly involved (Valk & van der Knaap, 1989).

THE DEVELOPING BRAIN

It is generally accepted that there exists a critical period during human brain ontogeny when neurogenesis is particularly vulnerable to either external insults or detrimental internal influences (Lauder & Krebs, 1986). The duration of a critical period varies for each organizational system and depends on such neurogenic events as cell proliferation, neuronal differentiation, gliogenesis, myelinogenesis, and synaptogenesis (Cowan, 1979). This concept of a critical period in regard to white matter seems best represented in the human brain by the sequence of neurobiological events occurring between the onset of the second trimester of pregnancy and the end of the third postnatal month (Morreale de Escobar, Escobar del Rey, & Ruiz-Marcos, 1983). It is generally contended that this period of development is characterized by very rapid cell division in the germinal layers, giving rise mainly to neuroblasts destined to provide the full complement of neurons present in the adult brain. The most active phase of forebrain neurogenesis takes place between 10 and 18 weeks gestation. The human brain "growth spurt" begins toward the end of the peak of active neuroblast multiplication and is characterized by a particularly rapid increase in brain weight, reflecting, in part, rapid multiplication and differentiation of glial cells. There is also a rapid growth of axonal and dendritic processes (although the number of neurons no longer increases during the most active part of the growth spurt), which establish neuronal circuitry and connections.

In humans, the main part of the brain growth spurt is postnatal and continues well into the second, and probably the third, year. The increase in brain weight, and in total number of both neurons and glia, is particularly rapid during the first 6 months following birth. During the first half of the brain growth spurt, oligodendroglia comprise most of the proliferating glial cells. These specialized glial cells are critical to the phase of rapid myelination, which occurs primarily during the second half of the brain growth spurt (Morreale de Escobar et al., 1983). Although insults incurred by the developing brain during active neurogenesis invariably cause gross malformations, the growth spurt represents a span of time when the brain would also be particularly vulnerable to the effects of malnutrition, metabolic disorders, or endocrine imbalance (Glorieux & LaVecchio, 1983).

Hormonal Influences

It is known that many hormones have unique effects on the developing brain. Such effects are referred to as either "early hormonal state" ("activational") or "organizational." Activational effects are viewed as behavioral manifestations of altered metabolic processes, altered sensitivity of peripheral sensory receptors, or alteration of CNS functions. Conversely, organizational effects occur as a result of permanent alteration of the endocrine system, either alone or in conjunction with the nervous system (Beckwith & Tucker, 1988). Leshner (1978) has presented one model hypothesizing the function of hormones during critical periods. He surmises that the concentrations of hormones during critical periods, or "neonatal surges," alter sensory receptors, general metabolic states, endocrine systems, and brain circuits to determine the pattern of responses available to the adult. Thus, neuroendocrine systems, once established, shape the responses of the organism to future situations.

Lauder and Krebs (1986) have elaborated on the concept of the critical period by proposing a hierarchy of internal regulatory signals, provided by neurotransmitters, neurohumors (neuronal substances such as peptides), and hormones, which is superimposed upon basic ontogenetic events. In their model, hormones are conceptualized as having a generalized influence on the underlying substrata of ontogenetic events and humoral regulatory influences. Support for this model is drawn from animal (primarily rat) studies demonstrating that proper levels of thyroid hormones, for example, are necessary for normal rates of germinal cell proliferation, cessation of cell division, formation of neurons from precursor cells, axonal and dendritic growth, neuronal migration, and formation of the correct number and types of synaptic relationships. Moreover, the release of norepinephrine appears to provoke the myelination of neural fibers (Beckwith & Tucker, 1988). Thus, it is possible that hormonal and humoral influences play a key role in the coordination of temporal events during nervous system development.

Teratology

In the field of teratogenesis, it is frequently observed that numerous and varied teratogenic agents exert their deleterious effects on the developing fetus through similar mechanisms. Several syndromes of uncertain etiology, characterized by both mental retardation (MR) and disorganization of brain structure, overlap substantially with the pattern of CNS damage resulting from prenatal alcohol exposure. They include primary microcephaly, as well as the Cornelia de Lange, DiGeorge, Dubowitz, and Rubinstein–Taybi syndromes. Differences in timing of similar insults, such as alcohol exposure, could differentially determine malformations. Thus, fetal alcohol exposure during one phase of embryological development may, for example, affect the upper limbs, as in the de Lange syndrome, or the heart, as in fetal alcohol syndrome (FAS). There is also evidence to suggest that characteristic facial malformations may be subject to the temporal factors of a given insult. Pratt and Doshi (1984) suggest that it may be valid to view some or all of these syndromes as a single entity that expresses the variable effects of a common mechanism. Differences in timing of the insult or interactions with other risk factors may account for the differential characteristic features, but each syndrome may result from several possible causes. The authors speculate that maternal alcoholism is likely to be the most common of these possible teratogenic agents.

Given that various teratogenic agents have like effects on the developing brain, the effects of fetal alcohol exposure can serve as an example of this type of damage to the integrity of the CNS. The range of malformation observed *in vivo* and during postmortem examination has encompassed severe CNS disorganization resulting from insults during the first trimester, including cortical disorganization, agenesis of the corpus callosum, and agenesis of the anterior commissure. These anomalies are presumed to be caused by focal destruction of cellular areas in the germinal matrices that give rise to these tissues. In addition, these abnormalities have been seen in conjunction with neuroglial heterotopias. This phenomenon suggests that, as well as being neurally toxic, teratogens may specifically interrupt the migration of cells from the germinal matrix to their proper destination. Abnormal glial migration is suggestive of abnormalities of oligodendroglial cells and myelin development during the rapid growth spurt (Lancaster, Phillips, Patsalos, & Wiggins, 1984). Hydrocephalus *ex vacuo* and periventricular leukomalacia have also been observed and are believed to be related to perinatal encephaloclastic processes (Clarren, 1986).

From knowledge of the temporal course of embryological development, it can be inferred that structural malformations of the cerebral cortex, corpus callosum, and anterior commissure would be incurred during the first 85 days of gestation, which encompass the periods of vast neural migration. Conversely, neuroglial heterotopias and cortical dysgenesis are more likely to develop during the second trimester. Lastly, cerebral white matter destruction is generally indicative of insults occurring during the third trimester (Clarren, 1986). Thus, the genetically couched course of embryology dictates that teratogens encountered early in gestation should produce a different pattern of brain malformation than late gestational exposure. Furthermore, prolonged teratogenic insults, such as consistent gestational alcohol exposure, would be expected to result in complex brain malformations arising in multiple "embryo-fetal" time periods.

CLASSIFICATION OF WHITE MATTER DISEASES

Once complete, the axon and its myelin sheath are dependent upon each other for survival. The axon requires the myelin sheath to conduct nerve impulses efficiently, and the myelin sheath deteriorates if the underlying axon is damaged, as is the case in Wallerian degeneration. Because of its very-long-chain fatty acids, mature myelin is quite stable and is largely unaffected by external agents. However, myelinogenesis is subject to damage or disruption from approximately the seventh gestational month to the end of the first postnatal year, primarily because of the relative ease of restricting the transport of the precursors of myelin into the brain. Moreover, once these precursors are in the brain, they are vulnerable until their actual incorporation as myelin. Enzyme systems and cofactors, which may be active only during myelination, are also susceptible to interruption. The extent of the damage incurred is dependent on both the severity and the timing of the insult during the process of myelination.

White matter diseases generally fall into two basic classifications. In myelinoclastic or demyelinating conditions, the formation and deposition of myelin proceeds in a normal fashion, only to be destroyed later in life. The diseases in this group are generally thought of as acquired, precipitated by adverse biological or environmental conditions. Multiple sclerosis (MS) is the best-known disease in this category. The second category consists of various dysmyelinating diseases. These are generally congenital disorders characterized by inborn errors of metabolism that interfere with the formation or maintenance of the myelin sheath (Bydder, 1990).

Myelinoclastic Diseases

In addition to MS, which is discussed in detail in Chapter 15 of this volume, numerous environmental factors and disease states are characterized by a considerable degree of demyelination. Iatrogenic causes of white matter damage include prophylactic intrathecal methotrexate treatment for acute lymphocytic leukemia, which is discussed in Chapter 11. White matter changes are also evident in radiation and anoxic damage (Bydder, 1990).

Numerous viral infections result directly in demyelination. Progressive multifocal leukoencephalopathy (PML) affects immunocompromised patients, such as those with carcinoma, leukemia, and other malignancies, as well as patients who are receiving immunosuppressive therapy (e.g., transplant patients). There are also several viral encephalitides, including the herpes virus, that are associated with demyelination. For example, subacute sclerosing panencephalitis (SSPE) has been linked to a prior exposure to the measles virus. Extensive white matter damage together with cerebral atrophy characterizes this disease, with deterioration continuing over a period of months or years (Bydder, 1990). Several other viral infections have been associated with demyelination, including postvaccinal encephalomyelitis, postinfectious encephalomyelitis, and postinfectious polyneuropathy or Guillain–Barré syndrome (Reitan & Wolfson, 1992).

A second way in which viral infections cause white matter change is through viral induced immune changes. For example, after exposure to vanceller influenza or other viruses, acute disseminated encephalomyelitis (ADE) may ensue, resulting in disseminated (though frequently symmetrical) cerebral changes. Other, less common causes of white matter damage include central pontine myelinolysis (CPM), Marchiafava–Bignami disease, and subcortical arteriosclerotic encephalopathy (SAE; Bydder, 1990).

Dysmyelinating Diseases

Although rare of their own accord, the leukodystrophies are among the most common of the dysmyelinating diseases and are discussed in detail in Chapter 12. "Leukodystrophy" is a general term referring to diffuse white matter disease, characterized by varying degrees of bilateral involvement of the hemispheres, with the cerebellum and brain stem typically being spared (Bydder, 1990). They include several familial diseases that manifest in infancy and childhood, as well as various conditions affecting the metabolism and deposition of myelin. The most common disease of this type is metachromatic leukodystrophy (MLD), an inherited autosomal recessive trait characterized by a genetically determined enzyme defect (Reitan & Wolfson, 1992).

Lipid storage diseases are another broad class of dysmyelinating diseases occurring primarily in children. These diseases are characterized by cerebral macular degeneration resulting from the accumulation of lipids in the ganglion cells of the retina. Upon examination, the fovea appears as a dark purple or cherry red spot because of the absence of ganglion cells. These diseases are classified on the basis of the stored material or the specific enzyme deficiency. Tay–Sachs disease and Niemann–Pick disease both involve an enzyme deficiency that contributes to the dysfunction of CNS myelin at an early age. Children affected with either of these conditions typically do not live past the age of 3–4 years (Reitan & Wolfson, 1992). Other less common dysmyelinating diseases include Anderson–Faby disease and Alexander disease (Bydder, 1990).

Myelin Damage

In a manner similar to that of the oligodendrocytes in the CNS, Schwann cells form the myelin sheath in the PNS. However, CNS myelin is more susceptible to injury than is PNS myelin. In the PNS the outer surface of a myelin sheath is covered by glial cytoplasm, affording some measure of protection. However, in the CNS the myelin sheath is in direct contact with other myelin sheaths, the surfaces of other glial cells and neurons, or the extracellular compartment. Therefore, such potentially hazardous substances as oxygen metabolites, lipid mediators, toxins, viruses, inflammatory cells, and cytokines may come in direct physical contact with the surface of the myelin sheath. CNS myelin is also vulnerable to injury because of the vast amount of myelin maintained by a single oligodendrocyte. Moreover, the thin oligodendroglial processes that transport the components necessary for the survival and maintenance of myelin are fragile and susceptible to injury. In addition, the type of demyelination known as Wallerian degeneration occurs when the axon substrate is damaged (Webster, 1993).

Some minor types of injury (e.g., electrolyte imbalance) may produce reversible changes in the myelin, characterized by a separation of the myelin lamellae and areas of swelling that remit during recovery. However, with severe injury the myelin sheath degenerates and is phagocytosed by macrophages, and to a small degree by astrocytes. This process is referred to as "primary demyelination" if the preponderance of axons remain intact, as is the case in MS, progressive multifocal leukoencephalopathy, and some viral infections of neurons (Webster, 1993).

During the active phase of myelination, each oligodendrocyte synthesizes more than three times its own weight of myelin per day. However, in adulthood myelin is a metabolically stable substance. Thus turnover is very slow, as is the production of myelin components. It does appear that new myelin is catabolized more quickly than older myelin. Therefore, myelin formed early in development is metabolically more stable than recently synthesized myelin (Valk & van der Knaap, 1989).

There is evidence to suggest that the process of myelin breakdown is similar across various causes of white matter pathology—Wallerian degeneration, encephalitic infections, or inherited metabolic diseases. Biochemical analysis of affected myelin reveals a consistent abnormal composition underlying the abnormalities specific to the particular disorder. For example, in a subgroup of peroxisomal disorders, such as adrenoleukodystrophy, there is an elevation of the very-long-chain fatty acids of the cholesterol esters. This pattern overlays the general characteristics of degenerating myelin, such as abnormal proportions of the various constituent lipids, in the context of a relatively normal ratio between the proteins and lipids. A dramatic rise in the amount of cholesterol, from approximately 27% of the total lipid content of normal myelin to over 50%, is characteristic of partially degraded myelin (Valk & van der Knaap, 1989).

However, the extent of myelin loss contributes more to the changes in the white matter as a whole than do changes in the biochemical composition of myelin. White matter changes are frequently reflected by an increased water content, as well as reduced lipid–protein ratios. There may be specific decreases in the major components of myelin, such as cholesterol, cerebroside, sulfatide, and ethanolamine phosphoglycerides. In addition, several diseases result in elevated cholesterol esters in the white matter, which is one marker of demyelination via phagocytosis of myelin.

WHITE MATTER AND AGING

Many compositional and morphological changes take place in the human brain with advancing age. In general, brain weight decreases and water content increases. Although some areas of the brain, such as the brain stem, show relatively little change, the cerebral cortex bears the telltale signs of aging. Levels of DNA and the number of neurons may be reduced by as much as 50% in some areas. Other familiar changes include the appearance of plaques and neurofibrillary tangles, as well as the loss of synapses and dendrites. Neurotransmitter systems, most notably those involving acetylcholine, are also adversely affected by increasing age. Of primary interest here is the reduction with age in the myelin content of white matter, subsequent to, in all probability, the degeneration of axons and the myelin sheath following a decline in the neuronal population. It would appear that these changes are not attributable to a primary process affecting myelin, as the lipid and protein composition of myelin remains relatively stable during aging (Valk & van der Knaap, 1989).

Diffuse white matter changes, referred to as leukoaraiosis (LA; Hachinski, Potter, & Merskey, 1987) or white matter hyperintensities (WMH), are in evidence on both CT and MRI. Common sites include deep cerebral areas, the basal ganglia, and the periventricular white matter, particularly at the horns of the lateral ventricles (Drayer, 1988). Various MRI studies have estimated that the prevalence of LA in healthy elderly individuals ranges from 11% to 89%. There is some suggestion that these white matter changes may be related to a decline in attention and speed of mental processing in this population. A comparison of neurologically normal elderly subjects with and without LA in the centrum semiovale and periventricular areas revealed that LA was correlated with slowing of distinct motor and attentional functions, as well as slowing of mental processing. These authors proposed that, in addition to elucidating some degree of the intellectual impairment commonly seen in the elderly, mild LA in these persons may be a harbinger of risk for further cognitive impairment (Ylikoski et al., 1993).

However, a study of healthy elderly individuals and patients with dementia of various etiologies revealed contradictory findings. Although

WMH were observed in some of the healthy aged subjects, they were not related to any combined or specific neuropsychological or global functioning test results. The relative volume of WMH was larger in the demented patients, and within that group it was larger in patients with vascular dementia than in patients with Alzheimer disease. Although WMH were not related to measures of intelligence and mental status, demented subjects with WMH were more impaired on specific neuropsychological measures than demented subjects without WMH. These deficits were interpreted as a general slowing in cognitive processes, as all affected measures were largely time-dependent. Pathology in the anterior and posterior periventricular regions, the watershed areas, was related most highly to cognitive impairment (Almkvist, Wahlund, Andersson-Lundman, Basun, & Backman, 1992). These results, combined with the correlation between degree of WMH with age and blood pressure, support the hypothesis that WMH are related to insufficient blood perfusion (Drayer, 1988).

SUMMARY

In this chapter, we have attempted to provide a general overview of the anatomical, structural, developmental, biochemical, and pathological characteristics of human CNS white matter. The three major types of white matter fibers are commissural fibers, which connect the two hemispheres; association fibers, which connect intrahemispheric cortical regions; and projection fibers, which course between the cortex and other areas of the brain and spinal cord. MRI has provided a high-resolution method of studying the temporal progression of myelination in the developing brain. The onset of myelination is important because it facilitates the transmission of neural impulses. In the CNS, myelination begins during the fifth month of gestation and continues rapidly during the first 2 years of life. In general, myelination proceeds in a posterior-to-anterior direction, with tracts typically becoming myelinated as they become functional.

Oligodendrocytes are responsible for the production and maintenance of the myelin sheath surrounding CNS axons. Myelin insulates axons and enhances impulse propagation by saltatory conduction. Demyelinating diseases are so devastating because they slow or block action potential conduction, causing deterioration in the ability to control behavior. Developing white matter is particularly vulnerable to noxious events between the onset of the second trimester of pregnancy and the first 3 months of postnatal life. During this time, the brain is also susceptible to the effects of teratogens, malnutrition, metabolic disorders, or endocrine imbalance. Evidence suggests that hormones influence the coordination of temporal events during nervous system development. Numerous teratogenic agents are known to affect the developing fetus adversely through similar mechanisms. The timing of the exposure to teratogens, rather than the nature of the particular noxious event, determines the nature of the resultant abnormalities.

CNS myelin is susceptible to injury because of the vast amount of myelin maintained by a single oligodendrocyte; the lack of protective cytoplasm in the outer surfaces of the sheath; and the fragility of the thin oligodendroglial processes that transport the components necessary for maintenance and nutrition. The integrity of the neural substrate is also critical to the survival of myelin. Regardless of the etiology, biochemical analysis of pathological myelin reveals a consistent abnormal composition on which the abnormalities intrinsic to the particular disorder are superimposed. White matter diseases can be classified as either myelinoclastic conditions which cause the destruction of once-normal myelin, or dysmyelinating conditions, which interfere with the actual formation or maintenance of the myelin sheath.

Whereas adults are most commonly afflicted with myelinoclastic diseases such as MS, dysmyelinating conditions often involving congenital metabolic errors that interfere with myelination are more common in children. Although mature myelin is largely impervious to insult, newly formed myelin is vulnerable from approximately the seventh gestational month to the end of the first postnatal year. The leukodystrophies, characterized by bilateral diffuse white matter disease, are among the most common of the dysmyelinating diseases. They include several inherited diseases (e.g., metachromatic leukodystrophy) that manifest in infancy and childhood, as well as various conditions affecting the metabolism and deposition of myelin. Lipid storage diseases (e.g., Tay–Sachs disease and Niemann–Pick disease) are also dysmyelinating conditions occurring primarily in children. The classification of these diseases is based on the material that accumulates or the specific enzyme deficiency.

With advancing age, there is a reduction in the myelin content of white matter; this is probably secondary to the degeneration of axons due to a decline in the neuronal population, rather than the result of a primary process affecting myelin. These diffuse white matter changes are commonly observed in deep cerebral areas, the basal ganglia, and the periventricular white matter of a large proportion of the healthy elderly, as well as in dementia patients. There are conflicting data regarding whether or not these white matter changes are related to a decline in attention and speed of mental processing in this population. However, the presence of white matter changes in the watershed areas of demented subjects does seem to be related to a general slowing in cognitive processes that has been attributed to hypoperfusion of the brain.

REFERENCES

Almkvist, O., Wahlund, L., Andersson-Lundman, G., Basun, H., & Backman, L. (1992). White-matter hyperintensity and neuropsychological functions in dementia and healthy aging. *Archives of Neurology, 49,* 626–632.

Barkovitch, A. J. (1991). Brain development: Normal and abnormal. In S. W. Atlas (Ed.), *Magnetic resonance imaging of the brain and spinal cord* (pp. 129–173). New York: Raven Press.

Barkovich, A. J., Kjos, B. O., Jackson, D. E., Jr., & Norman, D. (1988). Normal maturation of the neonatal and infant brain: MR imaging at 1.5T. *Radiology, 166,* 173–180.

Beckwith, B. E., & Tucker, D. M. (1988). Thyroid disorders. In R. E. Tarter, D. H. Van Thiel, & K. L. Edwards (Eds.), *Medical neuropsychology: The impact of disease on behavior* (pp. 197–221). New York: Plenum Press.

Bydder, G. (1990). Demyelinating disease and infection. In W. G. Bradley & G. Bydder (Eds.), *MRI atlas of the brain* (pp. 182–187). London: Raven Press.

Carpenter, M. B. (1985). *Core text of neuroanatomy* (3rd ed.). Baltimore: Williams & Wilkins.

Clarren, S. K. (1986). Neuropathology in fetal alcohol syndrome. In J. R. West (Ed.), *Alcohol and brain development* (pp. 158–166). New York: Oxford University Press.

Cowan, W. M. (1979). The development of the brain. In *The brain: A Scientific American book* (pp. 56–67). New York: W. H. Freeman.

Drayer, B. P. (1988). Imaging of the aging brain: I. Normal findings. *Radiology, 166,* 785–796.

Glorieux, J., & LaVecchio, F. A. (1983). Psychological and neurological development in congenital hypothyroidism. In J. H. Dussault & P. Walker (Eds.), *Congenital hypothyroidism* (pp. 411–430). New York: Marcel Dekker.

Hachinski, V. C., Potter, P., & Merskey, H. (1987). Leuko-araiosis. *Archives of Neurology, 44,* 21–23.

Koester, J. (1985). Functional consequences of passive membrane properties of the neuron. In E. R. Kandell & J. H. Schwartz (Eds.), *Principles of neural science* (2nd ed., pp. 66–74) New York: Elsevier.

Lancaster, F. E., Phillips, S. M., Patsalos, P. N., & Wiggins, R. C. (1984). Brain myelination in the offspring of ethanol-treated rats: *In utero* versus lactational exposure by crossfostering offspring of control, pairfed and ethanol treated dams. *Brain Research, 309,* 209–216.

Lauder, J. M., & Krebs, H. (1986). Do neurotransmitters, neurohumors, and hormones specify critical periods? In W. T. Greenough & J. M. Juraska (Eds.), *Developmental neuropsychobiology* (pp. 119–174). New York: Academic Press.

Leshner, A. I. (1978). *An introduction to behavioral endocrinology.* New York: Oxford University Press.

Martin, E., Kikinis, R., Zuerrer, M., Boesch, C. L., Briner, J., Kewitz, G., & Kaelin, P. (1988). Developmental stages of human brain: An MR study. *Journal of Computer Assisted Tomography, 12,* 917–922.

Morreale de Escobar, G., Escobar del Rey, F., & Ruiz-Marcos, A. (1983). Thyroid hormone and the developing brain. In J. H. Dussault & P. Walker (Eds.), *Congenital hypothyroidism* (pp. 85–126). New York: Marcel Dekker.

Pratt, O. E., & Doshi, R. (1984). Range of alcohol-induced damage in the developing central nervous system. In *Mechanisms of alcohol damage in utero* (Ciba Foundation Symposium No. 105, pp. 142–156). London: Pitman.

Raine, C. S. (1984). Morphology of myelin and myelination. In P. Morell (Ed.), *Myelin* (2nd ed., pp. 1–50). New York: Plenum Press.

Reitan, R. M., & Wolfson, D. (1992). *Neuroanatomy and neuropathology. A clinical guide for neuropsychologists* (2nd ed.). Tucson, AZ: Neuropsychology Press.

Ritchie, J. M. (1984). Physiologic basis of conduction in myelinated nerve fibers. In P. Morell (Ed.), *Myelin* (2nd ed., pp. 117–195). New York: Plenum Press.

Webster, H. deF. (1993). Myelin injury and repair. In F. J. Seil (Ed.), *Advances in neurology* (Vol. 59, pp. 67–73). New York: Raven Press.

Valk, J., & van der Knaap, M. S. (1989). *Magnetic resonance of myelin, myelination, and myelin disorders*. Berlin: Springer-Verlag.

Yakovlev, P. I., & Lecours, A. R. (1967). The myelogenetic cycles of regional maturation of the brain. In A. Minkowski (Ed.), *Regional development of the brain in early life* (pp. 3–69). Philadelphia: F. A. Davis.

Ylikoski, R., Ylikoski, A., Erkinjuntti, T., Sulkava, R., Raininko, R., & Tilvis, R. (1993). White matter changes in healthy elderly persons correlate with attention and speed of mental processing. *Archives of Neurology, 50,* 818–824.

3

Callosal Agenesis

Lisa A. Smith
Byron P. Rourke

Scientific accounts of the role of the corpus callosum (CC) in humans have changed dramatically throughout history. Originally, the structure was seen as playing a purely mechanical role (Chiarello, 1980). Vesalius (Clarke & O'Malley, 1968, cited in Chiarello, 1980) suggested that the structure was required in order to support the fornices and the ventricles, as well as to join the two sides of the brain. Later, the CC was given further responsibility: Some thought that it housed the imagination; others stated that they did not know what the function was, or else assigned to it no role at all (Chiarello, 1980). With the advent of surgery involving the sectioning of the CC to correct intractable epilepsy, modern-day clinicians thought themselves better able to understand the actual role played by this previously enigmatic portion of the human brain.

The deficits exhibited by commissurotomy patients would seem to allow scientists to pinpoint the role of the CC beyond a doubt. But, as in all scientific disciplines, new evidence always seems to arise that blurs the scientific lens. Humans who exhibit a congenital absence (or partial absence) of the CC do not exhibit the characteristic signs of commissurotomy patients. This lack of correlation between the two groups calls for further questioning of our views regarding the role(s) of this structure.

The purpose of the present chapter is to examine more closely the various aspects of callosal agenesis (hereafter including callosal dysgenesis). Throughout the chapter, references are made to the Nonverbal Learning Disabilities (NLD) model. There is a striking correspondence between certain aspects of callosal agenesis and Rourke's (1989) white matter model. Similarities are examined to provide the reader with an overview of how a disease process can lead an individual to exhibit characteristics of the NLD syndrome.

EMBRYOLOGY, ANATOMICAL DEVELOPMENT, AND PATHOLOGY

Topographic Organization of the Corpus Callosum

The CC contains fibers that connect both homotopic and heterotopic regions of the two hemispheres, although the majority connect homotopic areas. A study of the topography of this bundle of fibers has demonstrated that each lobe of the brain is represented by a portion of the CC. The rostral half consists of fibers originating in the frontal lobes, whereas the other three lobes utilize the caudal portion (Brodal, 1981). Parietal fibers occupy the most anterior portion of the caudal half, with temporal fibers next and occipital fibers crossing the median most caudally. Somatosensory fibers may even be represented somatotopically (Brodal, 1981).

Further information on CC topography was obtained by researchers studying brain pathology (De Lacoste, Kirkpatrick, & Ross, 1985). They studied brains that had acquired focal damage, and then observed the pattern of Wallerian degeneration. Despite some methodological difficulties, the findings support those of other researchers. De Lacoste et al. (1985) found that the rostrum and the genu of the CC were innervated by fibers from the inferior frontal and anterior inferior parietal regions of the cortex. The region of the temporal–parietal–occipital junction innervated the splenium and caudal portion of the body of the CC, and the superior parietal lobule and the occipital cortex selectively innervated the splenium (De Lacoste et al., 1985). The dorsal superior frontal cortex did not appear to innervate any portion of the CC. De Lacoste et al. (1985) suggest that this portion of the brain is "acallosal." However, the finding may simply be an artifact of their staining method. If, indeed, this portion of the cortex does not project fibers through the CC, such fibers may utilize the anterior commissure as an alternate route.

The topographic organization of the CC can be studied using evoked potentials (EPs) (Yu-ling et al., 1991). During surgery on persons with epilepsy about to undergo callosal section, different portions of the CC were stimulated, and the locations of EPs in the cortex were recorded. The location of the EPs suggested that the anterior portion of the CC projects primarily to the frontal poles; that the body projects to the frontal and temporal lobes; and that the caudal portion projects primarily to the parieto-occipital regions (Yu-ling et al., 1991).

Normal Callosal Development

The CC is the largest of the forebrain commissures, which consist of the CC, the anterior commissure, and the dorsal and ventral hippocampal commissures. All of the forebrain commissures develop from the lamina terminalis and the lamina reuniens, both of which are part of the rostral wall of the telencephalon (anterior to the chiasmatic plate) (Rakic & Yakovlev, 1968). The dorsal part of this wall thickens (lamina reuniens), while the ventral part does not (lamina terminalis).

Lemire, Loeser, Leech, and Alvord (1975) maintain that the lamina terminalis is inert, whereas the lamina reuniens is cellularly active. It is from the thick lamina reuniens portion that the forebrain commissures originate. This portion of the midline telencephalon is also called the commissural plate, since the fibers of the future CC cross at this anatomical locus. The commissural plate first differentiates when the embryo has reached approximately 39 days of gestation, and it is here that the forebrain commissures originate (Loeser & Alvord, 1968). The commissural plate (also called the massa commissuralis) acts as a passive bed for crossing fibers. It does not contain any callosal fibers (Chiarello, 1980), but contains only a small number of neuroblasts (Loeser & Alvord, 1968). At the 10th week of gestation, the dorsal and ventral portions of the lamina reuniens differentiate (Chiarello, 1980). The anterior commissure develops from the ventral portion, and the hippocampal commissure from the dorsal portion. Also arising from the dorsal portion are the CC, fornix, septum pellucidum, and cavum septi (Rakic & Yakovlev, 1968). There is debate as to exactly when the first callosal fibers appear; however, it seems that the first fibers of the CC begin to penetrate the commissural plate when the embryo is between the 11th and 13th weeks of gestation (Chiarello, 1980; Hewitt, 1962; Loeser & Alvord, 1968; Rakic & Yakovlev, 1968). The fornix and hippocampal commissure cross the midline of the massa commissuralis ventral to the fibers of the CC (Rakic & Yakovlev, 1968).

Growth of the CC follows the pattern and rate of growth of the cerebral hemispheres. Rakic and Yakovlev (1968) suggest that the CC is in its adult form (with the exception of length and thickness) in embryos of 18–20 weeks. However, Hewitt (1962) maintains that the rostrum does not appear until the embryo is 170 mm in length, and that even then the rostrum does not have an adult appearance before birth. It is only at birth that the splenium develops (Hewitt, 1962).

Generally, the CC develops in a rostral–caudal pattern (Schaefer et al., 1991), but there is question as to whether the rostrum or the splenium is the last to develop (Chiarello, 1980). Schaefer et al. (1991) suggest that the rostrum is the last to develop, despite the rostral–caudal pattern. However, as a result of this growth pattern, individuals who exhibit partial agenesis lack the posterior portion. This is a reflection of the embryological development of this structure. As a result, the few cases that have been reported of partial agenesis of the *anterior* CC have caused researchers some confusion.

Although preliminary investigations suggest that indeed these individuals were lacking the anterior portions of the CC (Barkovich, 1990; Schaefer et al., 1991), further study of these cases using magnetic resonance imaging (MRI) and pathological investigations have revealed that they did not lack the anterior CC. Upon autopsy, neuropathological study of one patient revealed that a fusion of the frontal lobes caused a displacement of the anterior portion of the CC. Thus, the entire callosum was present, but other structural defects hampered the view of the whole structure (Schaefer et al., 1991). Of the six patients with anterior agenesis reported by Barkovich (1990), closer examination revealed that two exhibited complete callosal agenesis but enlarged hippocampal commissures (which may have appeared to be callosal fibers), and the other four had intermediate forms of holoprosencephaly. (They appeared to have a splenium, but it was actually a dorsal interhemispheric commissure.) Thus, it is important for investigators to utilize all available technology when faced with patients who exhibit atypical presentations of well-known brain anomalies.

Growth of the CC continues to occur after birth. Streeter (1912, cited in Hewitt, 1962) indicates that as the child grows older, the CC, although it does grow caudally, does not do so continually from one end to the other. Rather, fibers are added interstitially as various areas of the cortex mature. The growth of the CC white matter parallels that of the cortical grey matter. Using MRI, Barkovich and Kjos (1988) were able to describe the normal growth pattern of the CC over the first year of life. Its appearance changes considerably throughout the first year. The genu exhibits a growth spurt during the second month after birth; the splenium shows a comparable growth spurt between 4 and 6 months. The CC resembles its adult form in the eighth postnatal month (Barkovich & Kjos, 1988).

Callosal fibers are not fully "operational" without myelin, and this process does not begin until the ninth month of gestation. Originally, only the midportion of the structure is affected (Valk & van der Knaap, 1989). By 1 year of postnatal age, the myelination of the CC is about 50% completed (Lemire et al., 1975). Other investigators suggest that this process begins in the splenium by 4 to 6 months of postnatal age, and that it progresses anteriorly throughout the first year, with the rostrum being the last portion to be myelinated (Byrd, Radkowski, Flannery, & McLone, 1990). Barkovich and Kjos (1988) noted that myelination of the splenium takes place at about 4 months of age, and myelination of the genu at about 6 months of age; however, there was individual variation. Once again, there appears to be some disagreement about the specifics of this process.

The rate of myelination slows after 2 years of age (Dietrich & Bradley, 1988), and is not completed until adulthood. Lemire et al. (1975)

point out that myelination begins later than other cellular differentiation and that it takes much longer to be completed. Some myelination still occurs in the second decade of life, and perhaps even longer. One can infer, then, that the CC does not function optimally until this process is complete.

More specific information about the rate of the myelination process of the CC may be gained in the near future with advances in the use of MRI. Dietrich and Bradley (1988), for example, point out that through the appropriate use of MRI, the clinician can follow the normal and abnormal progression of white matter maturation. Other investigators have indicated that MRI techniques (used with neonates) that allow for the visualization of the abnormal myelination process will permit physicians to predict neurological outcome (Guit, van de Bor, den Ouden, & Wondergem, 1990).

Abnormal Development in Callosal Agenesis

An extensive MRI study of 68 patients with various brain anomalies was completed by Barkovich and Norman (1988). The investigators used their knowledge of normal embryological development to make deductions about pathogenesis of callosal agenesis from their results. When they attempted "to correlate the degree of dysgenesis of the CC with associated anomalies of known chronology (such as migration anomalies), it soon became apparent that the timing did not coincide if the chronology of actual callosal formation was used" (Barkovich & Norman, 1988, p. 497). However, the other anomalies did correlate chronologically with the formation of the massa commissuralis or its precursor. Thus, insults during the formation of the CC itself are not as important as are insults to its precursors. If an insult occurs during the formation of the massa commissuralis, then callosal fibers will be unable to cross the midline. A very early insult to the lamina terminalis will cause total agenesis. Since development occurs in a rostral–caudal direction, partial agenesis will occur caudal to the point of insult. The later the insult, the greater the amount of CC that is able to form.

Although the extent of agenesis that an individual may exhibit varies greatly, it would appear that five types of embryological defects can lead to malformations in the CC. The diagnosis will depend upon the timing of the insult during gestation (Chiarello, 1980). The majority of this discussion is adapted from Lemire et al. (1975, p. 270).

1. An insult in the earliest stages of central nervous system (CNS) development will result in the failure of the midline telencephalon and vesicles to develop normally. Anatomically, this will result in a lack of

all forebrain commissures, a malpositioned hippocampus, and a single prosencephalic ventricle. The diagnosis in this case will be holoprosencephaly (Lemire et al., 1975). This is, quite obviously, the most severe type of callosal agenesis.

2. An insult before the 10th embryonic week will result in a failure of the lamina reuniens to develop normally (Chiarello, 1980). Anatomically, the individual will exhibit a lack of all forebrain commissures, the presence of Probst's bundle (to be discussed later), and a dorsal dilation of the third ventricle. The diagnosis will be total agenesis of the forebrain commissures.

3. If insult occurs in the 10th to 11th week (Chiarello, 1980), the dorsal portion of the lamina reuniens will fail to develop normally. Anatomically, in this case the anterior commissure will be spared, but the CC and the hippocampal commissures will fail to develop. Once again, Probst's bundle will be present, and there will be a dorsal dilation of the third ventricle. The diagnosis will be agenesis of the CC. Lemire et al. (1975) note that the latter presentation is the most common form of callosal agenesis. In this case, the two cerebral hemispheres are separate, with the exception of the anterior commissure and lamina terminalis.

4. An insult later in gestation will result in a defect only in the dorsal lamina reuniens. This form is often associated with a lipoma of the CC or a colloid cyst of the diencephalic roof. Anatomically, there is only focal absence of the CC (otherwise known as callosal dysgenesis). The anatomical abnormalities associated with agenesis will occur only in those areas that lack a portion of the callosum. The diagnosis will be focal agenesis.

5. A later-stage insult will result in cortical neuroblast abnormalities. Anatomically, the CC will appear membranous and will not contain axons. The diagnosis will be hypoplasia of the CC. This form of defect is often associated with agyria or mild arhinencephaly.

Jinkins, Whittemore, and Bradley (1989) suggest that the traditional classification system of simple and partial agenesis is inadequate to explain the morphology underlying such states. Using MRI, they found that the variety of morphologies exhibited in individuals with the disorder can best be described with three new terms outlining the three distinct categories of dysgenesis: "initiative agenesis," "hypogenesis," and "hypoplasia." Initiative agenesis describes a CC that is completely absent. Hypogenesis describes partial agenesis of varying degrees of caudal portions of the callosum, caused by the interruption of its development. Hypoplasia describes a CC that is present, but is focally or generally small in size. This state also includes a similar dysgenesis in the cerebral cortex (Jinkins et al., 1989). The authors provide embryological explanations to justify their new classification system.

Another anatomical finding is that the anterior commissure is often enlarged (if it is present at all) in agenic individuals. Chiarello (1980) suggests two explanations for this. First, the anterior commissure may act as an alternate pathway for callosal fibers. Fibers that would normally cross at the callosum are "forced" to seek an alternative route. Alternatively, Chiarello (1980) suggests that the CC plays a secondary role to the anterior commissure. Rather than simply serving as a compensatory mechanism when the callosum is absent, the enlarged anterior commissure may be a vestigial structure. Perhaps the fibers were originally meant to cross via the anterior commissure, but when the CC developed it took precedence over the anterior commissure.

Pathological examination of acallosal brains upon autopsy may provide further evidence of anatomical (or, rather, cellular) abnormalities. Shoumura, Ando, and Kato (1975) note that in two of their acallosal patients, the large pyramidal cells normally found in layer III of the cortex were difficult to detect, and that the number of smaller pyramidal cells was reduced in the region adjacent to the striatum. Animal studies have indicated that this particular area of the cortex is important for sending and receiving callosal fibers. Thus, if the cellular composition of this area in humans with callosal agenesis is compromised, then perhaps this area is also important in sending and receiving callosal fibers in humans. This study suggests that the origins of callosal agenesis may be found at the cellular level.

Three anatomical abnormalities are hallmarks of callosal agenesis. The first is Probst's bundle, a large fiber tract that runs anterior → posterior in acallosal brains, and consists of axons that do not cross the midline but terminate ipsilaterally (Lemire et al., 1975). It is located in the medial wall of each hemisphere, ventrolateral to the cingulum and dorsal to the fornix (Rakic & Yakovlev, 1968). Loeser and Alvord (1968) suggest that these fibers are not commissural fibers; they suggest that these fibers consist of what would normally be decussating axons crossing the callosum to connect heterotopic areas. In cases of partial agenesis of the CC, Probst's bundles occurs only in those focal areas where the callosum is absent. It is important to note, for later reference, that in terms of the Rourke (1989) model, this formation of the Probst's bundle directly affects the right ↔ left portion of the model. The commissural fibers that represent this portion of the model are not fully present. Only the decussating axons, connecting heterotopic areas, seem to be present in agenic individuals. Hence, skills and abilities relying on white matter that crosses the midline are expected to be impaired.

Other white matter tracts may also be affected in agenic individuals. Lewis, Reveley, David, and Ron (1988) suggest that the extension of the lateral ventricles upward (which occurs when the CC is absent) causes frontal and parietal white matter to be adversely affected. Other investigators suggest that deep white matter may be underdeveloped (Baierl, Markl, Thelen, & Laub, 1988). Thus, it is possible that individuals with callosal agenesis may exhibit compromised functioning of all white matter systems—affecting commissural, association, and projection fibers. If this be so, then all dimensions of the Rourke (1989) white matter model will be affected to some degree in cases of severe or complete agenesis.

The second distinct anatomical finding is a radial patterning of the sulci found in the medial portion of both hemispheres. In partial agenesis, such a pattern exists only in portions of the hemisphere where no callosum exists (Loeser & Alvord, 1968). It was speculated that this pattern may be a vestige of an earlier embryonic state. The radial pattern may occur in normal development, only to progress to the normal sulcal pattern with the growth of the CC. Lemire et al. (1975) take the position that this is not the case because such a radial pattern does not appear at any point in normal development. Also, sulcal development does not occur until after most of the development of the CC (Loeser & Alvord, 1968). The latter investigators suggest that such a pattern exists as a result of abnormal mechanical pressures that occur when the callosum does not develop. The patterns are therefore a reflection of physical forces, rather than constituting a vestige of a formal embryological stage.

The final anatomical hallmark of callosal agenesis is that lateral ventricles are abnormally shaped. The posterior horns are dilated because the forceps major is absent (Chiarello, 1980). This abnormality is a good indication to radiological investigators that agenesis exists. Whereas in the normal brain the medial walls of the lateral ventricles are side by side, in the acallosal brain the medial walls are "pushed" apart. In the acallosal brain the septum pellucidum is directed laterally; the roof of the third ventricle is dilated dorsally and protrudes between the septum pellucidum; and the foramen of Monro is elongated, allowing extensive communication between the lateral and third ventricles (Loeser & Alvord, 1968). (See Figure 3.1.) A differential diagnosis is hydrocephalus; however, this would be inaccurate. The shape of the ventricles results from mechanical forces caused by the lack of the callosum, rather than from excess cerebrospinal fluid or an obstruction.

Although the three major anatomical findings discussed above appear to be widely accepted as the major components of callosal agenesis, other investigators refer to "classical" findings occurring in *four* structures (Atlas et al., 1988). They suggest that the four anatomical anomalies are as follows: an enlarged and laterally rotated cingulate gyrus; a lateral callosal cistern filled with cerebrospinal fluid; Probst's bundles; and a frontal horn that is medially concave (Atlas et al., 1988).

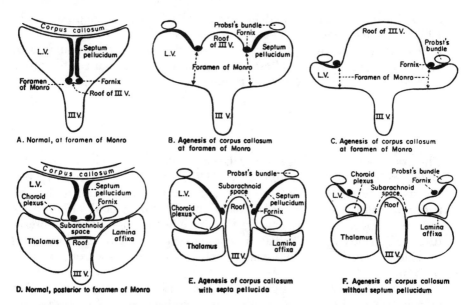

FIGURE 3.1. Schematic drawings of coronal sections of normal and acallosal brains. A, B, C: At level of foramen of Monro. A. Normal. B. Agenesis of corpus callosum with septa pellucida between fornices and Probst's bundles. C. Agenesis of corpus callosum with fornices apposed to Probst's bundles and no septa pellucida. Note the change in orientation of the septa pellucida and the preservation of anatomical relationships. D, E, F: Posterior to foramen of Monro. D. Normal. E. Agenesis of corpus callosum with septa pellucida. F. Agenesis of corpus callosum without septa pellucida. Note that subarachnoid space overlies the roof of the third ventricle even though the cavum velum interpositum is not present in an acallosal brain. The bare area of thalamus is also greatly reduced in the acallosal brain. From Loeser and Alvord (1968, p. 563). Copyright 1968 by Oxford University Press. Reprinted by permission.

EPIDEMIOLOGY

In their review of the literature, Serur, Jeret, and Wisniewski (1988) found that agenesis of the CC occurs with an incidence in the general population of 3–7 per 1000. They maintain that the incidence in the developmentally disabled population is higher, at 2–3 per 100. It is possible that the incidence in the general population may be an underestimate, because callosal agenesis can occur in individuals with normal levels of psychometric intelligence; such individuals are not likely to be referred to a medical facility for assessment. Lacey (1985) cites further evidence that the incidence is only 0.0005%. This figure was obtained from an unselected, random autopsy population. Because autopsy is not routinely performed on the entire population, the validity of this estimate is questionable.

Parrish, Roessmann, and Levinsohn (1979, cited in Ben Ari et al., 1989) reported that 62% of cases of agenesis of the CC are associated with anomalies in two other systems, and that 30% have anomalies in more than three systems. These investigators also maintained that other CNS anomalies occur in 85% of the agenesis population.

ETIOLOGY

The etiology of callosal agenesis is largely unknown (Lewis et al., 1988), and is probably diverse (Lemire et al., 1975). This is not surprising, given the five different levels of disorder and the severity falling under the rubric of callosal agenesis as discussed above. Jinkins et al. (1989) list a number of potential causal agents that have been proposed in the literature: "infectious agents, radiation, chemical agents, maternal hormones, nutritional deficiencies, hypoxia, and chromosomal and genetic factors" (p. 340).

Lemire et al. (1975) suggest that most cases of agenesis are a result of a defect in the lamina reuniens (the embryological structure from which the forebrain commissures develop). If this is the case, what causes the compromise of this structure to lead to the malformation of the CC? There are a number of indications that callosal agenesis is the result of a genetic anomaly. We discuss this in detail later.

Lemire et al. (1975) maintain that partial or focal agenesis may result from the presence of a lipoma or a colloid cyst of the diencephalic roof. This may or may not be a causal agent. Cysts occur in approximately 23% of cases of callosal agenesis, and interhemipheric cysts in approximately 7% of the affected individuals (Schwartz & Ghatak, 1990).

Mori (1992) describes four cases in which giant interhemispheric cysts were associated with agenesis of the CC. Such cysts are congenital. Thus, they may result from the same etiological agent as callosal agenesis, or may simply be coexisting anomalies. Schwartz and Ghatak (1990) note that cysts may occur later in development, resulting from a small vascular injury or from abnormal cell migration. Diagnosis often does not take place until adulthood because of the absence of obvious clinical symptoms.

A few other etiological explanations are suggested by Kolodny (1989). It is possible that early in embryogenesis, hyperglycinemia (a dysplastic process) may lead to structural abnormalities, including callosal agenesis. Also, a destructive process in which cerebral white matter is subjected to necrosis is possible. Lastly, toxic metabolites or a nutritional deficiency may cause injury to a CC during its formation. He cites Marchiafava–Bignami disease (a syndrome resulting from habitual use of cheap red wine) as evidence. Kolodny (1989) concludes that a dysplastic process is more likely than a destructive one, as evidenced by some patients presenting with nonketotic hyperglycinemia.

Animal studies have also led to different etiological origins. Hicks (1977) notes that rats exposed to X-rays during a critical period in the latter part of gestation did not develop a CC. This finding suggests that maternal exposure to radiation (at least in rats) may lead to structural abnormalities.

Byrd et al. (1990) suggest that agenesis of the CC can occur in both congenital and acquired forms, and that these forms have different etiological origins. The congenital form is explained above, but the acquired form must result from an already formed callosum being destroyed. The destruction may result from an insult acquired *in utero*. Byrd et al. (1990) state that this may produce an infarct in the anterior cerebral artery, leading to the destruction of the CC.

It is obvious, then, that no simple etiological explanation is possible. Callosal agenesis can exist in isolation or in combination with one or more other anomalies. As such, a simple explanation is insufficient to account for the many different mechanisms that may lead to agenesis.

OTHER MEDICAL FINDINGS AND ASSOCIATED ANOMALIES

The general opinion of clinicians in the field of neurology appears to be that individuals presenting with callosal agenesis exhibit either no or very few mild signs or symptoms that could be classified as neurologically abnormal (in contrast to findings to be discussed later). Rather, the presenting neurological symptoms are considered to be the results of the other associated brain anomalies (Loeser & Alvord, 1968; Mori, 1992).

In his study of the clinical features of agenesis, Lacey (1985) observed a trend with respect to age at diagnosis and presenting clinical characteristics. Children diagnosed in the neonatal period typically presented with macrocephaly, multiple congenital abnormalities, and seizures, whereas children diagnosed in adolescence (10–20 years) were typically referred because of learning, school-related, and behavioral problems. The age at diagnosis was related to the clinical prognosis: The younger the age at diagnosis (with the exception of children with macrocephaly and nothing else), the poorer the prognosis for future functioning. The young children often exhibited infantile seizures and multiple congenital anomalies that affected their later cognitive functioning. They were most often severely mentally retarded or developmentally delayed. These findings suggest that the agenesis per se is not the factor determining outcome; rather, the nature of other clinical symptoms is what may be crucial.

Thus, the clinical neurological picture of acallosal individuals is variable. In addition, the specific anomalies present depend on whether or not the individual in question has been diagnosed with a recognizable syndrome or simply has disorders resulting from some unknown cause. Callosal agenesis is a characteristic feature of Aicardi, Andermann, and Shapiro syndromes (Jeret, Serur, & Wisniewski, 1989). It is also present in some cases of (but is not necessarily characteristic of) the following syndromes: Dandy–Walker, Apert (Jeret et al., 1989; Gershoni-Baruch, Nachlieli, & Guilburd, 1991), and acrocallosal (Kolodny, 1989) syndromes. Agenesis of the CC has also appeared in combination with Ullrich–Turner syndrome (Kimura, Nakajima, & Yoshino, 1990) and with Miller–Dieker syndrome (Sharief, Craze, Summers, Butler, & Wood, 1991). Finally, various investigators have noted the presence of callosal agenesis in combination with other symptoms that are felt to represent new and previously unrecognized syndromes (Faye-Petersen, Ward, Carey, & Knisely, 1991; Lin & Gettig, 1990).

Agenesis of the CC has also been associated with other diseases and malformations, such as septo-optic dysplasia (Lahat, Strauss, Tadmor, & Bistritzer, 1992), Chiari II malformation (Mori, 1992), unlayered polymicrogyria (de Villemeur, Chiron, & Robain, 1992), hypothalamic disease (Page, Nussey, Jenkins, Wilson, & Johnson, 1989), and neurofibromatosis (Atlas et al., 1988), as well as double urinary collecting system, trigonocephaly, prominent philtrum, and clinodactyly (Ben Ari et al., 1989). Still other anomalies associated with agenesis are heterotopias, microgyria, abnormal cerebral fissures, porencephalic cyst, and hydrocephalus (Jacobson, 1989).

The neurological deficits exhibited by acallosal individuals are dependent upon the particular combinations of anomalies with which they present. The range of deficits can extend from subclinical signs to severe neurological compromise (Mori, 1992). Lewis et al. (1988) maintain that the most common presentation seems to be severe mental retardation with early (often focal) seizures. However, the seizures probably result from the other malformations with which agenesis is associated.

Byrd et al. (1990) found that when children with agenesis were grouped according to their associated anomalies, the clinical prognosis was best for children with isolated agenesis, and also for those with hydrocephalus who were shunted at or before the age of 3 months. The children with the poorest prognosis were those who demonstrated migrational disorders and those with hydrocephalus who were shunted after 6 months or who had multiple shunts and infections. Thus, agenesis alone does not result in a poor clinical prognosis.

GENETIC FINDINGS

As stated above, there is evidence that callosal agenesis is in some cases the result of a genetic anomaly. There are a number of syndromes with which this particular structural defect is associated. Serur et al. (1988), in a review of reported cases of callosal agenesis from 1968 to 1986, found 81 individuals who exhibited this structural anomaly in association with a chromosomal abnormality. They noted 32 different chromosome aberrations that led to, among other things, callosal agenesis. Such frequency of karyotype abnormalities led researchers to call for automatic chromosomal analysis or karyotyping of all affected individuals referred to medical facilities (Katafuchi et al., 1992; Serur et al., 1988).

Agenesis of the CC is characteristic of Aicardi syndrome, which includes the following: chorioretinal lacunar lesions (inflammation of choroid and retina of eye), infantile seizures, and agenesis of the CC (Donnenfeld et al., 1989). Patients also often exhibit costovertebral anomalies (Molina, Mateos, Merino, Epifanio, & Gorrono, 1989), such as hemivertebrae, scoliosis, and absent or malformed ribs (Donnenfeld et al., 1989). Choroid plexus abnormalities involving cysts have also been reported (Nielsen, Anvret, Flodmark, Furuskog, & Bohman-Valis, 1991).

The clinical picture of Aicardi syndrome must include the three symptoms cited above, but may also include other brain malformations and ophthalmological findings (Donnenfeld et al., 1989). In a study of Aicardi syndrome pathology in one young child, Font, Marines, Cartwright, and Bauserman (1991) found that the pathological abnormalities were evident exclusively in the brain and eyes. Developmental delay or mental retardation appears to be characteristic of children exhibiting this disorder. Donnenfeld et al. (1989) noted that all 18 of their subjects exhibited significant delays. Motor milestones were achieved late, and only 1 of the 18 subjects was able to use language (age range = 2 months to 10 years). Other studies note varying degrees of psychomotor impairment (Neidich, Nussbaum, Packer, Emanuel, & Puck, 1990). Life expectancy is short, as most children with this syndrome die before the age of 3 years (Font et al., 1991).

Some suggest that the disorder may arise as a result of maternal alcohol ingestion or first-trimester insults (Donnenfeld et al., 1989). The clinical and pathological evidence suggests that such an insult begins in the embryological stage when the CC is forming (Tagawa et al., 1989), probably during the fourth or fifth week of gestation (Font et al., 1991). Font et al. (1991) suggest that Aicardi syndrome is a result of a mutation of the X chromosome that occurs during meiosis.

The primary hypothesis surrounding the etiology of this disorder is that it is an X-linked dominant mutation on the short arm of the X chromosome. The syndrome occurs only in females and is alleged to be lethal in males, with the exception of one case of an individual with an XXY karyotype (Donnenfeld et al., 1989). It is not possible to offer support for this hypothesis as yet, because no reports of familial occurrence have appeared in the literature, with the exception of two sisters (not twins) who exhibited the syndrome (Molina et al., 1989). Despite the lack of data, much indirect evidence has been put forth to support the hypothesis; indeed, the X-linked etiology appears to be accepted in the medical field.

Because no parents of Aicardi children have received the same diagnosis, the genetic anomaly is thought to be a balanced *de novo* translocation of the distal short arm of the X chromosome—in other words, a new mutation rather than one passed familially from parent to child. The site of the translocation is thought to be at Xp22.3 (Donnenfeld et al., 1989). Support for the X-linked hypothesis comes from studies performed by Donnenfeld et al. (1989) and Neidich et al. (1990).

The information above suggests that callosal agenesis can be caused by a mutation in the X chromosome. Other evidence suggests that transmission of this structural anomaly occurs with an autosomal recessive inheritance. Callosal agenesis occurs in acrocallosal syndrome, which is postulated to occur as a result of autosomal recessive inheritance. The particular chromosome or gene locus has not been proposed.

The acrocallosal syndrome was first described by Schinzel in 1979 (Casamassima et al., 1989). Requirements for diagnosis are the presence of callosal agenesis, macrocephaly, craniofacial anomalies, polysyndactyly, and mental retardation (Gelman-Kohan, Antonelli, Ankori-Cohen, Adar, & Chemke, 1991). Other CNS disturbances have also been reported: arachnoid cyst, supratentorial cyst, partial absence of falx and tentorium, hypoplastic cerebellar hemispheres, Dandy–Walker malformation, micropolygyria, and optic atrophy (Cataltepe & Tuncbilek, 1992).

Although the autosomal recessive transmission of the syndrome is speculative, evidence supports this claim. A number of studies have reported parental consanguinuity (primarily first-cousin unions) (Cataltepe & Tuncbilek, 1992; Gelman-Kohan et al., 1991; Philip et al., 1988). Also, one consanguinous family has been reported in which the mother had four pregnancies (Cataltepe & Tuncbilek, 1992). One of these pregnancies resulted in a spontaneous abortion; another resulted in a child with anencephaly–polydactyly; and a third led to a child with the acrocallosal syndrome. The authors speculated that perhaps the child with anencephaly exhibited a severe form of disorder in the acrocallosal spectrum, and they pointed out the higher rate of spontaneous abortions in the literature of parents with acrocallosal children (23.4%).

Evidence for autosomal recessive inheritance is also found in other syndromes. A previously undescribed lethal syndrome of anomalies was presented by da-Silva (1988), in which three siblings demonstrated the following: hypoplastic CC, microcephaly, severe mental retardation, preauricular skin tag, camptodactyly, growth retardation, and recurrent bronchopneumonia. Because of the familial nature of this syndrome, da-Silva (1988) proposed autosomal recessive transmission. Agenesis of the CC was also reported in a case of an infant who exhibited caudal deficiency and polyasplenia anomalies (Rodriguez, Palacios, Omenaca, & Lorente, 1991).

Autosomal recessive transmission is the expected mode of inheritance for Toriello—Carey syndrome as well. In 1988, Toriello and Carey reported four cases of a syndrome involving the following: agenesis of the CC, telecanthus, short palpebral fissures, small nose with anteverted nares, Robin sequence, abnormal ears, redundant neck skin, laryngeal anomalies, cardiac defect, short hands, and hypotonia. Siblings of each sex were reported to exhibit the syndrome; thus an autosomal recessive inheritance was suggested (Toriello & Carey, 1988). Lacombe, Creusot, and Battin (1992) also described a patient who appeared to them to exhibit this same syndrome, with the addition of primitive cardiomyopathy. (Note the similarities to Williams syndrome as discussed in Chapter 6 of this volume.)

Finally, autosomal recessive transmission is the mode of inheritance for an inborn error of metabolism known as nonketotic hyperglycinemia (Rogers, Al-Rayess, O'Shea, & Ambler, 1991). White matter other than the CC is also compromised in this disorder (Dobyns, 1989).

Callosal agenesis occurs with greater frequency in individuals presenting with inborn errors of metabolism than it does in the normal population (Rogers et al., 1991). In a review of 194 cases of inborn errors of metabolism, 17% of the individuals had CC abnormalities. The frequency in the normal population is less than 1% (between 1 and 3 per 1000 children aged 1–7 years).

Agenesis of the CC has also been reported to arise as a result of autosomal dominant inheritance. Lynn, Buchanan, Fenichel, and Freemon (1980) reported a father—son case. The son was originally referred because of poor school performance. Extensive evaluations indicated that he and his father exhibited megalencephaly and agenesis of the CC. This was a case of familial callosal agenesis resulting from autosomal dominant inheritance. This case differs from the reported cases of autosomal recessive inheritance, in that callosal agenesis was the sole anomaly rather than being one aspect of a syndrome or collection of symptoms.

The evidence just reported thus suggests that callosal agenesis can be involved in syndromes arising from X-linked *de novo* mutations and from autosomal recessive familial inheritance. Callosal agenesis can also occur in isolation, resulting from an autosomal dominant familial inheritance. Other investigators have noted the presence of callosal agenesis in patients presenting with various types of trisomies (Atlas et al., 1988; Serur et al., 1988). These findings suggest that the development of the CC is controlled by a complex process, and is not simply dependent upon one gene locus or one chromosome.

IMAGING AND PRENATAL DIAGNOSIS

In many of the studies mentioned above, reference is made to the use of MRI. As these studies have already been discussed in the relevant sections of this chapter, a detailed description of the findings of imaging studies is not provided here.

Three primary imaging techniques are utilized by the medical profession at present to view the brain: computed tomography (CT), MRI, and ultrasound sonography (US). US is the only method that can aid physicians in prenatal diagnosis of this disorder, and this is discussed below. However, investigators agree that MRI is the method of choice for the diagnosis of agenesis after birth, because of its superior images of midline structures (Baierl et al., 1988; del Carpio-O'Donovan & Cardinal, 1990; Reinarz, Coffman, Smoker, & Godersky, 1988).

The use of US technology for expectant mothers provides clinicians with the opportunity to make diagnoses of agenesis before a child is born. The distinctive ventricles in acallosal individuals now allow radiologists to provide families with a (speculative) diagnosis of callosal agenesis *in utero*. Support for this claim is found in the work of a number of physicians (Bertino, Nyberg, Cyr, & Mack, 1988; Hilpert & Kurtz, 1990; Lockwood, Ghidini, Aggarwal, & Hobbins, 1988; Sandri et al., 1988; Vergani, Ghidini, Mariani, Greppi, & Negri, 1988).

Transabdominal US is now performed routinely on pregnant women. Although a clear view of the CC is not achieved on such a scan, recent research has suggested that a diagnosis of agenesis can be achieved using transverse scans, because of the ventricular abnormalities apparent in such individuals. Lockwood et al. (1988) note that the following can be observed: superior displacement and dilation of the third ventricle, lateral displacement of the frontal horns (the medial border has a concave appearance), and dilation of the posterior horns of the lateral ventricles. Bertino et al. (1988) obtained similar results. Sandri et al. (1988) suggest that the US examination should include a measurement of the distance between the bodies of the lateral ventricles. If the distance is very large, one can be more confident in the diagnosis. Sometimes the differential diagnosis includes hydrocephalus, which can be ruled out if there appears to be no progression in the ventriculomegaly over time (Vergani et al., 1988).

Upon finding abnormalities in transverse scans, radiologists may attempt to obtain coronal and sagittal scans. Although these views are more difficult to procure, because of the presentation of the fetus, they allow for a more certain diagnosis (Lockwood et al., 1988). The lateral displacement of the lateral ventricles is more easily observed on a coronal scan (Bertino et al., 1988). Most importantly, one may view the CC (or lack thereof) on sagittal and coronal views after the 20th week of gestation

(Vergani et al., 1988). The absence of a splenium on such views allowed Lockwood et al. (1988) to confirm their diagnoses.

The work of Hilpert and Kurtz (1990) has demonstrated that endovaginal US as opposed to transabdominal US, is a valuable alternative. Information gained from the transverse views of a transabdominal US allows only a speculative diagnosis. In fact, a number of differential diagnoses are possible, such as the following: agenesis of the CC, vein of Galen aneurysm, arachnoid cyst, lipoma of the CC, and teratoma. The coronal view obtained using endovaginal US allows for the confirmation of the absence of the CC.

Appropriate and careful use of US appears to be a valuable diagnostic tool. Lockwood et al. (1988) stress that the accurate diagnosis of callosal agenesis is important, in order to avoid any unnecessary obstetric intervention and to reassure parents.

LATERALITY, DICHOTIC, AND TACHISTOSCOPIC STUDIES

A number of neuropsychological studies have specifically addressed the issue of laterality and bilateral representation of function in acallosal individuals. Interest in this area was piqued by the lack of behavioral resemblance of acallosal patients to commissurotomy patients. It is widely accepted that commissurotomy patients behave in a manner that reveals the disconnectedness of their hemispheres. Indeed, the literature has termed this population "split-brain" patients. For current purposes, it will be assumed that the reader is aware of the characteristics of commissurotomy patients, since our main focus in this section is on the lack of similar characteristics in acallosal individuals. This discussion is limited, as we are interested in conveying a broad picture of acallosal individuals, rather than focusing on their split-brain characteristics (or lack thereof). Thus, the plethora of studies in this area is not discussed in detail.

When adults are deprived of their callosal connections through surgical intervention, they exhibit many deficits. However, acallosal individuals are amazingly adept at functioning normally (or almost normally) in their environments. Their brains appear to compensate for their anatomical constraints. The results of Lassonde, Sauerwein, Geoffroy, and Decarie (1986) highlight the plasticity of the young brain. Even commissurotomy patients could exhibit near-normal functioning when the surgical procedure occurred in early childhood. These patients exhibited less impairment than did their teenage counterparts. Lassonde et al. suggested that "it is highly probable that similar compensatory mechanisms are operating in agenic individuals and young callosotomized children" (1986, p. 963).

A review of the literature in this area reveals that there are many discrepancies in, and different interpretations of, the data. For instance, the results of dichotic listening studies are quite inconsistent and somewhat unreliable. Despite the difficulties, there appear to be some areas of agreement, particularly with respect to compensatory mechanisms utilized by acallosal individuals.

First, we address some of the studies utilizing the dichotic listening paradigm. Bryden and Zurif (1970) assessed the functioning of a 15-year-old acallosal boy on a dichotic digit recall task. The boy did not differ significantly from normal controls and did not demonstrate the strong laterality effect of commissurotomized patients. He did, however, exhibit left-ear dominance for the task. Saul and Gott (1976) tested two acallosal adults on a digit recall task. Both patients demonstrated a slight left-ear preference, but on a more demanding task (recall of phonemes), one of the patients demonstrated right-ear superiority. Lassonde, Lortie, Ptito, and Geoffroy (1981) tested two acallosal siblings on a dichotic recognition test for verbal and nonverbal material. Both individuals demonstrated a marked left-ear preference for both types of material. Finally, Bruyer, Dupuis, Ophoven, Rectem, and Reynaert (1985) also utilized a dichotic task with a 17-year-old male acallosal patient. Once again, inconsistent results were found. Their results demonstrated "a right hemisphere superiority in a phonemic dichotic task . . . but this superiority was not absolute: the performance of the right ear remained higher than the random level in the various situations" (Bruyer et al., 1985, pp. 427–428).

Studies of the visual functioning of acallosal individuals primarily employ tachistoscopic paradigms. Sauerwein and Lassonde (1983) tested two acallosal siblings on tachistoscopic tasks utilizing unilateral and bilateral presentation of verbal and nonverbal material. They found that their patients were able to cross-integrate bilaterally presented stimuli successfully, but that the speed of transmission time seemed to be slower than normal. Lassonde, Sauerwein, McCabe, Laurencelle, and Geoffroy (1988) tested six acallosal individuals on visual matching tasks and found that they were able to perform intra- and interhemispheric comparisons with a high level of accuracy, but that they again demonstrated slower-than-normal performance. Karnath, Schumacher, and Wallesch (1991) also examined visual comparison and naming tasks using the tachistoscope, and found that accuracy was dependent upon particular aspects of the visual stimulus. Performance was good when subjects were discriminating between grossly different stimuli, but it fell to chance levels when the stimuli were identical or very similar. Thus, it would appear that acallosal individuals are able to cross-integrate bilateral visual material, but that their performance level wanes if the task becomes more difficult.

Studies have also focused on the interhemispheric transfer of tactile information. Ettlinger, Blakemore, Milner, and Wilson (1972) noted that, in their study of four individuals with total agenesis and four with partial agenesis, both groups demonstrated no difference from normals in tactile transfer tasks. However, the total-agenesis group did perform below control levels on a cross-localization task. Dennis (1976) found similar results. Her two acallosal patients were able to perform interhemispheric tactile discrimination tasks well, but had particular difficulty with localization tasks. Sauerwein, Lassonde, Cardu, and Geoffroy (1981) also noted no deficits in tactile transfer tasks. There were also no deficits in learning of tactile forms as demonstrated with the Tactual Performance Test (TPT). In a further study of four acallosal individuals, Lassonde, Sauerwein, Chicoine, and Geoffroy (1991) demonstrated once again that such individuals do not have impaired interhemispheric communication with respect to tactile transfer. Their results differed from those above, however, in that they also found no impairment in cross-localization tasks.

It is clear that some inconsistencies are present in this literature. Despite these discrepancies, the following tentative conclusions can be drawn. First, on primarily dichotic listening tasks, there seems to be an absence of the strong laterality effect demonstrated in commissurotomy patients (although ear preference is variable). Second, acallosal individuals demonstrate a slower-than-normal speed of transmission on visual cross-integration tasks; also, accuracy declines as the tasks become more complex. Third, acallosal patients perform adequately on tactile transfer tasks, but may exhibit difficulties on tactile cross-localization tasks.

COMPENSATORY MECHANISMS

Behavioral Strategies

There has been some suggestion that acallosal individuals make use of behavioral strategies in order to perform as normal persons do on tasks requiring interhemispheric transfer. This strategy involves cross-cuing, which is "the use by one hemisphere of sensory information (e.g., visual cues) derived from responses (e.g., movements) initiated by the other hemisphere" (Ettlinger et al., 1972, p. 339). In their assessment of two acallosal siblings on the TPT, Sauerwein et al. (1981) noted that their subjects may have utilized a cross-cuing strategy in order to perform the transfer task. The authors suggested that "the fact that both patients were able to correctly recall the shapes and their location in the formboard task indicates that the shapes were familiar and that the subjects made use of visual imagery during learning and subsequent transfer" (p. 452).

However, they also noted that this strategy would not allow the subjects to "effect bilateral integration of tactile information" (p. 452).

Acallosal patients exhibit a number of abilities that split-brain patients do not, and these differences cannot be accounted for by cross-cuing (Ettlinger et al., 1972): (1) Acallosal individuals demonstrate normal ear asymmetries on dichotic tasks; (2) they can provide correct verbal responses to stimuli in the left visual field; (3) they can match colors across the vertical median; and (4) they can detect apparent movement across the vertical median (Ettlinger et al., 1972). Chiarello (1980) also notes that there is no need for acallosal individuals to develop such cross-cuing strategies in normal life, because they usually receive information bilaterally. Therefore, it appears that cross-cuing strategies may occur in some limited cases, but that this particular strategy does not account for good performance on a host of other tasks.

Bilateral Representation of Function

Almost all normal right-handed individuals have speech functions that appear to be subserved primarily by systems within the left hemisphere. Some argue that acallosal individuals do not have lateralized functions, and in fact that they possess bilateral representation of functions (including language). Saul and Gott (1976) reported on one adult acallosal individual who underwent sodium amytal testing that revealed bilateral speech representation. Chiarello (1980) also reminds us that acallosal individuals do not exhibit anomia for stimuli presented to the left hand or left visual field, as do commissurotomy patients. Ettlinger et al. (1972) note that bilateral representation of function would provide an adequate explanation for the fact that acallosal patients are able to write, draw, and construct with both hands.

Evidence contrary to the bilateral representation hypothesis is also presented. Such an explanation does not account for the lack of reduced ear asymmetries in acallosal individuals on dichotic tasks (Bryden & Zurif, 1970; Ettlinger et al., 1972). Also, Lassonde, Bryden, and Demers (1990) noted that their six acallosal subjects exhibited even greater laterality of function than did their IQ-matched normal controls. They interpreted their results by speculating "that constant interhemispheric communication, during the development of normal individuals with intact corpora callosa, leads to a diminution of the initial asymmetry. This can obviously not take place if the CC itself does not develop, and hence the initial asymmetry remains high in individuals with callosal agenesis" (Lassonde et al., 1990, p. 204).

Cook, Brugger, Regard, and Landis (1990) disagreed with Lassonde et al.'s (1990) choice of an IQ-matched control group, and suggested instead that control individuals of normal intelligence would have been a wiser choice: The lower IQ of the control group could have resulted from other neurological factors, whereas the acallosal subjects could have had lower IQs because of the lack of commissural fibers. Lassonde and Bryden (1990) replied that IQ matching was appropriate because the lack of a CC alone does not account for reduced IQ.

Reliance upon Ipsilateral Pathways

A number of studies suggest that acallosal individuals rely more heavily upon ipsilateral pathways as a compensatory mechanism for the lack of a callosum. Ettlinger et al. (1972) reported evidence for the development of ipsilateral motor control over time in commissurotomy patients. If this is the case, then it is conceivable that acallosal individuals could also rely on similar mechanisms. Ipsilateral involvement would help to explain why acallosal subjects demonstrate slower-than-normal crossed visual re- action times, and why they are able to write, draw, and construct with either hand. However, acallosal individuals probably do not rely on such mechanisms exclusively, because such an explanation does not account for their difficulty with cross-localization tasks (Ettlinger et al., 1972).

The majority of evidence for the reliance on ipsilateral pathways comes from studies assessing the tactile modality. Dennis (1976) performed an extensive study on two acallosal individuals. She found that they performed well on tasks of intra- and intermanual discrimination, but that they per- formed poorly on tasks of intra- and intermanual localization. The fact that "tactile localization is not further degraded on the intermanual task in [one subject] shows strikingly that it is not the process of intermanual transfer *per se* which is defective in complete callosal agenesis. Rather, the deficiency of the original unimanual perception of stimulus topography produces her inability to localize a stimulus across the body's midline" (p. 461). Milner (1983) points out that the poor tactile localization is explained by Dennis (1976) as "a consequence of an overdeveloped ipsilateral sensory pathway, which permits cross-integration (through a single hemisphere) at the cost of reduced sensory acuity" (p. 722).

Evidence for the use of ipsilateral pathways is also found in studies of commissurotomy patients. Lassonde et al. (1986) found that younger commissurotomized children were better at interhemispheric tactile transfer tasks than were their older counterparts. They hypothesize that younger children learn to rely on the ipsilateral connections of the extra- lemniscal, spinothalamic pathway. Older patients fare worse because the CC becomes myelinated with age, and they begin to rely more heavily on contralateral pathways. Similar results were found by Lassonde et al. (1991), who demonstrated that acallosal subjects performed well on intra-

and intermanual tasks, as well as on cross-localization tasks (in contrast to Dennis, 1976). The first study demonstrated that younger children rely more heavily on ipsilateral pathways. The results of the second study suggest that "congenital absence or section of the CC before completion of synaptic stabilization could *extend* the period of cerebral plasticity. Persisting connexions could be utilized to reinforce existing structures" (Lassonde et al., 1991, p. 493).

There are three limitations to this compensatory mechanism: First, reliance on ipsilateral systems results in difficulty with discrete willed movements, since ipsilateral motor systems control only gross movement and not the distal extremities. Second, difficulty with cross-localization persists (Dennis, 1976). Third, deficits in bimanual operations also persist (Sauerwein et al., 1981).

Use of Alternate Commissural Pathways

The majority of evidence for the reliance of acallosal individuals upon other commissural pathways comes from visual tachistoscopic studies and visual reaction time tasks. Before addressing these two lines of evidence, we consider the suggestion that auditory information crosses the midline via an alternate commissural pathway. Lassonde et al. (1981) found a right-hemisphere superiority in an acallosal subject for verbal and non-verbal material in a dichotic recognition task; this patient also demonstrated a slower-than-normal performance. The authors suggest that the slowness may have resulted from a limitation of the compensatory pathways. They suggest that the subject may have been utilizing a subcortical route for interhemispheric transfer.

With respect to tachistoscopic studies, Lassonde et al. (1988) found that acallosal subjects were able to perform intra- and interhemispheric comparisons at a high level of accuracy; they did, however, exhibit longer reaction times. Similar results were found in a young commissurotomized patient. Thus, the anterior commissure may be relied upon for visual transfer in these patients, but not in older commissurotomy patients. This is a plausible explanation, because the anterior commissure develops earlier in the embryo than does the CC. Again, the limitation is a slowing in reaction time.

Karnath et al. (1991) point out another limitation of the use of the anterior commissure. Their acallosal patient was adept at discriminating grossly different stimuli presented to either hemisphere, but performance reached only chance levels when the stimuli were identical or differed in only one feature. The greater demands of this task taxed the capacities of this compensatory mechanism. Their data suggest "that extracallosal commissures, in the case of [this patient] probably the anterior, are limited in their capacity of transferring and cross-integrating visual information" (p. 349).

Support for reliance upon extracallosal commissures is also found in visual reaction time experiments. Reynolds and Jeeves (1974) demonstrated that acallosal subjects exhibited a significant increase in the latency of crossed (hand response to opposite visual field stimulus) reaction time. Kinsbourne and Fisher (1971) found discrepant results, such that no latency difference between crossed and uncrossed stimulation was evident. However, two similar studies performed by Milner (1982) and Milner, Jeeves, Silver, Lines, and Wilson (1985) demonstrated that when acallosal individuals were asked to respond to a flash of light with their hand (same side as or different side from flash), they demonstrated faster performance in the uncrossed condition than in the crossed condition. This is consistent with the results of Reynolds and Jeeves (1974). In both of these studies, when the acallosal individuals were exposed to lights of different intensities, the lower intensities resulted in greater differences in reaction time between the crossed and uncrossed conditions. This argues for an alternative commissure explanation. The different intensities may yield different results because "the CUD [crossed–uncrossed difference] may reflect (at least in part) conduction time through a pathway sensitive to stimulus parameters, i.e., one composed of visually coded neurones" (Milner et al., 1985, p. 330). It is probably the anterior commissure and not the superior colliculus that takes on this role.

Conclusions

From this discussion of laterality studies, one can see that there are many discrepancies in the literature. Despite this, there seems to be a consensus that four compensatory mechanisms are all possible alternatives to the CC utilized by acallosal individuals. Opinion varies, but it would appear that behavioral strategies and bilateral representation of function are limited in their ability to explain the data. With respect to the other mechanisms, it would appear that the tactile modality relies upon ipsilateral pathways, and that the auditory and visual modalities rely upon alternate commissures or subcortical routes. Despite the success of these alternatives with respect to the absence of split-brain symptoms, there are limitations. And these limitations would appear to lead to the neuropsychological deficits that are discussed in the next section.

NEUROPSYCHOLOGICAL AND BEHAVIORAL STUDIES

Most behavioral studies of individuals with callosal agenesis have involved dichotic listening and tachistoscopic paradigms in an attempt to understand the lateralization of function in these individuals. These studies are valuable, in the sense that they provide us with information on how neural plasticity can allow a "damaged" brain to function at almost normal capacity. However, when interpreting this information, one must realize that the experimental situations depicted in these studies are highly artificial. Acallosal individuals do not live in a world of dichotically or tachistoscopically presented stimuli. Given this fact, we must attempt to assess the functioning of these individuals in more "normal" settings. Although neuropsychological tests do not mimic real life, they do provide clinicians with tools for assessing the skills and abilities of individuals, in order to predict how they will function in a natural environment.

The need for such neuropsychological investigations of acallosal patients is great, since some deficits go unnoticed by standard neurological examinations. Such investigations may lead one to assume that the absence of associated anomalies accompanying callosal agenesis also implies the absence of any behavioral pathology. Neuropsychological investigations illustrate that the absence of the CC leads to some alteration of normal behavior, no matter how subtle or slight. A discussion of such neuropsychological findings follows. Note that very few clinicians have put their acallosal clients through a full neuropsychological evaluation; rather, most studies focus solely on one or two specific areas of functioning. An attempt is made here to review these studies according to the area of functioning investigated. After this material is presented, the relationship of Rourke's NLD model to callosal agenesis is discussed.

Language and Verbal Functions

Dennis (1981) appears to have been the first individual to attempt an intensive study of the language capacities of an individual with callosal agenesis. She studied D. S. (age 27), who presented with complete agenesis. This female patient also exhibited other brain anomalies, as follows: hydrocephalus, Dandy–Walker syndrome, and a Dandy–Walker posterior fossa cyst. The patient was of normal psychometric intelligence. Dennis (1981) investigated the following language capacities: phonology (articulation and auditory discrimination); naming; fluency and automaticity; word and sentence comprehension; syntactic comprehension; sentence repetition; complex production; and metalinguistic and pragmatic comprehension.

D. S. was able to articulate English phonemes, and she was also able to identify these same sounds. She was able to name words in response to a picture or to a semantic cue, but was unable to provide appropriate words to rhyme, which Dennis (1981) cites as indicating limited access to a phonological retrieval system for common words. D. S. demonstrated good fluency and automatized naming. She performed at appropriate levels in her comprehension of single words, but she had difficulty comprehending the syntactic component of sentences. Further investigation into her syntactic deficits revealed that she had difficulty understanding passive affirmative sentences and negation. D. S. also had difficulty repeating sentences, presumably because of difficulty with the syntactical and lexical aspects of the sentences. When producing sentences, D. S. had trouble with the surface syntactical structure. Finally, she showed impaired metalinguistic and pragmatic comprehension.

Dennis (1981) concluded that D. S. demonstrated a deficit in the comprehension of the syntactic-pragmatic component of language. The performance of D. S. was similar to that of left hemidecorticates, and the "common impairment is in a language operation which is integrative—semantic, structural, and hierarchical" (p. 49). The integrative component of this functioning is worth noting. If left hemidecorticates also exhibit this pattern of functioning, then what is it that causes acallosal individuals to behave similarly when, presumably, their left hemisphere is intact? As stated earlier, in acallosal subjects, the dilation of the ventricles may lead to the deep white matter's being affected (Baierl et al., 1988; Lewis et al., 1988). As suggested by Rourke (1989), when the white matter association fibers in the left hemisphere are compromised, the prominent opercula of this hemisphere are unable to "communicate" properly with one another. When this situation is congenital, language is not expected to develop normally. Thus, the specific functions of each of the opercula in the "language" hemisphere would be "isolated" from one another. This would be expected to lead to a difficulty with the integrative functions of language, and is a possible explanation for the deficits exhibited by D. S.

Jeeves and Temple (1987) tested two adult acallosal subjects: B. F., a 20-year-old man who also presented with seizures, and K. C., a 22-year-old woman who also presented with a large frontal cyst. The following language functions were tested: visual naming, oral word fluency, sentence construction, cued-word retrieval, sentence repetition, and sentence comprehension. In addition to the syntactic–pragmatic difficulties exhibited by D. S., K. C. had difficulty retrieving words from semantic cues, constructing sentences, and comprehending active affirmative sentences (Jeeves & Temple, 1987). The different results do not necessarily contradict the explanation given by Dennis (1981), and could be explained by extracallosal damage. However, Dennis's (1981) interpretation is contradicted by the results of the other patient, B. F. He performed well on most tests, with the exception of two difficulties: He was not as good as controls at retrieving words from rhyme cues and at repeating pseudocleft sentences.

Jeeves and Temple (1987) attempted to replicate the testing conditions of Dennis (1981) by utilizing a subset of her tests. However, they suggested a different interpretation of her findings. Some of Dennis's findings suggested that D. S. also exhibited some phonological and semantic difficulties, in addition to the syntactic–pragmatic difficulties emphasized by Dennis herself. Thus, the language may be more compromised in acallosal individuals than was previously indicated.

Jeeves and Temple (1987) suggest that Dennis's (1981) explanation may have been too simplistic. One of their patients demonstrated difficulties in addition to those reported by Dennis, and the other demonstrated a specific deficit without the pattern reported by Dennis. The only language deficit exhibited by all three patients was the difficulty in retrieving words in response to rhyme. What, then, do these results tell us about the effects of agenesis on language development? How can we separate the effects of agenesis from the other brain anomalies exhibited by these persons? These questions must remain unanswered until further studies are performed that specifically address these issues. Jeeves and Temple (1987) suggest that in "the meantime it should be noted that failure to establish a specific language deficit in callosal agenesis does not mean that the callosum is not involved in normal language development" (p. 333).

The fact that the language deficit common to all three patients was a difficulty with rhyming led to a study that specifically addressed this issue. Temple, Jeeves, and Vilarroya (1989) assessed two more acallosal patients on a number of different rhyming tasks: S. B., a child who also presented with hypomelanosis syndrome of Ito, and K. W., a child who also exhibited corneal dystrophy. S. B. was tested on two occasions, at the age of 7 years, 9 months and at the age of 9 years, 5 months;. K. W. was tested only once, at the age of 13 years, 1 month. The following results were obtained.

At first testing, S. B. demonstrated impaired retrieval of words from rhyme cues, but this performance improved to within the normal range on the second testing occasion. K. W. also demonstrated an impaired retrieval of words from rhyme cues. S. B. demonstrated a mild visual anomia: She had difficulty retrieving words from visual cues. Both subjects exhibited difficulty detecting a word that did not rhyme with three other rhyming words, and in judging whether or not a pair of words did or did not rhyme. K. W. exhibited greater impairment on both of these tasks. When the subjects were tested for their ability to generate rhyming words (rhyme fluency), S. B. performed below control levels; however, her performance did improve over time. K. W. was also deficient at this task. When asked again to judge whether or not a pair of words rhymed, S. B. performed below control levels at first testing, but improved to within normal limits at second testing. K. W. demonstrated impaired performance on this task.

Both acallosal children demonstrated deficits in rhyming ability. These were pervasive deficits for K. W. and initially for S. B. The performance of S. B. improved over time in some areas, although her deficit in rhyme fluency was sustained. Obviously, this developmental change in S. B. suggests that the initial deficits may have reflected a developmental delay in performance rather than permanent deficits. The fact that K. W. also demonstrated deficits at an age that was even greater than the age of S. B. on her second testing complicates the picture. Since Jeeves and Temple (1987) reported rhyming difficulties in their adult acallosal subjects, it would seem that in the majority of those acallosal individuals tested (small though the sample may be), rhyming presents a problem. Temple et al. (1989) suggest that these deficits may reflect either problems of explicit phonological processing or deficits in acoustic matching. Further study utilizing musical notes and environmental sounds as stimuli would help determine which of these two explanations is more appropriate.

Temple, Jeeves, and Vilarroya (1990), using the same two patients mentioned above (S. B. and K. W.), attempted to assess reading ability. Single-word reading ability was comparable to that of age-matched controls for both children. However, both children, when compared to controls, were deficient at reading nonwords. S. B. improved slightly at reading nonwords with age, but her ability to read nonwords always fell below her ability to read words. It is interesting to note that even when K. W. was able to read nonwords, this appeared to be attributable to the use of analogy strategy rather than to a reliance upon phonological skills. For example, the nonword "polonel" would be compared to the real word "colonel," and then read accordingly.

Temple et al. (1990) maintain that these two children exhibited a deficit in explicit phonological processing. The results suggest that the rhyming deficits reported in the previous study (Temple et al., 1989) were also attributable to phonological processing problems rather than to acoustic matching problems. The investigators state that the findings of the 1990 study may suggest that this phonological processing problem hinders the normal development of the phonological reading route.

Sanders (1989) also assessed reading ability, but focused specifically on comprehension rather than word decoding. Sanders tested a 6-year-old acallosal girl, with psychometric verbal intelligence within normal limits, who also presented with some cerebellar agenesis. The first of the sentence comprehension tasks required her to match a sentence to the appropriate picture depicting the action, and the second required her to act out the action depicted in the sentence. Four sentence types were used: active; passive; relative clause where the subject of the matrix is the same as the subject of the clause (SS); and relative clause where the subject of the matrix is the object of the relative clause (SO). Examples of these four sentence types, respectively, are as follows:

1. (active) The unhappy boy is pushing the girl.
2. (passive) The unhappy girl is being pushed by the boy.
3. (SS) The boy who is pushing the girl is unhappy.
4. (SO) The girl whom the boy is pushing is unhappy.

The acallosal girl performed consistently below control levels on all but the SO sentence types on both the sentence–picture matching and the acting-out tasks. She functioned at a lower developmental reading level than did controls. She was able to discriminate between active and passive sentences. She could respond appropriately to most active sentences, but she seemed to guess randomly when attempting to understand passive sentences. Sanders (1989) notes that this performance represented an earlier stage in linguistic development in the acallosal child, and points out that the results could be consistent with either of two explanations: First, the performance of the acallosal child could simply have represented a developmental delay, since her performance was consistent with that of a younger child. Thus, it would be expected that she would reach the level of the controls, but at a slower pace. Or, second, her performance could represent a deficit that would not improve with time. In order to determine which explanation was correct, further testing of this child at a later age would be needed.

A limited number of language functions have been tested in these studies. More detailed and thorough investigations are needed before we can arrive at a clear picture of the language capabilities of acallosal individuals. For instance, Klouda, Robin, Graff-Radford, and Cooper (1988) report a case of a woman who had difficulty with the prosodic aspects of language after some of her callosal connections were severed. Rourke (1989) notes that prosody is also affected adversely in children exhibiting the NLD syndrome. Since acallosal individuals exhibit many NLD characteristics, it would seem worthwhile to explore further the nature of these prosodic deficits.

Visual-Perceptual and Tactile-Perceptual Functioning

The majority of the studies with acallosal patients have utilized tachistoscopic paradigms. As stated above, this is a highly artificial situation; it is important to examine the visual-perceptual functioning of these individuals in a more normalized setting. Dennis (1981), in her study of language functioning in a 27-year-old acallosal woman discussed above, also examined visual-perceptual functioning using a number of different tasks. D. S. was given a test of visual closure of incomplete line drawings, mazes, imagined rotations in space, and mental rotation of objects. All tasks were completed with no sign of impairment, suggesting that the absence of a CC in D. S. did not compromise her visual-perceptual functioning.

Meerwaldt (1983) examined a similar set of skills in an 8-year-old girl with agenesis. Specifically, Meerwaldt examined visual–spatial perception by means of the rod orientation test. The child had to orient a set of rods to match the position of a model, under two conditions: by visual inspection alone; and by tactile palpation alone (blindfolded), with one hand and then with the other. The visual task was performed without difficulty. However, significant difficulties were encountered on the tactile task with the right hand, but not with the left. Meerwaldt (1983) concluded that this child exhibited a right-hemisphere dominance for spatial perception. She was able to access the right-hemisphere systems when she used her left hand, but she was unable to access these systems properly when she used her right hand, suggesting a disturbance in interhemispheric transfer of tactile information. The generalizability of these results is limited for two reasons. First, a single subject was utilized. Second, the dichotic and tachistoscopic studies suggest that acallosal individuals will utilize other commissures, or will access ipsilateral pathways, or will simply have more bilaterally represented functions.

Ferris and Dorsen (1975) tested four individuals with agenesis of the CC who also presented with seizures. The intellectual functioning of these individuals was varied; however, all but one had Full Scale IQs in the mentally deficient range of functioning. These subjects are obviously not comparable to the majority of acallosal patients (with no other anomalies), who typically present with normal psychometric intelligence. Generalizability of the results is thus limited.

Ferris and Dorsen (1975) administered a number of different tests to these individuals. Each person was tested with the Halstead TPT. All patients scored below the level of frontal lobectomy patients as reported by Halstead (1947, cited by Ferris & Dorsen, 1975). Ferris and Dorsen (1975) noted that three of the patients "seemed unable to assess the shape or size of forms held in their hands or to recognize the similarity between the forms and the recesses in the board" (pp. 105–106). The strategy used seemed to be of the trial-and-error variety. Two patients did demonstrate a reduction in time taken between trials, indicating some transfer of learning. However, the performance of all patients was significantly impaired.

Russell and Reitan (1955) also assessed an acallosal patient with the TPT. This 19-year-old female patient presented with the following brain anomalies: absence of the posterior portion of the falx, maldeveloped cerebellum, and hydrocephalus. She required 44.7 minutes to place all 10 blocks—significantly more time than is normally required. (The cutoff score used for brain damage in the Reitan laboratory is 15 minutes.) She required a longer time to place the blocks on her second trial (left hand) than she did on the first attempt (right hand). This is an unusual pattern, since it implies that no bilateral transfer of learning has occurred (Russell & Reitan, 1955). Despite this finding, the patient was able to coordinate the movements of both hands together on the third trial, and did demonstrate some learning on the task.

Contradictory to the TPT results discussed above are those found by Sauerwein et al. (1981). They tested two siblings with borderline IQs using the TPT. Both subjects performed within normal limits.

These studies suggest that in most of the above-mentioned acallosal individuals, visual-perceptual functioning was intact; however, tactile-perceptual functioning presented particular difficulty. The tactile problems were most obvious when one hand only was required to complete the task without the aid of the other hand. A deficit in the bilateral transfer of tactile information is suggested.

Auditory-Perceptual Functioning

The majority of auditory-perceptual studies with acallosal subjects have utilized dichotic listening paradigms, as reviewed above. Few studies have assessed simple, bilateral auditory perception. The only study to assess this function, aside from that of Rourke (1987) (to be discussed later), was the study by Russell and Reitan (1955) discussed above. In their assessment of the 19-year-old female acallosal subject, they tested auditory perception using the Speech Sounds Perception Test and the Seashore Rhythm Test. Russell and Reitan (1955) report that her results were comparable with those obtained by Halstead's frontal lobectomy group, suggesting that she had difficulty distinguishing between phonemes, as well as trouble discriminating between rhythmic patterns. It should be noted that this individual was mentally deficient according to psychometric measures of intelligence; therefore, generalizability of these results to other acallosal individuals is questionnable.

Motor Skills

Russell and Reitan (1955) also tested their patient's simple motor skills with the Finger Oscillation Test (Tapping Test). They tested her dominant hand only, and found that her performance fell considerably below the mean obtained by Halstead's frontal lobectomy patients. Once again, it is not possible to generalize from such scant findings.

Chiarello (1980), in her review of 29 acallosal cases, noted that they often exhibited deficits in fine motor movements. Chiarello (1980) cited a study by Lehmann and Lampe (1970) that noted fine motor difficulties in acallosal patients, as well as epileptic controls. Dennis (1976) also noted that small "willed movements are deficient in the acallosals" (p. 464). Dennis (1976) suggested that these difficulties are the result of the fact that ipsilateral pathways control only gross arm and hand movements, and acallosal individuals demonstrate a tendency to rely more heavily on ipsilateral pathways than do individuals with intact brains.

Jeeves, Silver, and Jacobson (1988) also discuss motor functioning. They tested three acallosal subjects on a complex motor task that required the drawing of a straight line with both hands using separate dials. After extended practice, only one of the three reached the slower end of the normal range. They demonstrated better performance on the task when they were able to utilize visual feedback. The findings provide support for the "view that there *is* an inhibitory role for the callosum in the normal efficient control of bimanual motor output in the absence of visual feedback" (p. 850).

Visual–Spatial Skills

In her review of 29 acallosal cases, Chiarello (1980) notes that spatial–motor tasks yield the highest rate of deficit in these individuals. These deficient performances are seen specifically on tactile maze and form-board tasks, and are observed even when interhemispheric transfer is not necessary. She notes that unimanual stereognosis is not impaired in acallosal subjects, but that spatial localization and motoric precision are impaired. Perhaps "inaccurate performance might be due either to faulty spatial coding or to imprecision of fine motor control" (p. 145).

Memory and Attention

In her study of the 27-year-old female acallosal subject, Dennis (1981) also assessed memory and attention. She administered three auditory tasks (all utilizing word lists) to assess the following memory functions: recognition memory, memory for content, and memory for sequence. The subject, D. S., performed within normal limits on all three of these tasks. The attention task was an auditory discrimination task with the addition of different types of background noise (steady state, environmental/vocal, and vocal). When no noise was present, D. S. was able to perform the auditory discrimination task well; however, when background noise was introduced, her skill was compromised. In the steady-state condition, she performed worse than she did without noise, but still within the average range. However, when competing language was in the background, her performance became impaired. Therefore, in this particular patient, simple auditory attention was intact only when competing vocal noises were absent.

Ferris and Dorsen (1975) also assessed memory in their four acallosal patients. Visual memory and memory for tactile forms and locations were assessed using the Bender–Gestalt Test and the TPT, respectively. All four patients demonstrated a memory impairment for visual designs on the Bender–Gestalt. The results of the memory portion of the TPT also indicated a memory impairment for the spatial locations of the blocks, as three of the four patients tested on this measure received scores comparable to those of Halstead's frontal lobectomy patients. Russell and Reitan (1955) also indicated that their patient demonstrated impaired performance on TPT memory.

Problem Solving and Concept Formation

The results of Ferris and Dorsen (1975) and Russell and Reitan (1955) illustrate that acallosal individuals have impaired performance on the TPT, which is characterized as a measure of problem-solving ability. All but one of these five patients were mentally deficient on measures of psychometric intelligence. As such, the results are difficult to interpret.

Sauerwein et al. (1981) tested acallosal siblings who demonstrated performances on the TPT within normal ranges, suggesting that problem-solving skills were intact despite borderline IQs. Russell and Reitan (1955) also tested their patient on the Category Test, on which she demonstrated deficient performance. This suggests poor abstract or conceptual thinking, but again generalizability to other acallosal individuals is limited because of the low psychometric intelligence of this subject. Clearly, further testing of other acallosal subjects of average intelligence is required before any conclusions can be drawn.

Personality and Socioemotional Functioning

The only study (aside from that of Rourke, 1987) to report on any personality variables in acallosal individuals was the one by Russell and Reitan (1955). They administered the Minnesota Multiphasic Personality Inventory (MMPI), the Rorschach, and the Halstead Schematic Face Test to their 19-year-old female patient. The MMPI results suggested that she was experiencing depression and anxiety, and was emotionally unstable. The responses to the Rorschach were few and vague, and were suggestive of brain disorder. The patient obtained unusual results on the Halstead Schematic Face Test, which suggested that she "had not developed normally even in certain respects of categorizing not based on rational principles, perhaps as a result of her congenital brain anomaly" (Russell & Reitan, 1955, p. 212). Once again, note that this patient was functioning in the mentally deficient range. Thus, she cannot be considered to be representative of the entire acallosal population.

CALLOSAL AGENESIS AND THE NLD SYNDROME AND MODEL

A review of the NLD syndrome and model has been provided in Chapter 1; thus, a detailed description is not given here. However, there are some points that should be stressed.

It should be borne in mind that there are three types of white matter that can be destroyed or rendered dysfunctional in the brain: commissural fibers, association fibers, and projection fibers (Rourke, 1989). Various forms of neurological disease can affect each (and sometimes all) of these types of white matter. The white matter involvement in these particular forms of neurological disease may lead to the manifestation of the NLD syndrome.

Callosal agenesis is one such neurological disease. This particular disorder interferes with communication between the right and left hemispheres. Rourke (1988) points out that "such a disease would be expected to have a more profound effect upon the functioning of the right than the left cerebral hemisphere because of the right hemisphere's greater 'dependence' upon white-matter functioning, especially with regard to its apparent 'specialization' for the intermodal integration of novel stimuli" (p. 313). Rourke (1987) stressed that the NLD syndrome should be exhibited in acallosal individuals who exhibit no other demonstrable neurological disease. Given the fact that individuals with agenesis of the CC often present with additional brain anomalies, it is likely that the NLD syndrome will be evident in some of these individuals and not in others.

Research has indicated that in addition to callosal fibers, other white matter tracts can be affected in callosal agenesis (i.e., deep white matter) as a result of the dilation of the ventricles (Baierl et al., 1988; Lewis et al., 1988). Because the degree of white matter affected has a bearing on the likelihood that the NLD syndrome will be exhibited (Rourke, 1989), then the fact that extensive white matter involvment is found in acallosal individuals would seem to increase the chances that they will exhibit the NLD syndrome.

In our Windsor laboratory, we have investigated developmental trends apparent in individuals presenting with the NLD syndrome. The results of cross-sectional studies have suggested that age-related changes occur with NLD. In particular, these individuals seem to exhibit exacerbated symptoms over time if they are left to develop without remediation.

For instance, these individuals seem to be at a greater risk for socioemotional disturbances as they age. From these findings, one can infer that
similar developmental implications may be identifiable in acallosal individuals. A detailed review of the specific profile changes can be found
in the study by Casey, Rourke, and Picard (1991).

CASE STUDY OF AN ACALLOSAL CHILD PRESENTING WITH THE NLD SYNDROME

Rourke (1987) provides a detailed review of two full neuropsychological
assessments that were administered to a young girl (L. C.) who presented
with virtually complete agenesis of the CC, as well as a seizure disorder.
The case is also reviewed in Rourke's (1989) book under the pseudonym
"Mary." L. C. was 9 years of age at the first assessment and 11½ at the
second. This child appeared to exhibit all of the typical characteristics
of the NLD syndrome. The following is a brief review of the findings; a
more detailed delineation of the case can be found in Rourke (1987).

First Assessment

Tactile-Perceptual Skills

No simple tactile imperception was indicated. Tactile suppression was
exhibited with the left hand only. L. C. exhibited moderate to severe
impairment with both hands on tests of finger agnosia, finger dysgraphesthesia, and astereognosis for coins. Finger agnosia was somewhat more
marked on the left side.

Motor and Psychomotor Skills

L. C. was almost exclusively left-handed, right-footed, and left-eyed. Bilateral deficiencies were exhibited in grip strength, finger- and foot-tapping
speed, and psychomotor coordination under speeded conditions. She exhibited borderline static tremor with both hands, and mild to moderate
kinetic tremor. She exhibited severely impaired performance on a
speeded underlining test in the absence of virtually any requirement for
visual discrimination. In general, motoric deficiencies were somewhat
more marked with the left (dominant) hand. Her levels of performance
with each hand separately (especially the left hand) and with both hands
together on the TPT were severely impaired.

Visual–Spatial–Organizational Abilities

Very low scaled scores were obtained on the Wechsler Intelligence Scale
for Children (WISC) Picture Arrangement and Object Assembly subtests.

L. C. exhibited moderate impairment on a test of immediate memory for visual sequences. She had some difficulty with the Trail Making Test. She exhibited mild to moderate impairment on many subtests of the Underlining Test. She had trouble writing in cursive script, and her drawing of a complex key was immature and lacking in visual–spatial detail.

Nonverbal Problem Solving, Concept Formation, Hypothesis Testing, Benefiting from Informational Feedback

Overall performances on tests of various nonverbal reasoning capacities were severely impaired. L. C. exhibited difficulty dealing with cause-and-effect relationships. Her Performance IQ was 19 points below her Verbal IQ on the WISC. Throughout the testing sessions, there was much evidence of difficulty in dealing with humor and other forms of incongruity.

Rote Memory

L. C. obtained average or above-average scores on the WISC Information, Vocabulary, and Digit Span subtests. Her memory for sentences was normal. Her good performance on these tasks contrasted with her difficulty on memory tasks requiring more effortful processing (e.g., the last subtest of the Category Test, the memory component of the TPT, and the Target Test).

Adaptation to Novel, Complex Situations, Reliance on Rote Behaviors

On the Category Test and TPT (which involve the ability to adapt), L. C. exhibited clear evidence of perseveration and difficulties in applying problem-solving strategies to the tasks at hand in a flexible, adaptive fashion.

Reading, Spelling, and Arithmetic

L. C. obtained scores well above average on the Reading (word recognition) and Spelling subtests of the Wide Range Achievement Test (WRAT). Her score on the Arithmetic subtest was average, but was significantly below that obtained on the other two subtests. Arithmetic problems were also noted elsewhere in the examination.

Speech and Language Characteristics

Misspellings were almost exclusively of the phonetically accurate variety. L. C. performed at average levels on the Peabody Picture Vocabulary

Test and on tests of speech-sounds perception, auditory closure, verbatim sentence memory, and phonetically cued verbal fluency. She performed less well on verbal tasks that required some degree of verbal processing than on those of a more rote nature. Her ambient behavior in the testing situation was marked by much verbosity and by a clear tendency to seek information through verbal questioning rather than through exploration and experimentation.

Social Judgment, Social Interaction, Socioemotional Functioning

As indicated by her responses to the Personality Inventory for Children (PIC), L. C.'s mother saw her daughter as deficient in social relations with persons outside her immediate family, and as having a tendency toward an internalized form of psychopathology characterized by anxiety, social withdrawal, depression, and inappropriate social relations.

Second Assessment

The following changes were observed on the occasion of the second testing (2½ years later). L. C. exhibited drops in her WISC-R (vs. WISC) Verbal, Performance, and Full Scale IQs of 16, 15, and 16 points, respectively. She made some progress on WRAT Reading and Spelling, but no similar progress in Arithmetic. Finger agnosia and dysgraphesthesia were more marked, as was astereognosis for coins (but less so). Her performance on measures of static and kinetic steadiness became more normalized. She exhibited declines in sentence memory and verbal fluency; in these and in some other instances, L. C.'s performance in this second assessment became even more typical of the expected NLD syndrome pattern. Her cursive script improved. She did somewhat better on the Category Test, but her performance was still markedly impaired. Some worsening of her performance on the TPT was noted. Marginal advances were made on the Trail Making Test. Her personality profile, as indicated by the PIC, revealed markedly higher scores on the Adjustment, Intellectual Screening, and Development scales, and a lower score on the Hyperactivity scale.

Rourke (1987) notes that L. C.'s "profile of neuropsychological abilities and deficits fits the clinical features of the NLD syndrome quite precisely" (p. 228). What are needed now are further studies that utilize the same assessment measures to determine the functioning of acallosal individuals. An effort is made next to review the previously cited studies, in an attempt to determine whether and to what extent the patients in these studies exhibited symptoms of the NLD syndrome.

NLD CHARACTERISTICS OF ACALLOSAL INDIVIDUALS
AS INDICATED IN PREVIOUS STUDIES

We now attempt to provide a context for the neuropsychological findings discussed above in the context of the characteristics exhibited by L. C. in Rourke's (1987) case study. Not all areas discussed in L. C.'s case are addressed here because of the paucity of research. Very few complete neuropsychological evaluations have been administered; rather, investigators typically choose to examine only a few areas of functioning that are of interest to them. Many more complete assessments are required before any firm conclusions can be made about the connection of callosal agenesis to the NLD model. At the moment, we are speculating about the relationship between the two phenomena because of the logical fit with the state of the white matter in callosal agenesis and the effects of such compromised white matter hypothesized in the NLD/white matter model.

Attention

An area not specifically addressed in L. C.'s case is attention. The NLD model predicts that individuals with callosal agenesis will have intact verbal and visual attentional skills. In her study of a 27-year-old acallosal individual, Dennis (1981) indicated that D. S. performed well on an auditory discrimination task when there were no distracter variables present. This is consistent with the findings of Rourke (1987). However, Dennis (1981) also noted that the performance of D. S. was impaired on the same task when verbal distracters were included as background noise. Rourke (1987) did not test the limits of auditory attention with this procedure; thus, it is not possible to make the relevant comparison.

Tactile Perception

Tactile-perceptual skills have not been addressed in the literature, as they were with L. C.. When tactile functioning is tested, it is in the context of laterality studies, and usually includes tactile transfer tasks. Although acallosal subjects have performed within normal limits on these tasks, the findings from L. C.'s case suggest that more detailed testing of this modality might reveal finger agnosia, finger dysgraphesthesia, and astereognosis.

Motor Skills

In L. C.'s case, deficits were noted with respect to motor and psychomotor abilities. Indeed, this is one of the primary areas of deficit in the child with NLD. The findings of Jeeves et al. (1988) are consistent with this view. They found that three acallosal individuals demonstrated deficient performance on a motor task using both hands, and that their performance worsened in the absence of visual feedback. Ferris and Dorsen (1975) also tested complex psychomotor skills (and visual memory) using the Bender–Gestalt Test. Deficient performances were again exhibited, with the exception of one patient who possessed good coordination when drawing. Three of these four patients also exhibited poor psychomotor coordination when required to trace an object in a mirror.

Other Abilities

With the exception of L. C.'s case, visual–spatial–organizational abilities, as well as nonverbal problem solving and concept formation were not specifically assessed in the literature.

Memory

L. C. obtained average or above-average scores on tests of rote memory; indeed, this is an asset exhibited by children with NLD. Temple et al. (1989) found that the two acallosal subjects tested were able to retrieve words that were associated (paired) with another word. Dennis (1981) tested various types of memory for word lists and also found this to be an asset for D. S. Jeeves and Temple (1987) reported a previous testing of their subject K. C., during which she obtained a reduced Digit Span score on the WISC. Although this is a different test from those utilized by Dennis (1981), it does suggest that auditory memory may be impaired, which is contradictory to the predictions of the NLD model. Rourke (1987) maintains that those individuals in whom the pattern of assets and deficits of the NLD syndrome is most likely to be evident are those who exhibit uncomplicated callosal agenesis (i.e., free of other significant structural abnormalities of the brain). K. C. is reported to have had a left frontal cyst, which could have accounted for those areas of functioning that were discrepant from the typical NLD presentation.

Adaptation to Novelty, Reliance on Rote Behaviors

L. C. exhibited deficiencies in adaptation to novel, complex situations, as evidenced by her poor performance on the Category Test and TPT. Similar findings have been demonstrated in the literature cited above. It is important to note that the TPT is one of a subset of four neuropsychological tests that have been found to discriminate subjects with NLD from other learning-disabled and nonclinical children with high (>95%) accuracy (Harnadek & Rourke, 1994). Investigators who assessed acallosal patients on the TPT found that all subjects exhibited deficient performance (Ferris & Dorsen, 1975; Russell & Reitan, 1955). These findings are consistent with the predictions of the NLD model. Contradictory findings, however, were reported by Sauerwein et al. (1981). Two siblings performed within normal limits; however, localization memory was slightly impaired. These results are difficult to interpret because they do not appear consistent with other findings in the literature. The Category Test also taps these types of abilities. The acallosal subject tested by Russell and Reitan (1955) on this task performed poorly, thus again supporting the notion that acallosal individuals exhibit aspects of the NLD syndrome.

Reading

Although rote reading skills are preserved in children with NLD, they perform poorly on tests of reading comprehension. This was demonstrated by Dennis (1981), whose acallosal subject demonstrated deficient performance with verbal content and pragmatics, and also with reading comprehension (as measured by the ability to understand sentence syntax). Problems with content and reading comprehension were also noted by Jeeves and Temple (1987) and by Sanders (1989).

Language Skills

L. C., like other children with NLD, demonstrated good rote verbal and language skills, but she had difficulty with tasks requiring processing of this information. Dennis (1981) found that her patient performed better with phonology than semantics, and that she demonstrated deficient performance with verbal content and pragmatics. Because of their strong rote verbal skills, simple repetition is a task accomplished easily by children with NLD. Both Dennis (1981) and Jeeves and Temple (1987) reported that their acallosal patients had difficulty with the verbal repetition of sentences. Once again, this could be attributable in part to the other brain anomalies exhibited by these individuals. However, the most likely explanation seems to be the fact that the sentences used in the task in both of these studies included various grammatical forms. Dennis (1981) speculated that the deficits exhibited on this task could be attributed to the fact that her patient had difficulty comprehending the rules of syntax. When syntax is too complex, it hinders the repetition abilities of these individuals. It would appear, then, that these seemingly anomalous results do in fact coincide with the expected NLD pattern of assets and deficits.

Rourke (1989) also notes that the ability to make verbal associations is an asset for individuals with NLD. Dennis (1981) required her acallosal patient to make verbal associations in the naming task, which demanded that the patient provide a name to verbal cues. The patient performed well on this task.

Social Skills

Finally, children with NLD demonstrate deficient social skills and socio-emotional functioning. Russell and Reitan (1955) were the only investigators (besides Rourke, 1987) to administer personality measures. The results of the MMPI indicated that their acallosal subject was exhibiting signs of emotional instability—specifically, depression and anxiety.

The preceding discussion indicates that the studies reviewed here, which were not specifically testing for the presence of NLD symptomatology, did find that their acallosal patients exhibited some of the same characteristics as individuals with NLD. Although contradictions certainly exist, one cannot make firm conclusions about the applicability of the NLD model to callosal agenesis until studies test this notion more directly. However, at present, this line of research seems promising.

CONCLUSIONS

This extensive review of the neuropsychological literature on callosal agenesis has led us to a number of conclusions, which are as follows:

1. There is a clear demand for more studies in this area. In particular, there is a strong need for more systematic testing of *all* neuropsychological functions in acallosal individuals. If we are to understand how acallosal brains function, it is necessary to obtain neuropsychological profiles on many different individuals. Although studies focusing specifically on laterality issues are valuable, other areas of functioning are equally important to explore. A better understanding of the pattern of assets and deficits exhibited by these individuals will permit us to design intervention programs that will allow us to serve this population more effectively.

2. There are obvious problems of sample size in all of the studies reviewed. Although single-case studies are valuable, there is a need for studies utilizing larger groups of acallosal subjects, in order to examine the particular assets and deficits that are shared by these individuals.

The generalizability of single-case studies is extremely limited; thus, it is difficult to draw any firm conclusions about the profile of an acallosal individual.

3. There is a need to examine developmental aspects of this neurological disorder. From the NLD model, one can infer that acallosal children will behave differently in early childhood than they will in late childhood and adulthood (Casey et al., 1991). It would be beneficial to determine whether acallosal individuals also exhibit this developmental pattern. This has particular implications for treatment. Rourke (1989) stresses that when children with NLD are young it is better to attack the deficits, whereas when such children are older it is better to stress compensatory techniques.

4. The control groups used in all of these studies are inconsistent. At times, controls consisted of only two or three other individuals chosen at random from a population considered to be comparable; at other times, the "control groups" used were the norms established for a particular test. Different norms were used for different tests, leading to inconsistent controls. Clearly, there is a need for specific criteria for control groups. Should controls be matched on the basis of Verbal IQ, or on the basis of Verbal–Performance IQ discrepancy? These are questions that must be addressed if research in this area is to be comparable.

5. The effect of the extent of agenesis of the CC is considered in few studies. Some studies included patients with complete agenesis, whereas other studies included patients with only partial agenesis. It is unlikely that these two types of patients are comparable, except in the sense that they may represent varying degrees of dysfunction. Rourke (1989) stresses that the greater the amount of white matter affected, the more likely it is that a child will exhibit the NLD syndrome. Thus, to test the applicability of the NLD model, it is important to consider the amount of white matter affected, for theoretical as well as clinical reasons.

6. The comparability of studies is again hampered by the preponderance of associated brain anomalies that acallosal individuals frequently exhibit. Because studies have not controlled for these extra anomalies, it is very difficult to determine whether the behavioral symptoms present can be attributed to the lack of a CC or to some other brain anomaly. Rourke (1987) suggests that the acallosal individuals who are expected to exhibit the NLD syndrome are those who do not have any other significant structural anomaly. It is possible that other acallosal individuals also present with NLD in combination with other forms of dysfunction, but until we control for other anomalies, we will not be able to tease out any causal factors.

7. Some authors (e.g., Baierl et al., 1988; Lewis et al., 1988) have suggested that other white matter in addition to the CC is affected in some acallosal individuals. With the advent of more sophisticated imaging

techniques, it is now possible to examine these phenomena further. For instance, it would be interesting to perform an MRI study that compares the degree of white matter dysfunction with the degree of NLD symptomatology present.

It is clear, then, that this area of research has only just begun. Up to this point, studies have been fraught with methodological problems that make it difficult for any firm conclusions to be drawn. Despite the research-related difficulties, the areas on which we need to concentrate in the future are outlined above. The link between callosal agenesis and the NLD syndrome has now been suggested; theoretical arguments in favor of this connection seem firm. Now researchers in the field should take into account the suggestions listed above. If they do so, future studies should reveal whether, and to what extent, there are links between this brain anomaly and NLD.

REFERENCES

Atlas, S. W., Zimmerman, R. A., Bruce, D., Schut, L., Bilaniuk, L. T., Hackney, D. B., Goldberg, H. I., & Grossman, R. I. (1988). Neurofibromatosis and agenesis of the corpus callosum in identical twins: MR diagnosis. *American Journal of Neuroradiology*, 9, 598–601.

Baierl, P., Markl, A., Thelen, M., & Laub, M. C. (1988). MR imaging in Aicardi syndrome. *American Journal of Neuroradiology*, 9, 805–806.

Barkovich, A. J. (1990). Apparent atypical callosal dysgenesis: Analysis of MR findings in six cases and their relationship to holoprosencephaly. *American Journal of Neuroradiology*, 11, 333–339.

Barkovich, A. J., & Kjos, B. O. (1988). Normal postnatal development of the corpus callosum as demonstrated by MR imaging. *American Journal of Neuroradiology*, 9, 487–491.

Barkovich, A. J., & Norman, D. (1988). Anomalies of the corpus callosum: Correlation with further anomalies of the brain. *American Journal of Neuroradiology*, 9, 493–501.

Ben Ari, J., Shuper, A., Mimouni, M., Rosen, O., Grunebaum, M., & Merlob, P. (1989). Agenesis of the corpus callosum associated with double urinary collecting system, trigonocephaly, and other minor anomalies: A new association. *European Journal of Pediatrics*, 148, 787–788.

Bertino, R. E., Nyberg, D. A., Cyr, D. R., & Mack, L. A. (1988). Prenatal diagnosis of agenesis of the corpus callosum. *Journal of Ultrasound Medicine*, 7, 251–260.

Brodal, A. (1981). *Neurological anatomy: In relation to clinical medicine* (3rd ed.). New York: Oxford University Press.

Bruyer, R., Dupuis, M., Ophoven, E., Rectem, D., & Reynaert, C. (1985). Anatomical and behavioral study of a case of asymptomatic callosal agenesis. *Cortex*, 21, 417–430.

Bryden, M. P., & Zurif, E. B. (1970). Dichotic listening performance in a case of agenesis of the corpus callosum. *Neuropsychologia, 8*, 371–377.

Byrd, S. E., Radkowski, M. A., Flannery, A., & McLone, D. G. (1990). The clinical and radiological evaluation of absence of the corpus callosum. *European Journal of Radiology, 10*, 65–73.

Casamassima, A. C., Beneck, D., Gewitz, M. H., Horowitz, M. A., Woolf, P. K., Pettersen, I. M., & Shapiro, L. R. (1989). Acrocallosal syndrome: Additional manifestations. *American Journal of Medical Genetics, 32*, 311–317.

Casey, J. E., Rourke, B. P., & Picard, E. M. (1991). Syndrome of nonverbal learning disabilities: Age differences in neuropsychological, academic, and socioemotional functioning. *Development and Psychopathology, 3*, 329–345.

Cataltepe, S., & Tuncbilek, E. (1992). A family with one child with acrocallosal syndrome, one child with anencephaly–polydactyly, and parental consanguinity. *European Journal of Pediatrics, 151*, 288–290.

Chiarello, C. (1980). A house divided? Cognitive functioning with callosal agenesis. *Brain and Language, 11*, 128–158.

Cook, N. D., Brugger, P., Regard, M., & Landis, T. (1990). On the role of the corpus callosum in cerebral laterality: A comment on Lassonde, Bryden, and Demers. *Brain and Language, 39*, 471–474.

da-Silva, E. O. (1988). Callosal defect, microcephaly, severe mental retardation, and other anomalies in three sibs. *American Journal of Medical Genetics, 29*, 837–843.

De Lacoste, M. C., Kirkpatrick, J. B., & Ross, E. D. (1985). Topography of the human corpus callosum. *Journal of Neuropathology and Experimental Neurology, 44*, 578–591.

del Carpio-O'Donovan, R., & Cardinal, E. (1990). Agenesis of the corpus callosum and colloid cyst of the third ventricle: Magnetic resonance imaging of an unusual association. *Canadian Association of Radiologists Journal, 41*, 375–379.

Dennis, M. (1976). Impaired sensory and motor differentiation with corpus callosum agenesis: A lack of callosal inhibition during ontogeny? *Neuropsychologia, 14*, 455–469.

Dennis, M. (1981). Language in a congenitally acallosal brain. *Brain and Language, 12*, 33–53.

de Villemeur, T. B., Chiron, C., & Robain, O. (1992). Unlayered polymicrogyria and agenesis of the corpus callosum: A relevant association? *Acta Neuropathologica, 83*, 265–270.

Dietrich, R. B., & Bradley, W. G., Jr. (1988). Normal and abnormal white matter maturation. *Seminars in Ultrasound, CT, and MR, 9*, 192–200.

Dobyns, W. B. (1989). Agenesis of the corpus callosum and gyral malformations are frequent manifestations of nonketotic hyperglycinemia. *Neurology, 39*, 817–820.

Donnenfeld, A. E., Packer, R. J., Zackai, E. H., Chee, C. M., Sellinger, B., & Emanuel, B. S. (1989). Clinical, cytogenetic, and pedigree findings in 18 cases of Aicardi syndrome. *American Journal of Medical Genetics, 32*, 461–467.

Ettlinger, G., Blakemore, C. B., Milner, A. D., & Wilson, J. (1972). Agenesis of the corpus callosum: A behavioural investigation. *Brain, 95*, 327–346.

Faye-Petersen, O. M., Ward, K., Carey, J. C., & Knisely, A. S. (1991). Osteochondrodysplasia with rhizomelia, platyspondyly, callosal agenesis, thrombocytopenia, hydrocephalus, and hypertension. *American Journal of Medical Genetics, 40,* 183–187.

Ferris, G. S., & Dorsen, M. M. (1975). Agenesis of the corpus callosum: 1. Neuropsychological studies. *Cortex, 11,* 95–122.

Font, R. L., Marines, H. M., Cartwright, J., & Bauserman, S. C. (1991). Aicardi syndrome: A clinicopathologic case report including electron microscopic observations. *Ophthalmology, 98,* 1727–1731.

Gelman-Kohan, Z., Antonelli, J., Ankori-Cohen, H., Adar, H., & Chemke, J. (1991). Further delineation of the acrocallosal syndrome. *European Journal of Pediatrics, 150,* 797–799.

Gershoni-Baruch, R., Nachlieli, T., & Guilburd, J. N. (1991). Apert's syndrome with occipital encephalocele and absence of corpus callosum. *Child's Nervous System, 7,* 231–232.

Guit, G. L., van de Bor, M., den Ouden, L., & Wondergem, J. H. M. (1990). Prediction of neurodevelopmental outcome in the preterm infant: MR-staged myelination compared with cranial US. *Radiology, 175,* 107–109.

Harnadek, M. C. S., & Rourke, B. P. (1994). Principal identifying features of the syndrome of nonverbal learning disabilities in children. *Journal of Learning Disabilities, 27,* 144–154.

Hewitt, W. (1962). The development of the human corpus callosum. *Journal of Anatomy, 96,* 355–358.

Hicks, S. P. (1977). Introduction to embryogenic disorders. In E. S. Goldensohn & S. H. Appel (Eds.), *Scientific approaches to clinical neurology* (Vol. 1, pp. 552–571). Philadelphia: Lea & Febiger.

Hilpert, P. L., & Kurtz, A. B. (1990). Prenatal diagnosis of agenesis of the corpus callosum using endovaginal ultrasound. *Journal of Ultrasound Medicine, 9,* 363–365.

Jacobson, R. I. (1989). Congenital structural defects. In K. F. Swaiman (Ed.), *Pediatric neurology: Principles and practice* (Vol. 1, pp. 317–362). St. Louis: C. V. Mosby.

Jeeves, M. A., Silver, P. H., & Jacobson, I. (1988). Bimanual co-ordination in callosal agenesis and partial commissurotomy. *Neuropsychologia, 26,* 833–850.

Jeeves, M. A., & Temple, C. M. (1987). A further study of language function in callosal agenesis. *Brain and Language, 32,* 325–335.

Jeret, J. S., Serur, D., & Wisniewski, K. (1989). [Letter to the editor]. *Archives of Neurology, 46,* 10.

Jinkins, J. R., Whittemore, A. R., & Bradley, W. G. (1989). MR imaging of callosal and corticocallosal dysgenesis. *American Journal of Neuroradiology, 10,* 339–344.

Karnath, H. O., Schumacher, M., & Wallesch, C. W. (1991). Limitations of interhemispheric extracallosal transfer of visual information in callosal agenesis. *Cortex, 27,* 345–350.

Katafuchi, Y., Fukuda, T., Maruoka, T., Tokunaga, Y., Yamashita, Y., & Matsuishi, T. (1992). Partial trisomy 6p with agenesis of the corpus callosum and choanal atresia. *Journal of Child Neurology, 7,* 114–116.

Kimura, M., Nakajima, M., & Yoshino, K. (1990). Ullrich–Turner syndrome with agenesis of the corpus callosum. *American Journal of Medical Genetics*, *37*, 227–228.

Kinsbourne, M., & Fisher, M. (1971). Latency of uncrossed and of crossed reaction in callosal agenesis. *Neuropsychologia*, *9*, 471–473.

Klouda, G. V., Robin, D. A., Graff-Radford, N. R., & Cooper, W. E. (1988). The role of callosal connections in speech prosody. *Brain and Language*, *35*, 154–171.

Kolodny, E. H. (1989). Agenesis of the corpus callosum: A marker for inherited metabolic disease. *Neurology*, *39*, 847–848.

Lacey, D. J. (1985). Agenesis of the corpus callosum: Clinical features in 40 children. *American Journal of Diseases of Children*, *139*, 953–955.

Lacombe, D., Creusot, G., & Battin, J. (1992). New case of Toriello–Carey syndrome. *American Journal of Medical Genetics*, *42*, 374–376.

Lahat, E., Strauss, S., Tadmor, R., & Bistritzer, T. (1992). Infantile spasms in a patient with septo-optic dysplasia, partial agenesis of the corpus callosum and an interhemispheric cyst. *Clinical Neurology and Neurosurgery*, *94*, 165–167.

Lassonde, M., & Bryden, M. P. (1990). Dichotic listening, callosal agenesis and cerebral laterality. *Brain and Language*, *39*, 475–481.

Lassonde, M., Bryden, M. P., & Demers, P. (1990). The corpus callosum and cerebral speech lateralization. *Brain and Language*, *38*, 195–206.

Lassonde, M. C., Lortie, J., Ptito, M., & Geoffroy, G. (1981). Hemispheric asymmetry in callosal agenesis as revealed by dichotic listening performance. *Neuropsychologia*, *19*, 455–458.

Lassonde, M., Sauerwein, H., Chicoine, A.-J., & Geoffroy, G. (1991). Absence of disconnexion syndrome in callosal agenesis and early callosotomy: Brain reorganization or lack of structural specificity during ontogeny? *Neuropsychologia*, *29*, 481–495.

Lassonde, M., Sauerwein, H., Geoffroy, G., & Decarie, M. (1986). Effects of early and late transection of the corpus callosum in children: A study of tactile and tactuomotor transfer and integration. *Brain*, *109*, 953–967.

Lassonde, M., Sauerwein, H., McCabe, N., Laurencelle, L., & Geoffroy, G. (1988). Extent and limits of cerebral adjustment to early section or congenital absence of the corpus callosum. *Behavioral Brain Research*, *30*, 165–181.

Lemire, R. J., Loeser, J. D., Leech, R. W., & Alvord, E. C. (1975). *Normal and abnormal development of the human nervous system*. Hagerstown, MD: Harper & Row.

Lewis, S. W., Reveley, M. A., David, A. S., & Ron, M. A. (1988). Agenesis of the corpus callosum and schizophrenia: A case report. *Psychological Medicine*, *18*, 341–347.

Lin, A. E., & Gettig, E. (1990). Craniosynostosis, agenesis of the corpus callosum, severe mental retardation, distinctive facies, camptodactyly, and hypogonadism. *American Journal of Medical Genetics*, *35*, 582–585.

Lockwood, C. J., Ghidini, A., Aggarwal, R., & Hobbins, J. C. (1988). Antenatal diagnosis of partial agenesis of the corpus callosum: A benign cause of ventriculomegaly. *American Journal of Obstetrics and Gynecology*, *159*, 184–186.

Loeser, J. D., & Alvord, E. C. (1968). Agenesis of the corpus callosum. *Brain*, *91*, 553–570.

Lynn, R. B., Buchanan, D. C., Fenichel, G. M., & Freemon, F. R. (1980). Agenesis of the corpus callosum. *Archives of Neurology, 37*, 444–445.

Meerwaldt, J. D. (1983). Disturbances of spatial perception in a patient with agenesis of the corpus callosum. *Neuropsychologia, 21*, 161–165.

Milner, A. D. (1982). Simple reaction times to lateralized visual stimuli in a case of callosal agenesis. *Neuropsychologia, 20*, 411–419.

Milner, A. D., Jeeves, M. A., Silver, P. H., Lines, C. R., & Wilson, J. (1985). Reaction time to lateralized visual stimuli in callosal agenesis: Stimulus and response factors. *Neuropsychologia, 23*, 323–331.

Milner, D. (1983). Neuropsychological studies of callosal agenesis. *Psychological Medicine, 13*, 721–725.

Molina, J. A., Mateos, F., Merino, M., Epifanio, J. L., & Gorrono, M. (1989). Aicardi syndrome in two sisters. *Journal of Pediatrics, 115*, 282–283.

Mori, K. (1992). Giant interhemispheric cysts associated with agenesis of the corpus callosum. *Journal of Neurosurgery, 76*, 224–230.

Neidich, J. A., Nussbaum, R. L., Packer, R. J., Emanuel, B. S., & Puck, J. M. (1990). Heterogeneity of clinical severity and molecular lesions in Aicardi syndrome. *Journal of Pediatrics, 116*, 911–916.

Nielsen, K. B., Anvret, M., Flodmark, O., Furuskog, P., & Bohman-Valis, K. (1991). Aicardi syndrome: Early neuroradiological manifestations and results of DNA studies in one patient. *American Journal of Medical Genetics, 38*, 65–68.

Page, S. R., Nussey, S. S., Jenkins, J. S., Wilson, S. G., & Johnson, D. A. (1989). Hypothalamic disease in association with dysgenesis of the corpus callosum. *Postgraduate Medical Journal, 65*, 163–167.

Philip, N., Apicella, N., Lassman, I., Ayme, S., Mattei, J. F., & Giraud, F. (1988). The acrocallosal syndrome. *European Journal of Pediatrics, 147*, 206–208.

Rakic, P., & Yakovlev, P. I. (1968). Development of the corpus callosum and cavum septi in man. *Journal of Comparative Neurology, 132*, 45–72.

Reinarz, S. J., Coffman, C. E., Smoker, W. R. K., & Godersky, J. C. (1988). MR imaging of the corpus callosum: Normal and pathologic findings and correlation with CT. *American Journal of Radiology, 151*, 791–798.

Reynolds, D. M., & Jeeves, M. A. (1974). Further studies of crossed and uncrossed pathway responding in callosal agenesis: Reply to Kinsbourne and Fisher. *Neuropsychologia, 12*, 287–290.

Rodriguez, J. I., Palacios, J., Omenaca, F., & Lorente, M. (1991). Polyasplenia, caudal deficiency, and agenesis of the corpus callosum. *American Journal of Medical Genetics, 38*, 99–102.

Rogers, T., Al-Rayess, M., O'Shea, P., & Ambler, M. W. (1991). Dysplasia of the corpus callosum in indentical twins with nonketotic hyperglycinemia. *Pediatric Pathology, 11*, 897–902.

Rourke, B. P. (1987). Syndrome of nonverbal learning disabilities: The final common pathway of white-matter disease/dysfunction? *The Clinical Neuropsychologist, 1*, 209–234.

Rourke, B. P. (1988). The syndrome of nonverbal learning disabilities: Developmental manifestations in neurological disease, disorder, and dysfunction. *The Clinical Neuropsychologist, 2*, 293–330.

Rourke, B. P. (1989). *Nonverbal learning disabilities: The syndrome and the model.* New York: Guilford Press.

Russell, J. R., & Reitan, R. M. (1955). Psychological abnormalities in agenesis of the corpus callosum. *Journal of Nervous and Mental Disease, 121,* 205–214.

Sanders, R. J. (1989). Sentence comprehension following agenesis of the corpus callosum. *Brain and Language, 37,* 59–72.

Sandri, F., Pilu, G., Cerisoli, M., Bovicelli, L., Alvisi, C., & Salvioli, G. P. (1988). Sonographic diagnosis of agenesis of the corpus callosum in the fetus and newborn infant. *American Journal of Perinatology, 5,* 226–231.

Sauerwein, H., & Lassonde, M. C. (1983). Intra- and interhemispheric processing of visual information in callosal agenesis. *Neuropsychologia, 21,* 167–171.

Sauerwein, H. C., Lassonde, M. C., Cardu, B., & Geoffroy, G. (1981). Interhemispheric integration of sensory and motor functions in agenesis of the corpus callosum. *Neuropsychologia, 19,* 445–454.

Saul, R. E., & Gott, P. S. (1976). Language and speech lateralization by amytal and dichotic listening tests in agenesis of the corpus callosum. In D. O. Walter, L. Rogers, & J. M. Finzi-Fried (Eds.), *Conference on human brain function* (Brain Information Service Conference Report No. 42, pp. 138–141). Los Angeles: UCLA Brain Information Service/BRI Publications Office.

Schaefer, G. B., Shuman, R. M., Wilson, D. A., Saleeb, S., Domek, D. B., Johnson, S. F., & Bodensteiner, J. B. (1991). Partial agenesis of the anterior corpus callosum: Correlation between appearance, imaging, and neuropathology. *Pediatric Neurology, 7,* 39–44.

Schwartz, A. M., & Ghatak, N. R. (1990). Interhemispheric cysts in association with agenesis of the corpus callosum. *Clinical Neuropathology, 9,* 177–180.

Serur, D., Jeret, J. S., & Wisniewski, K. (1988). Agenesis of the corpus callosum: Clinical, neuroradiological, and cytogenetic studies. *Neuropediatrics, 19,* 87–91.

Sharief, N., Craze, J., Summers, D., Butler, L., & Wood, C. B. S. (1991). Miller-Dieker syndrome with ring chromosome 17. *Archives of Diseases in Childhood, 66,* 710–712.

Shoumura, K., Ando, T., & Kato, K. (1975). Structural organization of "callosal" OBg in human corpus callosum agenesis. *Brain Research, 93,* 241–252.

Tagawa, T., Mimaki, T., Ono, J., Tanaka, J., Imai, K., & Yabuuchi, H. (1989). Aicardi syndrome associated with an embryonal carcinoma. *Pediatric Neurology, 5,* 45–47.

Temple, C. M., Jeeves, M. A., & Vilarroya, O. (1989). Ten pen men: Rhyming skills in two children with callosal agenesis. *Brain and Language, 37,* 548–564.

Temple, C. M., Jeeves, M. A., & Vilarroya, O. O. (1990). Reading in callosal agenesis. *Brain and Language, 39,* 235–253.

Toriello, H. V., & Carey, J. C. (1988). Corpus callosum agenesis, facial anomalies, Robin sequence, and other anomalies: A new autosomal recessive syndrome. *American Journal of Medical Genetics, 31,* 17–23.

Valk, J., & van der Knaap, M. S. (1989). *Magnetic resonance of myelin, myelination, and myelin disorders.* Berlin: Springer-Verlag.

Vergani, P., Ghidini, A., Mariani, S., Greppi, P., & Negri, R. (1988). Antenatal
    sonographic findings of agenesis of corpus callosum. *American Journal of
    Perinatology, 5*, 105–108.
Yu-ling, T., Bing-huan, C., Jiong-da, Y., Jun, Z., Yi-chong, W., Song-hai, C.,
    Zhi-yu, W., & Qing-hai, L. (1991). Localization of functional projections
    from corpus callosum to cerebral cortex. *Chinese Medical Journal, 104*,
    851–857.

4

Asperger Syndrome

Ami Klin
Sara S. Sparrow
Fred R. Volkmar
Domenic V. Cicchetti
Byron P. Rourke

In 1943, Leo Kanner described 11 children with a congenital inability to relate emotionally to others. This condition, early infantile autism, has been the most intensively researched of all early childhood psychiatric disorders in the ensuing 50 years. Kanner's description has proved to be remarkably enduring, with its main components remaining virtually unchanged in the newest diagnostic systems utilized in the United States and other countries (Volkmar et al., 1994). Shortly after Kanner's report, Asperger (1944), an Austrian physician, also described a group of individuals—in this case, older children and adolescents—whose main disability involved difficulties relating to others and establishing friendships. An impressive revival of interest in Asperger's description followed the rediscovery of his paper by English-speaking researchers in the early 1980s (Wing, 1981). The resulting literature has explored primarily the issue of whether the two conditions—autism and Asperger syndrome (AS)—differ and, if so, what markers distinguish these two syndromes characterized by pervasive social disabilities. The development of the AS diagnostic concept is summarized in Table 4.1.

Until recently little progress had been made in the effort to elucidate this issue, for several reasons, including most prominently the lack of a consensual definition of AS. Recent attempts to codify AS for the use of clinicians and researchers in the *International Classification of Diseases*, 10th revision (ICD-10; World Health Organization [WHO], 1990) and the

TABLE 4.1. Historical Development of Diagnostic Concept

Asperger (1944)—"autistic psychopathy":
  All males, circumscribed interests, social deficits
  Cognitive skills within normal limits
  Language skills preserved
  Positive family history (fathers)

Wolff & Barlow (1979)—"schizoid personality in childhood"

Wing (1981)—"Asperger syndrome":
  Some females
  Occasionally observed with mild mental retardation
  Some language problems
  More complex family history
  Possible overlaps with autism

Subsequent developments:
  Inconsistencies in use
  Overlap with other diagnostic concepts (schizoid personality in childhood,
    NLD syndrome, developmental learning disability of right hemisphere,
    semantic–pragmatic disorder)
  DSM-IV and ICD-10 definitions

Diagnostic and Statistical Manual of Mental Disorders, fourth edition (DSM-IV; American Psychiatric Association [APA], 1994) have made possible the use of more stringent nosological criteria. Although the validity of AS is still a controversial issue (Klin & Volkmar, 1993), recent neuropsychological research (e.g., Klin, Volkmar, Sparrow, Cicchetti, & Rourke, in press) has begun to identify markers that appear to characterize AS vis-à-vis autism. Although this research effort has produced only tentative results to date, it appears that AS is characterized by a neuropsychological profile that closely mirrors Rourke's (1989) description of Nonverbal Learning Disabilities (NLD) syndrome, whereas the neuropsychological profile obtained in autism is in some respects the opposite.

This finding is of importance to both clinicians and researchers, because diagnosis, assessment, and treatment procedures, as well as the guidelines for biological research such as brain imaging, need to be adapted in order to explore more closely the distinct AS profile of strengths and weaknesses. In this regard, the research literature on NLD has proved to be an important starting point for the understanding of AS, given the degree of fitness of the NLD profile as a neurocognitive model of AS.

The present chapter includes a detailed description of AS, as well as some clinical guidelines for assessment and treatment. Given that AS is still characterized in contrast to autism, the various issues in diagnosis and natural course of the disorder are described with an effort to delineate the main areas of distinction. The question of whether AS and NLD are overlapping concepts cannot as yet be resolved, primarily because these terms have originated from different disciplines (psychiatry and neuropsychology, respectively). Although it is clear that many individuals with AS fulfill criteria for NLD, it is also clear that many individuals with an NLD profile do not exhibit the full clinical syndrome of AS. The degree to which AS and NLD—an in the same vein, autism unaccompanied by mental retardation—overlap cannot be resolved in our present state of knowledge; the answers must await further research in family genetics and biological correlates, as well as a more detailed characterization of the natural course of the conditions. This research is currently underway at the Yale Child Study Center, in a collaborative effort with the Learning Disabilities Association of America and the University of Windsor.

BACKGROUND

Autism has been widely recognized as the paradigmatic pervasive developmental disorder (PDD). Other diagnostic concepts with features somewhat similar to autism have been less intensively studied, and their validity, apart from strictly defined autism, is more controversial (Klin, 1994). One of these conditions was originally described by Asperger (1944); as noted above, Asperger provided an account of a number of cases whose clinical features resembled Kanner's (1943) description of autism (e.g., problems with social interaction and communication, and circumscribed and idiosyncratic patterns of interest). However, Asperger's description differed from Kanner's in that speech was less commonly delayed; motor deficits were more common; the onset appeared to be somewhat later; and all the initial cases occurred only in boys. Asperger also suggested that similar problems could be observed in family members, particularly fathers.

   This syndrome was essentially unknown in the English-language literature for many years. An influential review and series of case reports by Wing (1981) increased interest in the condition; since then, both the usage of the term in clinical practice and the number of case reports and research studies have been steadily increasing (Frith, 1991; Tantam, 1988). The commonly described clinical features of AS include (1) paucity of empathy; (2) naïve, inappropriate, one-sided social interaction, little ability to form friendships, and consequent social isolation; (3) pedantic and monotonic speech; (4) poor nonverbal communication; (5) intense absorption in circumscribed topics such as the weather, facts about TV stations, railway tables, or maps, which are learned in rote fashion and reflect poor understanding, conveying the impression of eccentricity; and (6) clumsy and ill-coordinated movements and odd posture (Wing, 1981).

Prevalence rates of at least 1 case in 10,000 have been suggested (Gillberg & Gillberg, 1989; Wing, 1981), although this estimate is not yet confirmed. Although Asperger originally reported the condition only in boys, reports of girls with the syndrome have now appeared. Nevertheless, boys are significantly more likely to be affected (Wing, 1991). Although most children with AS function in the normal range of intelligence, some have been reported to be mildly retarded. The apparent onset of the condition, or at least its recognition, is probably somewhat later than that of autism; this may primarily reflect the better-preserved language and cognitive abilities. It tends to be highly stable (Asperger, 1979), and the higher intellectual skills observed suggest a better long-term outcome than is typically observed in autism (Tantam, 1991).

RELATED DIAGNOSTIC CONCEPTS

Several similar diagnostic concepts originating from adult psychiatry, neuropsychology, neurology, and other disciplines share, to a great degree, the phenomenological aspects of AS. For example, Wolff and colleagues (Wolff & Barlow, 1979; Wolff & Chick, 1980) described a group of individuals with an abnormal pattern of behavior characterized by social isolation, rigidity of thought and habits, and an unusual style of communication. In agreement with Van Krevelen's (1971) discussion of Asperger's work, they characterized the condition as "schizoid personality in childhood." Unfortunately, a developmental account of this concept was not provided, making it difficult to ascertain the extent to which the individuals described may have also exhibited autistic-like symptomatology early in life. More generally, the conceptualization of AS as an unchanging personality trait does not take fully into account the developmental aspects of the disorder, which may prove to be of great importance for differential diagnosis.

In neuropsychology, a great deal of research has been devoted to Rourke's (1989) concept of the NLD syndrome. The main contribution of this line of research has been the attempt to delineate the implications for an individual's social and emotional development of a unique profile of neuropsychological assets and deficits that appears to have a deleterious impact on the person's capacity for socialization, as well as on the person's interactive and communicative styles. The neuropsychological characteristics of individuals with the NLD profile include deficits in tactile perception, psychomotor coordination, visual–spatial organization, nonverbal problem solving, and appreciation of incongruities and humor. Individuals with NLD also exhibit well-developed rote verbal capacities and verbal memory skills; difficulty in adapting to novel and complex situations; and overreliance on rote behaviors in such situations, relative deficits in mechanical arithmetic, as compared to proficiencies in single-word reading; poor pragmatics and prosody in speech; and significant deficits in social perception, social judgment, and social interaction skills. There are marked deficits in the appreciation of subtle and even fairly obvious nonverbal aspects of communication, which often result in other persons' social disdain and rejection. As a result, individuals with NLD show a marked tendency toward social withdrawal and are at risk for development of serious mood disorders (Rourke, Young, & Leenaars, 1989).

Many of the clinical features clustered together in NLD have also been described in the neurological literature as a form of "developmental learning disability of the right hemisphere" (Denckla, 1983; Weintraub & Mesulam, 1983). Children presenting with this condition have also been shown to exhibit profound disturbances in interpretation and expression of affect and in other basic interpersonal skills (Voeller, 1986). A familial link has also been suggested (Weintraub & Mesulam, 1983). Finally, an additional term researched in the literature, "semantic–pragmatic disorder" (Bishop, 1989), has also captured aspects of NLD and AS.

It is currently unclear whether these concepts describe different entities or (more probably), provide different perspectives on a heterogeneous yet overlapping group of individuals sharing at least some common phenomenological aspects. An important goal of current research is to seek convergence among the various discipline-specific accounts, in order to make use of different methodologies in the effort to validate the behaviorally defined concept of AS. However, in order to enhance comparability of studies, it is of paramount importance to establish consensual and stringent guidelines for the diagnosis of AS, particularly in regard to its similarities to related conditions.

CATEGORICAL DEFINITION AND CLINICAL DESCRIPTION

As defined in ICD-10 (WHO, 1990), the tentative criteria for AS follow the same format as the criteria for autism, and in fact overlap with them to some degree. The required symptomatology is clustered in terms of onset criteria, social and emotional criteria, and "restricted interests" criteria, with the addition of two common but not necessary characteristics involving motor deficits and isolated special skills, respectively. A final criterion involves the necessary exclusion of other conditions, most importantly autism or a subthreshold form of autism ("atypical autism/

PDD"). Interestingly, the ICD-10 definition of AS is offered with autism as its point of reference; hence some of the criteria actually involve the *absence* of abnormalities in some areas of functioning that are affected in autism. Table 4.2 summarizes the proposed ICD-10 diagnostic algorithm for AS.

The DSM-IV (APA, 1994) definition of AS (note that AS is called "Asperger disorder" there) is almost identical to the ICD-10 definition. There have been some modifications, however, which are summarized in Table 4.3. The impact of these slightly different definitions of AS on research studies utilizing the ICD-10 or DSM-IV diagnostic systems remains unclear. Let us proceed with a discussion of each one of the diagnostic criteria using the more comprehensive ICD-10 system as the basis for the description, and comparing the clinical presentation of individuals with AS to that of individuals with autism.

TABLE 4.2. Summary of the Proposed ICD-10 (WHO, 1990) Diagnostic Algorithm for AS

1. A lack of any significant general delay in language acquisition, cognitive development, adaptive functioning, or curiosity about the environment.
2. Qualitative impairments in reciprocal social interaction. Criteria as for autism—that is, abnormalities in three of the five areas listed:
   a. Nonverbal aspects of social interaction
   b. Development of peer relationships
   c. Seeking/offering comfort in times of distress
   d. Empathy
   e. Regulation of behavior according to social context
3. Restrictive, repetitive, and stereotyped patterns of behavior, interests, and activities. Criteria as for autism—that is, two of the six symptoms listed, though revision may reduce required number to only one symptom (most commonly item a):
   a. An encompassing preoccupation with stereotyped and restricted patterns of interest
   b. Attachments to unusual objects
   c. Adherence to nonfunctional routines or rituals
   d. Motor mannerisms
   e. Preoccupation with nonfunctional elements of play materials
   f. Distress over changes in small details of the environment
4. Two symptoms are suggestive of, but not required for, the diagnosis of AS:
   a. Delayed motor milestones and motor clumsiness
   b. Isolated special skill, often related to abnormal preoccupations
5. Exclusion of related disorders (most prominently autism and PDD-NOS).

Note. Adapted from WHO (1990).

TABLE 4.3. Current Differences between the DSM-IV (APA, 1994) and the ICD-10 (WHO, 1990) Definitions of AS

Criterion 1: In DSM-IV, this criterion is divided into language development and one item clustering other areas of development. The language item is further specified in terms of use of individual words by the age of 2 years, and use of phrases by the age of 3 years.

Criterion 2: In DSM-IV, ICD-10 item e ("regulation of behavior according to social context") is not included, and only two out of the four proposed are required.

Criterion 3: In DSM-IV, ICD-10 items b ("attachments to unusual objects") and f ("distress over changes in small details of the environment") are not included, and only one item of the four proposed is required.

Criterion 4 is not included in DSM-IV.

DSM-IV adds a criterion to the effect that the disorder should cause clinically important difficulty in work, social, or other important aspects of functioning.

Onset Criteria

In ICD-10, the individual's history must show "a lack of any clinically significant general delay" in language acquisition, cognitive development, and adaptive behavior. This contrasts with typical developmental accounts of autistic children, who show pervasive deficits and deviance in these areas prior to the age of 3 years, although this may not be true in the case of normal-IQ autistic children. Despite the use of "adaptive behavior" in the formulation of the criterion, it is apparently implied that deficits in social and emotional functioning and in play behavior do not rule out the AS diagnosis. This clarification has been made explicit in DSM-IV.

Although the onset criterion is in agreement with Asperger's account, Wing (1981) noted the presence of deficits in the use of language for communication, if not in the formal aspects of language, in some of her case studies. It is currently uncertain whether the lack of delays in the prescribed areas is a differential factor between AS and autism, or, alternatively, a simple reflection of the higher developmental level associated with the usage of the term AS.

Other common descriptions of the early development of individuals with AS include a certain precociousness in learning to talk ("He talked before he could walk"); a fascination with letters and numbers—in fact, the young child may even be able to decode words, although with little or no understanding ("hyperlexia"); and the establishment of attachment patterns to family members but inappropriate approaches to peers and other persons, rather than withdrawal or aloofness as in autism (e.g., the child may attempt to initiate contact with other children by hugging them or screaming at them, and then may be puzzled at their responses). Again, these behaviors are not uncommonly described for higher-functioning autistic children as well, albeit much more infrequently.

Qualitative Impairments in Reciprocal Social Interaction

In the second cluster of symptoms, the ICD-10 criteria for AS are identical to those for autism, requiring the presence of at least three of the following five symptoms: deficits in nonverbal aspects of social interaction (e.g., gaze and communicative gestures); impaired development of peer relationships; seeking comfort from and/or offering it to others in times of distress; empathy; and regulation of behavior according to social context.

Although the social criteria for AS and autism are identical, the former condition usually involves fewer symptoms and has a generally different presentation than does the latter. Individuals with AS are often socially isolated but are not unaware of the presence of others, even though their approaches may be inappropriate and peculiar (Wing, 1991). For example, they may engage an interlocutor (usually an adult), in one-sided conversation characterized by long-winded, pedantic speech about a favorite and often unusual and narrow topic. Also, although individuals with AS are often self-described "loners," they often express a great interest in making friendships and meeting people. These wishes are invariably thwarted by their awkward approaches and insensitivity to other persons' feelings, intentions, and nonliteral and implied communications (e.g., signs of boredom, haste to leave, and need for privacy). Chronically frustrated by their repeated failures to engage others and make friendships, some of these individuals develop symptoms of a mood disorder that may require treatment, including medication.

In regard to the emotional aspects of social transactions, individuals with AS may react inappropriately to, or fail to interpret the valence of, the context of affective interactions. They often convey a sense of insensitivity, formality, or disregard of other persons' emotional expressions. That notwithstanding, they may be able to describe correctly, in a cognitive and often formalistic fashion, other people's emotions, expected intentions, and social conventions; however, they are unable to act upon this knowledge in an intuitive and spontaneous fashion, and thus lose the tempo of interactions. Such poor intuition and lack of spontaneous adaptation are accompanied by marked reliance on formalistic rules of behavior and rigid social conventions. This presentation is largely responsible for the impression of social naiveté and behavioral rigidity so forcefully conveyed by these individuals.

Like the majority of the behavioral aspects used to decribe AS, at least some of these characteristics are also exhibited by higher-functioning autistic individuals, though again probably to a lesser extent. More typically, autistic persons are withdrawn and may seem to be unaware of and uninterested in other persons. Individuals with AS, on the other hand, are often eager (sometimes painfully so), to relate to others, but lack the skills to engage them successfully.

Qualitative Impairments in Communication

In contrast to autism, for which ICD-10 requires that a child exhibit at least two of the five criteria described in the cluster of communication impairments, none of these items is a requirement for AS. In fact, the presence of some of the listed symptoms may proscribe the diagnosis. The five communication symptoms included in the definition of autism involve delay or total lack of spoken language; failure to initiate or sustain conversation interchange; stereotyped and repetitive use of language (e.g., echolalia); abnormalities in prosody; and lack of pretend play.

Although significant abnormalities of speech are not typical of AS, at least three aspects of these individuals' communication skills are of clinical interest. First, though inflection and intonation may not be as rigid and monotonic as in autism, speech may be marked by poor prosody. For example, there may be a constricted range of intonation patterns that is used with little regard to the communicative function of the utterance (assertions of fact, humorous remarks, etc.). Second, speech may often be tangential and circumstantial, conveying a sense of looseness of associations and incoherence. Even though in some cases this symptom may be an indicator of a possible thought disorder (Dykens, Volkmar, & Glick, 1991), it is often the case that the lack of contingency in speech is a result of the one-sided, egocentric conversational style (e.g., unrelenting monologues about the names, codes, and attributes of innumerable TV stations in the country); failure to provide the background for comments and to clearly demarcate changes in topic; and failure to suppress the vocal output accompanying internal thoughts.

The third clinically interesting aspect of the communication patterns of individuals with AS is the marked verbosity observed, which some authors (Klin, 1994; Tantam, 1991) see as one of the most prominent differential features of the disorder. The child or adult with AS may talk incessantly, usually about a favorite subject, often with complete disregard for whether the listener might be interested, engaged, attempting to interject a comment, or trying to change the subject of conversation. Despite such long-winded monologues, the individual may never come to a point or conclusion. Attempts by the interlocutor to elaborate on issues of content or logic, or to shift the interchange to related topics, are often unsuccessful.

Despite the possibility that all of these symptoms may be accounted for in terms of significant deficits in pragmatics, skills, and/or insight into (and awareness of) other people's expectations, the challenge remains to understand this phenomenon developmentally as a strategy of social adaptation.

Restrictive, Repetitive, and Stereotyped Patterns of Behavior, Interests, and Activities

Although in the 1990 draft of ICD-10 the behavior pattern criteria for AS and autism are identical, requiring the presence of two of the six listed items, it appears that this rule may be changed in order to reduce the number required for AS from two symptoms to only one. DSM-IV has excluded two items that are uncommonly observed, and reduced the required number of criteria to one out of the four proposed. In ICD-10, however, the six criteria listed involve an encompassing preoccupation with restricted patterns of interest; attachments to unusual objects; adherence to nonfunctional routines or rituals; motor mannerisms (e.g., hand flapping); preoccupation with nonfunctional elements of play materials (e.g., their odor or texture); and distress over changes in small details of the environment.

In contrast to individuals with autism, in whom such symptoms may be very pronounced, individuals with AS are not commonly reported to exhibit them, with the exception of the first one listed. In the case of AS, this involves an all-absorbing preoccupation with an unusual and circumscribed topic, about which vast amounts of factual knowledge are acquired and all too readily demonstrated at the first opportunity in social interaction. It should be noted, however, that some case reports (e.g., Wing, 1981) have described the presence of motor mannerisms (e.g., toe walking and finger flicking) early in the lives of individuals with AS; these stopped later in life or would appear only in especially anxiety-provoking situations.

Motor Clumsiness and Isolated All-Absorbing Special Skill

In addition to the required criteria specified above, two other symptoms are given in ICD-10 as suggestive of AS but not necessary for the diagnosis. The first involves delayed motor milestones and presence of "motor clumsiness." These two symptoms, particularly clumsiness, are commonly mentioned in reports of AS (Tantam, 1991) and are in accordance with

Asperger's (1944) original description. Individuals with AS may have a history of delayed acquisition of motor skills, such as pedaling a bicycle, catching a ball, opening jars, climbing "monkey bars," and so on. They are often visibly awkward, exhibiting rigid gait patterns, odd posture, poor manipulative skills, and significant deficits in visual–motor coordination.

Although this presentation contrasts with the pattern of motor development in autistic children, for whom the area of motor skills is often a relative strength (Volkmar et al., 1987), it is similar in some respects to what is observed in older autistic individuals. Nevertheless, the commonality in later life may result from different underlying factors—for example, psychomotor deficits in the case of AS, and poor body image and sense of self in the case of autism. This highlights the importance of describing this symptom in developmental terms.

The second suggested symptom refers to an "isolated special skill, often related to abnormal preoccupations." Even though this formulation could encompass a wide range of "splinter skills" evidenced in individuals with PDD—from proficiency at assembling puzzles, drawing and musical abilities, to amassing vast amounts of factual knowledge about unusual subjects such as meteorology—there seems to be a pattern differentiating skills commonly exhibited by individuals with autism from those presented by individuals with AS. Manipulative, visual–spatial, and musical skills, as well as "savant talents," are more commonly described in autism; the amassing of factual information about an all-absorbing, circumscribed topic appears to be more typical in AS. This distinction may be necessary in order to specify the uniqueness of this behavior and its importance as a necessary requirement for the diagnosis of AS, as supported by several authors (Gillberg, 1989; Wing, 1991).

In regard to this symptom, although the actual topic may change from time to time (e.g., every 1 or 2 years), it may dominate the content of social interchange as well as the activities of an individual with AS, often immersing the whole family in the subject for long periods of time. Even though this symptom may not be easily recognized in childhood (because strong interests in dinosaurs or fashionable fictional characters are so ubiquitous among young children), it may become more salient later on as interests shift to unusual and narrow topics. This behavior is peculiar, in the sense that extraordinary amounts of factual information are often learned about very circumscribed topics (e.g., snakes, names of stars, maps, TV guides, train models, or railway schedules) without a genuine understanding of the phenomena involved.

DSM-IV does not include either of these items. The primary reasons for this exclusion are the current lack of an operationalized usage of the term "motor clumsiness" (Ghaziuddin, Tsai, & Ghaziuddin, 1992), and the absence to date of systematic knowledge of the "circumscribed interests" exhibited by individuals with AS (Klin, 1994).

Exclusionary Criteria

The ICD-10 definition of AS requires that the individual's presentation may not be attributable to other varieties of PDD or personality disorders. This requirement involves the validity of the concept, to which we now turn.

VALIDITY OF THE SYNDROME

Although AS may be differentiated from other PDDs on the basis of developmental/intellectual level (i.e., the vast majority of individuals with autism, Rett syndrome, and childhood disintegrative disorder are mentally retarded) and on the basis of severity of the social and communicative deficits (e.g., individuals with AS appear to be more affected than individuals for whom the diagnosis of PDD not otherwise specified [NOS] seems more appropriate) (Volkmar et al., 1994), its validity apart from higher-functioning autism (HFA) remains controversial (Klin, 1994; Wing, 1991). Studies to date have revealed lines of convergence and divergence between the two concepts. Disagreements about the validity of the category and the absence of "official" definitions of AS have meant that the concept is often used inconsistently by clinicians, who may employ it to refer to autistic persons with higher levels of intelligence, adults with autism, or even all "atypical" children who do not fulfill the criteria for autism. Clearly, such unspecific usage of the term needs to be avoided, but this of course can only be achieved if substantial progress is made in the validation of the concept in order to make possible a consensual, working definition of AS.

There is little disagreement over the fact that AS is on a continuum with autism, particularly in relation to the problems in the areas of social functioning and communication. For example, within the DSM-III-R (APA, 1987) diagnostic system, persons with AS either would meet criteria for autistic disorder or, less frequently, would be said to exhibit PDD-NOS. What is less clear is whether the condition is qualitatively different from, rather than just a milder form of, autism unaccompanied by mental retardation. Several studies (e.g., Ozonoff, Roger, & Pennington, 1991; Szatmari, Tuff, Finlayson, & Bartolucci, 1990) have attempted to identify discriminating criteria between the two conditions, with only mixed results to date. These studies involved primarily patterns of neurocognitive functioning, social cognition, associated neurobiological findings, and family history. Two factors appear to have contributed to a lack of clear results: First, an algorithm for the assignment of the diagnosis was often lacking; second, there was a great degree of circularity involved, as findings might have been a function of the diagnostic criteria adopted in the differential diagnosis of AS and HFA. Despite these problems, a few generalizations that lend some support to a qualitative differentiation between the two conditions may be made.

Clinical Presentation

As noted previously, even when developmental level is taken into consideration, severity of social deficits, abnormalities in language and communication, presence of stereotypies, motor clumsiness, and frequency and nature of special interests appear to help discriminate between AS and HFA (Volkmar et al., 1994). The question remains, however, as to whether these differences in phenomenological presentation reflect a contrast of degree or quality in presentation.

Onset and Early Development

Despite the commonly reported differences in onset patterns of AS and HFA, some case reports (Wing, 1981) have noted that at least a few individuals exhibited typical autistic behaviors early in life and yet had a presentation later in adolescence that was more compatible with a diagnosis of AS. These observations are very important, as they make a case for a continuity or at least an association between the two disorders. At present, however, the unavailability of longitudinal studies adopting operational definitions and quantitative methods renders it very difficult to make a case for convergence or divergence of symptomatology on the basis of developmental patterns alone. This issue is further confounded by the fact that a diagnosis of AS can be made more confidently for older children, when the most conspicuous symptoms—verbosity and circumscribed areas of interest—become more apparent. Hence, preschool children with social and emotional disabilities presenting to a clinic might often in the past have received a diagnosis of HFA or PDD NOS. Clearly, a heightened awareness and better definition of the diagnosis as well as more reliable information on profiles of early development of individuals with AS, are needed in the future.

Outcome

Several case reports have confirmed Asperger's (1979) observation that individuals with AS generally have a better outcome than do those with HFA (Rutter & Schopler, 1987). Whether this reflects a genuine difference in the course of the disorders or, alternatively, can be explained in terms of developmental/intellectual level alone is another important question that remains unanswered.

Family History

Substantiating to some extent Asperger's (1944) observation of high incidence of similar problems in the family members (particularly fathers) of individuals with AS, several anecdotal accounts and systematic studies (e.g., Burgoine & Wing, 1983; Gillberg & Gillberg, 1989) have found a very high frequency of AS symptoms, if not the full-blown diagnosis, in first-degree relatives (particularly fathers). Despite some recent findings revealing stronger genetic links in autism than were previously known (Rutter, 1992), both the increased rate and closer family proximity suggested for AS appear to contrast markedly with autism. However, family studies have also pointed to some lines of convergence between the two disorders; for example, some families had one member with AS and another with autism. Therefore, several unresolved questions await larger behavioral genetic studies.

Neurocognitive Profile

Although some studies have failed to identify differentiating patterns of neurocognitive functioning between AS and HFA (e.g., Ozonoff et al., 1991; Szatmari et al., 1990), at least one study (Klin et al., in press) of meticulously diagnosed individuals has identified some neuropsychological distinctions that were, at least to some extent, independent of the diagnostic criteria. In this study, groups of individuals with AS and HFA (of comparable chronological age and IQ) were compared in terms of their functioning in a variety of neuropsychological areas. Eleven of these areas discriminated between the two groups. Interestingly, some neuropsychological skills represented areas of strength in AS and weakness in HFA, whereas in regard to other skills the reverse pattern was obtained. Six areas of psychological deficit were predictive of a diagnosis of AS: both fine and gross motor skills, visual–motor integration, visual–spatial perception, nonverbal concept formation, and visual memory. Five areas of psychological deficit were predictive of a diagnosis of "not-AS": articulation, verbal output, auditory perception, vocabulary, and verbal memory (see Table 4.4). This study also revealed a pattern of Verbal–Performance IQ differential that contrasted in AS and HFA, with higher Verbal IQs than Performance IQs in AS and no significant Verbal–Performance IQ differetial in HFA. These findings are consistent with a great number of case reports (Gillberg, 1989; Wing, 1981) as well

TABLE 4.4. Eleven Areas of Neuropsychological Deficit Discriminating between HFA and AS

Predictive of AS	r_{phi}	Predictive of not-AS	r_{phi}
Fine motor skills	.61***	Articulation	−.58***
Visual–motor integration	.52**	Verbal output	−.58***
Visual–spatial perception	.50**	Auditory perception	−.54**
Nonverbal concept		Vocabulary	−.53**
formation	.50**	Verbal memory	−.35*
Gross motor skills	.48**		
Visual memory	.47**		

Note. Adapted from Klin et al. (in press). r_{phi} indicates extent of association between item and diagnosis. Items are rank-ordered by r_{phi} value.
 * $p < .05$. ** $p < .01$. *** $p < .001$.

as with at least one study involving individuals with AS (Volkmar et al., 1994), and several studies of individuals with HFA (Dawson, 1983; Lincoln, Courchesne, Kilman, Elmasian, & Allen, 1988).

Although these findings await replication, the approach adopted may prove to be of importance not only in the validation of AS, but also in terms of choice of intervention. In regard to validation issues, the neurocognitive patterns obtained in AS appear to follow very closely the cluster of neuropsychological assets and disabilities defining the concept of NLD (Rourke, 1989), which can serve as a neuropsychological model of the behaviorally defined psychiatric disorder. In regard to intervention issues, a divergence of patterns of neuropsychological abilities in AS and HFA would suggest different remediation approaches, as well as different possibilities for vocational training.

Faced with the complexities and circularities that currently characterize discussions of validity issues in AS, the researcher may justifiably feel motivated (and possibly daunted) by the challenge ahead. The clinician, however, needs to confront the more immediate and concrete challenge of assessment and planning for patients presenting at the clinic. The following are guidelines for clinical assessment and intervention involving individuals with AS.

ASSESSMENT

AS, like other types of PDD, involves delays and deviant patterns of behavior in multiple areas of functioning; these often require the input of professionals with different areas of expertise, particularly overall developmental functioning, neuropsychological features, and behavioral status. Hence the clinical assessment of individuals with AS is most effectively conducted by an experienced interdisciplinary team. A more comprehensive set of guidelines regarding the assessment of individuals with autism and other PDDs is provided elsewhere (Klin & Shepard, 1994). The following is a summary of the special areas of focus required in the assessment of individuals with AS.

A few principles should be made explicit prior to a discussion of the various areas of assessment. First, given the complexity of the condition, the importance of developmental history, and common difficulties in securing adequate services for children and individuals with AS, it is very important that parents be encouraged to observe and participate in the evaluation (Morgan, 1988). This guideline helps to demystify assessment procedures, provides the parents with shared observations that can then be clarified by the clinician, and fosters parental understanding of the condition. All of these can then help the parents evaluate the programs of intervention offered in their community.

Second, evaluation findings should be translated into a single coherent view of the individual. Easily understood, detailed, concrete, and realistic recommendations should be provided. When writing their reports, professionals should strive to express the implications of their findings for each patient's day-to-day adaptation, learning, and vocational training.

Third, many professionals' and officials' lack of awareness of AS, its features, and its associated disabilities often necessitates direct and continual contact between the evaluators and the various professionals securing and implementing the recommended interventions. This is particularly important in the case of AS, as most of these individuals have average Full Scale IQs, and are often not thought of as in need for special programming. Conversely, as AS becomes a more well-known diagnostic label, there is reason to believe that it is becoming a fashionable concept used in an often unwarranted fashion by practitioners who intend to convey only that their clients are currently experiencing difficulties in social interaction and in peer relationships. Because AS is a serious and debilitiating developmental syndrome impairing a person's capacity for socialization, and not a transient or mild condition, parents should be briefed regarding the present unsatisfactory state of knowledge about AS and the common confusions about use of the concept currently prevailing in the mental health community. Ample opportunity should be given to clarify misconceptions and establish a consensus about the patient's abilities and disabilities, which should not be simply assumed under the use of the diagnostic label.

In the majority of cases, a comprehensive assessment will involve the following components: history, psychological assessment, communication assessment, psychiatric examination, further consultation if needed, parental conferences, and recommendations.

History

A careful history should be obtained, including information related to pregnancy and neonatal period; early development and characteristics of development; and medical and family history. A review of previous records (including previous evaluations) should be performed, and the information should be incorporated and results compared in order to obtain a sense of the course of development. Several specific areas that should be directly examined because of their importance in the diagnosis of AS include a careful history of the onset/recognition of the problems; development of motor skills and language patterns; and areas of special interest (e.g., favorite occupations, unusual skills, collections). Particular emphasis should be placed on social development, including past and present problems in social interaction, patterns of attachment of family members, development of friendships, self-concept, emotional development, and mood presentation.

Psychological Assessment

The psychological assessment aims at establishing the overall level of intellectual functioning, profile of strengths and weaknesses, and style of learning. The specific areas to be examined and measured include neuropsychological functioning (e.g., motor and psychomotor skills, memory, executive functions, problem solving, concept formation, visual-perceptual skills); adaptive functioning (degree of self-sufficiency in real-life situations); academic achievement (performance in school-like subjects); and personality assessment (e.g., common preoccupations, compensatory strategies of adaptation, mood presentation).

The neuropsychological assessment of individuals with AS involves certain procedures of specific interest to this population. Whether or not a Verbal–Performance IQ discrepancy is obtained in intelligence testing, it is advisable to conduct a fairly comprehensive neuropsychological assessment, including measures of motor skills (coordination of the large muscles as well as manipulative skills and visual–motor coordination), visual-perceptual skills (gestalt perception, spatial orientation, parts–whole relationships, visual memory, facial recognition), concept formation (both verbal and nonverbal), and executive functions. A recommended protocol would include the measures used in the assessment of children with NLD (Rourke, 1989). Particular attention should be given to demonstrated or potential compensatory strategies; for example, individuals with significant visual–spatial deficits may translate the task or mediate their responses by means of verbal strategies or verbal guidance.

Hence, the patient should be questioned as to the strategy used to perform a task, if this is not clear.

Communication Assessment

The communication assessment aims to obtain both quantitative and qualitative information regarding the various aspects of the individual's communication skills. It should go beyond the testing of speech and formal language (e.g., articulation, vocabulary, sentence construction, and comprehension). The assessment should examine nonverbal forms of communication (e.g., gaze, gestures); nonliteral language (e.g., metaphor, irony, absurdities, and humor); suprasegmental aspects of speech (patterns of inflection, stress, and pitch); pragmatics (e.g., turn taking, sensitivity to cues provided by the interlocutor); and content, coherence, and contingency of conversation. Particular attention should be given to perseveration on circumscribed topics, metalinguistic skills (Tager-Flusberg, 1993), reciprocity, and rules of conversation (Grice, 1975).

Psychiatric Examination

The psychiatric examination should include observations of the patient during more and less structured periods—for example, while interacting with parents and while engaged in assessment by other members of the evaluation team. Specific areas for observation and inquiry include the patient's patterns of special interest and leisure time; social and affective presentation; quality of attachment to family members; development of peer relationships and friendships; capacities for self-awareness, perspective taking, and level of insight into social and behavioral problems; typical reactions in novel situations; and ability to intuit other persons' feelings and infer other persons' intentions and beliefs. Problem behaviors that are likely to interfere with remedial programming should be noted (e.g., marked aggression). The patient's ability to understand ambiguous, nonliteral communications (particularly teasing and sarcasm) should be examined, because misunderstandings of such communications may often elicit aggressive behaviors. Other areas of observation involve the presence of obsessions or compulsions, depression and panic attacks, integrity of thought, and reality testing.

Differential Diagnosis

The differential diagnosis of AS involves primarily autism without associated mental retardation (i.e., HFA), and PDD NOS in DSM-IV or atypical autism in ICD-10. Although some authors might include personality disorders characterized by significant deficits in socioemotional functioning (e.g., schizoid personality disorder), such diagnoses do not take into account the developmental factors of AS that may prove to be of great importance for an understanding of its pathogenesis and course.

As noted previously, the validity of AS is still very controversial, having several lines of convergence and divergence with HFA in particular. However, if strictly defined, AS differs from HFA in that the onset is usually later and the outcome more positive (see above). In addition, social and communication deficits are less severe; motor mannerisms are usually absent; circumscribed interests are more conspicuous; Verbal–Performance IQ differential usually favors the former in AS and is not significantly different in HFA; motor "clumsiness" is more frequently seen in AS; and family history of similar problems is more frequently ascertained in AS than in HFA.

The distinction between AS and PDD NOS is problematic, because the latter is essentially a residual category with no defining criteria. PDD NOS is used to describe a rather large and heterogeneous group of children who do not meet strict criteria for autism, but who exhibit a pattern of developmental and behavioral dysfunction similar to that observed in autism. Such children typically exhibit unusual sensitivities and affective responses in the presence of more differentiated social relatedness and better cognitive and communicative skills than most autistic children exhibit (Klin & Volkmar, 1993). The ICD-10 definition of atypical autism, despite its attempt to operationally define the areas of "atypicality" (e.g., age of onset, symptomatology), is also essentially a negative or subthreshold definition (i.e., not, or not quite, autism). From the information revealed in the very few attempts to study this population (Cohen, Paul, & Volkmar, 1986; Dahl, Cohen, & Provence, 1986), it is acceptable to conclude that if AS is strictly defined, it differs from the much more common PDD NOS in that social, emotional, and communicative deficits are more severe and outcome is poorer in AS; circumscribed interests and motor "clumsiness" are more pronounced in AS; and IQ range is probably more variable in PDD NOS. Empirical evidence substantiating some of these observations was obtained in the autism/PDD DSM-IV field trials (Volkmar et al., 1994).

TREATMENT AND INTERVENTION

The treatment of AS, like that of autism, is essentially supportive and symptomatic (Klin & Volkmar, 1993; Wing, 1981). Special educational services are sometimes helpful, although there is as yet very little reported experience on the effectiveness of specific interventions. Acquisition of basic skills in social interaction, as well as in other areas of adaptive functioning, should be encouraged. Supportive psychotherapy focused on problems of empathy, social difficulties, and depressive symptoms may be helpful, although it is usually very difficult for individuals with AS to engage in more intensive, insight-oriented psychotherapy.

Despite the paucity of published information on intervention strategies and issues, a few guidelines may be offered. These are based on informal observations made by experienced clinicians; on intervention strategies used with individuals with HFA (Mesibov, 1992; Van Bourgondien & Woods, 1992); and particularly on Rourke's (1989) suggested interventions for individuals with the NLD syndrome (see also the Appendix to this volume).

Securing Services

The authorities who decide on entitlement to services are usually unaware of the extent and significance of the disabilities in AS. Proficient verbal skills, overall IQ usually within the normal range, and a solitary lifestyle often mask outstanding deficiencies observed primarily in novel or otherwise socially demanding situations, thus making the very salient needs for supportive intervention less apparent. Thus, active participation by the clinician, together with parents and possibly an advocate, in forcefully pursuing the patient's eligibility for services is needed. The formalization of the diagnosis in ICD-10 and DSM-IV will certainly help in this effort. It appears that in the past, many individuals with AS were diagnosed as learning-disabled with eccentric features (Klin, Volkmar, & Sparrow, 1993)—a nonpsychiatric diagnostic label that is much less effective in securing services.

Learning

Skills, concepts, appropriate procedures, cognitive strategies, and so on may be more effectively taught to individuals with AS in an explicit and rote fashion using a parts-to-whole verbal instruction approach in which the verbal steps are presented in the correct sequence for the behavior to be effective. Additional guidelines should be derived from each individual's neuropsychological profile of assets and deficits. Specific intervention techniques should be similar to those usually employed for many subtypes of learning disabilities, with an effort to circumvent the identified difficulties by means of compensatory strategies, usually of a verbal nature. If significant motor and visual–motor deficits are corroborated during the evaluation, the individual should receive physical and occupational therapies. The latter should not only focus on traditional techniques designed to remediate motor deficits, but should also reflect an effort to integrate these activities with learning of visual–spatial concepts, visual–spatial orientation, and body awareness.

Adaptive Functioning

The acquisition of self-sufficiency skills in all areas of functioning should be given a high priority in any plan of intervention. The tendency of individuals with AS to rely on rigid rules and routines can be used to foster positive habits and enhance the persons' quality of life, as well as that of their family members. The teaching approach should follow closely the guidelines set forth above (see "Learning"), and should be practiced routinely in naturally occurring situations and across different settings in order to maximize generalization of acquired skills.

Maladaptive Behaviors

Specific problem-solving strategies, usually following a verbal algorithm, may be taught for handling the requirements of frequently occurring, troublesome situations (e.g., ones involving novelty, intense social demands, or frustration). Training is usually necessary for recognizing situations as troublesome and for selecting the best available learned strategy to use in such situations.

Social and Communication Skills

Social and communication skills are possibly best taught by a communication specialist with an interest in pragmatics in speech. Alternatively, social training groups may be used if there are enough opportunities for individual contact with the instructor and for the practicing of specific skills. Teaching may include the following: (1) appropriate nonverbal behavior (e.g., the use of gaze for social interaction, monitoring, and patterning of voice inflection), which may involve imitative drills, working with a mirror, and so forth; (2) verbal decoding of nonverbal behaviors of others; (3) processing of visual information simultaneously with auditory information (in order to foster integration of competing stimuli and to facilitate the creation of the appropriate social context of the interaction); and (4) social awareness, perspective-taking skills, and correct interpretation of ambiguous communications (e.g., nonliteral language).

Vocational Training

Often adults with AS may fail to meet entry requirements for jobs in their area of training (e.g., a college degree) because of their poor interview skills, or may fail to maintain a job because of their social disabilities, eccentricities, or anxiety attacks. Having failed to secure skilled employment, sometimes these individuals may be helped by well-meaning friends or relatives to find a manual job. As a result of their typically very poor visual–motor skills, they may once again fail, and this can have devastating emotional effects. It is important, therefore, that individuals with AS be trained for and placed in jobs for which they are not neuropsychologically impaired, and in which they will enjoy a certain degree of support and shelter. It is also preferable that these jobs not involve intensive social demands.

Social Contact and Self-Help/Support

Because individuals with AS are usually self-described as "loners," despite an often intense wish to make friends and have a more active social life, there is a need to facilitate social contact within the context of an activity-oriented group (e.g., church communities, hobby clubs, and self-help/support groups). The little experience available with self-help and support groups suggests that individuals with AS enjoy the opportunity to meet others with similar problems and may develop relationships centering around an activity or subject of shared interest.

Pharmacotherapy

Although little information about pharmacological interventions with individuals with AS is available, a conservative approach based on the evidence from autism should probably be adopted (Campbell, Anderson, Green, & Deutsch, 1987). In general, pharmacological interventions with young children are probably best avoided. The best-studied agents (i.e., the tranquilizers) have some utility in selected cases and in regard to specific maladaptive behaviors, but their many side effects (particularly sedation) may prove problematic. These agents may be indicated in some situations, but are typically used with older individuals, and even then at the lowest effective dose and for the shortest period of time. Nevertheless, specific medication may be indicated if AS is accompanied by debilitating depressive symptoms, severe obsessions and compulsions, or a thought disorder.

SUMMARY

As with autism, there has recently been a true fascination with the diagnostic concept of AS; this fascination is reflected in both an impressive upsurge of research work and a growing usage of the term in clinical practice. The reason appears to be twofold: (1) the age-old intrigue about the basis for socialization, and (2) the less than satisfactory utility of currently available psychiatric concepts intended to cover the range of expressions of social disabilities, in terms of both severity and quality of impairment. Although various lines of neurobiological work have attempted to unravel the biological correlates of social skills, the NLD syndrome and model is unique in its attempt to explore the range of phenotypic expressions related to a very specific neuropsychological profile of assets and deficits. Beyond establishing helpful guidelines for intervention in AS and possibly providing validity markers to be used in the differential diagnosis of the PDDs disorders without accompanying mental retardation, the NLD approach suggests a more general research strategy that is badly needed in the field of research on psychiatric conditions involving deficits in socialization. This approach strives to define an initial marker and to delineate the developmental courses, strategies of adaptation, range of symptomatology, and family aggregation associated with it. Such inductive methodology promises to help us bridge the current gap separating underlying neurobiological mechanisms and the behavioral syndromes thought to result therefrom.

REFERENCES

American Psychiatric Association (APA). (1987). *Diagnostic and statistical manual of mental disorders* (3rd ed., rev.). Washington, DC: Author.

American Psychiatric Association (APA). (1994). *Diagnostic and statistical manual of mental disorders* (4th ed.). Washington, DC: Author.

Asperger, H. (1944). Die "Autistischen Psychopathen" im Kindesalter. *Archiv für Psychiatrie und Nervenkrankheiten, 117*, 76–136.

Asperger, H. (1979). Problems of infantile autism. *Communication, 13*, 45–52.

Bishop, D. V. M. (1989). Autism, Asperger's syndrome and semantic–pragmatic disorder: Where are the boundaries? *British Journal of Disorders of Communication, 24*, 107–121.

Burgoine, E., & Wing, L. (1983). Identical triplets with Asperger's syndrome. *British Journal of Psychiatry, 143*, 261–265.

Campbell, M., Anderson, L. T., Green, W. H., & Deutsch, S. I. (1987). Psychopharmacology. In D. J. Cohen & A. Donnellan (Eds.), *Handbook of autism and pervasive developmental disorders* (pp. 545–565).

Cohen, D. J., Paul, R., & Volkmar, F. R. (1986). Issues in the classification of pervasive developmental disorders: Toward DSM-IV. *Journal of the American Academy of Child and Adolescent Psychiatry, 25*, 213–220.

Dahl, K., Cohen, D. J., & Provence, S. (1986). Clinical and multivariate approaches to nosology of the pervasive developmental disorders. *Journal of the American Academy of Child and Adolescent Psychiatry, 25*, 170–180.

Dawson, G. (1983). Lateralized brain dysfunction in autism: Evidence from the Halstead–Reitan Neuropsychological Battery. *Journal of Autism and Developmental Disorders, 13*, 269–286.

Denckla, M. B. (1983). The neuropsychology of social–emotional learning disabilities. *Archives of Neurology, 40*, 461–462.

Dykens, E., Volkmar, F. R., & Glick, M. (1991). Thought disorder in high-functioning autistic adults. *Journal of Autism and Developmental Disorders, 21*, 291–321.

Frith, U. (Ed.). (1991). *Autism and Asperger syndrome.* Cambridge, England: Cambridge University Press.

Ghaziuddin, M., Tsai, L. Y., & Ghaziuddin, N. (1992). A reappraisal of clumsiness as a diagnostic feature of Asperger syndrome. *Journal of Autism and Developmental Disorders, 22*, 651–656.

Gillberg, C. (1989). Asperger's syndrome in 23 Swedish children. *Developmental Medicine and Child Neurology, 31*, 520–531.

Gillberg, I. C., & Gillberg, C. (1989). Asperger syndrome: Some epidemiological considerations. *Journal of Child Psychology and Psychiatry, 30*, 631–638.

Grice, H. P. (1975). Logic and conversation. In R. Cole & J. Morgan (Eds.), *Syntax and semantics: Speech acts* (pp. 85–102). New York: Academic Press.

Kanner, L. (1943). Autistic disturbances of affective contact. *Nervous Child, 2*, 217–253.

Klin, A. (1994). Asperger syndrome. *Child and Adolescent Psychiatry Clinics of North America, 3*, 131–148.

Klin, A., & Shepard, B. (1994). Psychological assessment of autistic children. *Child and Adolescent Psychiatry Clinics of North America, 3*, 53–70.

Klin, A., & Volkmar, F. R. (1993). The pervasive developmental disorders. In J. D. Noshpitz (Ed.), *Basic handbook of child psychiatry* (2nd ed., pp. 236–256). New York: Basic Books.

Klin, A., Volkmar, F. R., & Sparrow, S. S. (1993, March). *Higher functioning autism and Asperger's syndrome: Validity and neuropsychological aspects.* Paper presented at the biennial meeting of the Society for Research in Child Development, New Orleans.

Klin, A., Volkmar, F. R., Sparrow, S. S., Cicchetti, D. V., & Rourke, B. P. (in press). Validity and neuropsychological characterization of Asperger syndrome. *Journal of Child Psychology and Psychiatry.*

Lincoln, A. J., Courchesne, E., Kilman, B. A., Elmasian, R., & Allen, M. (1988). A study of intellectual abilities in high-functioning people with autism. *Journal of Autism and Developmental Disorders, 18*, 505–524.

Mesibov, G. B. (1992). Treatment issues with high-functioning adolescents and adults with autism. In E. Schopler & G. B. Mesibov (Eds.), *High-functioning individuals with autism* (pp. 143–156). New York: Plenum Press.

Morgan, S. (1988). The autistic child and family functioning: A developmental–family systems perspective. *Journal of Autism and Developmental Disorders, 18*, 263–278.

Ozonoff, S., Roger, S. J., & Pennington, B. F. (1991). Asperger's syndrome: Evidence of an empirical distinction from high-functioning autism. *Journal of Child Psychology and Psychiatry, 32,* 1107–1122.

Rourke, B. P. (1989). *Nonverbal learning disabilities: The syndrome and the model.* New York, Guilford Press.

Rourke, B. P., Young, G. C., & Leenaars, A. A. (1989). A childhood learning disability that predisposes those afflicted to adolescent and adult depression and suicide risk. *Journal of Learning Disabilities, 22,* 169–185.

Rutter, M. (1992, May). *Autism: Genetic aspects.* Paper presented at the 4th Congress, Autism Europe, Den Haag, Holland.

Rutter, M., & Schopler, E. (1987). Autism and pervasive developmental disorders: Concepts and diagnostic issues. *Journal of Autism and Developmental Disorders, 17,* 159–186.

Szatmari, P., Tuff, L., Finlayson, M. A. J., & Bartolucci, G. (1990). Asperger's syndrome and autism: Neurocognitive aspects. *Journal of the American Academy of Child and Adolescent Psychiatry, 29,* 130–136.

Tager-Flusberg, H. (1993). What language reveals about the understanding of minds in children with autism. In S. Baron-Cohen, H. Tager-Flusberg, & D. J. Cohen (Eds.), *Understanding other minds: Perspectives from autism* (pp. 138–157). Oxford: Oxford University Press.

Tantam, D. (1988). Annotation: Asperger's syndrome. *Journal of Child Psychology and Psychiatry, 29,* 245–255.

Tantam, D. (1991). Asperger syndrome in adulthood. In U. Frith (Ed.), *Autism and Asperger syndrome* (pp. 147–183). Cambridge, England: Cambridge University Press.

Van Bourgondien, M.E., & Woods, A.V. (1992). Vocational possibilities for high-functioning adults with autism. In E. Schopler & G. B. Mesibov (Eds.), *High-functioning individuals with autism* (pp. 227–242). New York: Plenum Press.

Van Krevelen, D. A. (1971). Early infantile autism and autistic psychopathy. *Journal of Autism and Childhood Schizophrenia, 1,* 82–86.

Voeller, K. K. S. (1986). Right-hemisphere deficit syndrome in children. *American Journal of Psychiatry, 143,* 1004–1009.

Volkmar, F. R., Klin, A., Siegel, B., Szatmari, P., Lord, C., Campbell, M., Freeman, B. J., Cicchetti, D. V., & Rutter, M., Kline, W, Buitelaar, J., Hattab, Y., Fombonne, E., Fuentes, J., Werry, J., Stone, W., Kerbeshian, J., Hoshino, Y., Bregman, J., Loveland, K. Szymanski, L., & Towbin, K. (1994). Field trial for autistic disorder in DSM-IV. *American Journal of Psychiatry, 151,* 1361–1367.

Volkmar, F. R., Sparrow, S. S., Goudreau, D., Cicchetti, D. V., Paul, R., & Cohen, D. J. (1987). Social deficits in autism: An operational approach using the Vineland Adaptive Behavior Scales. *Journal of the American Academy of Child and Adolescent Psychiatry, 26,* 156–161.

Weintraub, S., & Mesulam, M. M. (1983). Developmental learning disabilities of the right hemisphere: Emotional, interpersonal, and cognitive components. *Archives of Neurology, 40,* 463–468.

Wing, L. (1981). Asperger's syndrome: A clinical account. *Psychological Medicine, 11,* 115–130.

Wing, L. (1991). The relationship between Asperger's syndrome and Kanner's autism. In U. Frith (Ed.), *Autism and Asperger syndrome* (pp. 93–121). Cambridge, England: Cambridge University Press.

Wolff, S., & Barlow, A. (1979). Schizoid personality in childhood: A comparative study of schizoid, autistic, and normal children. *Journal of Child Psychology and Psychiatry, 20,* 19–46.

Wolff, S., & Chick, J. (1980). Schizoid personality in childhood: A controlled follow-up study. *Psychological Medicine, 10,* 85–100.

World Health Organization (WHO). (1990, May). *International classification of diseases* (10th revision): *Chapter V. Mental and behavioral disorders (including disorders of psychological development): Diagnostic criteria for research.* Geneva: Author.

5

Velocardiofacial Syndrome

Katy B. Fuerst
Catherine B. Dool
Byron P. Rourke

The velocardiofacial (VCF) syndrome was first described in 12 children by Shprintzen et al. (1978), although a familial case had been reported previously by Strong (1968). VCF syndrome is a recurrent-pattern congenital malformation syndrome (Golding-Kushner, Weller, & Shprintzen, 1985). A "recurrent-pattern" syndrome occurs when similar patterns of multiple anomalies are present in more than one related or unrelated individuals (Siegel-Sadewitz & Shprintzen, 1982). VCF syndrome is thought to be a common syndrome of clefting with unknown genesis, although autosomal dominant inheritance is probable (Golding-Kushner, Weller, & Shprintzen, 1985). Other common features of this disorder include heart defects, characteristic facies, and learning disabilities. Numerous minor anomalies occur with some variability.

FEATURES OF THE VCF SYNDROME

Phenotypic Features

The phenotypic spectrum of the VCF syndrome is broad. The more common features include overt and submucous clefting of the palate, cardiac anomalies, characteristic dysmorphic facies, learning disabilities, and velopharyngeal insufficiency (Lipson et al., 1991). Those afflicted often have slender hands and digits and are of relatively small stature for chronological age, secondary to microsomia that is not attributable to the severity of cardiac disease (Shprintzen, Goldberg, Young, & Wolford, 1981).

Craniofacial Abnormalities

Clefts, usually limited to the soft palate, were originally thought to be an almost invariable feature of the VCF syndrome (Shprintzen et al., 1981; Williams, Shprintzen, & Goldberg, 1985). However, since the patients were mainly diagnosed through craniofacial centers, an ascertainment bias may have been operating (Gorlin, Cohen, & Levin, 1990; Meinecke, Beemer, Schinzel, & Kushnick, 1986). If other centers reported a lower incidence of cleft palate, it would indicate greater variability of clinical expression of this syndrome than was previously appreciated (Lipson et al., 1991; Meinecke et al., 1986).

The pharyngeal musculature is often hypotonic in children with the VCF syndrome. As a result, incomplete closure of the velum and pharyngeal wall occurs. When coupled with a cleft palate, this frequently results in speech that is severely hypernasal with articulation errors. A history of nasal regurgitation during feeding in the first year of life is also common. Pharyngeal flap surgery for the repair of the velopharyngeal insufficiency is often necessary. In many cases, this is an effective treatment and results in considerable improvement in speech intelligibility, perhaps especially when the surgery is performed early in childhood (Lipson et al., 1991).

In the VCF syndrome, the typical facies is characterized by all or some of the following features: vertically long face; a long, prominent nose with a broad, squared root (bridge) and deficient alae (lateral wall of nostril); malar (cheek or cheekbone) flattening; small mandible (lower jaw) accompanied by retrognathia (retruded mandible); myopathic facies (secondary to hypotonic facial musculature), often associated with narrow, downward slanting or almond-shaped palpebral fissures; minor malformations and prominence of the auricles (the pinna, or external ear); and abundant scalp hair (Golding-Kushner et al., 1985; Gorlin et al., 1990; Lipson et al., 1991; Smith, 1988). Conductive hearing loss secondary to cleft palate is relatively common, as are frequent episodes of serous otitis media (Shprintzen et al., 1981). Subtle changes in facial appearance are reported with age. Older patients tend to develop a broad bulbar tip to the nose (Lipson et al., 1991). The cranial base has been found to be flatter than normal (a condition referred to as platybasia). Platybasia results in the abnormal position of the facial bones in relation to the neurocranium, and may account for such facial features as the retrognathia, malar flatness, prominent nasal root, and velopharyngeal insufficiency (Arvystas & Shprintzen, 1984).

Cardiovascular Abnormalities

Between 42% and 85% of patients with VCF syndrome have single or combined cardiac abnormalities (Lipson et al., 1991; Meinecke et al.,

1986; Young, Shprintzen, & Goldberg, 1980). Frequently observed abnormalities include ventricular septal defects (VSDs), a right-sided aortic arch, and tetralogy of Fallot (Young et al., 1980). Tetralogy of Fallot includes VSDs, a malpositioned aorta, pulmonic stenosis, and right ventricular hypertrophy. Over one-third of all patients will require surgical repair of their heart defects (Shprintzen et al., 1978; Young et al., 1980).

Other Vascular Abnormalities

Other vascular abnormalities have been documented in patients with VCF syndrome. In some patients, the internal carotid arteries have been found to be enlarged, tortuous, and medially displaced. Medial displacement in the posterior pharyngeal wall has sometimes prevented pharyngeal flap surgery for correction of the velopharyngeal insufficiency, necessitating treatment with a prosthetic speech device instead (MacKenzie-Stepner et al., 1987; D'Antonio & Marsh, 1987). In over 30% of cases, tortuosity of the retinal vessels has also been found (Mansour, Wang, Goldberg, & Shprintzen, 1987).

Endocrine, Immunological, and Other Abnormalities

A history of neonatal hypocalcemia was found in approximately 13% to 20% of cases with the VCF syndrome (Lipson et al., 1991; Goldberg, Motzkin, Marion, Scrambler, & Shprintzen, 1993). It was almost invariably transient, with no further symptoms or complications (Goldberg et al., 1993). Hypoparathyroidism has been found in 8% of cases at one center (Lipson et al., 1991) and in a single patient with short stature at another center (Goldberg et al., 1993). Small or absent thymus (10%), tonsils (50%), and adenoids (85%) have been reported (Gorlin et al., 1990), as have T-cell anomalies (Lipson et al., 1991). Patients with VCF syndrome may also manifest overt or subclinical features of the Di George anomaly, a developmental defect that results in cardiac, thymic, and parathyroid disorders (Goldberg et al., 1993; Lipson et al., 1991; Stevens, Carey, & Shigeoka, 1990).

Less frequent anomalies include abdominal hernias (inguinal and umbilical), scoliosis, and the Robin sequence (Golding-Kushner et al., 1985). The Robin sequence, a triad of micrognathia (small jaws, particularly the lower jaw), U-shaped cleft palate, and glossoptosis (dropping of the tongue), can occur either as an isolated series of malformations or in conjunction with recurrent-pattern congenital malformation syndromes (Shprintzen et al., 1981). Short stature (below the 5th centile) has been reported in between one-third and two-thirds of cases (Shprintzen et al., 1978; Lipson et al., 1991). However, it has been suggested that when parental height is taken into account, a much smaller percentage of patients show true short stature (Goldberg et al., 1993).

Genetics

It is strongly suspected that a genetic component is inherent in the VCF syndrome. Reports of familial cases have included two apparently affected mothers with affected daughters, an affected mother with an affected son, one affected mother with both an affected son and daughter, and one case of male-to-male transmission (indicating autosomal dominant, rather than X-linked, inheritance). Autosomal dominant inheritance is also supported by similar severity of expression between male and female patients. However, no chromosomal anomalies have been associated with the syndrome. A small number of chromosome studies have been performed, yielding normal karyotypes (Lipson et al., 1991; Shprintzen et al., 1981; Williams et al., 1985). Most cases reported in the literature have been sporadic, suggesting a high spontaneous mutation rate. However, careful examinations of family members of persons diagnosed with VCF syndrome have revealed milder clinical expressions of the disorder, suggesting perhaps a lower mutation rate than was previously thought (Meinecke et al., 1986).

Teratogens

No common environmental agent or teratogen has been implicated in the etiology of the VCF syndrome. Shprintzen et al. (1981) reviewed the pregnancy histories in their sample, and detected four unaffected mothers who had been given progestational agents (i.e., substances used in birth control pills) during the early first trimester. In addition, one mother was an operating room nurse who had been exposed to anesthetic gases during pregnancy. The possible teratogenic effects of these substances in relation to VCF syndrome is unknown. Given that no consistent etiology is apparent, it is probable that the syndrome results from heterogeneous causes and that nongenetic phenocopies (i.e., similar in appearance to the cases resulting from a genetic anomaly, but causally related instead to environmental factors) account for some percentage of the sporadic cases (Lipson et al., 1991).

Epidemiology

The incidence of VCF syndrome in the general population is not known. It appears likely that many cases of this recently recognized syndrome are overlooked, because many of the reported anomalies are minor and occur with some frequency in the general population (Goldberg et al., 1993). Between 5% and 8% of children with cleft palate referred to craniofacial centres were identified as having VCF syndrome (Lipson et al., 1991; Shprintzen, Siegel-Sadewitz, Amato, & Goldberg, 1985). Thus, it is thought to be the most common syndrome of clefting (Shprintzen et al., 1985).

Differential Diagnosis

Diagnosis of VCF syndrome is difficult because of the minor nature of many of the structural anomalies and the variable expression of the disorder. Therefore, a "gestalt" approach to diagnosis must be taken (Williams et al., 1985). The diagnosis of the VCF syndrome must be made through the exclusion of other chromosomal, teratogenic, and genetic conditions. Specifically, it must be distinguished from other disorders with cardiac and craniofacial involvement. Syndromes included in the differential diagnosis include trichorhinophalangeal syndrome (similar facies), Stickler syndrome (cleft palate, retrognathia, and short stature), fetal alcohol syndrome (FAS; cleft palate, short stature, mental retardation, and cardiac anomalies), myotonic dystrophy (similar facies, hypernasal speech, and Robin sequence), Prader–Willi syndrome (similar facies and hypotonia), Noonan syndrome (facial, cardiac, and cognitive involvement), and Williams syndrome (cardiac, facial, and cognitive involvement) (Lipson et al., 1991; Shprintzen et al., 1981; Young et al., 1980).

The DiGeorge syndrome, also referred to as the DiGeorge sequence or anomaly, was originally thought to be a distinct disorder and also one that must be ruled out before making a diagnosis of VCF syndrome. The DiGeorge anomaly involves developmental defects of the third and fourth pharyngeal pouches (early embryological structures associated with the pharynx, just behind the oral cavity), resulting in thymic and parathyroid hypoplasia, as well as cardiac defects (Stevens et al., 1990). It has been reported in association with at least 18 different disorders, including FAS and VCF syndrome (Lammer & Opitz, 1986). It has been proposed that the DiGeorge anomaly is not a distinct syndrome, but rather a developmental field defect arising from heterogeneous causes as a component of several distinct disorders (Carey, 1980). (A "developmental field defect" is a causally heterogeneous malformation pattern resulting from a group of embryonic cells that form a single developmental unit.) Stevens et al. (1990) have supported this hypothesis by documenting the coexistence of VCF syndrome and the DiGeorge anomaly. Additional support comes from the observation of hypocalcemia, hypoparathyroidism, and T-cell dysfunction in patients with VCF syndrome. It is possible that many reported cases of the DiGeorge sequence were actually cases of the VCF syndrome manifesting the DiGeorge anomaly (Lipson et al., 1990).

Neurological Involvement and Neuroimaging

Approximately 4% of reported cases have microcephaly, suggesting possible central nervous system (CNS) involvement (Goldberg et al., 1993; Williams et al., 1985). However, there have been few reports of neuroimaging studies in this population. Magnetic resonance imaging (MRI) scans of four patients were reported as normal (Shprintzen, Goldberg, Golding-Kushner, & Marion, 1992). Neuropathological data are not available.

Embryology

The nature and origin of the congenital cardiac defects in the VCF syndrome may provide important clues about the pathogenesis of the disorder. These aorticopulmonary septal, or conotruncal, defects— tetralogy of Fallot, aberrant subclavian artery, and a double-outlet right ventricle—have been related to defective proliferation and migration of the neural crest. The noncardiac malformations of the VCF syndrome may originate from the same error in early embryogenesis (Thomas & Frias, 1987). (A comprehensive presentation of human embryology is beyond the scope of this discussion. The interested reader may consult the numerous works in this area for a complete discussion of the processes involved.)

Similar congenital heart defects may result from a variety of developmental mechanisms operating during early embryogenesis. These include the following: (1) abnormal proliferation and migration of cells from branchial arch mesenchyme and the neural crest, (2) changes in the proportion of right and left heart blood flow, (3) defects in programmed cell death, and (4) abnormal cellular matrix formation (Clark, 1985). Studies employing the chick embryo have demonstrated that cardiac defects consistently resulted from the ablation of premigratory neural crest cells from the cranial region of the neural fold. It is inferred that the defects were caused either by the absence of the neural crest or by their defective interaction with cardiac mesenchyme. Although several different defects resulted, the most common, known as conotruncal defects, were VSDs, a single outflow vessel originating from the right ventricle, and a single outflow vessel overriding the ventricular septum. Thymic hypoplasia often accompanied these defects (Kirby, Gale, & Stewart, 1983). Reduction or absence of the thymus in experimental animals has also been demonstrated subsequent to ablation of the premigratory neural crest (Bockman & Kirby, 1984). The cardiac neural crest migrates into the pharyngeal arches 3, 4, and 6, which in turn contribute to the development of the aortic arch and outflow tracts, where they form the aorticopulmonary septum and populate the truncal folds. The thymus also develops from pharyngeal arches 3 and 4 (Lipson et al., 1991).

Conotruncal defects in humans include supracristal VSD, aorticopulmonary window, double-outlet right ventricle, tetralogy of Fallot, transposition of the great vessels, truncus arteriosus communis, and pulmonary atresia with VSD. Many of these defects are associated with different malformation syndromes, including the DiGeorge syndrome. These relationships have been explained by anomalies in the development and migration of the neural crest (Thomas & Frias, 1987). In addition to the cardic derivatives described above, neural crest cells contribute to the formation of the tongue, thymus, thyroid, and parathyroid glands, as well as to the development of the skeleton and soft tissues of the face and branchial arches (Noden, 1986). The five pairs of branchial, or visceral, arches form the lateral and ventral walls of the pharynx of the embryo. They are important in the formation of structures of the face and neck. For example, the maxillary and mandibular processes, which form the upper and lower jaws, are derivatives of the first branchial arch. Taken together, these facts provide support for an embryological basis for the VCF syndrome.

Further support comes from an analysis of the ocular features observed in the VCF syndrome (Mansour et al., 1987). These include retinal vascular tortuosity, posterior embryotoxon (opacity of the cornea), narrow palpebral fissure, suborbital discoloration, small optic nerves, iris nodules, and cataracts. Retinal vascular tortuosity is thought to characterize many genetic and acquired disorders, including FAS and VCF syndrome. It may involve the large or small vessels of either the arterial or venous systems. Prominent tortuosity of both the venous and arterial vascular trees was found in 36% of patients with VCF syndrome examined by Mansour et al. In these cases, the retinal vascular tortuosity was found to be associated intrinsically with the syndrome and not secondary to the heart disease or to other known etiologies. Posterior embryotoxon, also thought to be attributable to abnormal neural crest migration, was present in 23% of the cases. In addition, narrow palpebral fissures may be related to the integrity of the connective tissue of the eyelid, which derives from the neural crest as well. These findings suggest a primary developmental anomaly of neural crest derivatives in the pathogenesis of the syndrome.

NEUROPSYCHOLOGICAL ASSETS AND DEFICITS

Although learning disabilities or mental retardation have been almost invariably found in VCF syndrome, only one study has specifically addressed the cognitive abilities of these children (Golding-Kushner et al., 1985). This was a retrospective, cross-sectional study of 26 children assessed at a craniofacial center. Although further prospective neuropsychological studies of children with VCF are necessary in order to delineate the natural history and prognosis of this disorder, this initial study and several case reports suggest a number of similarities in the neuropsychological, academic, and psychosocial presentations of the VCF syndrome and the Nonverbal Learning Disabilities (NLD) syndrome. The neuropsychological assets and deficits of children with VCF syndrome are described in this section; the next section presents a comparison of the VCF and NLD syndromes.

Sensory and Perceptual Abilities

It is not yet clear whether the visual- and tactile-perceptual abilities of children with VCF syndrome are impaired. Golding-Kushner et al. (1985) noted that all of the children "failed" a "perceptual screening test". This test included the assessment of bilateral integration and tactile discrimination, praxis, and visual–spatial or visual-perceptual skills (involving completion of form boards, block construction, and geometric designs). There is no indication whether performance was poor on all components of the test, nor whether this test had been standardized so that performance could be compared to appropriate norms. Also, the visual tasks were quite complex and drew on skills beyond perceptual abilities (e.g., constructional abilities).

Motor and Psychomotor Skills

Hypotonia is frequently seen during infancy in children with VCF syndrome (Lipson et al., 1991; Smith, 1988). As an apparent consequence, motor milestones may be slightly delayed in some children (Meinecke et al., 1986; Shprintzen et al., 1978). According to parental report, the mean age at which children with VCF syndrome walked was 17 months, with only 27% walking before the age of 15 months. Minor difficulties with coordination persisted into adolescence, and graphomotor performance was noted to be poor (Golding-Kushner et al., 1985).

Attention and Memory

Simple auditory attention span, as measured by digit span, was found to be intact. Anecdotal report suggests that these children have an excellent ability to learn rote verbal material, though this was not formally assessed (Golding-Kushner et al., 1985). The visual and tactile attention and memory abilities of children with VCF syndrome have yet to be studied.

Concept Formation and Problem Solving

The concept-formation and problem-solving abilities of children with VCF syndrome have not been formally assessed, but anecdotal reports suggest that this is a significant area of deficiency. These children have been noted to remain "concrete" in their thinking as they grow older. Their problem-solving skills have been found to be poor relative to their verbal memory. They appear unable to apply a problem-solving process learned in one context to another involving novel stimuli. In keeping with these conceptual difficulties, older children with VCF have been noted to appreciate humor only rarely, and to perform poorly on the Verbal Absurdities subtest of the Detroit Tests of Learning Aptitude (Golding-Kushner et al., 1985).

Intelligence

In the Golding-Kushner et al. (1985) study, 17 children received psychometric intelligence assessments. The tests administered varied between the different age groups. The 4-year-olds obtained mean IQs of 87 on the mainly verbal Stanford–Binet and 84 on the Leiter International Performance Test. The older children were assessed with the Wechsler Intelligence Scale for Children—Revised (WISC-R). The 8-year-olds obtained a mean WISC-R Verbal IQ of 76 and a mean Performance IQ of 79. The 13-year-olds obtained a mean Verbal IQ of 79 and a mean Performance IQ of 70.

As the authors acknowledge, meaningful comparisons cannot be made between the scores of the younger group and the two older groups, as the different tests may well assess different abilities. Certainly, given the cross-sectional nature of the study, conclusions about deterioration in intellectual abilities over time are not warranted. However, in two cases, children were followed longitudinally from preschool into the elementary grades. Drops in IQ scores of approximately 10 points were noted in these cases (Golding-Kushner et al., 1985); however, the authors do not indicate whether this involved both Verbal and Performance IQs. If, as has been suggested, children with VCF syndrome remain concrete in their thought with little ability to generalize to novel situations, then it would be expected that these two children's "performance" skills had fallen progressively further behind their rote verbal abilities, relative to those of controls.

Language Skills

Significant speech and language delay has been reported in children with VCF syndrome (Lipson et al., 1991; Shprintzen et al., 1978). Many were initially diagnosed following referrals because of hypernasal speech (Shprintzen et al., 1978). Their voice quality throughout childhood has been described as low-volume and monotonic, although these children appear able to modify their pitch when requested to do so. Virtually identical results were found even for children without middle-ear pathology (Golding-Kushner et al., 1985).

Children in the youngest age group (4 years) in the Golding-Kushner et al. (1985) study scored within normal limits on all subtests of the Illinois Test of Psycholinguistic Abilities. However, children in the 8-year-old group scored within the normal range on only two tests: those for auditory sequential memory (digit span) and manual expression. On other tests, that required increased processing and reasoning ability, they scored approximately two standard deviations below the mean. However, it must be emphasized again that conclusions about developmental changes in ability cannot be made on the basis of these cross-sectional data. It may well be that the 8-year-old group simply had more significant cognitive deficits. In fact, their receptive vocabulary scores, as measured by the Peabody Picture Vocabulary Test, were slightly lower than those of the 4-year-olds and the 13-year-olds

Despite obtaining language scores within normal limits, the youngest children were described as exhibiting some deficiencies in spontaneous speech. Their utterances were reduced in length and complexity, and they were noted to rely to a great extent on nonverbal communication. At 8 years of age, children's language was marked by immature syntax and grammar, a reduced expressive vocabulary, and concreteness (Golding-Kushner et al., 1985; Shprintzen et al., 1978).

Academic Achievement

Simple reading skills appear to be intact. The youngest children in the study by Golding-Kushner et al. (1985) showed normal letter-naming ability, while the two older groups of children exhibited normal single-word reading on the Wide Range Achievement Test—Revised (WRAT-R). However, despite normal word decoding, the older children demonstrated somewhat poorer reading comprehension. Written spelling was within normal limits for the 13-year-old group, and was slightly poorer for the 8-year-olds. This difference might be attributable to difficulties with the copying task included as part of the WRAT-R Spelling subtest for the 8-year-old children: This task requires visual-perceptual and graphomotor skills.

Arithmetic skills were impaired at all ages. The youngest group exhibited poor numerical awareness on the Leiter scales, and the two older groups exhibited poor written calculation skills on the WRAT-R Arithmetic subtest relative to their WRAT-R single-word reading skills (Golding-Kushner et al., 1985). It is reported that children with VCF syndrome can often function adequately in a normal classroom with remedial help (Shprintzen et al., 1978).

Psychosocial Aspects

At all ages, children with VCF syndrome in the Golding-Kushner et al. (1985) study were noted to have bland affect, with little facial expression. However, they were easily able to vary their expression on request. Poor social competence was also noted. Their interactions with others were found to be deficient in terms of quantity and quality. Their behavior tended toward extremes, with the children being either disinhibited or shy. However, they also tended to be affectionate, and presented with no serious behavioral control problems or bizarre behavior (Golding-Kushner et al., 1985). Lipson et al. (1991) also found social withdrawal to be common, and felt that it might be secondary to the frustration experienced by many of the children because of their poor speech intelligibility. Following pharyngoplasty, improved confidence and ability were reported in some of these socially withdrawn children.

Recent reports (Goldberg et al., 1993; Shprintzen et al., 1992) suggest that some 10% of patients with VCF syndrome may go on to develop psychiatric disorders. Although a wide range of psychiatric diagnoses have been reported, the most common symptoms described are those associated with depression and anxiety disorders. These include disturbed mood, severe vegetative symptoms, disturbed appetite, fatigue, and low self-esteem, as well as poor concentration and decision-making ability (Goldberg et al., 1993).

COMPARISON TO THE NLD SYNDROME

Neurocognitive Assets and Deficits in the Two Syndromes

Although many aspects of the cognitive abilities of children with the VCF syndrome remain to be explored, certain similarities between the

neuropsychological assets and deficits of these children and those characteristic of the NLD syndrome are notable. Speech and language were
found to be delayed in both groups. Whereas children with NLD have
been noted to go on to develop a high volume of speech output (Rourke,
1989), this has not been found in the VCF syndrome. However, it might
be argued that the cleft palates and/or velopharyngeal insufficiency so
frequently seen in VCF syndrome are contributing factors. In terms of
expressive language, a tendency toward concreteness has been noted in
both syndromes. However, there is some suggestion that children with
the VCF syndrome may have additional language problems not seen in
the NLD syndrome, as the grammar and syntax of the former have been
reported to be deficient. Both groups demonstrate strengths in the area
of intact auditory attention span, as well as ease in learning rote verbal
material.

Similar patterns of academic performance are seen in both groups,
although it is not clear whether the same extremes in terms of assets and
deficits are exhibited in the VCF syndrome. In both syndromes, single-
word reading is significantly better developed than is reading comprehension. In the NLD syndrome, phonemic abilities, as seen in the ability to
decode words and to spell, have been described as being overdeveloped
(Rourke, 1989). It is not known whether children with the VCF syndrome
also demonstrate overdeveloped phonemic skills. Both groups of children
tend to show deficits in mechanical arithmetic and mathematical reasoning. In the NLD syndrome, these have long been seen as outstanding
deficits (Strang & Rourke, 1985). The same level of impairment was not
evident in the children with VCF syndrome who have been studied.
Both groups of children demonstrate similar deficits in problem solving,
concept formation, and appreciation of incongruities. In both disorders,
these problems become more marked with age, probably secondary to
changing developmental demands (Casey, Rourke, & Picard, 1991).

It is not clear whether children with the VCF syndrome demonstrate
deficits in tactile and visual perception, or, secondary to these perceptual
deficits, poor attention and memory abilities for information presented
in these modalities. This is the profile seen in the NLD syndrome (Rourke,
1989). Certainly, on the basis of measures of psychometric intelligence,
the marked deficits on Performance subtests relative to Verbal subtests
that is so frequently seen in NLD was not evident in the profiles of the
children with VCF syndrome studied by Golding-Kushner et al. (1985).

Although socioemotional functioning has only recently been examined in children with the VCF syndrome, the evidence suggests that, like
children with the NLD syndrome, they demonstrate significant impairments in social interaction. In the NLD syndrome, it has been argued
that the primary neuropsychological deficits (e.g., visual-perceptual impairments, problems with novel situations) contribute to their poor social

skills (Rourke, 1989). Lipson et al. (1991) suggested that the social withdrawal in young children with VCF syndrome might result at least partly from their impaired ability to communicate with others. It might also be the case that their concreteness, reasoning difficulties, and problems with countenancing novelty contribute to their poorer social interaction skills. Recently there have been reports that some children with VCF syndrome show evidence of psychopathology as they grow older. Although further information is needed in this area, the most recent report (Goldberg et al., 1993) suggests that internalized psychopathology is often seen. It has been well documented in the NLD syndrome that as these children get older, increasing evidence of similar types of emotional problems become evident (Rourke, 1989; Rourke & Fuerst, 1991).

Is There Evidence of Dysfunctional or Dysmorphic White Matter in the VCF Syndrome?

A review of the literature pertaining to the VCF syndrome has not yielded any hard evidence of white matter pathology. However, it has been demonstrated that those afflicted manifest psychological and behavioral characteristics of the NLD syndrome during childhood. It is reasonable to propose that another, as yet unidentified component of the VCF syndrome may well involve pathology of CNS white matter. Two lines of evidence may be used to propose converging hypotheses in support of this view.

First, the vast majority of defects of CNS ontogeny can be described in terms of the orderly development of the fetal brain. Both the simultaneity and sequence of events are critical, as many different processes occur during any given window of time. The concept of a critical period of heightened vulnerability of the fetus to noxious stimuli is also important. Interestingly, it is not the nature of the teratogen, but rather its timing in relation to embryogenic events, that determines the type of malformation produced. Animal studies have shown that this is the case for viral diseases, drugs, radiation, fever, and malnutrition (Menkes, 1990). The results of the studies reviewed above have supported the embryological basis for the VCF syndrome by demonstrating that the dysmorphic structures are susceptible during the same ontogenetic time frames. However, exactly when during embryogenesis this occurs has not been speculated upon. In order to support the white matter model, a reasonable argument that the primordium of white matter is vulnerable to insult at the same point in development must be presented.

It would not appear to be a primary defect in the integrity of the myelin that results in white matter dysfunction, because the process occurs late in the development of the fetus. Myelinogenesis begins at the end of the first trimester; however, it occurs for the most part postnatally, continuing through the third or fourth year of life (Menkes, 1990). The functional integrity of the white matter may also be disrupted during the period of cellular proliferation and migration. During approximately the seventh and eighth weeks of gestation, undifferentiated germinal cells of the neural tube begin to proliferate. These include medulloblasts, which are precursors for neurons and oligodendroglia (cells that will eventually form CNS myelin). Cells also begin to migrate from the matrix zone to form the surrounding mantle zone (grey matter), which in turn develops cellular processes that extend laterally to form the marginal zone (white matter; Menkes, 1990).

However, these processes also occur much later than those suspected in the embryogenesis of the defects characterizing the VCF syndrome. Although the cardiac and ocular defects are thought to arise from abnormal migration of the neural crest, the animal studies suggest that a primary neural crest defect is involved. Thus, it seems that the most plausible time of origin of white matter dysfunction concurrent with facial and cardiac anomalies would be during early embryogenesis, possibly during the fourth week. During this time, many simultaneous processes occur, including the formation of the primordia for facial structures, viscera, and the telencephalon. Anomalies of these events that are reliant on neural induction are known to produce secondary anomalies of proliferation or migration (Menkes, 1990). It is possible that this is the mechanism by which cerebral white matter pathology arises in VCF.

The second line of evidence that could implicate the involvement of white matter pathology in the VCF syndrome comes from the observation of VCF syndrome concurrent with holoprosencephaly in one case study. This infant was born at 38 weeks gestation following a normal pregnancy. The facial appearance was characteristic of severe holoprosencephaly, and an ultrasound scan of the brain confirmed this diagnosis. In addition, an echocardiogram revealed the features of tetralogy of Fallot. A postmortem examination following death at 32 days confirmed alobar holoprosencephaly and tetralogy of Fallot. Chromosome analysis yielded a normal 46XY karyotype. Family history suggested that this infant had VCF syndrome. An older sister had died at the age of 3 months. Although no postmortem examination of the sister was conducted, records indicated that she had severe congenital heart disease and mildly dysmorphic facial features, including a retruded mandible. Moreover, the mother had undergone a total correction of tetralogy of Fallot at the age of 12 years. She also had a large submucous cleft palate, facial features and narrow fingers characteristic of VCF syndrome, and an IQ of 77 (Wraith, Super, Watson, & Phillips, 1985).

The authors suggested that a concomitant of VCF syndrome may be the variable expression of holoprosencephaly. The two conditions have several facial and palatal features in common. In holoprosencephaly, the facial features occur as a consequence of the brain malformation and vary from very gross abnormalities to mild hypotelorism, microcephaly, and midfacial hypoplasia with or without midline clefting of the lip and palate. The degree of facial malformation does not necessarily correspond to the severity of the holoprosencephaly. Thus, mild degrees of holoprosencephaly may account for the mild mental deficits and learning disabilities, as well as the facial features of VCF syndrome (Wraith et al., 1985). Given that holoprosencephaly is associated with varying degrees of dysgenesis of the corpus callosum even in its mildest form, this evidence would be in accord with the propositions of the white matter model. Recent advances in MRI technology suggest that the conclusions drawn by these authors may be accurate.

Milder degrees of callosal dysgenesis are very difficult to identify without coronal or sagittal images, which are readily attainable with MRI. This technology has revealed a much higher incidence of callosal dysgenesis in conjunction with other brain malformations than was previously suspected. The commisural plate forms between the 8th and 16th gestational weeks, whereas the corpus callosum proper forms between approximately the 12th and 20th weeks. During this time, the entire brain is developing; hence, the association between brain and callosal abnormalities is not surprising. These frequently include Chiari II and Dandy–Walker malformations, interhemispheric arachnoid cysts, neuronal migration anomalies, encephaloceles, and midline facial anomalies. Thus, it has been recommended that the corpus callosum should be carefully examined in infants and children presenting with seizure disorders, developmental delay, or facial dysmorphism (Barkovich, 1991).

The corpus callosum is formed in an orderly and sequential manner beginning anteriorly with the genu and proceeding posteriorly with the body, splenium, and rostrum (see Chapter 3 of this volume). Thus, an interruption in normal brain development will result in the anterior portion being formed and the posterior portion being absent or dysplastic. The one exception to this rule is holoprosencephaly. In the past, this disorder was thought to result from a defect in the cleavage of the prosencephalon into the diencephalon and telencephalon, as well as a failure of cleavage of the telencephalon into the two cerebral hemispheres. However, it is now thought to result from the lack of forebrain induction (Barkovich, 1991). This process occurs during the fourth week of gestation and involves the elaboration of foregut entoderm into the primordium for facial structures. It is activated by the rostral neural tube, the primordium for the telencephalon, and by cephalic mesoderm, the primordium for facial bone and skull (Menkes, 1990).

Several observations support this hypothesis. For example, the prefrontal cortex, normally comprising the bulk of the frontal lobes, is absent in holoprosencephaly. In addition, both the pituitary gland and the hypo-thalamus are usually poorly formed and hypofunctional. The olfactory system also tends to be unformed. When facial anomalies are present, they result from a lack of induction of the midline aspects of the face. In short, holoprosencephaly can be seen as a condition in which the most rostral midline segments of both the brain and face fail to develop or develop improperly (Barkovich, 1991).

The severity of holoprosencephaly is variable. Three types, referred to as alobar, semilobar, and lobar, represent a continuum of brain and facial anomalies, with alobar being the most severe and lobar holopro-sencephaly presenting as nearly normal. Alobar holoprosencephaly usu-ally results in spontaneous abortion. In general, those afflicted have severe midline facial deformities and lack any grossly recognizable normal cerebral structures. Those with semilobar holoprosencephaly typically have normal or mildly dysmorphic facies. The interhemispheric fissure and falx cerebri are usually formed posteriorly but absent anteriorly, as is the corpus callosum. Holoprosencephaly is the only condition where the normal anterior-to-posterior development of the corpus callosum is disrupted. Therefore, it is unclear whether this structure is merely a "pseudosplenium." Other anomalies include continuity of the cerebral cortex between the hemispheres, a rudimentary hippocampal formation, large and incompletely formed temporal horns of the lateral ventricles, and absence of the septum pellucidum (Barkovich, 1991).

The lobar form of holoprosencephaly may be the most interesting in terms of the possibility of white matter dysfunction in the VCF syn-drome. The anomalies in this condition are subtle and may be easily overlooked, particularly if they are not accompanied by any facial abnor-malities. The interhemispheric fissure and the falx cerebri extend fron-tally, but the falx is usually dysplastic. The formation of the frontal horns ranges from normal to very rudimentary. MRI reveals mild dysplasia of the genu of the corpus callosum and absence of the septum pellucidum. The hippocampal formations and temporal horns of the lateral ventricles are nearly, if not entirely, normal. Some degree of dysplasia of the frontal lobes will be apparent with careful examination (Barkovich, 1991).

SUMMARY

There is some evidence to suggest that the learning disabilities and psy-chosocial characteristics of children afflicted with the VCF syndrome may result from cerebral abnormalities. Although these deficits have been noted on several occasions, their cause has not been previously speculated upon. In the past, physicians and other caregivers have been concerned with the more practical issues of respiration and speech. However, it is becoming increasingly important to delineate more accurately the full spectrum of disorders such as the VCF syndrome, in order to assist in providing an accurate prognosis and appropriate intervention. It is now recognized that, despite relatively normal language and psychometric intelligence level before the age of 6 years, children with the VCF syndrome should be considered as being at high risk for NLD and other learning disabilities. Although MRI findings from four VCF children do not suggest white matter pathology (Shprintzen et al., 1992), a study incorporating MRI and neuropsychological examinations of a larger sample of these individuals may demonstrate findings that are consistent with the notion that these children manifest the NLD syndrome as a result of white matter perturbations.

REFERENCES

Arvystas, M., & Shprintzen, R. J. (1984). Craniofacial morphology on the velo-cardio-facial syndrome. *Journal of Craniofacial Genetics and Developmental Biology, 4*, 39–45.

Barkovich, A. J. (1991). Brain development: Normal and abnormal. In S. W. Atlas (Ed.), *Magnetic resonance imaging of the brain and spinal cord* (pp. 129–173). New York: Raven Press.

Bockman, D. E., & Kirby, M. L. (1984). Dependence of thymus development on derivatives of the neural crest. *Science, 223*, 498–500.

Carey, J. C. (1980). Spectrum of the DiGeorge "syndrome." *Journal of Pediatrics, 96*, 955–956.

Casey, J. E., Rourke, B. P., & Picard, E. M. (1991). Syndrome of nonverbal learning disabilities: Age differences in neuropsychological, academic, and socioemotional functioning. *Developmental Psychopathology, 3*, 329–345.

Clark, E. B. (1985). Mechanisms in the pathogenesis of congenital heart defects. *Proceedings of the Greenwood Genetics Center, 4*, 80.

D'Antonio, L. L., & Marsh, J. L. (1987). Abnormal carotid arteries in the velocardiofacial syndrome. *Plastic and Reconstructive Surgery, 80*, 471–472.

Goldberg, R., Motzkin, B., Marion, R., Scrambler, P. J., & Shprintzen, R. J. (1993). Velo-cardio-facial syndrome: A review of 120 patients. *American Journal of Medical Genetics, 45*, 313–319.

Golding-Kushner, K. J., Weller, G., & Shprintzen, R. J. (1985). Velo-cardio-facial syndrome: Language and psychological profiles. *Journal of Craniofacial Genetics and Developmental Biology, 5*, 259–266.

Gorlin, R. J., Cohen, M. M., & Levin, L. S. (1990). Velocardiofacial syndrome (Shprintzen syndrome, Sedlackova syndrome). In *Syndromes of the head and neck* (3rd ed., pp. 740–742). New York: Oxford University Press.

Kirby, M. L., Gale, R. F., & Stewart, D. E. (1983). Neural crest cells contribute to normal aortopulmonary septation. *Science, 220*, 1059–1061.

Lammer, E. J., & Opitz, J. M. (1986). The DiGeorge anomaly as a developmental field defect. *American Journal of Medical Genetics Supplement, 2*, 113–127.

Lipson, A. H., Yuille, D., Angel, M., Thompson, P. G., Vandervoord, J. G., & Beckenham, E. J. (1991). Velocardiofacial (Shprintzen) syndrome: An important syndrome for the dysmorphologist to recognize. *Journal of Medical Genetics, 28*, 596–604.

MacKenzie-Stepner, K., Witzel, M. A., Stringer, D. A., Lindsay, W. K., Munro, I. R., & Hughes, H. (1987). Abnormal carotid arteries in the velocardiofacial syndrome: A report of three cases. *Plastic and Reconstructive Surgery, 80*, 347–351.

Mansour, A. M., Goldberg, R. B., Wang, F. M., & Shprintzen, R. J. (1987). Ocular findings in the velo-cardio-facial syndrome. *Journal of Pediatric Ophthalmology and Strabismus, 24*(5), 263–266.

Meinecke, P., Beemer, F. A., Schinzel, A., & Kushnick, T. (1986). The velo-cardio-facial (Shprintzen) syndrome: Clinical variability in eight patients. *European Journal of Pediatrics, 145*, 539–544.

Menkes, J. H. (1990). *Textbook of child neurology* (4th ed.). Philadelphia: Lea & Febiger.

Noden, D. N. (1986). Origins and patterning of craniofacial mesenchymal tissues. *Journal of Craniofacial Genetics and Developmental Biology* (Suppl. 2), 115–131.

Rourke, B. P. (1989). *Nonverbal learning disabilities: The syndrome and the model.* New York: Guilford Press.

Rourke, B. P., & Fuerst, D. R. (1991). *Learning disabilities and psychosocial functioning: A neuropsychological perspective.* New York: Guilford Press.

Shprintzen, R. J., Goldberg, R. B., Golding-Kushner, K. J., & Marion, R. W. (1992). Late-onset psychosis in the velo-cardio-facial syndrome. *American Journal of Medical Genetics, 42*, 141–142.

Shprintzen, R. J., Goldberg, R. B., Lewin, M. L., Sidoti, E. J., Berkman, M. D., Argamaso, R. V., & Young, D. (1978). A new syndrome involving cleft palate, cardiac anomalies, typical facies, and learning disabilities: Velo-cardio-facial syndrome. *Cleft Palate Journal, 5*(1), 56–62.

Shprintzen, R. J., Goldberg, R. B., Young, D., & Wolford, L. (1981). The velo-cardio-facial syndrome: A clinical and genetic analysis. *Pediatrics, 67*(2), 167–172.

Shprintzen, R. J., Siegel-Sadewitz, V. L., Amato, J., & Goldberg, R. B. (1985). Anomalies associated with cleft lip, cleft palate or both. *American Journal of Medical Genetics, 20*, 585–595.

Siegel-Sadewitz, V., & Shprintzen, R. J. (1982). The relationship of communication disorders to syndrome identification. *Journal of Speech and Hearing Disorders, 47*, 338–354.

Smith, D. W. (1988). Shprintzen syndrome (velo-cardio-facial syndrome). In K. L. Jones (Ed.), *Smith's recognizable patterns of human malformation* (4th ed., p. 224). Philadelphia: W. B. Saunders.

Stevens, C. A., Carey, J. C., & Shigeoka, A. O. (1990). DiGeorge anomaly and velocardiofacial syndrome. *Pediatrics, 85*(4), 526–530.

Strang, J. D., & Rourke, B. P. (1985). Arithmetic disability subtypes: The neuropsychological significance of specific arithmetic impairment in childhood. In B. P. Rourke (Ed.), *Neuropsychology of learning disabilities: Essentials of subtype analysis* (pp. 167–186). New York: Guilford Press.

Strong, W. B. (1968). Familial syndrome of right sided aortic arch, mental deficiency, and facial dysmorphism. *Journal of Pediatrics*, *73*, 882–888.

Thomas, I. T., & Frias, J. L. (1987). The heart in selected congenital malformations. A lesson in pathogenic relationships. *Annals of Clinical and Laboratory Science*, *17*(4), 207–210.

Williams, M. A., Shprintzen, R. J., & Goldberg, R. B. (1985). Male to male transmission of the velo-cardio-facial syndrome: A case report and review of 60 cases. *Journal of Craniofacial Genetics and Developmental Biology*, *5*, 175–180.

Wraith, J. E., Super, M., Watson, G. H., & Phillips, M. (1985). Velo-cardio-facial syndrome presenting as holoprosencephaly. *Clinical Genetics*, *27*, 408–410.

Young, D., Shprintzen, R. J., & Goldberg, R. B. (1990). Cardiac malformations in the velocardiofacial syndrome. *American Journal of Cardiology*, *46*, 643–648.

6

Williams Syndrome

Peter E. Anderson
Byron P. Rourke

Williams syndrome (WS) is a rare disorder that has been identified several times by researchers approaching the problem from different perspectives. The following discussion reflects this diversity.

HISTORY OF WS

Independent teams of endocrinologists published a number of papers in 1952 describing a disorder that was named "idiopathic infantile hypercalcemia" (Fanconi, Girardet, Schlesinger, Butler, & Black, 1952; Lightwood, 1952; Payne, 1952). At this point, two types of the disorder were delineated. The milder type, or Lightwood type, of idiopathic infantile hypercalcemia presented with symptoms such as anorexia, vomiting, loss of weight, constipation, and colic (Lightwood, 1952). These symptoms were thought to be caused by the hypercalcemia. In accordance with this theory, a modification of the infant's diet was recommended, in which the intake of calcium and vitamin D were limited. These steps usually resulted in the cessation of symptoms.

The severe type, or Fanconi type, of idiopathic infantile hypercalcemia (Fanconi et al., 1952) also presented with hypercalcemic symptoms (i.e., those of the Lightwood type) that were mitigated with dietary modifications. In addition to these symptoms, however, more serious symptoms were noted, including renal impairment, osteosclerosis (i.e., hardening of bones with increased heaviness), stenoses of major arteries, and moderate to severe mental retardation (Arnold, Yule, & Martin, 1985; Udwin, Yule, & Martin, 1986). The early researchers also made reference to the facial characteristics of these individuals, shortly thereafter termed "elfin facies" (Lowe, Henderson, Park, & McGreal, 1954). This combination of characteristics includes a medial eyebrow flare (i.e., eyebrow hair growth pattern toward the nose); short palpebral fissures (i.e., the opening between the eyelids); either lacy or stellate (i.e., star-like) patterns in the iris; a depressed nasal bridge with anteverted nares; a long, smooth philtrum; and thick lips with an open mouth posture. The ears have also been described as low-set, but Joseph and Parrott (1958) contended that the head posture (extended) could lead to this impression.

In 1961, a team of cardiologists from New Zealand (Williams, Barratt-Boyes, & Lowe) described a syndrome characterized by supravalvular aortic stenosis. On the basis of a number of features of one patient, including facial characteristics and deficient mental abilities, Williams correctly predicted the presence of supravalvular aortic stenosis in three additional patients. Beuren, another cardiologist, also reported several cases of the syndrome, resulting in periodic use of the identifier "Williams–Beuren syndrome" (e.g., Beuren, Apitz, & Harmjanz, 1962; Beuren, Schulze, Eberle, Harmjanz, & Apitz, 1964).

Black and Bonham Carter (1963) used the phrase "elfin facies" in conjunction with WS when they emphasized the association between aortic stenosis and the facies characteristic of Fanconi type idiopathic infantile hypercalcemia. Garcia, Friedman, Kaback, and Rowe (1964) provided the first definitive link between the two disorders, presenting a case to establish the association as a clinically recognizable syndrome. Martin, Snodgrass, and Cohen (1984) also compared the clinical features of Fanconi type idiopathic infantile hypercalcemia and WS. The results of this investigation indicated that there is most likely a common genetic abnormality. However, hypercalcemia, while being linked to the underlying disorder, is seen as being expressed with variable frequency and penetration (Udwin, 1990). Jones and Smith (1975) also reported that hypercalcemia, if present, is of a transient nature.

To sum up, this disorder was first identified in the 1950s as idiopathic infantile hypercalcemia. At this time it was also recognized that two types existed, one milder (the Lightwood type), and one more severe in nature (the Fanconi type). Cardiologists in the 1960s identified a disorder on the basis of supravalvular aortic stenosis, later noting the similarities between these patients and those with Fanconi type infantile hypercalcemia.

EPIDEMIOLOGY

As mentioned, WS is a rare disorder, although perhaps not as rare as previously thought (Martin et al., 1984). Fraser, Kidd, Kooh, and Paunier (1966), using data published by the British Paediatric Association Committee on Hypercalcaemia, found that for all forms of hypercalcemia, there was a prevalence rate of 1 per 20,000 live births. When only Fanconi type idiopathic infantile hypercalcemia was considered, the prevalence rate decreased to 1 per 100,000–200,000 live births. These authors noted that similar statistics were not available in North America at that time. However, on the basis of available medical records and knowledge of symptoms of the disorder (e.g., supravalvular aortic stenosis and confirmed hypercalcemia), an estimate of 1 per 150,000 live births was reached. This is most likely an underestimate, as it is commonly accepted that hypercalcemia, if present in WS, is transient (Jones & Smith, 1975). Therefore, if the testing for such a condition were not performed at the proper time, such a child would not be diagnosed with the disorder.

Martin et al. (1984) reported that the incidence of idiopathic infantile hypercalcemia in Great Britain is approximately 1 per 47,000 live births, while Greenberg (1989, 1990) estimated it to be between 1 in 20,000 and 1 in 50,000 live births. The increase in awareness of this disorder relative to previous years was found to be due, at least in part, to the efforts of groups such as the Infantile Hypercalcaemia Foundation (United Kingdom). Beuren et al. (1964), discussing the increase in the early 1960s, credited the publication of more detailed studies on this disorder. Feature articles and special issues on WS in a number of journals (e.g., *American Journal of Medical Genetics*, Supplement 6, 1990; Burn, 1986; Shepherd & Goel, 1990) continue to play a role in increasing awareness of WS.

LABORATORY STUDIES

Laboratory studies have tended to focus, at least in the initial stages, on the causes of hypercalcemia. Russo, Chamany, Klemish, Hall, and Murray (1991) pointed out that calcium levels in the blood are regulated by three mechanisms: vitamin D, calcitonin, and parathyroid hormone. The first two of these are discussed in the WS literature.

The link with vitamin D surfaced early, and was supported by research using an animal model (Friedman & Roberts, 1966). These investigators reported that supravalvular aortic stenoses were present when pregnant rabbits were exposed to megadoses of vitamin D. Thus, the initial treatment for idiopathic infantile hypercalcemia consisted of dietary modification. For example, in Great Britain, dietary supplements supplied by the government in the 1950s were found to have 10 times the amount of recommended vitamin D. When the diets of individuals with idiopathic hypercalcemia were modified to restrict the intake of vitamin D, the reported problems were mitigated.

However, as Jones (1990) outlined, it is difficult to draw conclusions from this research because the level of severity of symptoms was not reported. Thus, it is possible that these early "cures" were associated with individuals presenting with the mild form of idiopathic infantile hypercalcemia. As mentioned previously, Jones (1990; Jones & Smith, 1975) reported that hypercalcemia is not thought to be a predominant symptom of WS, and that if it is present, it tends to be transient in nature.

Approximately 10 years after the first documentation of idiopathic infantile hypercalcemia, calcitonin was discovered (Jones, 1990), providing a new avenue for research related to hypercalcemia—that of a deficiency in the production or release of calcitonin. A serendipitous finding was the discovery of calcitonin gene-related peptide (CGRP), a peptide produced by the same gene that produces calcitonin. This led to the speculation that an abnormality in the production of these two substances could be related to some of the symptomatology of WS—that is, calcitonin to the hypercalcemic symptoms and CGRP to the other symptoms (Culler, Jones, & Deftos, 1985).

Culler et al. (1985) examined the relationship between impaired calcitonin secretion and the ability to rid the body of a calcium bolus. Five patients with WS, who at the time of the study had normal serum calcium levels, were found to clear the bolus at a rate slower than that of normal controls, supporting an earlier finding (Forbes, Bryson, Manning, Amirhakimi, & Reina, 1972). Culler et al. (1985) concluded their studies by stating that although the calcitonin deficiency can explain the tendency to develop hypercalcemia, it does not explain the many other symptoms of the disorder.

Jones (1990) explained the potential significance of the link between WS and calcitonin/CGRP as follows. Calcitonin sites in the body tend to be the bones and kidneys (note that individuals with WS experience difficulties with both), whereas CGRP sites are much more heavily concentrated in the cardiovascular and central nervous systems. If we consider some of the classic symptoms of WS (i.e., supravalvular aortic stenosis; pulmonary and peripheral stenoses; hypertension; moderate to severe mental retardation; and abnormalities of hearing, speech, and behavior), the potential significance of the CGRP connection grows.

Reiss, Feinstein, Rosenbaum, Borengasser-Caruso, and Goldsmith (1985) described two children with WS and associated autism who also exhibited hyperserotonemia. These investigators proposed that WS is a disorder in which elevated serotonin levels may play a role—a finding that August and Realmuto (1989) contested. August and Realmuto described two children with WS who had blood serotonin levels in the normal range, and suggested that hyperserotonemia was associated with autism rather than with WS. In other words, August and Realmuto inferred from the elevated blood levels of serotonin that the children studied by Reiss et al. (1985) had autism as a primary disorder, and that WS was a secondary disorder. The view that hyperserotonemia is associated with autism is tentatively supported by Piven et al. (1991), but, as August and Realmuto (1989) concluded, further studies of blood serotonin levels in WS with and without autism are needed to clarify the question.

Other laboratory studies have examined the various symptoms of WS. For example, Ingelfinger and Newburger (1991) examined the prevalence of renal difficulties in a sample of WS individuals. They found renal or renovascular abnormalities in approximately one-half of their sample. Daniels, Loggie, Schwartz, Strife, and Kaplan (1985) found that hypertension in patients with WS is often attributable to peripheral vascular abnormalities. These authors also speculated concerning the "unusually tortuous" retinal vessels of the patients described by Williams et al. (1961). More specifically, they stated that this may be related to systemic hypertension, which could reflect an intrinsic vascular disease.

Voit et al. (1991) investigated potential reasons for reported early fatigue (e.g., Morris, Demsey, Leonard, Dilts, & Blackburn, 1988). In patients with WS who complained of weakness and a tendency to fatigue, Voit et al. found an increase in lipid storage. They also found decreased muscle carnitine concentration in several of their patients.

Hotta et al. (1990) reported on the ocular symptoms of three patients with WS; they concluded that changes in retinal vessels and the iris (i.e., the lacy or stellate pattern) are not often seen in individuals with other diseases, and as such should be useful markers for WS. Holstromm, Almond, Temple, Taylor, and Baraitser (1990) photographed the eyes of a number of children with WS, and found that the stellate iris pattern was present in slightly more than half of this sample. They also noted that although the pattern is quite evident in light-eyed children (e.g., those with blue eyes), it is much more difficult to distinguish in individuals with darker-colored eyes.

Finally, as the last example of laboratory research on WS, Preus (1984b) developed an objective method for the diagnosis of WS. Beginning with phenotypic similarities among a group of patients, and using cluster analysis to identify subgroups within the sample, Preus developed a diagnostic index that had an expected accuracy rate of 99%. This index includes 50 characteristics typically associated with WS; individuals are classified according to the presence or absence of these symptoms. On the basis of the final score, an individual is classified as having WS or not having WS. Preus also discussed a 40 item diagnostic index for use with infants that had an expected accuracy rate of 98.8%. Greenberg (1989, 1990) has noted, however, that these indices are thought to disregard several important features of the disorder; they are also quite cumbersome to use, especially for those not trained in clinical genetics.

In conclusion, early research investigating WS focused on the hypercalcemic symptoms, whereas the role of calcitonin and CGRP in WS emerged only in later work. Several investigators reported impaired clearance of a calcium bolus (presumably as a result of the impaired production or release of calcitonin). The calcitonin and CGRP lead promises to be of great importance in the future research in WS, especially CGRP, which is much more active in the cardiovascular and central nervous systems.

POSTMORTEM FINDINGS

There is a paucity of postmortem studies of the central nervous systems of individuals with WS. However, steps are being taken to alter this situation. Much of the necropsy research has focused on nephrocalcinosis and other kidney-related symptoms (related to hypercalcemia). These studies tended to predominate in the 1950s, before the emphasis on the cardiovascular symptoms (in the 1960s).

For example, Joseph and Parrott (1958) reported the autopsy results of a 23-month-old female with severe idiopathic infantile hypercalcemia. According to these investigators, the infant's kidneys weighed 15 grams (as compared to a normal weight of 45 grams), and the heart weighed 75 grams (as compared to a normal weight of 55 grams). The left ventricle was also hypertrophied in a concentric manner. The brain was observed to be normal except for a complete blockage of the right lateral sinus by an antemortem clot. The skull was normal, with a slight thickening of the basiphenoid and the bone forming the upper wall of the orbits. When the results of this autopsy were discussed in relation to previously published reports, the investigators focused on the kidney related findings.

The 1960s was the decade when Williams et al. (1961) and Beuren et al. (1962, 1964) published their reports, as well as the decade when the cardiovascular symptoms of idiopathic infantile hypercalcemia became the focus of attention. For instance, Rashkind, Golinko, and Arcasoy (1961) reported the autopsy results of a 19-month-old male, focusing on the cardiac findings. The heart was found to be slightly heavier than normal, with biventricular hypertrophy, but no evidence of calcification in and around the heart. Rashkind et al. (1961) also reported that the parathyroids and thyroid were normal. Their summarizations of other studies were limited to discussions of the prevalence of hypercalcemia, heart and kidney findings, and blood pressure.

Hutchins, Mirvis, Mendelsohn, and Bulkley (1978) reported the autopsy findings of a 30-year-old man with idiopathic infantile hypercalcemia, beginning with the cardiac findings. Discussion of the central nervous system was limited to the mention of an intracerebral hemorrhage, apparently the result of a ruptured aneurysm in the right middle cerebral artery quite close to the site of the hemorrhage. There was marked cerebral edema and necrosis of the cerebellar tonsils. The parathyroids were normal at both gross and microscopic levels, but the parafollicular cells (C cells) within the thyroid gland evidenced increased calcitonin-containing cells. The investigators interpreted this last finding as possibly attributable to increased thyrocalcitonin activity, and speculated that this was related to persistent (rather than transient) hypercalcemia and calcitonin overproduction. Culler et al. (1985) provided a reinterpretation of these findings, suggesting that the difference in C cells was related to an abnormality in the production or release of calcitonin.

Most recently, Kawai et al. (1993) have reported their autopsy results of an adolescent with WS who died of an intracerebral hemorrhage. The results included a description of a "complicated cerebrovascular network," as well as narrowed vessels in the circle of Willis. It was also noted that this case was complicated by the presence of moyamoya disease, which is characterized by the narrowing of the large cerebral arteries and the enlargement of the smaller collateral arteries.

GENETICS

Early in the history of WS, researchers considered possible genetic causes. At the simplest level, Beuren et al. (1964) reported that there were 46 chromosomes, and that no chromosome seemed abnormal in structure or length.

Teams of researchers have also examined the possibility of a simple genetic defect resulting in the hypercalcemic symptoms of WS. Hitman, Garde, Daoud, Snodgrass, and Cohen (1989), for example, investigated 13 families that each had one member with WS. They found no indication of a major rearrangement of the short arm of chromosome 11 (where the calcitonin/CGRP gene is located). Russo et al. (1991) replicated this result. Russo et al. also focused on the white blood cell DNA of the children with WS, in an attempt to determine whether a mutation in the calcitonin/CGRP gene might be responsible for the hypercalcemic symptoms (a mutation that occurred after conception, and therefore would not be transmitted by either parent). Like Hitman et al. (1989), they found no evidence of a large deletion or rearrangement of the gene. These investigators summarized their findings by stating that mutations may exist within the calcitonin/CGRP gene itself, or that another locus may account for the deficient levels of calcitonin in WS.

Reports of monozygotic twins with WS have also fueled research and debate about the genetic basis of WS. Murphy, Greenberg, Wilson, Hughes, and DiLiberti (1990) examined two sets of monozygotic twins with WS and reviewed the information pertaining to two other sets previously reported. According to these investigators, concordance in monozygotic twins, and no reported cases of concordance in dizygotic twins, add support to the likelihood of a genetic contribution to the genesis of WS. For example, Hokama and Rogers (1991) described a case of WS in one dizygotic twin, and suggested that this provides evidence for an autosomal dominant mutation. Cortada, Taysi, and Hartmann (1980) reported a mother and daughter with WS, but this was later found to be a case of Noonan syndrome (Preus, 1984a). Also, Bellugi, Wang, and Jernigan (1994) reported a case of a father and son with WS, offering yet more support for a genetic basis for WS. Greenberg (1990) referred to a possible autosomal dominant pattern for the disorder, but emphasized that there is most likely a high frequency of new mutations.

Burn (1986), reviewing the literature on WS, described several genetic studies that have indicated a deletion of 15p, a balanced translocation of 9;17, and a deletion of the long arm of chromosome 4 (e.g., Jefferson, Burn, Gaunt, Hunter, & Davison, 1986). Burn also included a summary of a study by Grimm and Wesselhoeft (1980), who attempted to determine the possible links between familial supravalvular aortic stenosis and WS. These investigators concluded that these clinical phenotypes are on a continuum, representing the variable penetrance and expression of the same gene. With reference to the earlier findings reported by Burn (1986), the possibility that each of these cases of WS may have been a phenocopy is left open.

There have also been a number of recently published reports in which attempts have been made to discuss the gene or genes thought to be involved in WS. A number of chromosomes have been implicated, including chromosomes 1, 2, 4, and 11 (Tupler et al., 1992), chromosome 6 (Bzduch & Lukacova, 1989), chromosomes 13 and 18 (Colley, Thakker, Ward, & Donnai, 1992), and the 21st and X chromosomes (Telvi et al., 1992). It is the view of Murphy et al. (1990) that progress is being made in this area, and that there is reason for confidence that a locus for the syndrome will soon be identified.

Most recently, preliminary results of a research project examining the genetic basis of WS have been reported ("Gene for Williams Syndrome Discovered," 1994). In all cases studied in this project to date, a microdeletion on chromosome 7 has been found, involving an elastin gene. These investigators are of the opinion that this microdeletion may account for some of the features of the syndrome (e.g., the facial features, joint problems, heart disease, and hernias), but not for others (e.g., the hypercalcemia, learning difficulties, and behavioral problems).

DIFFERENTIAL DIAGNOSES

Although there appear to be relatively few disorders that are commonly confused with WS (Jones, 1988), Greenberg (1989) mentioned that "common" misdiagnoses include Coffin-Lowry and Noonan syndromes (e.g., Preus, 1984a). Greenberg (1989) also cautioned that the greater danger is that WS will go undiagnosed, with the symptoms being dismissed as individual symptoms, not as part of a syndrome. For example, the hypercalcemic symptoms can be dismissed as colic, and the cardiac symptoms as pure supravalvular aortic stenosis (i.e., this can be an isolated autosomal dominant condition; Schmidt et al., 1989).

The many developmental delays that are part of WS (e.g., delays in height, weight, head circumference, language, cognition), as well as the characteristic facies, combine to provide a picture of a child much younger than his or her chronological age, with the potential effect of masking the delays. In other words, a child with WS who is 4 years of age (and is characterized by these delays and facies) may appear to be between 2 and 3 years of age, and therefore not delayed in comparison to apparent age-mates. Greenberg (1989) also mentioned potential difficulties in diagnosing WS in African-American, Hispanic, and other ethnic groups whose members characteristically have eyes of a darker color, thus masking the common stellate iris pattern.

MEDICAL/NEUROLOGICAL FINDINGS

Numerous and varied medical complications are associated with WS, including those of a cardiovascular nature. For example, Williams et al. (1961) focused on supravalvular aortic stenosis, whereas Daniels et al. (1985) reported peripheral vascular anomalies; both of these can result in hypertension. Terhune, Buchino, and Rees (1985) related these cardiovascular anomalies to a significant increase in risk for myocardial infarcts.

Furthermore, von Arnim and Engel (1964) reported exaggerated tendon reflexes, a finding echoed in later publications (e.g., Bellugi, Bihrle, Jernigan, Trauner, & Doherty, 1990; Trauner, Bellugi, & Chase, 1989). Trauner et al. (1989) also reported a preponderance of dolichocephaly (i.e., a skull with a long anteroposterior diameter), as well as assorted other neurological abnormalities (e.g., gross and fine motor dysfunction, cerebellar dysfunction, and oral–motor dysfunction). According to Jones and Smith (1975), mild microcephaly is common in individuals with WS (approximately 25th centile), and their voices are often described as low and hoarse, or "metallic."

Dilts, Morris, and Leonard (1990) found that a sample of subjects with WS exhibited poor strength, balance, and coordination, as well as impaired motor planning. They also noted a tendency toward hypotonia in early childhood, and increasing hypertonia and joint limitations in older childhood. Furthermore, these problems appear to continue into adolescence (Kaplan, Kirschner, Watters, & Costa, 1989) and adulthood (Morris & Carey, 1990; Morris, Leonard, Dilts, & Demsey, 1990).

Dilts et al. (1990) also found that most of their subjects were described as hypersensitive, especially to auditory input. Klein, Armstrong, Greer, and Brown (1990), tabulating results from a questionnaire survey, found that 95% of their subjects exhibited hyperacusis (i.e., supersensitive auditory acuity). In the same study, they reported a prevalence rate of 61% for the presence of otitis media (i.e., inflammation of the middle ear) in patients with WS. The otitis media reported tended to be recurrent; this typically leads to hearing loss. This fact makes the extremely high prevalence of hyperacusis in these individuals even more intriguing.

A general growth deficiency is widely reported (Jones & Smith, 1975; Morris et al., 1988; Pankau, Partsch, Gosch, Oppermann, & Wessel, 1992). Pankau et al. (1992), presenting data on 165 patients, described an average birth length, followed by growth rates at the 3rd centile for males and females. This was followed by a growth spurt between the ages of 11 and 13 years of age for males (resulting in average height at the 10th centile), and a growth spurt between the ages of 10 and 12 years of age for females (resulting in average height at the 25th centile). After the growth spurt, both male and female growth rates slowed once again, with both sexes reaching an average final height at the 3rd centile. Morris et al. (1988) also reported a low-normal height (3rd centile) relative to the averaged height of the two parents.

Morris et al. (1988) have referred to a "catch-up pattern" in relation to the head size of individuals with WS. Their sample is described as having had microcephaly (approximately 2nd centile) during the first 4 years. After this point, there appeared to be a "catch-up period" to approximately the 25th centile. According to Morris et al., this pattern is not known in other microcephalic conditions, and thus could be of diagnostic significance.

In adults, lordosis and limitation of joint movement are common (Kaplan et al., 1989; Morris & Carey, 1990; Morris et al., 1988). Morris et al. (1988) also noted a tendency toward obesity in adults. Facial characteristics are thought to endure, with the most noticeable changes being the addition of a broad brow with a prominent supraorbital ridge and bitemporal narrowness (Morris et al., 1990).

To sum up, there is considerable evidence to suggest that WS is a disorder affecting multiple systems. More specifically, WS is characterized by a variety of medical and neurological sequelae, including growth deficiencies (coupled with a catch-up period for some aspects), joint limitations, and a wide range of neurological abnormalities.

DEVELOPMENTAL EFFECTS ON EXPRESSION OF WS

Overall, the literature on WS is quite circumscribed at this time. More-over, researchers in the past have tended to focus on the difficulties with, as well as the possible etiological roles played by, the endocrine and cardiovascular systems of these individuals. As a result, current knowledge about the effects of development or maturation on the expression of this disorder is somewhat limited. Also, with the exception of the recent past, very little emphasis seems to have been placed on the neuro-psychological profile of assets and weaknesses commonly associated with WS.

Morris et al. (1988) attempted to provide a natural history of the disorder and, in doing so, suggested that the facies (typically the group of characteristics most noticeable, and thus most linked to WS) is not readily identifiable at birth. Nevertheless, some parents retrospectively recalled that their affected children were "queer-looking" at birth (Joseph & Parrott, 1958). Morris et al. (1988) found that the mean age of diagnosis was 6.4 years, although for individuals under the age of 16, the mean age at diagnosis was 4.0 years. A series of infant photographs reviewed by the investigators showed that facial features of most children were discernible as WS in nature by age 4 months, and that the "obvious" WS facies was evident by age 18 months (Morris et al., 1988). On the basis of these findings, these authors concluded that the disorder could be diagnosed by the age of 2 years.

Morris et al. (1988) also reported that most parents found the first 12 months to be "miserable." More specifically, many of these parents reported that their children with WS had a number of problems relating to constipation, feeding, vomiting, and colic, all of which may have been associated with hypercalcemia. In addition, these parents indicated that much of their time was occupied with frequent visits to pediatricians and other specialists (mean of 9.6 visits to a pediatrician in the first 12 months, excluding well-child care).

Udwin et al. (1986) examined the age at diagnosis and the psychological profile of children with idiopathic infantile hypercalcemia. Their results were not statistically significant, but they did note a trend toward poorer performances on tasks involving visual–spatial and motor abilities for children diagnosed at a later chronological age. Significant effects were found in relation to total behavioral deviance on the Rutter teacher scale and to hyperactivity subscale scores on the Rutter teacher and parent scales. This suggests that earlier identification of the disorder may be beneficial in terms of the identification and attempted remediation of (nonverbal) cognitive and behavioral symptoms.

Morris et al. (1988) reported delays in weight gain and normal growth, as well as delays in reaching developmental milestones (walking independently on average at 21.0 months, talking on average at 21.6 months). These findings were supported by Lopez-Rangel, Maurice, McGillivray, and Friedman (1992) and by Thal, Bates, and Bellugi (1989). Morris et al. (1988) also suggested that these delays could contribute to delays in the diagnosis of WS (i.e., as noted above these children may look much younger than their actual chronological age and thus may not appear to be delayed).

Morris et al. (1988) reported academic difficulties by the first grade in virtually all of their sample of children with WS, as well as difficulties in adaptive skills and visual–motor integration (e.g., noting tentativeness for walking on slight grades or stairs). Joint limitations were also noted to begin in childhood.

Morris et al. (1990) noted that the deficits evident in childhood continued into adolescence and adulthood, and that in most cases they increased with increasing task demands, although Lopez-Rangel et al. (1992) reported that problems varied greatly from patient to patient. The cardiovascular and hypertensive symptoms also remained problematic, as did a host of other medical concerns discussed above (see Greenberg, 1990, and Morris et al., 1990). Joint limitations became more problematic, and kyphoscoliosis and lordosis were common. As a result of their deficits, the majority of these individuals were found to live with their parents or in an institutional setting into adulthood. These findings, especially those related to the social and behavioral limitations, are echoed by Udwin (1990; Bradley & Udwin, 1989).

In conclusion, the mean age at which a diagnosis of WS can be made appears to be decreasing, with some investigators concluding that the disorder can be diagnosed by 2 years of age. The age at diagnosis is of some importance, as the results of one study suggests a tendency for visual-spatial and motor abilities to be less developed in children receiving a later rather than an earlier diagnosis. Significant delays in weight gain and growth, and in reaching developmental milestones, are also frequently reported. Deficits in academic and adaptive functioning are evident in childhood and continue into adolescence and adulthood. Indeed, a majority of adults with WS have been found to be unable to live in an independent setting.

NEUROIMAGING AND NEUROPHYSIOLOGICAL FINDINGS

Concerning findings from neuroimaging studies, the Salk Institute for Biological Studies has recently published a number of articles and chapters delineating morphological differences between the brains of individuals with WS, and normal controls, and in some cases individuals with Down syndrome as well. The following reasons were given for using age- and IQ-matched Down syndrome controls in these studies: Down syndrome is relatively well characterized in the literature as being a syndrome with generalized "psychomotor retardation with language, motor, and cognitive skills all appropriate for . . . developmental levels" (Trauner et al., 1989, p. 166). This stands in contrast to individuals with WS, who exhibit similar levels of gross intelligence (i.e., Full Scale IQ of approximately 50), but a radically different overall neurocognitive profile.

An example of such a study is that conducted by Wang, Doherty, Hesselink, and Bellugi (1992), who examined magnetic resonance imaging scans of groups of normal controls, subjects with WS, and subjects with Down syndrome to search for discernible differences in the morphology of the corpus callosum. A thorough description of the procedure is provided by Wang, Doherty, et al. (1992). The results of this procedure demonstrated that the corpus callosum in subjects with WS, though smaller than that in control subjects, was similar in shape. In the subjects with Down syndrome, however, the corpus callosum was found to be shorter and therefore more circular than the corpus callosum in either of the other groups. Wang, Doherty, et al. (1992) also reported that, commensurate with the relative linguistic strengths of the group with WS versus the group with Down syndrome (the subjects with WS typically demonstrated better language skills), the width of the rostral fifth of the corpus callosum was more preserved in the subjects with WS.

Moreover, Jernigan and Bellugi (1990) described scans of these same subjects, focusing on cerebral and cerebellar size differences. Using a method developed by Jernigan, Press, and Hesselink (1990), they found that the average cerebral volumes of the groups with WS and Down syndrome were significantly smaller than that of the normal controls (approximately 80% for WS and 77% for Down syndrome; Bellugi et al., 1990). A trend toward brachycephaly was noted for the subjects with Down syndrome, and a trend toward dolichocephaly for the subjects with WS. In both cases, the smaller cerebral volume corroborates reports of microcephaly.

When the average cerebellar volumes of these groups of subjects were examined, a similar picture was noted for the subjects with Down syndrome, with the volume being 69% of the volume of the normal control subjects. The cerebellar volume of the subjects with WS was significantly larger than that of the subjects with Down syndrome, being approximately 99% of the cerebellar volume of the normal control subjects. This disparity resulted in a significant difference in the cerebellum-to-cerebrum ratio between the group with WS and the other two groups.

Jernigan and Bellugi (1990) then compared measurements of the cerebellar vermal areas of the normal controls and the subjects with WS. They found that the vermal areas I through V were low normal in the subjects with WS relative to the controls, but that the vermal areas VI and VII were significantly larger than those of the controls. The vermal ratio (I through V to VI and VII) was also larger in the subjects with WS than in the normal controls.

These results were then related to findings concerning the vermal areas of autistic subjects. The opposite pattern is characteristic of individuals with autism, that is, hypoplasia of VI and VII. Hypotheses were proffered concerning the significance of these findings with respect to the different neurobehavioral patterns (e.g., strength of language abilities in WS relative to autism; see also Wang, Hesselink, Jernigan, Doherty, & Bellugi, 1992).

As a base for these hypotheses, Jernigan and Bellugi (1990) drew on a theoretical paper by Leiner, Leiner, and Dow (1986), in which the latter authors argued that the role of the cerebellum may well extend beyond that which is typically depicted in neuroanatomy textbooks (i.e., control of motor function). More specifically, according to Leiner et al. (1986), phylogenetic and ontogenetic evidence suggests that the increased size of the neocerebellar vermi (VI and VII) in humans, relative to speechless primates, can be linked to the development of speech. Evidence from positron emission tomography scans during verbal processing tasks has further supported the involvement of areas VI and VII in linguistic tasks (Leiner, Leiner, & Dow, 1989). The results of other studies also suggest that it is likely that the cerebellum plays a contributory role in mental processes (e.g., Bracke-Tolkmitt et al., 1989).

Jernigan, Bellugi, Sowell, Doherty, and Hesselink (1993) further examined the scans of these subjects and reported that some frontal and temporal limbic structures (i.e., uncus, amygdala, hippocampus, and parahippocampal gyrus) appeared to be spared relative to other structures. These findings are interesting, given the (over)sociability of individuals with WS.

Bellugi and colleagues (U. Bellugi, personal communication, August 29, 1993; Bellugi et al., 1994) have recently reported the acquisition of a brain specimen from an individual with WS for analysis. Thus, additional information concerning the central nervous system of individuals with WS is forthcoming.

Finally, Neville, Mills, and Bellugi (1994) presented various findings utilizing an event related potential (ERP) technique. The subjects with WS and controls in this study were divided by age. Neville et al. first reported that the brainstem auditory ERPs were similar for WS and control subjects. Stimuli were then presented in the auditory and visual modalities. Although the ERPs produced by the visual stimuli in subjects with WS were similar to those of the controls, the ERPs produced by the auditory stimuli were less refractory (i.e., they demonstrated increased amplitude at fast repetition rates). These results were interpreted to suggest that the visual system of individuals with WS is similar to that of controls, but that the auditory system is different. On the basis of their ERP findings, the authors suggested that the initial stages of auditory language processing in individuals with WS are conducted by systems other than those used by normal individuals. They also hypothesized that the unusually high auditory sensitivity of individuals with WS may be responsible for the "island of sparing" (i.e., their linguistic skills).

It is important to note that Neville et al. (1994) suggested caution in the interpretation of these findings, due in part to the limited number of subjects with WS at each age. Nevertheless, these authors believe that these findings could be utilized in an attempt to develop further working hypotheses.

In conclusion, reports have indicated that the corpus callosum in individuals with WS is smaller than that in normal controls, although the rostral fifth is relatively preserved (in keeping with better-developed language skills in WS than in Down syndrome). The cerebral volume of individuals with WS was significantly lower than that of normal controls, but the cerebellar volume was virtually identical. Within the cerebellum, the neocerebellar vermi were significantly better developed in the subjects with WS, leading the investigators to speculate about the relation of this finding to preserved language functioning. Finally, the preliminary results of ERP studies, comparing individuals with WS with age-matched normal controls, suggests that the visual systems were similar in these two groups. However, the auditory systems of the subjects with WS were found to differ from those of the controls.

NEUROPSYCHOLOGICAL FINDINGS

Typical neuropsychological findings, when available, are presented in a manner similar to that of Rourke (1989). To begin with, there does not appear to be any pertinent information relating to tactile-perceptual skills.

Findings presented relating to the category of motor and psychomotor skills seem to indicate that, relative to controls matched for age, sex, and various measures of global intelligence or linguistic abilities, individuals with WS perform significantly more poorly on tests demanding more complex skills, but not on those requiring more basic skills. For example, MacDonald and Roy (1988) compared children with WS to a clinical control group matched for age, sex, and Peabody Picture Vocabulary Test—Revised (PPVT-R) Standard Score. They reported similar performances on the Finger-Tapping Test, but significantly poorer performances for the children with WS on the Grooved Pegboard Test. Bennett, LaVeck, and Sells (1978), using the McCarthy Scales of

Children's Abilities, noted that there were no differences between children with WS and controls selected on the basis of referral for problems of a developmental nature on several of the subscales (Verbal, Memory, and Quantitative subscales). However, these authors reported that the performance of the subjects with WS was significantly weaker than that of the controls on the Motor subscale, consisting of gross and fine motor tasks. Likewise, Pagon, Bennett, LaVeck, Stewart, and Johnson (1987), using the Bruininks–Oseretsky Test of Motor Proficiency (a measure of both gross and fine motor abilities), reported that individuals with WS performed at or below the 3rd centile.

There has been a considerable amount of research concerning the visual–spatial–organizational abilities of individuals with WS. For example, poor performances were noted on various measures of visual–spatial abilities by MacDonald and Roy (1988; Target Test) and by Bennett et al. (1978; Perceptual Performance subscale of the McCarthy Scales). Pagon et al. (1987) utilized the Developmental Test of Visual–Motor Integration, a task requiring the subject to copy designs that follow a "developmental gradient of difficulty" (Spreen & Strauss, 1991), and noted that each child with WS performed in a manner below his or her academic achievement age. Likewise, Crisco, Dobbs, and Mulhern (1988) found that the subjects with WS performed in a deficient manner on several subtests (e.g., Visual Memory, Visual Reception, Visual Closure) of the Illinois Test of Psycholinguistic Abilities.

Inferences can also be drawn concerning other results. For example, differences between Verbal and Performance scores on the Wechsler Intelligence Scale for Children—Revised (WISC-R) can be indicative of the relative levels of verbal and visual–spatial–organizational abilities in individuals with WS. The majority of studies of WS have reported the Full Scale IQ of subjects with WS to range from mildly to severely mentally retarded; thus, it would be expected that both Verbal and Performance Scale scores could be rather depressed. However, the verbal abilities of children with WS are often found to be significantly better developed than their performance abilities (e.g., Udwin et al., 1986; Udwin, Yule, & Martin, 1987), suggesting more poorly developed visual–spatial–organizational abilities.

Bellugi and colleagues have utilized a variety of instruments to investigate the visual–spatial abilities of individuals with WS. They have noted that the visual–spatial ability pattern of children with WS is somewhat fragmented. For example, Bellugi, Sabo, and Vaid (1988) reported that subjects with WS performed poorly on the Block Design subtest of the WISC-R, on the Developmental Test of Visual–Motor Integration, and on the Judgement of Line Orientation Test. These findings are in keeping with those outlined earlier (i.e., weak visual–spatial abilities in individuals with WS). However, further investigation revealed several "islands of sparing." For example, average performances were noted on several tests of facial recognition (Mooney Faces Test, Benton Test of Facial Recognition). The sparing of facial recognition is echoed by Udwin and Yule (1991).

When Bellugi, Marks, Bihrle, and Sabo (1988) requested subjects with WS to produce freehand drawings of a number of items (e.g., elephant, bicycle; Boston Diagnostic Aphasia Examination), another interesting discrepancy was noted. The verbal descriptions produced by the subjects as they "talked their way through" the task were quite rich and accurate. The actual drawings, however, were quite poor and particularly deficient in the integration of the parts.

The Delis Hierarchical Processing Task was used to provide another dimension of the visual–spatial abilities of individuals with WS (Bihrle, Bellugi, Delis, & Marks, 1989). This task requires the individual, after a delay, to reproduce a number of large stimuli, such as a letter of the alphabet or a simple shape (e.g., a square or triangle), that are comprised of small local forms (e.g., a letter of the alphabet or a simple shape). Examples of such stimuli would be a capital M made up of z's or a large triangle made up of small squares. Using children with Down syndrome as a control group, Bellugi and colleagues found striking differences between the performances of these two groups. Specifically, the subjects with WS tended to produce the local forms (e.g., the z's) to the exclusion of the global form (e.g., the M), whereas the subjects with Down syndrome tended to produce the global form (e.g., the M) to the exclusion of the local forms (e.g., the z's). These investigators state that this interesting pattern of visual–spatial abilities, with both deficits and islands of sparing, is uncommon enough that it may be a hallmark of WS, and perhaps could be of diagnostic use.

Nonverbal problem solving or concept formation is an important aspect of adequate neuropsychological functioning, but one that has not been intensively examined to date among individuals with WS. The findings of research conducted by Bellugi, Bihrle, Neville, Jernigan, and Doherty (1992) indicated that subjects with WS performed very poorly on the Category Test. Also, as mentioned earlier, individuals with WS performed poorly on the Block Design subtest of the WISC-R, a subtest that is thought to require some form of nonverbal problem-solving ability for successful completion.

Rote memory skills represent another area of neuropsychological functioning that is not widely discussed in the WS literature. When such information is presented, subjects with WS have tended to perform in the moderately to severely impaired range of functioning (e.g., Bennett et al., 1978; Crisco et al., 1988; MacDonald & Roy, 1988; Udwin & Yule, 1991).

Like many other domains of functioning, the area of adaptation to novel, complex situations has not been studied extensively in a formal sense. Some evidence seems to suggest that this may not be an area of strength for individuals with WS. For example, the information obtained from parent-completed measures indicated that children with WS were prone to overfriendliness with others, especially in the context of language and topics of conversation (e.g., Udwin & Yule, 1990, 1991). It would seem that whereas "normal" persons learn to tailor their conversation to situations, treating each individual as a new situation, subjects with WS do not appear to do so in many cases. That is, individuals with WS do not appear to modulate or adapt their behavior to a new person or situation. Moreover, at least one report has indicated that subjects with WS fail to demonstrate adaptation to a situation that is identical to one with which they are familiar. Bellugi et al. (1994) related the experience of requesting such a subject to tell and retell a story to the same individual. They noted that there was very little change in the method of recounting the story, despite the listener's having previously witnessed the telling of the tale.

Because reading, spelling, and arithmetic skills are sometimes associated with supposed precocious linguistic abilities in this population, these areas have been more carefully explored than other areas. Generally speaking, these skills tend to be poorly developed in subjects with WS, as assessed by a variety of measures of academic functioning (e.g., MacDonald & Roy, 1988; Pagon et al., 1987). For example, MacDonald and Roy (1988) reported that Wide Range Achievement Test—Revised (WRAT-R) scores for Reading, Spelling, and Arithmetic were significantly lower for children with WS than for their controls (e.g., between two and three standard deviations below the mean). Pagon et al. (1987) also reported extremely low scores for their subjects with WS on an achievement test (using the test norms as a reference group); furthermore, eight of the nine children with WS recorded their lowest or next-to-lowest score on the Mathematics subtest. Udwin et al. (1987) reported that approximately one-half of their sample with WS was unable to register a basal level of performance on tests of reading and spelling (Neale Analysis of Reading Ability, Vernon Graded Word Spelling Test). Of those subjects able to record at least a basal score (mean age of approximately 12 years), reading and spelling achievement levels were more than 4 years lower than one would expect.

Speech and language characteristics are significant dimensions of the unusual neuropsychological profile of WS; hence, there is a plethora of relevant information in this area. A number of researchers, for example, refer to the receptive language skills of individuals with WS. MacDonald and Roy (1988) reported a moderately impaired performance on the PPVT-R (approximately two standard deviations below the mean). Bellugi and colleagues, as part of a large, ongoing study of WS, reported receptive language scores lower than the chronological age of their subjects, but higher than the mental age of each subject. Arnold et al. (1985), comparing expressive and receptive language skills, found the former to be better developed than the latter in their sample of subjects with WS. They also found the receptive language skills of these subjects to be several years behind their chronological age.

Bellugi and her colleagues have undertaken a comprehensive exploration of the linguistic capabilities of individuals with WS, going beyond gross measures such as Verbal IQ (e.g., Bellugi, Marks, et al., 1988). Following the Piagetian theory that cognitive concepts need to be mastered before complex language is possible, these researchers administered a number of tasks that, if completed successfully, demonstrate mastery of the concrete operational stage of cognitive development. Bellugi, Marks, et al. (1988) found that adolescents with WS were routinely unable to succeed with tasks of seriation/insertion and conservation/reversibility. Therefore, it was with some surprise that they discovered areas of strength with certain linguistic devices. For example, these adolescents demonstrated a capacity to understand complex sentences (e.g., a reversible passive sentence—"The horse is chased by the man"), as well as to detect and correct grammatically incorrect sentences. Again, these linguistic tasks were performed at a much higher level than their performances on nonverbal cognitive tasks would lead one to expect.

Finally, Udwin and Yule (1990) attempted to determine the aptness of the "cocktail party speech" descriptor, and discovered that approximately 37% of a group of children with WS had this characteristic. Language samples from this subgroup of children were then compared with samples from children with WS who did not display cocktail party speech. The former subgroup (i.e., the children with cocktail party speech) produced a significantly greater number of utterances, intelligible utterances, and utterances containing clichés, idioms, social (filler) phrases, and irrelevant personal experiences. However, Udwin and Yule (1990) concluded that the "content of their speech is by no means meaningless, repetitive, or superficial, since a significantly greater proportion of their speech also serves complex communicative purposes" (p. 111).

Udwin and Yule (1990) went on to compare the language of a group of 20 children with WS to that of controls matched for age, sex, social class, and Verbal IQ. The group with WS again produced significantly more utterances containing idioms and social phrases. Udwin and Yule also noted that 70% of this group displayed an "overfamiliar" manner with the experimenter, relative to only 15% of the control group.

These authors concluded that hyperverbal speech is not characteristic of all individuals with WS, but is characteristic of some. When WS children were compared to matched controls, few differences were noted, the main ones involving social aspects of language (e.g., overfamiliarity, greater use of adult vocabulary, and social phrases) that contributed to an overall sense of a "glib" or facile use of language. Udwin and Yule (1990) posited that these vocabulary and stylistic differences, in conjunction with severe deficits in other areas of functioning, combine to produce the illusion of an "unusual command of language" (von Arnim & Engel, 1964).

Finally, socioemotional functioning is an area in which individuals with WS tend to experience difficulties, as shown by parent and teacher responses on questionnaires and by anecdotal evidence. Pagon et al. (1987) asked the parents of nine children with WS (ages 10–20) to complete the Achenbach Child Behavior Checklist. Common behavioral problems (i.e., those endorsed by seven or more of nine parents) involved immaturity, inattentiveness, clumsiness, talkativeness, and a tendency to be argumentative.

Udwin and colleagues have routinely assessed the socioemotional functioning of the children with WS they have studied (Arnold et al., 1985; Udwin & Yule, 1991; Udwin et al., 1986, 1987). On the Rutter parent and teacher Scales, 83% of the children exceeded the cutoff score for disturbed behavior, either at school, at home, or in both venues (Arnold et al., 1985). These authors also reported a prevalence rate of 87% for hyperactivity at home and/or school. In addition, both parents and teachers described these children as solitary, and parents were of the opinion that their children with WS were not liked by other children.

Udwin and Yule (1991), comparing children with WS to controls matched on age, sex, social class, and Verbal IQ, found that the children with WS had significantly higher Deviant scores and total raw scores on the Rutter teacher scale. Udwin et al. (1987) examined the items constituting the Neurotic subscale on both Rutter scales, and found a significant difference between groups: A greater number of children with WS were described as being worried, fussy, tearful, and complaining of aches and pains.

Udwin (1990) described the findings of a survey of the caretakers of 119 adults with WS, and suggested that the difficulties noticed in childhood remained and, indeed, were exacerbated with increasing age. With respect to social interactions and social judgment, 67% of these caretakers reported that these areas remained problematic for the adults with WS. For example, these individuals were found to have difficulties making and keeping friends of their own age. Indeed, even as adults they reportedly preferred the company of those older than themselves. Udwin reported that only 14% of these adults were currently in a relationship, that only one (0.8%) was married, and that only 8.5% were capable of managing their own leisure time. In excess of 60% of the caregivers reported continued restlessness and inattention, as well as worrying, fearfulness, irritability, and attention-seeking behavior. In addition, more than 70% reported that a major concern was the safety of the individuals with WS, because they showed a tendency toward overfriendliness and a lack of restraint in communications with others (e.g., strangers).

To sum up, individuals with WS have been found to perform better on measures of simple motor functioning than on tasks of complex motor functioning. Poor performances have also been noted on a variety of tasks measuring the visual–spatial–organizational abilities of these subjects in the context of preserved facial recognition. Although few studies have investigated nonverbal problem solving or concept formation and rote memory functioning in individuals with WS, some evidence suggests that these abilities are poorly developed. Information concerning the ability of these individuals to adapt to novel, complex situations has come from anecdotal reports for the most part; these reports are suggestive of a deficiency in this area of functioning. All aspects of academic achievement are very weak, with scores on measures of arithmetic ability consistently reported as being lower than those on measures of reading and spelling ability. Speech and language characteristics have been the target of many investigations. Although both receptive and expressive language skills are below what would be expected relative to mental age, expressive language has been reported as being the better developed of the two. Hyperverbal speech has been determined to be a characteristic of some individuals with WS, with noticeable characteristics including various social aspects of language. Finally, socioemotional difficulties have been consistently reported among these individuals in both home and school settings. There is evidence to suggest that these difficulties continue throughout adolescence and into adulthood.

RELATIONSHIP TO THE WHITE MATTER MODEL

In comparing the neuropsychological profile of WS with that of the Nonverbal Learning Disabilities (NLD) syndrome and with the white matter model, it is of paramount importance to focus on the *pattern* of assets and deficits, rather than simply the level of functioning in each skill/ability domain. With this caveat in mind, we turn to a discussion of the findings in infancy and childhood.

Rourke (1987, 1988, 1989) has provided a list of characteristics or abilities in which children with the NLD syndrome are expected to be deficient, several of which are applicable to children with WS. For example, the delayed achievement of developmental milestones predicted by Rourke is supported by the findings of Morris et al. (1988; average age of walking independently, 21.0 months; average age of talking, 21.6 months) and Thal et al. (1989; two children, ages 23 and 66 months, at the one-word stage of language). Dilts et al. (1990), in a paper defining a behavioral phenotype for WS, reported that many parents described their WS children as very cautious while traversing slopes, stairs, or uneven surfaces, as well as unable to use common tools (e.g., a kitchen knife for spreading or cutting); these accounts corroborate Rourke's prediction of noticeable psychomotor clumsiness in children with NLD (Pagon et al., 1987; see Strang & Rourke, 1985, p. 314, and Anonymous, 1985, for delay of specific psychomotor skills such as tying shoes). Dilts et al. (1990) also noted the similarity of this phenotype to the "nonverbal–perceptual–organizational–output disability" described by Strang and Rourke (1985).

Rourke (1987, 1989) has also postulated the delayed acquisition of self-help skills, an early and consistent finding in children with WS. Arnold et al. (1985) described their sample of 42 children (mean age of 10 years, 4 months) as deficient in independent skills, and thus overly dependent on adults for assistance. In addition to these difficulties, the NLD model predicts significant complications with peer interactions (Rourke, 1982; Rourke & Strang, 1983); this is strongly and consistently supported in the work of Udwin and colleagues (Arnold et al., 1985; Udwin & Yule, 1991; Udwin et al., 1986, 1987).

Udwin and Yule (1990) supported previous anecdotal and parental reports by finding that the language of children with WS tends to be of the cocktail party variety (37% of their sample), making up in verbosity for what it seems to lack in content. Bellugi et al. (1992) also mentioned the tendency of subjects with WS to provide extremely lengthy, somewhat anecdotal responses to items on the Vocabulary subtest of the WISC-R. Moreover, according to Udwin and Yule (1990), these children tended to speak rather formally, with noticeable adult intonations. This observation, in conjunction with the often-noted tendency to be overfriendly with others, especially adults (e.g., Udwin & Yule, 1990), is also similar to manifestations of the NLD syndrome (e.g., see Sparrow, 1991).

There is evidence to suggest that the pattern of abilities and weaknesses observed in individuals with NLD persists into adolescence and adulthood (Bieliauskas, 1991; DeLuca, 1991; Rourke & Fisk, 1992; Rourke, Young, Strang, & Russell, 1986). This is consistent with reports in the WS literature; indeed, it is argued that the deficits are thought to become more apparent and more debilitating with age, especially in relation to situations where judgment and reasoning are required (Morris et al. 1990; Udwin, 1990). Older persons with WS typically live with parents or in an institutional setting, and are remarkably deficient in adaptive living skills (Bradley & Udwin, 1989; Udwin, 1990).

Rourke's (1989) observation of the paucity of formal operational thought with respect to the NLD syndrome is certainly supported by the work of Bellugi (Bellugi, Marks, et al., 1988). These authors demonstrated that three adolescents with WS had yet to master basic tasks associated with the concrete operational stage of cognitive development.

Rourke (1989) has provided a complete discussion of the neuropsy-chological assets and deficits of an individual exhibiting the NLD syndrome, many of which are similar to the assets and deficits of an individual with WS. For example, the verbal skills of children with WS generally tend to be somewhat better developed than their nonverbal or performance skills (Udwin et al., 1987). Their relative facility with rote material (Udwin et al., 1987) and verbal memory (Bennett et al., 1978; Udwin & Yule, 1991) has also been noted. More specific language abilities have been demonstrated to be well developed, at least in relation to the overall pattern of abilities and deficits (e.g., verbal reception—Bellugi et al., 1990; verbal associations—Bellugi et al., 1990; Udwin et al., 1987; verbal output—Udwin & Yule, 1990). Pagon et al. (1987) have reported that the performance of subjects with WS on reading subtests of academic achievement tests was better than their performance on arithmetic subtests, a major prediction in the NLD model. Udwin et al. (1987) also reported early graphomotor difficulties in children with WS, consistent with expectations of the NLD model.

Other deficits that appear to be present in children with NLD and WS include deficits in visual perception (Bihrle et al., 1989; MacDonald & Roy, 1988), as well as visual attention (Crisco et al., 1988). Visual or visual–spatial memory is also an area of weakness for children with WS (Crisco et al., 1988; Udwin & Yule, 1991), although the latter authors found that tasks that are easily coded in a verbal manner are better handled than those that do not lend themselves to this—another prediction of Rourke (1989). Bellugi et al. (1992) noted the tendency of subjects with WS to verbalize visual–spatial tasks spontaneously (e.g., drawing tasks), although the final result remained remarkably poor. Complex psychomotor skills (Bennett et al., 1978; MacDonald & Roy, 1988) and concept formation are also deficient (Bellugi et al., 1992) in individuals with WS.

Bellugi et al. (1990) described subjects with WS as having difficulty with oral–motor praxis, and Udwin et al. (1987) reported that these individuals often demonstrate a good use of phonology. Both of these findings are in keeping with the predictions of the NLD model.

In contrast to the profile of children with NLD, children with WS seem to possess adequate abilities in the area of prosody (Reilly, Klima, & Bellugi, 1991). Reilly et al. (1991) also reported that many other storytelling techniques were employed by children with WS, including voice modulation, character speech (i.e., providing speech for characters in a wordless story), and describing the internal states of characters. However, it is important to bear in mind that the tendency (or need?) to use such storytelling techniques as voice modulation remained abnormally high, suggesting a lack of adaptation on the part of the children with WS. Also, these children may simply have been mimicking the prosody of others, rather than using prosody to convey meaning.

Finally, in relation to socioemotional or adaptational abilities, it is well documented that children with WS have deficiencies in social competence (Arnold et al., 1985; Udwin et al., 1986, 1987), in emotional stability (Arnold et al., 1985), and in making and keeping friends (Dilts et al. 1990). These children have also been described by both teachers and parents as hyperactive, immature, clumsy, and talkative (Arnold et al., 1985; Udwin et al., 1986, 1987; Udwin & Yule, 1991).

Another link to the NLD/white matter model relates directly to the findings of Wang and colleagues concerning the corpus callosum in subjects with WS. It will be recalled that there was a pattern of irregularity relative to normal controls, with the callosum in subjects with WS being smaller than that of the controls but similarly shaped. The relative smallness suggests some compromising of this crucial bridge between the hemispheres.

Rourke posits a link between these manifestations and deficient functioning of right-hemisphere systems (Rourke, 1982, 1989). A good deal of information exists concerning differential deficits of left-hemisphere-damaged and right-hemisphere-damaged patients, some of which suggests that the visual–spatial deficits of individuals with WS are similar to those of right-hemisphere-damaged patients. For example, the performance of children with WS on the Delis Hierarchical Processing Task was very similar to that of patients with damaged right hemispheres (Delis, Kiefner, & Fridlund, 1988; Delis, Kramer, & Kiefner, 1988; Delis, Robertson, & Efron, 1986). Both groups (children with WS and right-hemisphere-damaged patients) exhibited a tendency to focus on the local forms (e.g., the small z's making up the global form of an M) to the exclusion of the global form.

Evidence presented by Stiles-Davis (1988) and Stiles and Nass (1989) concerning the pattern of errors on visual–spatial tasks (e.g., the Block Design subtest of the WISC-R) again demonstrated the similarities between the performance of children with WS and individuals with right-hemisphere damage. Both groups of patients in this case demonstrated an inability to maintain the gestalt of the design (e.g., the 2×2 matrix), similar to their performances on the Delis Hierarchical Processing Task. Stiles-Davis (1988) also found that the drawings of children with a right-hemisphere injury lacked "cohesion," and that the parts were "scattered around the page" instead of being "configured into a coherent whole" (p. 262). This description is very similar to those of the drawings of children with WS, reported by Bellugi and her colleagues (e.g., Bellugi et al., 1990).

In conclusion, when one takes the absolute level of functioning of these individuals into consideration and focuses on the pattern of assets and deficits, there is strong evidence for relating the NLD syndrome to WS. This evidence includes various developmental delays, seemingly precocious language abilities, verbal abilities that are better developed than visual–spatial abilities, and deficiencies in social functioning. In addition, the major connective structure (i.e., band of white matter) between the cerebral hemispheres, the corpus callosum, has been documented as being smaller than that of matched controls. Finally, the performance of individuals with WS on several tasks of visual-spatial functioning has been reported as very similar to the performances of individuals with right-hemisphere damage.

TREATMENT

With the plethora of medical complications associated with WS, one can imagine that potential treatment regimens are quite numerous. When one recalls that the initial discovery of the disorder was linked to hypercalcemia, it should come as no surprise that early treatment focused on controlling the dietary intake of vitamin D and calcium. Fraser et al. (1966) provided readers with several dietary options, including milk with the calcium removed, a milk substitute (e.g., soybean milk), and a strained lamb mixture to insure adequate protein intake without increasing dietary vitamin D or calcium. Meyerson and Frank (1987), however, cautioned against using a soft-food diet for extended periods of time, because of the possibility of further delaying prespeech feeding skills. Furthermore, they recommended that if a soft-food diet is followed, it should be supplemented with a training program that emphasizes the development of sucking, swallowing, and chewing, to assist in the continued evolution of these skills.

Morris et al. (1990) characterized WS as a progressive multisystem disorder and followed this with a host of recommendations concerning treatment. Among other things, visual acuity and ophthalmological evaluations were recommended, as was preventive dentistry to minimize the risk of severe malocclusion. Both cardiac difficulties and hypertension are persistent, and consequently must be monitored. Because of the commonality of peripheral stenoses, it is recommended that blood pressure be taken in all four limbs annually. Hypertension, if present and severe enough, would suggest the use of hypertensive medications. Gastrointestinal complaints should receive prompt attention, especially if complaints of constipation are consistent (Bradley & Udwin, 1989). Renal functions should also be monitored quite closely, as nephrocalcinosis and renal failure are quite common. Finally, in relation to hypercalcemia, there is a tendency to develop ectopic calcium deposits as well as secondary hyperparathyroidism, resulting in the need for dietary restrictions and possibly thyroid medication. Greenberg (1990), summarizing many of these recommendations, has presented a table of suggested assessments, as well as suggested frequencies of assessment for infancy, childhood, and adolescence/adulthood.

As for psychological treatments, Morris et al. (1988) have suggested that psychoeducational testing be routinely completed, to insure the appropriate educational intervention. Udwin et al. (1987) recommended that remediation be based on the individual's strengths, a position echoed by Dilts et al. (1990). Udwin et al. (1987) also suggested that specific remediation may be necessary in the areas of visual perception, spatial orientation, numeracy, pencil control, and attending ability. It may be possible to use the superior spoken language of the individual with WS by encouraging "talking-through" exercises. Training that utilizes computers, rather than paper-and-pencil exercises, is also an option. In teaching the child with WS to read, it will probably be beneficial to use a phonics approach, given that this will permit the building of skills on a strength (spoken language), as opposed to reading approaches that emphasize visual skills.

Meyerson and Frank (1987) encouraged training children with WS in the appropriate use of language. This could include an emphasis on the metapragmatic uses of language (e.g., the importance of varying one's linguistic style with different listeners, the maintenance of topics, and the initiation of new topics). In addition, these authors advised that one should include a focus on the development of the skills necessary to make concise and accurate responses, as well as turn taking. Because individuals with WS tend to enunciate quite clearly, direct articulation therapy is typically not necessary.

Many researchers also address the needs of parents/caregivers of individuals with WS. For example, Meyerson and Frank (1987) encouraged caregivers to consider attempting to identify those stimuli to which their children with WS appear to be hypersensitive (i.e., hyperacusis), and to make efforts to delay the performance of noisy activities (e.g., vacuuming, cutting the lawn) until these children are not present. Alternatively, filtered ear protection is presented as an option, as is the selection of quieter home appliances (Klein et al., 1990). Caregivers are also encouraged to be vigilant for hearing loss due to otitis media; the effects of conductive hearing loss on language development can be severe, especially in children with below-average psychometric intelligence.

Tomc, Williamson, and Pauli (1990) warn of the potentially detrimental effects of early descriptions of individuals with WS. Tomc et al. (1990) reported the findings of a survey study indicating that children with WS are much more likely to be viewed as "difficult," among other things, and that anticipatory parental counseling should attempt to lessen the incongruity between the course of the disorder and the early descriptions of temperament. Examples of early descriptions of these children include those provided by von Arnim and Engel (1964), who described them as "polite, open and gentle" (p. 367), and Beuren et al. (1962), who reported that "all have the same kind of friendly nature—they love everyone, are loved by everyone, and are very charming" (p. 1235).

Udwin (1990) provided many insights for treatment based on the survey of the caregivers of 119 adults with WS (ages 16 to 38). For example, establishing closer links with available social services is advised, including the use of respite care. Given the long-term prospects for individuals with WS, planning for occupational settings should be considered well in advance of their leaving school, and should take into consideration the unique neuropsychological profile of these individuals. Also, because one of the deficiencies of individuals with WS is in the area of judgment of social situations (e.g., overfriendliness, especially with strangers), Udwin advised that related intervention occur early, to prevent (as much as possible) difficulties and dangers in later childhood, adolescence, and adulthood.

Finally, a comment recalling the potential difficulties involved with the correct and timely diagnosis of WS is in order. Given the developmental and medical manifestations of WS, it seems reasonable to implement a treatment program, utilizing the recommendations above, as well as those suggested by Rourke (see the Appendix to this volume), for those presenting with these manifestations. Indeed, such procedures should be invoked on the basis of the developmental and medical manifestations of this disorder alone, regardless of the current diagnosis.

REFERENCES

Anonymous. (1985). Case history of a child with Williams syndrome. *Pediatrics*, *75*, 962–968.

Arnold, R., Yule, W., & Martin, N. (1985). The psychological characteristics of infantile hypercalcaemia: A preliminary investigation. *Developmental Medicine and Child Neurology*, *27*, 49–59.

August, G. J., & Realmuto, G. M. (1989). Williams syndrome: Serotonin's association with developmental disabilities. *Journal of Autism and Developmental Disorders*, *19*, 137–141.

Bellugi, U., Bihrle, A., Jernigan, T., Trauner, D., & Doherty, S. (1990). Neuropsychological, neurological, and neuroanatomical profile of Williams syndrome. *American Journal of Medical Genetics* (Suppl. 6), 115–125.

Bellugi, U., Bihrle, A., Neville, H., Jernigan, T., & Doherty, S. (1992). Language, cognition, and brain organization in a neurodevelopmental disorder. In M. Gunnar & C. Nelson (Eds.), *Developmental behavioral neuroscience* (pp. 201–232). Hillsdale, NJ: Erlbaum.

Bellugi, U., Marks, S., Bihrle, A., & Sabo, H. (1988). Dissociation between language and cognitive functions in Williams syndrome. In D. Bishop & K. Mogford (Eds.), *Language development in exceptional circumstances* (pp. 177–189). London: Churchill Livingstone.

Bellugi, U., Sabo, H., & Vaid, J. (1988). Spatial deficits in children with Williams syndrome. In J. Stiles-Davis, M. Kritchevshy, & U. Bellugi (Eds.), *Spatial cognition: Brain bases and development* (pp. 273–298). Hillsdale, NJ: Erlbaum.

Bellugi, U., Wang, P., & Jernigan, T. (1994). Williams syndrome: An unusual neuropsychological profile. In S. Broman & J. Grafman (Eds.), *Atypical cognitive deficits in developmental disorders: Implications for brain function* (pp. 23–56). Hillsdale, NJ: Erlbaum.

Bennett, F. C., LaVeck, B., & Sells, C. J. (1978). The Williams elfin facies syndrome: The psychological profile as an aid in syndrome identification. *Pediatrics, 61,* 303–306.

Beuren, A. J., Apitz, J., & Harmjanz, D. (1962). Supravalvular aortic stenosis in association with mental retardation and a certain facial appearance. *Circulation, 26,* 1235–1240.

Beuren, A. J., Schulze, C., Eberle, P., Harmjanz, D., & Apitz, J. (1964). The syndrome of supravalvular aortic stenosis, peripheral pulmonary stenosis, mental retardation and similar facial appearance. *American Journal of Cardiology, 13,* 471–483.

Bieliauskas, L. A. (1991). Case studies of adults with nonverbal learning disabilities. In B. P. Rourke (Ed.), *Neuropsychological validation of learning disability subtypes* (pp. 370–376). New York: Guilford Press.

Bihrle, A. M., Bellugi, U., Delis, D., & Marks, S. (1989). Seeing either the forest or the trees: Dissociation in visuospatial processing. *Brain and Cognition, 11,* 37–49.

Black, J. A., & Bonham Carter, R. E. (1963). Association between aortic stenosis and cases of severe infantile hypercalcaemia. *Lancet, ii,* 745–749.

Bracke-Tolkmitt, R., Linden, A., Canavan, A. G. M., Rockstroh, B., Scholz, E., Wessel, K., & Diener, H.-C. (1989). The cerebellum contributes to mental skills. *Behavioral Neuroscience, 103,* 442–446.

Bradley, E. A., & Udwin, O. (1989). Williams' syndrome in adulthood: A case study focusing on psychological and psychiatric aspects. *Journal of Mental Deficiency Research, 33,* 175–184.

Burn, J. (1986). Williams syndrome. *Journal of Medical Genetics, 23,* 389–395.

Bzduch, V., & Lukacova, M. (1989). Interstitial deletion of the long arm of chromosome 6(q22.2q23) in a boy with phenotypic features of Williams syndrome. *Clinical Genetics, 35,* 230–231.

Colley, A., Thakker, Y., Ward, H., & Donnai, D. (1992). Unbalanced 13;18 translocation and Williams syndrome. *Journal of Medical Genetics, 29,* 63–65.

Cortada, X., Taysi, K., & Hartmann, A. F. (1980). Familial Williams syndrome. *Clinical Genetics, 18,* 173–176.

Crisco, J. J., Dobbs, J. M., & Mulhern, R. K. (1988). Cognitive processing of children with Williams syndrome. *Developmental Medicine and Child Neurology, 30,* 650–656.

Culler, F. L., Jones, K. L., & Deftos, L. J. (1985). Impaired calcitonin secretion in patients with Williams syndrome. *Journal of Pediatrics, 107,* 720–723.

Daniels, S. R., Loggie, J. M. H., Schwartz, D. C., Strife, J. L., & Kaplan, S. (1985). Systemic hypertension secondary to peripheral vascular anomalies in patients with Williams syndrome. *Journal of Pediatrics, 106,* 249–251.

Delis, D. C., Kiefner, M. G., & Fridlund, A. J. (1988). Visuospatial dysfunction following unilateral brain damage: Dissociations in hierarchical and hemispatial analysis. *Journal of Clinical and Experimental Neuropsychology, 10,* 421–431.

Delis, D. C., Kramer, J. H., & Kiefner, M. G. (1988). Visuospatial functioning before and after commissurotomy: Disconnection in hierarchical processing. *Archives of Neurology, 45,* 462–465.

Delis, D. C., Robertson, L. C., & Efron, R. (1986). Hemispheric specialization of memory for visual hierarchical stimuli. *Neuropsychologia, 24,* 205–214.

DeLuca, J. W. (1991). Case studies of adolescents with nonverbal learning disabilities. In B. P. Rourke (Ed.), *Neuropsychological validation of learning disability subtypes* (pp. 356–369). New York: Guilford Press.

Dilts, C. V., Morris, C. A., & Leonard, C. O. (1990). Hypothesis for development of a behavioral phenotype in Williams syndrome. *American Journal of Medical Genetics* (Suppl. 6), 126–131.

Fanconi, G., Girardet, P., Schlesinger, B., Butler, N., & Black, J. A. (1952). Chronische hypercalcaemie, kominiert mit osteosklerose, hyperasotaemie, minderwuchs and kongenitalen missbildungen. *Helvetica Paediatrica Acta, 7,* 314–334.

Forbes, G. B., Bryson, M. F., Manning, J., Amirhakimi, G. H., & Reina, J. C. (1972). Impaired calcium homeostasis in the infantile hypercalcemic syndrome. *Acta Paediatrica Scandinavica, 61,* 305–309.

Fraser, D., Kidd, B. S. L., Kooh, S. W., & Paunier, L. (1966). A new look at infantile hypercalcemia. *Pediatric Clinics of North America, 13,* 503–525.

Friedman, W. F., & Roberts, W. C. (1966). Vitamin D and the supravalvular aortic stenosis syndrome: The transplacental effects of vitamin D on the aorta of the rabbit. *Circulation, 34,* 77–86.

Garcia, R. E., Friedman, W. F., Kaback, M. M., & Rowe, R. D. (1964). Idiopathic hypercalcemia and supravalvular aortic stenosis: Documentation of a new syndrome. *New England Journal of Medicine, 271,* 117–120.

Gene for Williams syndrome discovered. (1994, Spring). *Canadian Association for Williams Syndrome Newsletter,* pp. 1–3.

Greenberg, F. (1989). Williams syndrome. *Pediatrics, 84,* 922–923.

Greenberg, F. (1990). Williams syndrome professional symposium. *American Journal of Medical Genetics* (Suppl. 6), 85–88.

Grimm, T., & Wesselhoeft, H. (1980). The genetic aspects of Williams-Beuren syndrome and the isolated form of the supravalvular aortic stenosis: Investigation of 128 families. *Zeitschrift für Kardiologie, 69,* 168–172.

Hitman, G. A., Garde, L., Daoud, W., Snodgrass, G. J. A. I., & Cohen, R. D. (1989). The calcitonin–CGRP gene in the infantile hypercalcaemia/Williams–Beuren syndrome. *Journal of Medical Genetics, 26,* 609–613.

Hokama, T., & Rogers, J. G. (1991). Williams syndrome in one dizygotic twin. *Acta Paediatrica Japonica, 33,* 678–680.

Holstromm, G., Almond, G., Temple, K., Taylor, D., & Baraitser, M. (1990). The iris in Williams syndrome. *Archives of Disease in Childhood, 65,* 987–989.

Hotta, Y., Kishishita, H., Wakita, M., Inagaki, Y., Momose, T., & Kato, K. (1990). Ocular findings of Williams syndrome. *Acta Paediatrica Scandinavica, 79,* 869–870.

Hutchins, G. M., Mirvis, S. E., Mendelsohn, G., & Bulkley, B. H. (1978). Supravalvular aortic stenosis with parafollicular cell (C-cell) hyperplasia. *American Journal of Medicine, 64,* 967–973.

Ingelfinger, J. R., & Newburger, J. W. (1991). Spectrum of renal anomalies in patients with Williams syndrome. *Journal of Pediatrics, 119,* 771–773.

Jefferson, R. D., Burn, J., Gaunt, K. L., Hunter, S., & Davison, E. V. (1986). A terminal deletion of the long arm of chromosome 4[46,XX,del(4)(q33)] in an infant with phenotypic features of Williams syndrome. *Journal of Medical Genetics, 23,* 474–480.

Jernigan, T. L., & Bellugi, U. (1990). Anomalous brain morphology on magnetic resonance images in Williams syndrome and Down syndrome. *Archives of Neurology, 47,* 529–533.

Jernigan, T. L., Bellugi, U., Sowell, E., Doherty, S., & Hesselink, J. R. (1993). Cerebral morphologic distinctions between Williams and Down syndromes. *Archives of Neurology, 50,* 186–191.

Jernigan, T. L., Press, G. A., & Hesselink, J. R. (1990). Methods for measuring brain morphologic features on magnetic resonance images. *Archives of Neurology, 47,* 27–32.

Jones, K. L. (1988). *Smith's recognizable patterns of human malformation* (4th ed.). Philadelphia: W. B. Saunders.

Jones, K. L. (1990). Williams syndrome: An historical perspective of its evolution, natural history, and etiology. *American Journal of Medical Genetics* (Suppl. 6), 89–96.

Jones, K. L., & Smith, D. W. (1975). The Williams elfin facies syndrome: A new perspective. *Journal of Pediatrics, 86,* 718–723.

Joseph, M. C., & Parrott, D. (1958). Severe infantile hypercalcaemia with special reference to the facies. *Archives of Disease in Childhood, 33,* 385–395.

Kaplan, P., Kirschner, M., Watters, G., & Costa, M. T. (1989). Contractures in patients with Williams syndrome. *Pediatrics, 84,* 895–899.

Kawai, M., Nishikawa, T., Tanaka, M., Ando, A., Kasajima, T., Higa, T., Tanikawa, T., Kagawa, M., & Momma, K. (1993). An autopsied case of Williams syndrome complicated by moyamoya disease. *Acta Paediatrica Japonica— Overseas Edition, 35,* 63–67.

Klein, A. J., Armstrong, B. L., Greer, M. K., & Brown, F. R. (1990). Hyperacusis and otitis media in individuals with Williams syndrome. *Journal of Speech and Hearing Disorders, 55,* 339–344.

Leiner, H. C., Leiner, A. L., & Dow, R. S. (1986). Does the cerebellum contribute to mental skills? *Behavioral Neuroscience, 100,* 443–454.

Leiner, H. C., Leiner, A. L., & Dow, R. S. (1989). Reappraising the cerebellum: What does the hindbrain contribute to the forebrain? *Behavioral Neuroscience, 103,* 998–1008.

Lightwood, R. (1952). Idiopathic hypercalcaemia in infants with failure to thrive. *Archives of Disease in Childhood, 27,* 302–303.

Lopez-Rangel, E., Maurice, M., McGillivray, B., & Friedman, J. M. (1992). Williams syndrome in adults. *American Journal of Medical Genetics, 44,* 720–729.

Lowe, K. G., Henderson, J. L., Park, W. W., & McGreal, D. A. (1954). The idiopathic hypercalcaemic syndromes of infancy. *Lancet, ii,* 101–110.

MacDonald, G. W., & Roy, D. L. (1988). Williams syndrome: A neuropsychological profile. *Journal of Clinical and Experimental Neuropsychology, 10*, 125–131.

Martin, N. D. T., Snodgrass, G. J. A. I., & Cohen, R. D. (1984). Idiopathic infantile hypercalcaemia—a continuing enigma. *Archives of Disease in Childhood, 59*, 605–613.

Meyerson, M. D., & Frank, R. A. (1987). Language, speech and hearing in Williams syndrome: Intervention approaches and research needs. *Developmental Medicine and Child Neurology, 29*, 258–262.

Morris, C. A., & Carey, J. C. (1990). Three diagnostic signs in Williams syndrome. *American Journal of Medical Genetics* (Suppl. 6), 100–101.

Morris, C. A., Demsey, S. A., Leonard, C. O., Dilts, C., & Blackburn, B. A. (1988). Natural history of Williams syndrome: Physical characteristics. *Journal of Pediatrics, 113*, 318–326.

Morris, C. A., Leonard, C. O., Dilts, C., & Demsey, S. A. (1990). Adults with Williams syndrome. *American Journal of Medical Genetics* (Suppl. 6), 102–107.

Murphy, M. B., Greenberg, F., Wilson, G., Hughes, M., & DiLiberti, J. (1990). Williams syndrome in twins. *American Journal of Medical Genetics* (Suppl. 6), 97–99.

Neville, H. J., Mills, D. L., & Bellugi, U. (1994). Effects of altered auditory sensitivity and age of language acquisition on the development of language-relevant neural systems: Preliminary studies of Williams syndrome. In S. Broman & J. Grafman (Eds.), *Atypical cognitive deficits in developmental disorders: Implications for brain function* (pp. 67–83). Hillsdale, NJ: Erlbaum.

Pagon, R. A., Bennett, F. C., LaVeck, B., Stewart, K. B., & Johnson, J. (1987). Williams syndrome: Features in late childhood and adolescence. *Pediatrics, 80*, 85–91.

Pankau, R., Partsch, C. J., Gosch, A., Oppermann, H. C., & Wessel, A. (1992). Statural growth in Williams-Beuren syndrome. *European Journal of Pediatrics, 151*, 751–755.

Payne, W. W. (1952). The blood chemistry in idiopathic hypercalcaemia. *Archives of Disease in Childhood, 27*, 302–303.

Piven, J., Tsai, G., Nehme, E., Coyle, J. T., Chase, G. A., & Folstein, S. E. (1991). Platelet serotonin, a possible marker for familial autism. *Journal of Autism and Developmental Disorders, 21*, 51–59.

Preus, M. (1984a). Differential diagnosis of the Williams and the Noonan syndromes. *Clinical Genetics, 25*, 429–434.

Preus, M. (1984b). The Williams syndrome: Objective definition and diagnosis. *Clinical Genetics, 25*, 422–428.

Rashkind, W. J., Golinko, R., & Arcasoy, M. (1961). Cardiac findings in idiopathic hypercalcemia of infancy. *Journal of Pediatrics, 58*, 464–469.

Reilly, J., Klima, E. S., & Bellugi, U. (1991). Once more with feeling: Affect and language in atypical populations. *Development and Psychopathology, 2*, 367–391.

Reiss, A. L., Feinstein, C., Rosenbaum, K. N., Borengasser-Caruso, M. A., & Goldsmith, B. M. (1985). Autism associated with Williams syndrome. *Journal of Pediatrics, 106*, 247–249.

Rourke, B. P. (1982). Central processing deficiencies in children: Toward a developmental neuropsychological model. *Journal of Clinical Neuropsychology*, *4*, 1–18.

Rourke, B. P. (1987). Syndrome of nonverbal learning disabilities: The final common pathway of white-matter disease/dysfunction? *The Clinical Neuropsychologist*, *1*, 209–234.

Rourke, B. P. (1988). The syndrome of nonverbal learning disabilities: Developmental manifestations in neurological disease, disorder, and dysfunction. *The Clinical Neuropsychologist*, *2*, 293–330.

Rourke, B. P. (1989). *Nonverbal learning disabilities: The syndrome and the model*. New York: Guilford Press.

Rourke, B. P., & Fisk, J. L. (1992). Adult presentations of learning disabilities. In R. F. White (Ed.), *Clinical syndromes in adult neuropsychology: The practitioner's handbook* (pp. 451–473). New York: Elsevier.

Rourke, B. P., & Strang, J. D. (1983). Subtypes of reading and arithmetical disabilities: A neuropsychological analysis. In M. Rutter (Ed.), *Developmental neuropsychiatry* (pp. 473–488). New York: Guilford Press.

Rourke, B. P., Young, G. C., Strang, J. D., & Russell, D. L. (1986). Adult outcomes of central processing deficiencies in childhood. In I. Grant & K. M. Adams (Eds.), *Neuropsychological assessment of neuropsychiatric disorders* (pp. 244–267). New York: Oxford University Press.

Russo, A. F., Chamany, K., Klemish, S. W., Hall, T. M., & Murray, J. C. (1991). Characterization of the calcitonin/CGRP gene in Williams syndrome. *American Journal of Medical Genetics*, *39*, 28–33.

Schmidt, M. A., Ensing, G. J., Michels, V. V., Carter, G. A., Hagler, D. J., & Feldt, R. H. (1989). Autosomal dominant supravalvular aortic stenosis: Large three-generation family. *American Journal of Medical Genetics*, *32*, 384–389.

Shepherd, R. C., & Goel, K. M. (1990). Picture of the month—paediatrics: Williams syndrome. *Scottish Medical Journal*, *35*, 47.

Sparrow, S. S. (1991). Case studies of children with nonverbal learning disabilities. In B. P. Rourke (Ed.), *Neuropsychological validation of learning disability subtypes* (pp. 349–355). New York: Guilford Press.

Spreen, O., & Strauss, E. (1991). *A compendium of neuropsychological tests: Administration, norms, and commentary* . New York: Oxford University Press.

Stiles, J., & Nass, R. (1989). *Spatial grouping activity in young children with congenital right or left hemisphere brain injury* . Unpublished technical report.

Stiles-Davis, J. (1988). Spatial dysfunctions in young children with right cerebral hemisphere injury. In J. Stiles-Davis, M. Kritchevshy & U. Bellugi (Eds.), *Spatial cognition: Brain bases and development* (pp. 251–272). Hillsdale, NJ: Erlbaum.

Strang, J. D., & Rourke, B. P. (1985). Adaptive behavior of children who exhibit specific arithmetic disabilities and associated neuropsychological abilities and deficits. In B. P. Rourke (Ed.), *Neuropsychology of learning disabilities: Essentials of subtype analysis* (pp. 302–328). New York: Guilford Press.

Telvi, L., Pinard, J.M., Ion, R., Sinet, P. M., Nicole, A., Feingold, J., Dulac, O., Pompidou, A., & Ponsot, G. (1992). De novo t(X; 21)(q28; q11) in a girl with phenotypic features of Williams–Beuren syndrome. *Journal of Medical Genetics, 29,* 747–749.

Terhune, P. E., Buchino, J. J., & Rees, A. H. (1985). Myocardial infarction associated with supravalvular aortic stenosis. *Journal of Pediatrics, 106,* 251–254.

Thal, D., Bates, E., & Bellugi, U. (1989). Language and cognition in two children with Williams syndrome. *Journal of Speech and Hearing Research, 32,* 489–499.

Tomc, S. A., Williamson, N. K., & Pauli, R. M. (1990). Temperament in Williams syndrome. *American Journal of Medical Genetics, 36,* 345–352.

Trauner, D. A., Bellugi, U., & Chase, C. (1989). Neurologic features of Williams and Down syndromes. *Pediatric Neurology, 5,* 166–168.

Tupler, R., Maraschio, P., Gerardo, A., Mainieri, R., Lanzi, G., & Tiepolo, L. (1992). A complex chromosome rearrangement with 10 breakpoints: Tentative assignments of the locus for Williams syndrome to 4q33 → q35.1. *Journal of Medical Genetics, 29,* 253–255.

Udwin, O. (1990). A survey of adults with Williams syndrome and idiopathic infantile hypercalcaemia. *Developmental Medicine and Child Neurology, 32,* 129–141.

Udwin, O., & Yule, W. (1990). Expressive language of children with Williams syndrome. *American Journal of Medical Genetics* (Suppl. 6), 108–114.

Udwin, O., & Yule, W. (1991). A cognitive and behavioral phenotype in Williams syndrome. *Journal of Clinical and Experimental Neuropsychology, 13,* 232–244.

Udwin, O., Yule, W., & Martin, N. (1986). Age at diagnosis and abilities in infantile hypercalcaemia. *Archives of Disease in Childhood, 61,* 1164–1167.

Udwin, O., Yule, W., & Martin, N. (1987). Cognitive abilities and behavioral characteristics of children with idiopathic infantile hypercalcaemia. *Journal of Child Psychology and Psychiatry, 28,* 297–309.

Voit, T., Kramer, H., Thomas, C., Wechsler, W., Reichmann, H., & Lenard, H. G. (1991). Myopathy in Williams–Beuren syndrome. *European Journal of Pediatrics, 150,* 521–526.

von Arnim, G., & Engel, P. (1964). Mental retardation related to hypercalcaemia. *Developmental Medicine and Child Neurology, 6,* 366–377.

Wang, P. P., Doherty, S., Hesselink, J. R., & Bellugi, U. (1992). Callosal morphology concurs with neurobehavioral and neuropathological findings in two neurodevelopmental disorders. *Archives of Neurology, 49,* 407–411.

Wang, P. P., Hesselink, J. R., Jernigan, T. L., Doherty, S., & Bellugi, U. (1992). Specific neurobehavioral profile of Williams' syndrome is associated with neocerebellar hemispheric preservation. *Neurology, 42,* 1999–2002.

Williams, J. C. P., Barratt-Boyes, B. G., & Lowe, J. B. (1961). Supravalvular aortic stenosis. *Circulation, 24,* 1311–1318.

7

de Lange Syndrome

Katherine D. Tsatsanis
Byron P. Rourke

de Lange syndrome (DLS) is a dysmorphogenic disorder characterized by multiple congenital abnormalities and, in most instances, severe cognitive limitations. The characteristic features of DLS include microcephaly, growth failure, distinctive facies, anomalies of development of the hands and feet (ranging from micromelia to phocomelia), and excessive growth of hair (hirsutism) of the lanugo type. Less frequent findings include ocular abnormalities, congenital heart defects, and seizure disorders. The diagnosis of this syndrome is based solely on clinical grounds; as yet, there are no biochemical or chromosomal markers for DLS. Although there has been a concerted effort to uncover the etiology of DLS, no known factor has been found to play a causative role in its origin. Many investigators support a genetic basis for the disorder, and a great deal of research has been focused on the genetic aspects of DLS. However, no consistent pattern of chromosomal abnormality has been identified, and most karyotypes appear normal.

In this chapter, a comprehensive review of the DLS research literature and findings is presented. In the final sections, a relationship among DLS, Nonverbal Learning Disabilities (NLD), and white matter dysfunction is advanced. Specifically, it is proposed that individuals who are mildly affected with DLS exhibit a pattern of neuropsychological assets and deficits very similar to the pattern evident in the developmental presentation of the NLD syndrome. An altered pattern of axonal connection is thought to underlie the pattern of deficits observed in both DLS and the NLD syndrome. In addition to a continuing interest in a genetic etiology for the disorder, an emphasis in the areas of neuropsychology and pathophysiology in future DLS research is likely to yield interesting developments.

HISTORICAL NOTE

In 1933, Cornelia de Lange, a Dutch pediatrician, described two girls with a disorder that she called "typus degenerativus Amstelodamensis," naming it after the city in which she worked (Berg, McCreary, Ridler, & Smith, 1970; de Lange, 1933; Filippi, 1989). An earlier description (Brachmann, 1916) of a similar condition in a neonate has also been reported. In recognition of Brachmann's study, Opitz (1985) has proposed the eponym "Brachmann–de Lange" for this syndrome. Although Brachmann's case was described in detail, the pathological aspects of the study were rather limited, and there exists some uncertainty that the case was an example of the syndrome described by de Lange (Berg et al., 1970; McArthur & Edwards, 1967). Moreover, de Lange's contributions to both the description and identification of this syndrome are undeniably more profound. Thus, in accord with several other authors, the eponym "de Lange syndrome" (DLS) is used in this chapter.

EPIDEMIOLOGY

Reports of DLS appear from a range of ethnic groups and have an essentially global distribution (Berg et al., 1970; Motl & Opitz, 1971). In their monographic study of DLS, Berg et al. (1970) accounted for 248 cases worldwide. Although the exact number of DLS cases to date is difficult to determine, it has been remarked that over 300 have been reported and described in the literature (de Die-Smulders, Theunissen, & Schrander-Stumpel, 1992).

DLS has an estimated incidence of 1 per 10,000 live births (Opitz, 1985). Determination of the true incidence of DLS is rendered extremely difficult by the fact that there is no clinical (e.g., biochemical or chromosomal) marker for the disorder (Opitz, 1985). The empirical risk of recurrence in siblings of an affected child has been estimated to be between 2% and 5% (Pashayan, Whelan, Guttman, & Fraser, 1969).

An extensive investigation of DLS in Denmark has yielded a prevalence figure of 0.5 per 100,000 (Beck, 1976), and an incidence figure of 1 per 50,000 for the years 1967–1982 (Beck & Fenger, 1985). The frequency of DLS among siblings was found to be 5.5% (Beck, 1976). It is important to note that these numbers represent minimum figures. The manner in which the patients were traced was biased toward severely mentally retarded individuals, and the authors noted that cases were brought to their attention after the study was completed.

There does not appear to be an effect for gender in DLS, as both males and females are equally affected with the disorder (Beck, 1976; Berg et al., 1970; de Die-Smulders et al., 1992; Filippi, 1989). In addition, neither birth order nor parental age at the time of birth seems to be a significant factor in DLS (Berg et al., 1970; Filippi, 1989; Hawley, Jackson, & Kurnit, 1985).

MEDICAL FINDINGS

This section details the most common clinical findings in DLS. These findings represent the contributions of several sources (Berg et al., 1970; Filippi, 1989; Hawley et al., 1985; Jackson, Kline, Barr, & Koch, 1993; Joubin, Pettrone, & Pettrone, 1982; Kurlander & DeMyer, 1967; McArthur & Edwards, 1967; Preus & Rex, 1983) and are presented here in summary form. Studies that have contributed specific findings are cited specifically in the text.

Craniofacial Features

The facial features of individuals with DLS are quite distinctive. They include confluent eyebrows (synophrys), well-defined and high-arched brows, long upturned eyelashes, a small nose with anteverted nostrils, and a long and/or protruding philtrum. The lips are thin and downturned, producing a carp-like mouth or grim facies. The ears are usually low-set, the neck is often short or webbed, and the mandible may be small. Dental abnormalities, with late eruption of widely spaced teeth as well as cleft palate, are also prevalent features of DLS patients.

Skeletal Charcateristics

Various skeletal abnormalities are prominent in DLS. Deformities of the hands and feet, and a substantial reduction in bone age, are consistently reported. The hands are usually small, with short and tapered fingers; a short, incurved fifth finger (clinodactyly); and a low-set, proximally placed thumb. A transverse palmar (simian) line is often present. There is limited elbow extension, often secondary to subluxation or dislocation of the radial head. Gross deformities of the upper limbs range from oligodactyly (subnormal number of fingers) to micromelia (small or short limbs) and phocomelia (poor or absent development of the proximal portions of the extremities). The feet are also small, and partial webbing (syndactyly) of the second and third toes is common. Braddock et al. (1993) examined 16 individuals with DLS and reported the presence of 13 pairs of ribs in 9 cases. They suggest that an extra rib pair may be a key diagnostic finding in this syndrome.

Growth and Development

Short stature, low weight, and microcephaly (all usually below the 3rd centile) are principal manifestations of DLS. The birth weight of individuals with DLS is quite low. These children are often born weighing under 2500 grams, although the pregnancies are of normal duration. In their survey of 277 patients with DLS, Kline, Barr, and Jackson (1993) reported birth weights below the 5th centile in 68% of the cases. The mean birth height and weight for both sexes were found to be at or below the 5th centile. The height and weight of individuals with DLS tend to remain low, as severe growth failure and delayed physical development are consistent features of DLS.

Gastrointestinal Complications

Both structural and functional abnormalities of the gastrointestinal (GI) tract have been reported with frequency in patients with DLS. GI complications probably contribute to the small weight and size of children with DLS. They are also related to the increased morbidity and mortality found in this syndrome (Cates, Billmire, Bull, & Grosfeld, 1989). Berg et al. (1970) note that GI complications are the second most common cause of death in children with DLS.

Feeding problems are not uncommon, including the following: regurgitation; projectile vomiting; sucking, chewing, and swallowing difficulties; and lack of interest in food (Bull, Fitzgerald, Heifetz, & Brei, 1993; Cates et al., 1989; Jackson et al., 1993; Rosenbach, Zahavi, & Dinari, 1992). These difficulties may be associated with severe gastroesophageal reflux, which is a frequently reported problem in DLS (Bull et al., 1993; Cates et al., 1989; Filippi, 1989; Jackson, 1992; Jackson et al., 1993; Rosenbach et al., 1992). Gastroesophageal reflux may present with secondary esophagitis, anemia, and chronic or acute aspiration, and thus is clinically significant in the treatment of DLS patients (Bull et al., 1993; Filippi, 1989; Jackson, 1992).

Cardiovascular Defects

Congenital heart defects are found in 20–30% of patients with DLS (Berg et al., 1970; Filippi, 1989; Hawley et al., 1985; Jackson et al., 1993). The nature of these defects is wide-ranging, but ventricular and atrial septal defects appear to be most common.

Endocrine Deficiencies

Multiple endocrine deficiencies have been reported in patients with DLS (France, Crome, & Abraham, 1969; Hillman, Hammond, Noé, & Reiss,

1968; Kousseff, Thomson-Meares, Newkirk, & Root, 1993; Schlesinger, Clayton, Bodian, & Jones, 1963; Schwartz, Schwartz, Kousseff, Bercu, & Root, 1990; Tonini & Marinoni, 1990); however, this is not a consistent finding (Hart, Jaslow, & Gomez, 1965).

Tests of endocrine function in four children with DLS revealed evidence of hypopituitarism (Schlesinger et al., 1963). Thyroid deficiency was suspected in three cases, and adrenocortical insufficiency was present in varying degrees in all four children.

France et al. (1969) conducted a study of endocrine function in nine individuals with DLS. Although no uniform dysfunction was revealed, in six cases there was evidence to suggest a selective or isolated deficiency in thyroid-stimulating hormone (TSH) secretion by the pituitary. It was further suggested that this deficiency involved a problem in the hypothalamus. A role for hypothalamic lesions in hypertrichosis was also advanced by France and colleagues.

An examination of hypothalamic–pituitary function in five patients with DLS revealed two instances of human growth hormone (HGH) deficiency (Schwartz et al., 1990). In addition, three patients displayed low plasma concentrations of insulin-like growth factor 1 (IGF-1), which is thought to be related to postnatal growth retardation—a characteristic feature of DLS. Adrenal and thyroid functions were reported to be essentially normal in these patients. In a second study (Kousseff et al., 1993), 5 of 12 patients with DLS who received endocrine evaluations showed compromised endocrine function. Four patients were found to demonstrate HGH deficiency (two of whom were previously reported by Schwartz et al., 1990), and a fifth patient displayed low plasma concentrations of IGF-1 (Kousseff et al., 1993).

Hillman et al. (1968) also investigated HGH values in three children with DLS. In two patients the levels were relatively high, despite short stature and low weight. The authors suggested a peripheral undersensitivity to endogenous HGH to explain their finding. They also proposed that this undersensitivity may have its origins in reduced thyroid function.

A case of a child with DLS who displayed multiple pituitary deficiency (panhypopituitarism) has also been reported (Tonini & Marinoni, 1990). Replacement therapy was found to improve growth and allow partial psychomotor advances.

The results of the endocrine studies reveal no consistent abnormality in functioning in children with DLS. However, the findings do seem to suggest a role for the pituitary gland in the expression of the disorder.

Ophthalmological Anomalies

There is no particular ocular abnormality that presents as a defining or typical feature of DLS. However, a wide range of ocular anomalies is present in these children. Ophthalmological examinations of children with DLS have revealed occurrences of photophobia without apparent ocular cause (thought to be a behavioral manifestation), ptosis, nystagmus, horizontal strabismus, chronic conjunctivitis, and myopia (Barr et al., 1971; Filippi, 1989; Jackson et al., 1993; Levin, Seidman, Nelson, & Jackson, 1990).

Otological Manifestations

Hearing loss has been reported sporadically in the DLS literature (Filippi, 1989; Hawley et al., 1985; Jackson et al., 1993; Sataloff, Speigel, Hawkshaw, Epstein, & Jackson, 1990). In their study of otolaryngological manifestations in 45 patients with DLS, Sataloff et al. (1990) found that 30% of their sample exhibited stenotic external auditory canals, 50% had serious otitis media, 24% displayed mild hearing loss, 24% had moderate hearing loss, and 52% demonstrated severe hearing loss. It is interesting to note that only 6% of these children had been evaluated previously for hearing loss. This suggests that hearing deficiencies may be underreported in the DLS literature.

Children with DLS are predisposed to hearing loss for several reasons. These include the presence of cleft palate and other midfacial developmental aberrations, as well as the chronic otitis media (Sataloff et al., 1990). Each of these factors is typically associated with hearing loss.

Other Features

Excessive hair growth (hirsutism) of the lanugo type is a distinctive feature of DLS. The areas that are typically affected are the forehead, upper lip, forearms, shoulders, and midline of the back (Preus & Rex, 1983). It is also interesting to note that children with DLS frequently have dark brown or black hair color (Berg et al., 1970; Filippi, 1989).

A characteristic vocal quality is noted in the crying of DLS children. The cry is typically described as a feeble, low-pitched, growling sound.

Other common anomalies include genital abnormalities. Undescended testes are often present in males, and hypoplastic genitalia is common in females. These findings are interpreted to suggest a dysfunction in gonadotropin secretion in DLS.

PRENATAL FINDINGS

Although no biochemical markers have been identified, three reports of antepartum abnormalities in maternal fluids/serum signify a promising direction for diagnostic and etiological considerations in DLS.

First, there is evidence to suggest a possible etiological relationship between low levels of 5-hydroxyindole-3-acetic acid (5-HIAA) and DLS (Lacourt, Arendt, Cox, & Béguin, 1977). Lacourt et al. (1977) observed an exceptionally low level of 5-HIAA in the amniotic fluid of a woman who subsequently gave birth to a child with DLS. The low 5-HIAA value was thought to reflect abnormalities in fetal neurological development. That is, 5-HIAA is an end product of serotonin metabolism, and thus low levels of 5-HIAA may indicate low levels of serotonin. A role for serotonin in fetal development and nervous system functioning has been recognized. In the context of DLS, it is also interesting to note that serotonin is related to both hypothalamic and pituitary function (Delitala, 1989; Greenberg & Coleman, 1973).

Furthermore, in their study of 11 patients with DLS, Greenberg and Coleman (1973) found that 9 individuals demonstrated low blood serum levels of serotonin. A relationship between low serotonin levels and hyperactive or aggressive behavior was also found. The authors note, however, that patients with DLS are part of a subgroup of a large array of children who show low serotonin levels in association with hyperactive behavior.

The complete absence of pregnancy-associated plasma protein A (PAPPA) has been observed in the maternal serum and placental tissue of a woman who gave birth to a child with DLS (Westergaard et al., 1983). PAPPA is a large glycoprotein that is produced by the placenta and secreted into the maternal circulation (Westergaard et al., 1983). The maternal serum level of PAPPA typically increases exponentially until term. Although the precise biological function of PAPPA is not known, low serum levels of PAPPA in the first trimester have been associated with chromosomal abnormalities in the fetus and increased risk of miscarriage (Silahtaroglu, Tümer, Kristensen, Sottrup-Jensen, & Tommerup, 1993; Westergaard et al., 1983). Silahtaroglu et al. (1993) have localized the gene for PAPPA to chromosome 9q33.1. If indeed PAPPA is a causative agent in DLS, a role for chromosome 9 in the genesis of this syndrome is suggested.

There have been at least four reports of individuals with DLS who demonstrate an abnormality of chromosome 9, although this is rare. One case of a ring chromosome 9 abnormality (Barr et al., 1971) and two cases of a pericentric inversion of chromosome 9 (Berg et al., 1970; Breslau, Disteche, Hall, Thuline, & Cooper, 1981) have been observed. However, it was noted that this type of inversion has an incidence of 1–2% in the normal population (Breslau et al., 1981). In addition, Hersh et al. (1985) reported a case of a young woman with features resembling DLS who had a chromosomal abnormality characterized by dup(4p)-del(9p). Her mother and two siblings demonstrated the same balanced translocation; however, they were not affected with DLS. A maternal aunt and uncle also presented with many of the features of DLS. Chromosomal data, obtained via high-resolution banding techniques, were not available for the aunt and uncle.

Bruner and Hsia (1990) described a case of DLS that was identified at 15 weeks' gestation by a low maternal serum alphafetoprotein (MSAFP) value. They note that low MSAFP levels in pregnancies are often a marker of fetal chromosomal abnormalities.

There is evidence to suggest a possible connection between DLS and maternal fluid/serum levels of serotonin, PAPPA, and MSAFP. Each of these findings merits further observation and exploration, in order (1) to determine whether one of these substances may serve as a biochemical marker for DLS, and (2) to clarify their role in the development and manifestation of the syndrome.

NEUROPATHOLOGY: POSTMORTEM STUDIES

Reports of neuropathological changes associated with DLS are scarce. In particular, there is a notable absence of neuroimaging studies in the DLS literature. Several postmortem studies have been reported, and the results of these are detailed below. The neuropathological findings derived from autopsy reports do not indicate a pathognomonic neuropathological attribute for DLS; however, a wide range of anomalies is found upon autopsy in both central nervous system (CNS) and peripheral nervous system structures of individuals with DLS.

Abnormalities of the pituitary, thyroid, and adrenal glands have been commonly reported. A reduction or complete absence of basophil cells in the pituitary gland was present in four cases of DLS (France et al., 1969; Schlesinger et al., 1963). An account of a distinctive anomaly of the pituitary gland was presented by Björklöf and Brundelet (1965). They described the study of a woman with DLS in whom the greater part of the pituitary gland was occupied by a large cyst in the region of the Rathke cleft. The cyst produced compression hypoplasia of the anterior and posterior lobes of the pituitary gland. In addition, the thyroid and adrenal glands were observed to be small and clearly underdeveloped. Hypoplasia (or a reduction in size) of the thyroid gland was a frequent finding in the autopsy reports (France et al., 1969; Hart et al., 1965; McArthur & Edwards, 1967; Schlesinger et al., 1963). In addition, hypoplasia of the adrenal glands was present in three cases (Hart et al., 1965; Schlesinger et al., 1963).

Direct involvement of the hypothalamus is relatively infrequent. In the autopsy case of a young woman with DLS presented by Sato et al. (1986), a tumor that grew from the hypothalamus to the optic nerve and posterior lobe of the hypophysis was revealed. The tumor also involved the wall of the right lateral ventricle, the corpus callosum, and the caudate nucleus. Normal levels of HGH-producing cells, but reduced numbers of cells producing TSH and follicle-stimulating hormone (FSH), were found. The brain was atrophic but the cerebellum was relatively well developed.

Microcephaly, decreased numbers of neurons, increased numbers of astrocytes, and diffuse cortical gliosis were commonly found (Barr et al., 1971; Beck & Fenger, 1985; France et al., 1969; McArthur & Edwards, 1967; Schlesinger et al., 1963). Anomalies in white matter development were also reported with some frequency (Barr et al., 1971; Björklöf & Brundelet, 1965; France et al., 1969; Schlesinger et al., 1963). The implications of these findings are considered later in the section on white matter dysfunction.

GENETICS

An extensive body of research has been devoted to uncovering evidence for a genetic etiology for DLS. DLS clearly shares the main features of autosomal chromosome disorders: (1) intrauterine and postnatal growth deficiency; (2) a specific pattern of dysmorphic signs, especially of the facies, genitalia, and distal limbs; (3) multiple malformations; and (4) impaired mental development (Schinzel, 1983). In addition, common malformations include the following: cleft palate; malrotation of the gut; esophageal atresia; malformation of the heart, kidney, and urinary tract; hypoplasia of the thumb; and brain malformation. The majority of these malformations are also present in DLS. Although a genetic basis for DLS is suspected, a consistent chromosomal aberration or pattern of inheritance has yet to be identified.

Chromosomes

In the majority of cases of DLS, no chromosomal abnormality is detected, and normal karyotypes are revealed even with the use of precise techniques (Breslau et al., 1981; Filippi, 1989; Hawley et al., 1985; Merikangas, Merikangas, Katz, & Pan, 1977; Preus & Rex, 1983). Beck and Mikkelsen (1981) undertook an analysis of chromosome abnormalities in patients with DLS, using a sophisticated technique (methotrexate prometaphase) that should detect minute chromosome abnormalities. The karyotypes of all 31 patients were found to be normal.

In those cases in which chromosomal abnormalities have been found, the nature of the aberrations has varied. In a review of abnormal chromosome findings in the DLS literature from 1963 to 1972, Beck and Mikkelsen (1981) found the following: cases of excess chromosomal fragments; partial trisomies (including chromosomes 3, 5, 9, and 13); other chromosomal rearrangements (e.g., translocations); and loss of chromosomal material.

An etiological connection between DLS and a partial duplication of the long arm of chromosome 3 has been speculated by several investigators. Ireland, English, Cross, Houlsby, and Burn (1991) reported the case of an infant who presented with the typical features of DLS and was revealed, upon chromosome analysis, to have a balanced reciprocal translocation between the long arm of chromosomes 3 and 17. Specifically, a *de novo* translocation with breakpoints at bands 3q26.3 and 17q23.1 was indicated. These authors proposed that the gene for DLS is located at 3q26.3.

Furthermore, the clinical presentation of individuals with dup(3q) syndrome is somewhat similar to that of DLS. Indeed, a large family with DLS described by Falek, Schmidt, and Jarvis (1966) was shown to exhibit a dup(3q) karyotype, and this is now considered to reflect the phenotypic expression of dup(3q) syndrome (Opitz & Smith, 1966; Wilson, Dasouki, & Barr, 1985). In addition, a case of ring chromosome 3 in association with features of DLS has been reported (Lakshminarayana & Nallasivam, 1990). Although a superficial resemblance exists among dup(3q) syndrome, ring 3 syndrome, and DLS, it is generally acknowledged that these syndromes represent distinct clinical entities.

Pattern of Inheritance

The majority of cases of DLS are thought to occur sporadically in families with an otherwise normal medical history. In a survey of 64 families that each had a member with DLS, no recurrences were found among 100 siblings and family histories were unremarkable (Hawley et al., 1985). In this context, it is important to bear in mind that a familial pattern is not easily identified in this syndrome, because individuals with DLS are unlikely to reproduce. Nevertheless, evidence has amounted to suggest that the syndrome is transmitted in either an autosomal recessive or an autosomal dominant fashion. A chromosomal basis for the syndrome has not been revealed in any of these cases.

Familial cases of DLS have been reported, but no clear pedigree pattern has emerged from these reports. Kumar, Blank, and Griffiths (1985) described an extended family in which several members were identified as having DLS. The segregation pattern was suggestive of an autosomal dominant gene with variable expression.

Several reports of features of DLS in both parent and child are also suggestive of an autosomal dominant inheritance pattern (Bankier,

Haan, & Birrell, 1986; Beck, 1974; de Die-Smulders et al., 1992; Leavitt, Dinno, & Davis, 1985; Robinson, Wolfsberg, & Jones, 1985). De Die-Smulders et al. (1992) observed that in these cases the parent displayed mild manifestations of the disorder as compared to the proband, and that both were found to exhibit a milder expression of DLS than the classical case. The parents demonstrated normal to mildly or moderately impaired performance on psychometric intelligence tests, and no parent was found to have upper-limb malformations. The children were more severely affected than were their parents, but did not display reduction deformities of the forearms or gross internal anomalies (the more severe expressions of DLS; de Die-Smulders et al., 1992). In addition, it is interesting to note that in each of these reports, the mother was the transmitting parent.

In other instances, DLS has been found to reoccur in siblings with (nonconsanguineous) parents who appear healthy (Beratis, Hsu, & Hirschhorn, 1971; Fryns et al., 1987; Lieber, Glaser, & Jhaveri, 1973). In the cases described by Fryns et al. (1987) and Lieber et al. (1973), the children were observed to manifest a severe form of DLS with significant upper-limb defects; three of the four children died at an early age. The three siblings with DLS reported by Beratis et al. (1971) were severely affected but did not show major upper-limb deformities; one child died at an early age. Cases of DLS in the offspring of phenotypically normal consanguineous parents have also been reported (Berg et al., 1970; Naguib, Teebi, Al-Awadi, & Marafie, 1987). Together, these reports provide support for an autosomal recessive pattern of inheritance for DLS that appears to be associated with a severe manifestation of the disorder.

Cases of monozygotic twins concordant for the syndrome (Barr et al., 1971; Berg et al., 1970) also suggest a familial pattern of inheritance. Two instances of twins discordant for DLS—male dizygotic (Stevenson & Scott, 1976) and female monozygotic (Carakushansky & Berthier, 1976)—have been reported. Carakushansky and Berthier (1976) argue that their findings are suggestive of (1) a postzygotic new mutation of a dominant gene, or (2) chromosomal or mitotic instability in which early cleavage divisions are followed by subsequent reunion of chromosome fragments.

The results of the foregoing studies do not illuminate the genetic underpinnings of DLS. Neither a consistent chromosomal abnormality nor a pattern of inheritance has been identified. Most cases of DLS appear to occur sporadically, which suggests that they arise from spontaneous mutations. However, cases of familial occurrence of DLS provide evidence for autosomal dominant transmission. In addition, Opitz (1985) has advanced an argument for an autosomal recessive pattern of inheritance. He proposes that DLS arises from inheritance of an autosomal recessive gene that, in its homozygous state, shows a high prenatal lethality. This would explain a segregation ratio of one order of magnitude less than expected under the recessive hypothesis (Opitz, 1985).

An interest in novel genetic mechanisms such as genomic imprinting has also been expressed (Punnett & Zakai, 1990; Wilson, 1991). The significance of genomic imprinting with respect to DLS probably pertains to the following three aspects: First, genomic imprinting involves the differential expression of genetic material, depending upon parental origin (Hall, 1990). In this respect, it is interesting to note that the majority of individuals demonstrating mild DLS are female. In addition, parental transmission typically involves a mother with mild DLS. Genomic imprinting also implies a critical period in development. In particular, the stage during which germline cells are formed is considered to be a sensitive period. It is thought that genetic information can be marked at this time, temporarily changing it to permit differential expression (Hall, 1990). Thus, if the intact regions of a chromosome homologous to deletions are imprinted, the intact chromosome need not carry recessive mutations. The imprinted genes should, in fact, behave like recessive genes (Punnett & Zakai, 1990).

The inconsistency of the genetic findings suggests that a multifactorial determination of DLS cannot be dismissed. Chromosomal abnormalities may be features of the syndrome, but these need not be the primary causative agents in its etiology. On the other hand, it is also conceivable that abnormalities in chromosomal structure are as yet too minute to detect, or may involve a complex mechanism of transmission that has yet to be identified. Further refinements of knowledge in this area are dependent upon increasingly sophisticated techniques in genetic research.

TERATOGENS

There is no evidence to suggest that exposure to consistent teratogenic agents is responsible for DLS. Surveys of children with DLS have not revealed any common teratogens or environmental agents (Barr et al., 1971; Berg et al., 1970; Filippi, 1989; Hawley et al., 1985).

VARIABILITY

Although individuals with DLS demonstrate a characteristic phenotype and distinctive constellation of minor anomalies, there appears to be a wide range of variability in the expression of the disorder. In addition to pointing to a wider phenotypic variability in DLS, the studies cited below raise questions about the timing and sequence of events involved in the development of DLS.

There are several reports of mild DLS in which the phenotypic expression becomes more apparent with age (Greenberg & Robinson, 1989; Pashayan, Levy, & Fraser, 1970; Passarge, Mecke, & Altrogge, 1971). In the case presented by Pashayan et al. (1970), the child had features suggestive of Turner syndrome at 9 months of age, but at 21 months exhibited the characteristic appearance of DLS. In a second case (Passarge et al., 1971), a child who showed some of the features of the *cri du chat* syndrome at ages 8 and 11 months had developed the typical expression of DLS by 21 months of age. These reports suggest that a gradual evolution of DLS may exist in some cases, and that the critical period for expression of the phenotype lies between 9 and 21 months of age. It is interesting to note that this period overlaps with a postnatal spurt in brain growth characterized by increased dendritic processes, synaptogenesis, and myelination.

On the basis of clinical impression, Hawley et al. (1985) suspected the existence of a mild expression of DLS associated with a higher birth weight. They examined this hypothesis by dividing their subjects into two groups, low (under 2268 grams) and high (over 2268 grams) birth weight. They found that a lower birth weight was correlated with a more severe expression of DLS. In particular, the low-birth-weight group demonstrated more significant upper-limb malformations, more severe hearing loss, and more severely limited psychomotor development. The low-birth-weight children were also observed to experience difficulty obeying simple commands and performing self-help skills. A relationship between lower birth weight and more severe impairment of motor and language skills was also observed by Goodban (1993). Similarly, Barr et al. (1971) found that birth weight and severity of upper-limb involvement were predictive of expression of DLS. In particular, there was a tendency for patients with higher IQs to have had higher birth weights and less impaired development of the upper extremities. Moreover, our survey of the case reports of children mildly affected with DLS (e.g., with IQs in the borderline to average range) showed that, with one exception, all of the children had a birth weight greater than 2268 grams.

Reports of autosomal dominant transmission provide further evidence to suggest that there are varying degrees of severity in the expression of DLS. As noted, these cases are striking because DLS is consistently found to be manifested in a milder form in the parent than in the proband, and both are found to exhibit a milder expression of DLS compared to "classical cases" (de Die-Smulders et al., 1992). Thus, de Die-Smulders et al. (1992) propose that there are at least two clinical variants of DLS: (1) a severe form that is characterized by severely limited growth and cognitive development, distinctive facies, and major upper-limb malformations; and (2) a milder form that presents a more subtle expression of the disorder in all respects, including growth, cognitive functioning, and facies, and is not characterized by a limb reduction defect.

The existence of a range of severity in the phenotypic expression of DLS has been increasingly recognized (Berg et al., 1970; Hawley et al., 1985; Jackson, 1992; Opitz, 1985; Preus & Rex, 1983). It has been argued that DLS is homogeneous in "type" but variable in "amount"; that is, subgroups within this disorder are not apparent, but its expression does appear to lie on a continuum of severity (Hawley et al., 1985; Preus & Rex, 1983). However, Van Allen et al. (1993) report that clinical geneticists at the 1991 D. W. Smith Workshop on Malformations and Morphogenesis reached a consensus that "mild" DLS represents a distinct entity, although the minimal diagnostic criteria for this syndrome have not been agreed upon. In their paper, Van Allen et al. (1993) propose a provisional classification system for DLS and outline criteria for Type I ("classic"), Type II ("mild"), and Type III ("phenocopies") DLS. The issue of phenotypic variability is a prominent topic in the current DLS literature and has been recently addressed by several authors (e.g., Leroy et al., 1993; Moeschler & Graham, 1993; Saul, Rogers, Phelan, & Stevenson, 1993; and Selicorni et al., 1993).

It is difficult to gauge the limits of variability of a disorder when neither its cause nor a clinical marker for it has been identified. However, in addition to the evidence cited above, there are several reasons to expect variable expression in a disorder such as DLS. First, if DLS does indeed have its origins in a chromosomal aberration, it can be expected to show the wide variability in the nature and severity of expression that is generally typical of chromosomal syndromes (Jones, 1988). Furthermore, as patients may exhibit chromosomal aberrations involving more (or less) than the critical segment, features of this syndrome may overlap with those of other conditions. Finally, a disorder of this complexity is likely to have a multifactorial etiology which in turn engenders the potential for a varied range of expression.

DIFFERENTIAL DIAGNOSIS

Diagnosis of DLS is made on the basis of a constellation of clinical features. As yet, no biochemical or genetic markers have been identified by which to confirm or exclude diagnosis.

Berg et al. (1970) listed 15 clinical findings that they judged to be most salient in diagnosis. More recently, Preus and Rex (1983) have constructed a diagnostic index made up of 30 features that they consider to distinguish most accurately individuals with and without DLS. However, this classification system is likely to be biased against individuals who are mildly affected with DLS (Opitz, 1985). A rather simple index using 11 metacarpal and phalangeal measurements from radiographs has also been proposed (Halal & Preus, 1979).

DLS has been found to share similar features with several other congenital disorders. A discussion of these findings follows.

Although, as noted earlier, there is a striking overlap in the phenotypic expression of dup(3q) syndrome and DLS, these are considered to be distinct syndromes that are clinically distinguishable. Several authors have delineated the similarities and differences between the dup(3q) syndrome and DLS (Breslau et al., 1981; Francke & Opitz, 1979; Wilson et al., 1985). There is some overlap in the facial characteristics (e.g., hirsutism, anteverted nostrils, downturned corners of the mouth, short and/or webbed neck), but intrauterine growth retardation, a prominent philtrum, proximally placed thumbs, oligodactyly, phocomelia, and partial webbing of toes 2 and 3 are more frequent in DLS. Dup(3q) syndrome is characterized to a greater extent by craniosynostosis, cleft palate, and urinary tract anomalies (Steinbach et al., 1981; Wilson et al., 1985). In addition, convulsions, hypertelorism (abnormal width between the eyes), eye and palate anomalies, and renal and cardiac abnormalities are more commonly found in dup(3q) syndrome (Breslau et al., 1981; Steinbach et al., 1981). It is also notable that Steinbach and colleagues (1981) found no significant difference between dup(3q)del(3p) and the dup(3q) syndrome.

A case of ring chromosome 3 with features of DLS has also been described (Lakshminarayana & Nallasivam, 1990). Although instances of ring 3/del(3p) chromosome abnormalities are few in number, the concordant features in these patients suggest the existence of a distinct syndrome (Wilson, Pooley, & Parker, 1982). The clinical features of these patients include mental retardation; prenatal and postnatal growth retardation; microcephaly; hypertonia; digital anomalies; and a characteristic facies with ptosis, epicanthal folds, broad nasal root, downturned corners of the mouth, and dysplastic ears (Wilson et al., 1982).

Fryns (1986) proposes that the diagnosis of Coffin–Siris syndrome be considered, particularly in mild cases of DLS. It was his impression that the patients described in three studies (Leavitt et al., 1985; Mosher, Schulte, Kaplan, Buehler, & Sanger, 1985; Robinson et al., 1985) who displayed the typical facies of DLS but near-average intelligence were examples of the Coffin–Siris syndrome. This syndrome is characterized by mild to moderate growth deficiency and microcephaly; general hirsutism of the lumbar region and the arms; and a coarse facies with full lips (Jones, 1988). Clinodactyly of the first finger, and hypoplasia or absence of the terminal phalanges of the fifth (and, eventually, fourth and third) rays of the hands and feet, are also present (Fryns, 1986).

A case has also been reported of a woman who was diagnosed with Rubinstein–Taybi syndrome at 14 years of age and, upon re-examination

22 years later, was determined to have DLS (Partington, 1990). Characteristic features of Rubinstein–Taybi syndrome include short stature, broad thumbs and toes, a degree of microcephaly, and distinctive facies (including slanted palpebral fissures, hypoplastic maxilla, and beaked nose) (Jones, 1988; Nyhan & Sakati, 1976).

Heckmann et al. (1991–1992) described a case of a 5-year-old girl who was diagnosed with DLS at 1 year of age but was found at postmortem to have Leigh syndrome. This child demonstrated some of the typical facial features of DLS, as well as other characteristic anomalies (e.g., microcephaly and growth retardation). Postmortem examination revealed partial agenesis of the corpus callosum, optic atrophy, decreased myelination of the internal capsule, small cerebral peduncles, and necrotic lesions characteristic of Leigh syndrome. Leigh syndrome is a rapidly progressive encephalomyelopathy of infancy or childhood that is thought to be inherited in an autosomal recessive manner. The diagnostic criteria are neuropathological and include degeneration of grey matter, predominantly in the diencephalon and brain stem. The lesions are characterized by necrosis, myelin destruction, astrocytosis, and capillary proliferation (Heckmann et al., 1991–1992; Urion, Konkel, & Korf, 1994). The syndrome may be related to biochemical defects in the pyruvate decarboxylase system (Bergsma, 1979).

Although Heckmann et al. are not aware of any other case linking Leigh syndrome to DLS, some patients with Leigh syndrome have been reported to exhibit facial features resembling those in fetal alcohol syndrome (Heckmann et al., 1991–1992). This finding is particularly interesting when viewed in conjunction with Opitz's (1985) warning that infants with fetal alcohol syndrome can be misdiagnosed as having DLS.

The results of these studies reveal an overlap in the phenotypic expression of several syndromes of variable etiology and inheritance. In part, complications arise in the diagnosis of DLS because the limits of the syndrome are not well defined, and diagnosis rests on the clinical manifestation of the disorder.

NEUROPSYCHOLOGICAL LITERATURE

There is a relative paucity of studies examining the neuropsychological assets and deficits of children with DLS. Aspects of their cognitive and psychosocial functioning have been addressed in case reports, but these tend not to be detailed. The results of a comprehensive neuropsychological assessment have been reported in only one instance (Stefanatos & Musikoff, 1994).

Moderate to severe mental retardation has traditionally been considered an integral part of DLS. However, there are several reports of individuals who demonstrate the typical characteristics of the syndrome but obtain scores in the average to borderline range on tests of psychometric intelligence (Beck, 1976; Brylewski, 1978; Cameron & Kelly, 1988; Gadoth, Lerman, Garty, & Shumuelewitz, 1982; Halal & Silver, 1992; Leavitt et al., 1985; McIntire & Eisen, 1965; Pashayan et al., 1969; Robinson et al., 1985; Saal, Samango-Sprouse, Rodnan, Rosenbaum, & Custer, 1993; Stefanatos & Musikoff, 1994). A bias in the DLS literature is introduced on two accounts when children demonstrating the severe form of DLS alone are studied. First, this approach precludes a consideration of mild manifestations of the disorder; in such cases, the potential for clinical variability is overlooked. Second, a failure to analyze atypical forms of DLS limits the potential for identifying a pattern of neuropsychological performance that may characterize these children to a greater or lesser extent. If cases of severe cognitive limitation alone are considered, a recognizable pattern of performance is unlikely to emerge.

As noted earlier, support has recently emerged for the notion of a continuum of severity in the expression of DLS. Therefore, in this section, the cognitive characteristics and psychosocial functioning of children with both severe ("classical") and mild (sometimes referred to as "atypical") DLS are addressed. Because this literature consists largely of fragments of information found in case reports and anecdotal information (e.g., reports of clinical impression), the findings are reported here in summary form. However, the results of an exhaustive neuropsychological assessment (Stefanatos & Musikoff, 1994) are presented in detail, in order to yield a more complete picture of a case of mild DLS.

Severe DLS

Children with severe DLS exhibit moderate to severe mental retardation, severely impaired psychomotor development, and little expressive language (Abraham & Russell, 1968; Barr et al., 1971). Although they are able to perform some general self-help tasks, individuals with DLS typically require assisted care (Beck, 1987). The vocalizations of children with severe DLS often consist of low-pitched cries and dysphonic grunts. Young adults have been found to demonstrate meaningful speech, but their vocalizations are marked by a harsh, hoarse, and dysphonic quality (Fraser & Campbell, 1978). Children with severe DLS are typically nonsocial and rarely express any emotion (Abraham & Russell, 1968; Barr et al., 1971; Johnson, Ekman, Friesen, Nyhan, & Shear, 1976). Their facial expression may be described as mask-like. These children have also been reported to engage in repetitious self-stimulatory activity and self-mutilating behavior (Berg et al., 1970; Greenberg & Coleman, 1973; Johnson et al., 1976).

Mild DLS

Children with mild DLS function in the average to mildly impaired range. Their psychomotor development is typically delayed (de Die-Smulders et al., 1992; Halal & Silver, 1992; Mosher et al., 1985; Robinson et al., 1985), and they show more impairment in gross motor than in fine motor skills (Cameron & Kelly, 1988; Halal & Silver, 1992; Leavitt et al., 1985). Visual–motor (Beck, 1976; Gadoth et al., 1982; Moeschler & Graham, 1993) and visual–spatial abilities (Halal & Silver, 1992) are reported to be deficient, although Saal et al. (1993) observed relatively well-developed perceptual skills in their patient with DLS. In addition, these children are found to exhibit difficulties in maintaining attention and concentration (Cameron & Kelly, 1988; Gadoth et al., 1982; Halal & Silver, 1992). Language development is generally delayed. Although children with mild DLS may experience difficulties with both the expressive and receptive aspects of language, their receptive language skills are typically more advanced than are their expressive skills (Beck, 1976; Brylewski, 1978; Cameron & Kelly, 1988; Halal & Silver, 1992; Leavitt et al., 1985; McIntire & Eisen, 1965; Moeschler & Graham, 1993). In a survey of the speech and language skills of 116 individuals with DLS, Goodban (1993) observed the following: (1) Language production was markedly inferior to language comprehension; (2) individuals with well-developed vocabulary skills did not display expected levels of syntactic skills; and (3) almost all DLS individuals, including those who demonstrated well-developed vocabulary skills, were quiet and talked very little. In several instances (Brylewski, 1978; Cameron & Kelly, 1988; McIntire & Eisen, 1965), speech and language skills have been found to improve with age and remediation.

It is also important to note the role of hearing loss, a common characteristic of DLS, in the context of language development. Sataloff et al. (1990) found a relationship between degree of hearing loss and language development in children with DLS: Specifically, children with better hearing also demonstrated better language development. This finding was confirmed by Goodban's (1993) survey of the speech and language skills of individuals with DLS. Moreover, Sataloff et al. (1990) noted that of their sample of 45 patients with DLS, only 3 had been evaluated previously for hearing loss, although 34 demonstrated moderate or severe hearing loss. This finding underscores the importance of examining hearing in children with DLS. Hearing loss may be one of the most significant factors in the delay of language skills in children with DLS, and yet it is seldom recognized. Furthermore, it is conceivable that hearing loss leads to the misdiagnosis of attention deficit or poor concentration.

The concept-forming and problem-solving abilities of children with mild DLS have not been addressed in any detail. There is but one instance of a child who was reported to experience difficulty in abstract thinking (Gadoth et al., 1982). The generally young age of these children precludes any comment regarding their academic achievement. However, retrospective studies of adults with suspected DLS contain consistent reports of difficulties in school learning (Halal & Silver, 1992; Leavitt et al., 1985; Mosher et al., 1985; Robinson et al., 1985).

In terms of psychosocial functioning, these children are often characterized as shy and withdrawn (Brylewski, 1978; Halal & Silver, 1992; McIntire & Eisen, 1965). In one report, a child was described by his mother as having considerable difficulty in adapting to new persons or new situations and as withdrawing from social interactions in general (Halal & Silver, 1992). In addition, the parents of a 6-year-old boy with mild DLS noted behavioral problems that included a preference for rigid routines and rigid thinking (Bay, Mauk, Radcliffe, & Kaplan, 1993). This behavior worsened as the boy began to display explosive, aggressive outbursts. A behavioral rating scale placed him within the mild to moderate range of autism. Jackson (1992) remarks that children mildly affected with DLS often demonstrate a strong preference for a structured environment, and that they exhibit marked behavioral and psychosomatic reactions to disruptions of their normal daily routines.

Case Report: Atypical DLS

Stefanatos and Musikoff (1994) have presented the results of a comprehensive neuropsychological assessment of a 14-year-old female with DLS. These findings are described in detail below.

Results of psychometric intelligence testing showed performance within the borderline range; however, there was a striking disparity between verbal and performance measures. A Verbal IQ within the normal range was obtained, whereas the subject's Performance IQ was 61.

Examination of motor skills demonstrated bimanual weakness, slowing, and incoordination (which was somewhat more prominent with the left hand). Gross motor skills were also found to be deficient.

This young girl demonstrated relative impairment on measures requiring visual-perceptual, visual–spatial–organizational, and visual–motor skills. She experienced particular difficulty on tasks involving attention to visual details, visual–spatial problem solving, and visual–constructional skills.

Performance on language measures was consistently within average limits. However, the girl did have difficulty generating words when provided with phonemic cues.

The subject's rote memory for a series of digits was above average, and she exhibited average immediate and delayed recall for verbal material. She demonstrated significant impairment on a nonverbal memory task involving a complex visual figure.

Assessment of academic achievement revealed average performance on single-word spelling and single-word oral reading, but depressed mechanical arithmetic scores. The difficulty in mechanical arithmetic was thought to be related to deficiencies in visual–motor, visual–spatial, and organizational abilities underlying mathematical skills.

In terms of psychosocial functioning, this young girl was described as well behaved and of strong character. However, she was socially immature and showed interest in activities that were generally appropriate for younger children. In addition, she was described as remarkably shy and withdrawn.

Relationship of DLS to the NLD Syndrome

The pattern of neuropsychological assets and deficits displayed by children with mild DLS shares virtually all of the clinical features of the syndrome of NLD (Rourke, 1989).

The primary neuropsychological deficits displayed by children with NLD are in tactile perception, visual perception, and complex motor skills, as well as in the ability to deal effectively with novel material. These deficits are hypothesized to eventuate in deficient tactile and visual attention, as well as restricted exploratory behavior. There are no accounts of the performance of children with mild DLS on tactile-perceptual tasks. However, psychomotor skills are consistently found to be delayed in these children. In addition, they are reported to demonstrate significantly impaired visual-perceptual, visual–motor, and visual–spatial–organizational skills. Attention to visual detail has also been found to be severely impaired; there are other reports of limited concentration and attention in these children as well. Although their ability to deal with novel material has not been specifically addressed, Jackson (1992) has remarked that children with mild DLS require a structured environment and are adverse to disruptions in their daily routine—characteristics of children who experience significant difficulties in dealing with novelty.

The secondary deficits of the NLD syndrome are seen to lead to memory problems for information delivered through the tactile and visual modalities, and to deficits in concept formation and problem solving. Relative assets are found in the auditory and verbal realm, specifically with respect to auditory perception, rote verbal material, and memory and attention for auditory and verbal information. Memory, concept formation, and problem solving have not been widely addressed in the DLS literature. However, significantly impaired memory for complex visual information, in the presence of average to above-average rote memory and memory for verbal material, were demonstrated in the case described by Stefanatos and Musikoff (1994).

Many dimensions of speech and language in children with NLD are thought to reflect their more basic neuropsychological assets, including auditory perception, attention, and memory. Thus, these children are found to display well-developed phonological skills, verbal repetition, verbal reception, and verbal storage. Various linguistic deficits (e.g., repetitive, rote speech; poor psycholinguistic pragmatics; minimal speech prosody; and reliance on language for social relating, information gathering, and relief from anxiety) are proposed to arise from primary and secondary deficits in the child with NLD.

There are many aspects of speech and language development in children with mild DLS that remain to be explored. In general, however, these children are reported to display delayed development of language and to show more advanced receptive than expressive language skills. There is also evidence to suggest that their speech and language improve with age. Indeed, the young girl described by Stefanatos and Musikoff (1994) performed consistently within average limits on verbal measures. Children with mild DLS have not been observed to produce large volumes of verbal output, as is characteristic of children with NLD.

It is important to note that several aspects of DLS are likely to have an impact on language development. Various abnormalities of the speech mechanism have been reported, including a small mandible, anteverted nostrils, small nose, wide space between the mouth and nose, downturned lips, cleft palate and poor palatal function, and malspaced teeth. Moore (1970) further notes that other anomalies may be significant in impaired speech production, including short thick neck, webbing of the neck, poor feeding habits, sucking and swallowing difficulties, regurgitation, and general muscular hypotonia. Moreover, hearing loss is a characteristic feature of DLS and has been shown to play a significant role in language development. Thus, it is likely that the area of least overlap between DLS and the NLD syndrome would lie in the domain of speech output.

In the academic realm, children with NLD are found to experience difficulty in mechanical arithmetic, mathematics, reading comprehension, and science. Relative strengths are found in word decoding, spelling, and verbatim memory. The reports of academic achievement in children with DLS are limited because of their typically young age. However, in the report by Stefanatos and Musikoff (1994), a 14-year-old girl with DLS was found to demonstrate the pattern of academic performance characteristic of NLD—that is, well-developed single-word oral reading and spelling, but deficient mechanical arithmetic skills.

Children with NLD are also found to display disturbed psychosocial and emotional functioning, typically of an internalized nature. Shyness, social withdrawal, and social immaturity are reported both for children with DLS and for those with NLD. The more severe emotional problems documented in older individuals with NLD have not been reported in individuals with DLS. However, the research on this area of functioning in DLS is quite limited.

Summary

An area of clinical concern with DLS is the widening of accepted diagnostic criteria and greater recognition of the wide clinical variability of the syndrome (Jackson, 1992). Traditionally, there has been a tendency to recognize only the more severe variant of DLS; however, there has been increasing appreciation of the existence of a mild form of DLS. These children typically demonstrate mildly delayed growth, an absence of limb reduction abnormalities, more subtle facial characteristics, and cognitive functioning in the normal to mildly or moderately impaired range. The importance of considering individuals with more subtle expressions of DLS lies in the possibility of uncovering other manifestations of the syndrome. One contribution in this respect may be the striking resemblance between the pattern of neuropsychological assets and deficits and of socioemotional functioning shown by children with mild DLS, and that shown by children displaying the developmental manifestations of the NLD syndrome.

WHITE MATTER INVOLVEMENT

In addition to a characteristic pattern of neuropsychological assets and deficits, a relationship between NLD and white matter dysfunction has been hypothesized (Rourke, 1989). Specifically, it is proposed that damage to white matter may explain some of the common neuropsychological, linguistic, academic, and psychosocial/adaptive deficits that are features of the NLD syndrome. Although detailed investigations of white matter involvement have not been carried out for individuals who exhibit DLS, there is evidence to suggest a role for white matter dysfunction in the expression of DLS.

DLS represents a dysmorphogenic disorder characterized by multiple malformations and deformations. Morphogenesis is thought to be guided by genetic information, and the entire process is considered to be programmed in a precisely timed and orderly manner that leaves little room for deviation from a preordained course (Jones, 1988). A defect in morphogenesis is likely to affect the development of brain structures and the formation and migration of neurons (Lyon & Beaugerie, 1988). The overall results are, therefore, a reduction in numbers of neurons and abnormalities in the arrangement of cortical neurons. These anomalies, in turn, are thought to affect the formation and organization of axonal connections in the brain—that is, to affect the development of white matter pathways.

DLS is diagnosed on the basis of a pattern of clinical features. However, the principal phenotypical developmental defect in DLS is growth deficiency, which is prenatal in its onset and continues into postnatal life. Growth deficiency may reflect a genetically determined abnormality in development that also yields multiple secondary effects. This proposed primary disturbance in growth manifests itself in small stature and microcephaly, and may be responsible for generating the dysmorphic features associated with DLS (Villee & Najjar, 1994).

Fetal defects that arise early in gestation from the effects of a chromosome abnormality are found to interfere with cell growth, may cause a reduction in cell numbers and may affect cell migration (Lyon & Beaugerie, 1988; Villee & Najjar, 1994). There is a range of evidence to suggest the primacy of delayed maturation and impaired development in DLS. Several characteristic features of DLS that are indicative in this respect are hirsutism of the lanugo type, cleft palate, ventricular septal defects, syndactyly, undescended testes, and pelvic kidney. Each of these defects represents a deviation in the normal process of morphogenesis and is suggestive of underdevelopment. Lanugo hair that typically covers the body of the fetus is characteristic of premature births. Cleft palate represents inadequate growth of the palatal shelves, and septal defects involve a failure of growth in masses of connective tissue. Syndactyly may reflect a failure in the process of controlled cell death that is involved in the demise of tissue between the digits to allow separation of the fingers and toes. Undescended testes and pelvic kidney represent an embryonic pattern of development that is retained instead of the adult formation (Patten, 1968).

Further evidence is provided by the results of autopsy studies, which have revealed a wide range of anomalies present in the nervous system structures of individuals with DLS. Abnormalities in the pituitary gland, including the complete absence of basophil cells, have been described. Hypoplasia of the thyroid gland and of the adrenal glands has been found with some frequency. Hypoplastic tissue structures are underdeveloped and typically reduced in size. A cyst in the Rathke pouch was observed in one report (Björklöf & Brundelet, 1965). Cells from the Rathke pouch normally become interspersed with those of the anterior lobe of the pituitary, but in some cases remnants may persist at the boundary of the posterior lobe of the pituitary; these result in small cysts (Greenspan & Baxter, 1994).

Decreased numbers of neurons, increased numbers of astrocytes, and diffuse cortical gliosis are also commonly observed. Reduced numbers of neurons could result from an insufficiency in the production of neurons, exaggeration of the normal phenomenon of spontaneous cell death, or an arrest of cell growth (Lyon & Beaugerie, 1988). Anomalies in white matter development are reported with some frequency. The white matter anomalies observed indicate slowed maturation, underdevelopment, and possible degeneration of myelin.

Microcephaly is also consistently found in individuals with DLS. Microcephaly may be characterized both by a decreased number of neurons (neuronal proliferation) and by abnormal configurations (migration anomalies) (Menkes, 1990). In DLS, abnormalities of neurogenesis are more prevalent than are anomalies associated with abnormal cell migration. This finding may reflect the fact that cellular differentiation is controlled by DNA activity, whereas cellular migration is controlled by metabolic mechanisms (Menkes, 1990), and there is little evidence to suggest that DLS is a metabolic disorder. It is also notable that primary microcephaly is associated with dysmorphic facial features and with various neurosensorial and visceral defects (Lyon & Beaugerie, 1988). A direct linear relationship between severity of microcephaly and intelligence has also been demonstrated (Menkes, 1990). Thus, several features of DLS may in fact be associated with primary microcephaly.

The normal features that occur during morphogenesis include proper migration of the cells to predetermined locations, regulated rate of cell division, controlled cell death, and mechanical forces. An aberration in any of these features could lead to abnormal fetal development (Jones, 1988). Thus, a malformation (e.g., microcephaly) could lead to deformations (e.g., characteristic facies) because the mechanical forces are altered. The manifestations of DLS may be associated with a defect of a primary genetic determination in any or all of these systems. The fundamental outcome of this defect in morphogenesis is thought to be a disorder of growth that manifests itself in short stature and microcephaly. In addition, however, there are resultant secondary effects that probably have an impact on fetal development and on the expression of DLS.

The genetic potential for growth and development is also dependent upon an adequate supply of oxygen, certain nutrients and vitamins, and hormones (Jones, 1988). Jones (1988) notes that severe problems in the development and function of the brain, pituitary gland, thyroid gland, lungs, heart, liver, intestines, or kidneys usually do not have an adverse effect on prenatal growth. However, each of these problems can increase the likelihood of serious postnatal growth deficiency. Cells require an adequate supply of oxygen, nutrients, and water for growth, and this may be compromised by organ defects. Children with DLS display numerous organ anomalies, and there is strong evidence of poor nutrition resulting from GI abnormalities (such as gastroesophageal reflux), as well as compromised cardiovascular functioning and increased susceptibility to infection in DLS.

In addition, an argument can be advanced for the role of endocrine dysfunction in the expression of DLS. The hypothalamus and pituitary glands regulate the function of several endocrine glands, including the thyroid gland, adrenal glands, and gonads (Greenspan & Baxter, 1994). Factors from the hypothalamus regulate the synthesis and release of hormones from the anterior pituitary gland. The anterior pituitary hormones include TSH, adrenocorticotropic hormone (ACTH), FSH, luteinizing hormone (LH), and HGH. These hormones act on specific target tissues in the body to influence the production and release of the final hormones, which include thyroid hormone, glucocorticoids, sex hormones, and IGF-1 (Villee & Najjar, 1994). A review of the endocrine studies shows no consistent abnormality of functioning in DLS. However, a role for pituitary function in the expression of DLS is suggested by the findings. Children with DLS have been reported to demonstrate thyroid deficiency, adrenocortical insufficiency, deficiency in TSH secretion, HGH deficiency, and low levels of IGF-1.

Hypoplasia of the pituitary, thyroid, and adrenal glands is a frequent finding in the autopsy studies. Hypoplasia involves poor development of the gland and can lead to a reduction in size. The consequences of underdevelopment and reduced size of the gland are impaired synthesis and secretion of hormones. Irregularities in the basophil cells of the pituitary gland are also frequently reported. Basophil cells are found in the anterior lobe of the pituitary gland. Thyrotrophs (TSH-secreting cells), corticotrophs (ACTH-secreting cells), and gonadotrophs (LH- and FSH-secreting cells) originate from basophil cells (Greenspan & Baxter, 1994). An absence or reduction of the number of basophil cells in the pituitary gland is likely to have an impact upon the secretion of the anterior pituitary hormones, including TSH, ACTH, LH, and FSH. Reduced production of hormones by the pituitary gland may in turn lead to inadequate development of the thyroid and adrenal glands (Crowley, 1974; Greenspan & Baxter, 1994). Pituitary defects may also account for the usual presence of undescended testes in males with DLS (Gray & Skandalakis, 1972; Jones, 1988).

FSH and LH, secreted by the anterior pituitary gland, stimulate the fetal gonads to produce estradiol or testosterone during the first months of pregnancy (Greenspan & Baxter, 1994; Villee & Najjar, 1994). Thus, a reduction in the production or secretion of these hormones may decrease stimulus to early testicular development. Finally, although there is little evidence to suggest a role for HGH in fetal growth, this pituitary hormone is thought to be necessary for normal growth postnatally (Villee & Najjar, 1994).

Defects in the endocrine glands affect the release of hormones that are essential for growth and maturation. IGF-1 and insulin may play a significant role in fetal growth (Greenspan & Baxter, 1994; Villee &

Najjar, 1994). In addition, IGF-1 is involved in the regulation of stem cell growth and differentiation (Villee & Najjar, 1994). Glucocorticoids, in excess, inhibit growth and bone maturation by decreasing cell proliferation and the synthesis of RNA, protein, and collagen (Greenspan & Baxter, 1994). Glucocorticoids are also found to accelerate the development of a number of systems and organs (such as the lungs, liver, and GI tract) in fetal and differentiating tissues (Greenspan & Baxter, 1994).

Thyroid hormone is thought to be a significant factor in the maturation of the CNS. Adequate levels of thyroid hormone are required for normal prenatal development of the CNS (Crowley, 1974; Greenspan & Baxter, 1994). Specifically, this hormone has been found to be necessary for cell proliferation, neuronal differentiation, axonal and dendritic growth, gliogenesis, myelinogenesis, and synaptogenesis (Lauder & Krebs, 1986). In addition to influencing tissue growth and brain maturation, thyroid hormone affects growth at the pituitary level by regulating the synthesis and secretion of HGH (Villee & Najjar, 1994). Thyroid hormone also regulates the rate of fetal metabolic processes and has a marked positive effect on the heart, cardiac output, and gut motility (Greenspan & Baxter, 1994).

The hypothalamus develops endocrine function by 6 to 7 gestational weeks, and the anterior pituitary gland is functional at 7 to 8 weeks. The fetal thyroid gland begins to secrete thyroid hormone by 10 to 12 gestational weeks and is fully active at 20 weeks (Greenspan & Baxter, 1994). This development coincides with the beginning of a spurt in brain growth. This spurt, which continues well into the second year of life, is characterized by a phase of rapid multiplication of glial cells, differentiation of neurons and glial cells, and the rapid growth of axonal and dendritic processes that permit the establishment of neuronal circuits and connections (Jones, 1988; Menkes, 1990; Morreale de Escobar, Escobar del Rey, & Ruiz-Marcos, 1983).

Although most neurons are present at birth, few fiber tracts are completely myelinated at birth; the period of most rapid myelination occurs within the first 2 years of life (Dietrich & Bradley, 1988; Menkes, 1990; Rourke, Bakker, Fisk, & Strang, 1983). In addition, it has been shown that the growth spurts that take place in the brain postnatally occur without a concurrent increase in neuronal proliferation; that is, cell proliferation and migration are complete at birth. Instead, the growth of dendritic processes, synaptogenesis, and myelination is thought to account for these postnatal increases in brain weight (Kolb & Fantie, 1989). These findings suggest that the development of axonal connections and of white matter pathways, as well as the process of myelination, is far from complete in the brain of the newborn.

Thus, it is conceivable that an effect of developmental defects in the infant with DLS is the alteration of white matter formation. The late specification of neuronal connectivity suggests that environmental factors are more likely to exert an influence on white matter pathways. Menkes (1990) notes that CNS myelination is particularly vulnerable to malnutrition, which can be the cause of a reduction in myelin synthesis and dendrite density, and of a proliferation of oligodendrocytes. Furthermore, impaired endocrine function doubtless affects CNS maturation and white matter development postnatally.

In addition, it is important to acknowledge that grey and white matter anomalies are associated with the proposed primary aspect of DLS—a defect in morphogenesis leading to growth deficiency and manifesting itself in short stature and microcephaly. These prenatal defects in neuronal proliferation and migration may lead to both structural and functional reorganization in the brain: Alternate pathways and connections may be formed to compensate for these primary deficits. In the first instance, the development and organization of axonal connections depend upon the number and location of cortical neurons. Furthermore, dendritic arborization and synaptic development are related to early cell migration (Menkes, 1990).

To sum up, two mechanisms have been proposed to play a role in the expression of DLS: (1) a primary growth deficiency of genetic origin, which presents with short stature, microcephaly, and multiple deformations, and (2) secondary effects of poor organ and endocrine development, affecting nutrition, oxygen requirements, and hormone production and secretion. Thus, a genetic determination *in utero* is proposed for the disorder, and this is thought to be exacerbated postnatally by structural and functional complications. In either case, an influence on CNS development and maturation, affecting both grey and white matter, is probable. It is hypothesized that an altered pattern of synaptic connection and axonal projections is generated by both the primary and secondary mechanisms involved in the expression of DLS. Moreover, this anomalous pattern of white matter development is thought to account for features of the NLD syndrome—that is, to be related to a specific pattern of neuropsychological assets and deficits. Variations in the severity of dysmorphogenesis in DLS are probably also reflected in variations in the severity of expression of the deficits of the NLD syndrome.

FUTURE DIRECTIONS

The variable expression of complex disorders such as DLS makes diagnosis a difficult enterprise. As yet, the boundaries of the syndrome have not been well defined; this underscores the need for more far-reaching research in this area. In particular, future directions in DLS research should include extensive imaging and postmortem studies. Detailed neuroanatomical study is fundamental to uncovering pathophysiological changes in the disorder. In addition, there is evidence to suggest that an association exists between DLS and hypothalamic–pituitary dysfunction. Further neuropathological studies are needed to investigate the role of endocrine function in the development of DLS. It has also been proposed that poor maturation of structure and function of organ systems, particularly of the CNS, is involved in DLS. Further exploration concerning how these defects contribute to the expression of DLS would appear to be particularly worthwhile. Technological advances, particularly in the area of genetic research, are also likely to yield interesting new developments in the definition of the syndrome and its etiology.

The recognition of clinical syndromes is also enhanced by comprehensive neuropsychological examination. Expanding the syndrome definition of DLS, particularly with respect to the severity of expression of cognitive factors, will help to generate a wider range of cases for study. An examination of these "atypical" cases may reveal previously unidentified expressions of the disorder, which may in turn contribute to our understanding of its nature and origins.

In addition, there have been reports of unaffected children born to parents displaying DLS (Halal & Silver, 1992; Mosher et al., 1985; Robinson et al., 1985). The appearance of these children was not suggestive of DLS (although they typically displayed a few isolated features), and development appeared to be taking place in an age-appropriate manner. It would be interesting to conduct more rigorous neuropsychological evaluations of these children, in order to determine whether they manifest the NLD syndrome. These children may in fact represent the mildest extreme on a continuum of severity in this disorder. In general, more extensive neuropsychological assessment of a wide range (i.e., with respect to severity of expression) of children with DLS at varying ages is needed, to define the limits of the disorder more clearly.

DLS probably has its origins in a variety of factors of variable significance. The combination of factors in any individual case may be different, and thus may engender a slightly different expression of the disorder. The recognition of clinical syndromes by physical, radiological/imaging, and neuropsychological examination becomes an important endeavor, because it permits the identification of unifying principles that may enhance our conception of the syndrome and gauge the limits of its variability. The NLD/white matter hypothesis is interesting in this respect, because it affords another avenue by which to distinguish DLS. Moreover, it represents a view in which pathophysiological and neuropsychological findings may be integrated to account for the total expression of this and other disorders.

CONCLUSION

The phenotype of DLS is, almost without exception, identical to the "developmental" presentation of NLD. The neuropsychological assets and deficits in the mild presentation of DLS are virtually the same as those posited as typical of NLD. What remain to be determined are (1) the dynamic interactions of the assets and deficits in DLS, and (2) the precise role that white matter perturbations may play in this developmental mix. Of course, the mediating role of hormonal influences in the developmental scenario that eventuates in DLS appears to be an extremely important dimension to investigate. These complex interactional systems, in conjunction with the phenotypical physical anomalies in the craniofacial and cardiac realms, would suggest strongly that the link between the NLD behavioral phenotype and other neurodevelopmental disorders with these same features (e.g., velocardiofacial syndrome, Williams syndrome, etc.; see other chapters in this book) do, in fact, describe a final common pathway of white matter disease and dysfunction. Only further research, guided by such hypotheses, will resolve these complex issues.

REFERENCES

Abraham, J. M., & Russell, A. (1968). de Lange syndrome: A study of nine examples. *Acta Paediatrica Scandinavica, 57*, 339–353.

Bankier, A., Haan, E., & Birrell, R. (1986). Familial occurrence of Brachmann–de Lange syndrome [Letter to the editor]. *American Journal of Medical Genetics, 25*, 163–165.

Barr, A. N., Grabow, J. ., Matthews, C. G., Grosse, F. R., Motl, M. L., & Opitz, J. M. (1971). Neurologic and psychometric findings in the Brachmann–de Lange syndrome. *Neuropädiatrie, 3*(1), 46–66.

Bay, C., Mauk, J., Radcliffe, J., & Kaplan, P. (1993). Mild Brachmann–de Lange syndrome: Delineation of the clinical phenotype, and characteristic behaviors in a six-year-old boy. *American Journal of Medical Genetics, 47*, 965–968.

Beck, B. (1974). Familial occurrence of Cornelia de Lange's syndrome. *Acta Paediatrica Scandinavica, 63*, 225–231.

Beck, B. (1976). Epidemiology of Cornelia de Lange's syndrome. *Acta Paediatrica Scandinavica, 65*, 631–638.

Beck, B. (1987). Psycho-social assessment of 36 de Lange patients. *Journal of Mental Deficiency Research, 31*, 251–257.

Beck, B., & Fenger, K. (1985). Mortality, pathological findings and causes of death in the de Lange syndrome. *Acta Paediatrica Scandinavica, 74*, 765–769.

Beck, B., & Mikkelsen, M. (1981). Chromosomes in the Cornelia de Lange syndrome. *Human Genetics, 59*, 271–276.

Beratis, N. G., Hsu, L. Y. F., & Hirschhorn, K. (1971). Familial de Lange syndrome: Report of three cases in a sibship. *Clinical Genetics, 2*, 170–176.

Berg, J. M., McCreary, B. D., Ridler, M. A. C., & Smith, G. F. (1970). *The de Lange syndrome*. Oxford: Pergamon Press.

Bergsma, D. (Ed.). (1979). *Birth defects compendium* (2nd ed.). New York: Alan R. Liss.

Björklöf, K., & Brundelet, P .J. (1965). Typus degenerativus Amstelodamensis (Cornelia de Lange first syndrome): Congenital hypopituitarism due to a cyst of Rathke's Cleft? *Acta Paediatrica Scandinavica, 54*, 275–287.

Brachmann, W. (1916). Ein fall von symmetrischer monodaktylie durch ulnadefekt, mit symmetrishcer flughautbildung in den ellenbogen sowie anderen abnormalitaten. *Jahrbuch für Kinderheilkunde und Physische Erziehung, 84*, 225–235.

Braddock, S. R., Lachman, R. S., Stoppenhagen, C. C., Carey, J. C., Ireland, M., Moeschler, J. B., Cunniff, C., & Graham, J. M. (1993). Radiological features in Brachmann–de Lange syndrome. *American Journal of Medical Genetics, 47*, 1006–1013.

Breslau, E. J., Disteche, C., Hall, J. G., Thuline, H., & Cooper, P. (1981). Prometaphase chromosomes in five patients with the Brachmann–de Lange syndrome. *American Journal of Medical Genetics, 10*, 179–186.

Bruner, J. P., & Hsia, Y. E. (1990). Prenatal findings in Brachmann–de Lange syndrome. *Obstetrics and Gynecology, 76*(5, Pt. 2), 966–968.

Brylewski, J. (1978). A typical case of Cornelia de Lange's syndrome. *British Medical Journal, i*, 756.

Bull, M. J., Fitzgerald, J. F., Heifetz, S. A., & Brei, T. J. (1993). Gastrointestinal abnormalities: A significant cause of feeding difficulties and failure to thrive in Brachmann–de Lange syndrome. *American Journal of Medical Genetics, 47*, 1029–1034.

Cameron, T. H., & Kelly, D. P. (1988). Normal language skills and normal intelligence in a child with de Lange syndrome. *Journal of Speech and Hearing Disorders, 53*, 219–222.

Carakushansky, G., & Berthier, C. (1976). The de Lange syndrome in one of twins. *Journal of Medical Genetics, 13*, 404–406.

Cates, M., Billmire, D. F., Bull, M. J., & Grosfeld, J. L. (1989). Gastroesophageal dysfunction in Cornelia de Lange syndrome. *Journal of Pediatric Surgery, 24*(3), 248–250.

Crowley, L. V. (1974). *An introduction to clinical embryology*. Chicago: Year Book Medical.

de Die-Smulders, C., Theunissen, P., & Schrander-Stumpel, C. (1992). On the variable expression of the Brachmann–de Lange syndrome. *Clinical Genetics, 41*, 42–45.

de Lange, C. (1933). Sur un type nouveau dégénération (typus Amstelodamensis). *Archives de Médecine des Enfants, 36*, 713–719.

Delitala, G. (1989). Clinical neuropharmacology in the management of disorders of the pituitary and hypothalamus. In L. J. DeGroot (Ed.), *Endocrinology* (2nd ed., Vol. 1, pp. 454–502). Philadelphia: W. B. Saunders.

Dietrich, R. B., & Bradley, W. G. (1988). Normal and abnormal white matter maturation. *Seminars in Ultrasound, CT, and MR, 9*(3), 192–200.

Falek, A., Schmidt, R., & Jarvis, G. (1966). Familial de Lange syndrome with chromosome abnormalities. *Pediatrics, 37*(1), 92–101.

Filippi, G. (1989). The de Lange syndrome: Report of 15 cases. *Clinical Genetics, 35*, 343–363.

France, N. E., Crome, L., & Abraham, J. M. (1969). Pathological features in the de Lange syndrome. *Acta Paediatrica Scandinavica, 58*, 470–480.

Francke, U., & Opitz, J. M. (1979). Chromosome 3q duplication and the Brachmann–de Lange syndrome (BDLS). *Journal of Pediatrics, 95*, 161–162.

Fraser, W. I., & Campbell, B. M. (1978). A study of six cases of de Lange Amsterdam dwarf syndrome, with special attention to voice, speech and language characteristics. *Developmental Medicine and Child Neurology, 20*, 189–198.

Fryns, J. P. (1986). On the nosology of the Cornelia de Lange and Coffin–Siris syndromes. *Clinical Genetics, 29*, 263–264.

Fryns, J. P., Dereymaeker, A. M., Hoefnagels, M., D'Hondt, F., Mertens, G., & van den Berghe, H. (1987). The Brachmann–de Lange syndrome in two siblings of normal parents. *Clinical Genetics, 31*, 413–415.

Gadoth, N., Lerman, M., Garty, B.-Z., & Shumuelewitz, O. (1982). Normal intelligence in the Cornelia de Lange syndrome. *Johns Hopkins Medical Journal, 150*, 70–72.

Goodban, M. T. (1993). Survey of speech and language skills with prognostic indicators in 116 patients with Cornelia de Lange syndrome. *American Journal of Medical Genetics, 47*, 1059–1063.

Greenberg, A., & Coleman, M. (1973). Depressed whole blood serotonin levels associated with behavioral abnormalities in the de Lange syndrome. *Pediatrics, 52*(5), 720–723.

Greenberg, F., & Robinson, L. K. (1989). Mild Brachmann–de Lange syndrome: Changes of phenotype with age. *American Journal of Medical Genetics, 32*, 90–92.

Greenspan, F. S., & Baxter, J. D. (1994). *Basic and clinical endocrinology* (4th ed.). Norwalk, CT: Appleton & Lange.

Gray, S. W., & Skandalakis, J. E. (1972). *Embryology for surgeons*. Philadelphia: W. B. Saunders.

Halal, F., & Preus, M. (1979). The hand profile in de Lange syndrome: Diagnostic criteria. *American Journal of Medical Genetics, 3*, 317–323.

Halal, F., & Silver, K. (1992). Syndrome of microcephaly, Brachmann–de Lange-like facial changes, severe metatarsus adductus, and developmental delay: Mild Brachmann–de Lange syndrome? *American Journal of Medical Genetics, 42*, 381–386.

Hall, J. G. (1990). Genomic imprinting: Review and relevance to human diseases. *American Journal of Human Genetics, 46*, 857–873.

Hart, Z. H., Jaslow, R. I., & Gomez, M. (1965). The de Lange syndrome. *American Journal of Diseases of Children, 109*, 325–332.

Hawley, P. P., Jackson, L. G., & Kurnit, D. M. (1985). Sixty-four patients with Brachmann–de Lange syndrome: A survey. *American Journal of Medical Genetics, 20*, 453–459.

Heckmann, H., Ang, L. C., Casey, R., George, D. H., Lowry, N., & Shokeir, M. H. K. (1991–1992). Leigh's disease with clinical manifestations of Cornelia de Lange syndrome. *Pediatric Neurosurgery, 17*(4), 192–195.

Hersh, J. H., Dale, K. S., Gerald, P. S., Yen, F. F., Weisskopf, B., & Dinno, N. D. (1985). Dup(4p)del(9p) in a familial mental retardation syndrome. *American Journal of Diseases of Children*, *139*, 81–84.

Hillman, J. C., Hammond, J., Noé, O., & Reiss, M. (1968). Endocrine investigations in De Lange's and Seckel's syndromes. *American Journal of Mental Deficiency*, *73*, 30–33.

Ireland, M., English, C., Cross, I., Houlsby, W. T., & Burn, J. (1991). A *de novo* translocation t(3;17)(q26.3;q26.1) in a child with Cornelia de Lange syndrome. *Journal of Medical Genetics*, *28*, 639–640.

Jackson, L. G. (1992). de Lange syndrome. *American Journal of Medical Genetics*, *42*, 377–378.

Jackson, L. G., Kline, A. D., Barr, M. A., & Koch, S. (1993). de Lange syndrome: A clinical review of 310 individuals. *American Journal of Medical Genetics*, *47*, 940–946.

Johnson, H. G., Ekman, P., Friesen, W., Nyhan, W. L., & Shear, C. (1976). A behavioral phenotype in the de Lange syndrome. *Pediatric Research*, *10*, 843–850.

Jones, K. L. (Ed.). (1988). *Smith's recognizable patterns of human malformation* (4th ed.). Philadelphia: W.B. Saunders.

Joubin, J., Pettrone, C. F., & Pettrone, F. A. (1982). Cornelia de Lange's syndrome. *Clinical Orthopaedics and Related Research*, *171*, 180–185.

Kline, A. D., Barr, M., & Jackson, L. G. (1993). Growth manifestations in the Brachmann–de Lange syndrome. *American Journal of Medical Genetics*, *47*, 1042–1049.

Kolb, B., & Fantie, B. (1989). Development of the child's brain and behavior. In C. Reynolds & E. Fletcher-Janzen (Eds.), *Handbook of clinical child neuropsychology* (pp. 17–39). New York: Plenum Press.

Kousseff, B. G., Thomson-Meares, J., Newkirk, P., & Root, A. W. (1993). Physical growth in Brachmann–de Lange syndrome. *American Journal of Medical Genetics*, *47*, 1050–1052.

Kumar, D., Blank, C. E., & Griffiths, B. L. (1985). Cornelia de Lange syndrome in several members of the same family. *Journal of Medical Genetics*, *22*, 296–300.

Kurlander, G. J., & DeMyer, W. (1967). Roentgenology of the Brachmann–de Lange Syndrome. *Radiology*, *88*, 101–110.

Lacourt, G. C., Arendt, J., Cox, J., & Béguin, F. (1977). Microcephalic dwarfism with associated low amniotic fluid 5-hydroxyindole-3-acetic acid (5HIAA): Report of a case of Cornelia de Lange syndrome. *Helvetica Paediatrica Acta*, *32*, 149–154.

Lakshminarayana, P., & Nallasivam, P. (1990). Cornelia de Lange syndrome with ring chromosome 3. *Journal of Medical Genetics*, *27*, 405–406.

Lauder, J. M., & Krebs, H. (1986). Do neurotransmitters, neurohumors, and hormones specify critical periods? In W. T. Greenough & J. M. Juraska (Eds.), *Developmental neuropsychobiology* (pp. 119–174). Orlando, FL: Academic Press.

Leavitt, A., Dinno, N., & Davis, C. (1985). Cornelia de Lange syndrome in a mother and daughter. *Clinical Genetics*, *28*, 157–161.

Leroy, J. G., Persijn, J., Van de Weghe, V., Van Hecke, R., Oostra, A., De Bie, S., & Craen, M. (1993). On the variability of the Brachmann–de Lange syndrome in seven patients. *American Journal of Medical Genetics, 47,* 983–991.

Levin, A. V., Seidman, D. J., Nelson, L. B., & Jackson, L. G. (1990). Ophthalmologic findings in the Cornelia de Lange syndrome. *Journal of Pediatric Ophthalmology and Strabismus, 27*(2), 94–102.

Lieber, E., Glaser, J. H., & Jhaveri, R. (1973). Brachmann–de Lange syndrome: Report of two cases in a sibship. *American Journal of Diseases of Children, 125,* 717–718.

Lyon, G., & Beaugerie, A. (1988). Congenital developmental malformations. In M. I. Levene, M. J. Bennett, & J. Punt (Eds.), *Fetal and neonatal neurology and neurosurgery* (pp. 229–248). Edinburgh: Churchill Livingstone.

McArthur, R. G., & Edwards, J. H. (1967). de Lange syndrome: Report of 20 cases. *Canadian Medical Association Journal, 96*(17), 1185–1198.

McIntire, M. S., & Eisen, J. D. (1965). The Cornelia de Lange syndrome: A case report with mild mental retardation. *American Journal of Mental Deficiency, 70,* 438–442.

Menkes, J. H. (1990). *Textbook of child neurology* (4th ed.). Philadelphia: Lea & Febiger.

Merikangas, J. R., Merikangas, K., Katz, L., & Pan, S. (1977). Chromosome banding study of the Cornelia de Lange syndrome. *Human Genetics, 39,* 217–219.

Moeschler, J. B., & Graham, J. M. (1993). Mild Brachmann–de Lange syndrome: Phenotypic and developmental characteristics of mildly affected individuals. *American Journal of Medical Genetics, 47,* 969–976.

Moore, M. V. (1970). Speech, hearing, and language in de Lange syndrome. *Journal of Speech and Hearing Disorders, 35,* 66–69.

Morreale de Escobar, G., Escobar del Rey, F., & Ruiz-Marcos, A. (1983). Thyroid hormone and the developing brain. In J. H. Dussault & P. Walker (Eds.), *Congenital hypothyroidism* (pp. 85–126). New York: Marcel Dekker.

Mosher, G. A., Schulte, R. L., Kaplan, P. A., Buehler, B. A., & Sanger, W. G. (1985). Brief clinical report: Pregnancy in a woman with the Brachmann–de Lange syndrome. *American Journal of Medical Genetics, 22,* 103–107.

Motl, M. L., & Opitz, J. M. (1971). Studies of malformation syndromes XXVA: Phenotypic and genetic studies of the Brachmann–de Lange syndrome. *Human Heredity, 21,* 1–16.

Naguib, K. K., Teebi, A. S., Al-Awadi, S. A., & Marafie, M. J. (1987). Brachmann–de Lange syndrome in sibs. *Journal of Medical Genetics, 24,* 627–629.

Nyhan, W. L., & Sakati, N. O. (1976). *Genetic and malformation syndromes in clinical medicine.* Chicago: Year Book Medical.

Opitz, J. M. (1985). Editorial comment: The Brachmann–de Lange syndrome. *American Journal of Medical Genetics, 22,* 89–102.

Opitz, J. M., & Smith, D. W. (1966). Familial de Lange syndrome with chromosome abnormalities. *Pediatrics, 37*(6), 1028–1029.

Partington, M. W. (1990). Rubinstein–Taybi syndrome: A follow-up study. *American Journal of Medical Genetics* (Suppl. 6), 65–68.

Pashayan, H., Levy, E. P., & Fraser, F. C. (1970). Can the de Lange syndrome always be diagnosed at birth? *Pediatrics*, *46*(6), 940–942.

Pashayan, H., Whelan, D., Guttman, S., & Fraser, F.C. (1969). Variability of the de Lange syndrome: Report of 3 cases and genetic analysis of 54 families. *Journal of Pediatrics*, *75*(5), 853–858.

Passarge, E., Mecke, S., & Altrogge, H. C. (1971). Cornelia de Lange syndrome: Evolution of the phenotype. *Pediatrics*, *48*(5), 833–836.

Patten, B. M. (1968). *Human embryology* (3rd ed.). New York: McGraw-Hill.

Preus, M., & Rex, A. P. (1983). Definition and diagnosis of the Brachmann–de Lange syndrome. *American Journal of Medical Genetics*, *16*, 301–312.

Punnett, H. H., & Zakai, E. H. (1990). Old syndromes and new cytogenics. *Developmental Medicine and Child Neurology*, *32*, 820–831.

Robinson, L. K., Wolfsberg, E., & Jones, K. L. (1985). Brachmann–de Lange syndrome: Evidence for autosomal dominant inheritance. *American Journal of Medical Genetics*, *22*, 109–115.

Rosenbach, Y., Zahavi, I., & Dinari, G. (1992). Gastroesophageal dysfunction in Brachmann–de Lange syndrome. *American Journal of Medical Genetics*, *42*, 379–380.

Rourke, B. P. (1989). *Nonverbal learning disabilities: The syndrome and the model.* New York: Guilford Press.

Rourke, B. P., Bakker, D. J., Fisk, J. L., & Strang, J. D. (1983). *Child neuropsychology: An introduction to theory, research, and clinical practice.* New York: Guilford Press.

Saal, H. M., Samango-Sprouse, C. A., Rodnan, L. A., Rosenbaum, K. N., & Custer, D. A. (1993). Brachmann–de Lange syndrome with normal IQ. *American Journal of Medical Genetics*, *47*, 995–998.

Sataloff, R. T., Speigel, J. R., Hawkshaw, M., Epstein, J. M., & Jackson, L. (1990). Cornelia de Lange syndrome: Otolaryngologic manifestations. *Archives of Otolaryngology—Head and Neck Surgery*, *116*, 1044–1046.

Sato, A., Kajita, A., Sugita, K., Izumi, T., Fukuyama, Y., Funata, N., & Okeda, R. (1986). Cornelia de Lange syndrome with intracranial germinoma. *Acta Pathologica Japonica*, *36*(1), 143–149.

Saul, R., Rogers, C., Phelan, M.C., & Stevenson, R.E. (1993). Brachmann–de Lange syndrome: Diagnostic difficulties posed by the mild phenotype. *American Journal of Medical Genetics*, *47*, 999–1002.

Schinzel, A. (1983). *Catalogue of unbalanced chromosome aberrations in man.* Berlin: Walter de Gruyter.

Schlesinger, B., Clayton, B., Bodian, M., & Jones, K. V. (1963). Typus degenerativus Amstelodamensis. *Archives of Disease in Childhood*, *38*, 349–357

Schwartz, I. D., Schwartz, K. J., Kousseff, B. G., Bercu, B. B., & Root, A. W. (1990). Endocrinopathies in Cornelia de Lange syndrome. *Journal of Pediatrics*, *117*(6), 920–923.

Selicorni, A., Lalatta, F., Livini, E., Briscioli, V., Piguzzi, T., Bagozzi, D. C., Mastroiacovo, P., Zampino, G., Gaeta, G., Pugliese, A., Cerutti-Mainaroli, P., Guala, A., Zelante, L., Stabile, M., Belli, S., Freschini, P., Gianotti, A., & Scarano, G. (1993). Variability of the Brachmann–de Lange syndrome. *American Journal of Medical Genetics*, *47*, 977–982.

Silahtaroglu, A. N., Tümer, Z., Kristensen, T., Sottrup-Jensen, L., & Tommerup, N. (1993). Assignment of the human gene for pregnancy-associated plasma protein A (PAPPA) to 9q33.1 by fluorescence in situ hybridization to mitotic and meiotic chromosomes. *Cytogenics and Cell Genetics, 62*, 214–216.

Stefanatos, G. A., & Musikoff, H. (1994). Specific neurocognitive deficits in Cornelia de Lange syndrome. *Journal of Developmental and Behavioral Pediatrics, 15*(1), 39–43.

Steinbach, P., Adkins, W. N., Jr., Caspar, H., Dumars, K. W., Gebauer, J., Gilbert, E. F., Grimm, T., Habedank, M., Hansmann, I., Herrmann, J., Kaveggia, E. G., Langenbeck, U., Meisner, L. F., Najatzadeh, T. M., Opitz, J. M., Palmer, C. G., Peters, H. H., Scholz, W., Tavares, A. S., & Wiedeking, C. (1981). The dup(3q) syndrome: Report of eight cases and review of the literature. *American Journal of Medical Genetics, 10*, 159–177.

Stevenson, R. E., & Scott, C. I. (1976). Discordance for Cornelia de Lange syndrome in twins. *Journal of Medical Genetics, 13*, 402–404.

Tonini, G., & Marinoni, S. (1990). Neonatal-onset panhypopituitarism in a girl with Brachmann–de Lange syndrome. *American Journal of Medical Genetics, 36*, 102–103.

Urion, D. K., Konkel, R. J., & Korf, B. (1994). Neurology. In M. E. Avery, & L. R. First (Eds.), *Pediatric medicine* (2nd ed., pp. 755–804). Baltimore: Williams & Wilkins.

Van Allen, M. I., Filippi, G., Siegel-Bartelt, J., Yong, S.-L., McGillivray, B., Zuker, R. M., Smith, C. R., Magee, J. F., Ritchie, S., Toi, A., & Reynolds, J. F. (1993). Clinical variability within Brachmann–de Lange syndrome: A proposed classification system. *American Journal of Medical Genetics, 47*, 947–958.

Villee, D., & Najjar, S. (1994). Endocrinology. In M. E. Avery & L. R. First (Eds.), *Pediatric medicine* (2nd ed., pp. 887–1011). Baltimore: Williams & Wilkins.

Westergaard, J. G., Chemnitz, J., Teisner, B., Poulsen, H. K., Ipsen, L., Beck, B., & Grudzinskas, J. G. (1983). Pregnancy-associated plasma protein A: A possible marker in the classification and prenatal diagnosis of Cornelia de Lange syndrome. *Prenatal Diagnosis, 3*, 225–232.

Wilson, G. N. (1991). Cornelia de Lange syndrome with ring chromosome 3. *Journal of Medical Genetics, 28*, 143.

Wilson, G. N., Dasouki, M., & Barr, M., Jr. (1985). Further delineation of the dup(3q) syndrome. *American Journal of Medical Genetics, 22*, 117–123.

Wilson, G. N., Pooley, J., & Parker, J. (1982). The phenotype of ring chromosome 3. *Journal of Medical Genetics, 19*, 471–473.

8

Early Hydrocephalus

Jack M. Fletcher
Bonnie L. Brookshire
Timothy P. Bohan
Michael E. Brandt
Kevin C. Davidson

Hydrocephalus is a condition caused by a variety of etiologies that increase the volume of cerebrospinal fluid (CSF) in the ventricular system. This disorder is always secondary to some other pathological event or structural anomaly. For example, children with aqueductal stenosis (AS) do not reabsorb CSF adequately because there is a blockage in the normal CSF circulatory pattern at the aqueduct of Sylvius. AS is often accompanied by other central nervous system (CNS) anomalies, particularly partial agenesis of the corpus callosum. Spina bifida (SB) is a defect in neural tube closure. It is associated with the Arnold–Chiari malformation, which involves neuropathological changes in the cerebellum and hindbrain. This malformation introduces a barrier to CSF outflow from the ventricular system to the subarachnoid. SB is also often associated with other CNS anomalies, particularly corpus callosum deficits. The congenital abnormalities in AS and SB result from early disruptions in neuroembryogenesis. The neural tube closes by the fourth gestational week; the corpus callosum is formed between weeks 8 and 12; and the aqueduct of Sylvius develops between weeks 12 and 16 (Barkovich, 1990). Hence, these multiple anomalies indicate a prolonged rather than a brief disruption in neuroembryogenesis during the first trimester and the early part of the second trimester. There are other congenital causes of hydrocephalus, such as the Dandy–Walker syndrome (see McCullough, 1990).

Other etiologies of hydrocephalus do not reflect congenital abnormalities. Premature infants with intraventricular hemorrhage (IVH) can develop hydrocephalus as a result of blockage of CSF reabsorptive mechanisms. The hemorrhages are in the germinal matrix and parenchyma, and may result in the development of porencephalic cysts. Specific neurological deficits are related to the laterality and severity of the hemorrhage and the resulting porencephalic cyst. These destructive lesions occur in what would normally be the late second- and early third-trimester period (Volpe, 1989). Hence, premature infants have late gestational disruptive lesions, rather than the early gestational anomalies that are seen in patients with SB and AS. Corpus callosum abnormalities may be present because of destructive lesions.

Other etiologies that lead to hydrocephalus are largely postnatal, including meningitis, traumatic brain injury, and a variety of other cerebral insults. In young children the cerebral sutures are not fully fused, so that the skull expands to accommodate ventricular swelling; this expansion leads to the enlarged head (macrocephaly) commonly associated with hydrocephalus. Macrocephaly does not always accompany hydrocephalus in older children, because their cerebral sutures are fused. The disorder results as a consequence of other disease processes that obstruct CSF flow. For example, a tumor can exert pressure on the ventricular system, leading to increased CSF and ventricular dilation. Infectious diseases (e.g., meningitis, Reye syndrome) can lead to general brain swelling, increased intracranial pressure, and hydrocephalus.

CLASSIFICATION

Traditional View

Hydrocephalus has traditionally been classified according to whether (1) the etiology is congenital or postnatal, (2) the condition is communicating or noncommunicating, and (3) the condition is uncomplicated (i.e., only hydrocephalus) or complicated (i.e., hydrocephalus in association with other clinical problems) (see Menkes, 1985). Most congenital forms of hydrocephalus (about 70%) of all cases are noncommunicating, representing obstruction within the ventricular system (usually at the fourth ventricle). The largest category of noncommunicating hydrocephalus is SB, representing dysraphic conditions of the spine with associated brain changes. There are different types of dysraphic lesions. SB occulta is the most common type, occurring in 5% of the population. It is associated with a normal spina cord and brain, but incomplete vertebral arches (Liptak et al., 1988). SB meningocele represents a normal spinal cord with abnormal arches and protrusion of the meninges into soft tissue.

Brain abnormalities are rare in association with SB meningocele. The most severe type of spinal dysraphism is SB meningomyelocele, which is three times more frequent than SB meningocele and has a population rate of 0.4–1.0 per 1000 live births (Liptak et al., 1988). Approximately 95% of children with SB meningomyelocele have a Chiari malformation, and 80–90% develop progressive hydrocephalus, necessitating shunting (Bohan et al., 1994).

Other noncommunicating types of hydrocephalus involve AS and the Dandy–Walker syndrome, both of which represent defects that antedate birth. AS accounts for 20% of all cases of hydrocephalus (Menkes, 1985). It is possible that AS is a mild form of neural tube defect, but some cases seem to be genetically transmitted (Menkes, 1985). Hydrocephalus results from restriction in the size of the aqueduct, blocking CSF flow. The relatively rare Dandy–Walker syndrome is characterized by a failure of the cerebellar midline to develop, with fourth-ventricle occlusions that block CSF flow (McCullough, 1990).

Hydrocephalus that occurs after birth is usually communicating, representing 30% of all cases. In communicating hydrocephalus, obstruction occurs in the subarachnoid spaces, where CSF flow is blocked as it leaves the fourth ventricle to enter the subarachnoid areas. In older children, subarachnoid hemorrhage from CNS trauma (e.g., head injury) can lead to communicating hydrocephalus. Infectious diseases such as meningitis can block CSF flow at the level of the subarachnoid spaces (McCullough, 1990).

Perhaps the most common cause is IVH (Volpe, 1989). IVH does not always lead to hydrocephalus, as reflected by different systems for grading the severity of hemorrhage. For example, Papile et al. (1978) identified four levels of IVH severity. Grade I IVH represents isolated bleeding in one or both germinal matrices; Grade II IVH consists of a rupture of the germinal matrix with bleeding into the lateral ventricles, but no ventricular swelling; Grade III IVH represents a rupture of the germinal matrix complicated by lateral ventricle swelling; and Grade IV IVH refers to dilated, blood-filled ventricles, with the hemorrhage of the germinal matrices extending into adjacent brain parenchyma. Hydrocephalus results primarily from Grades III and IV IVH. The incidence of IVH has been declining (Volpe, 1989), but many children with Grade III and IV IVH will show progressive ventricular dilation, necessitating the need for intervention (spinal taps, pharmacology). Shunting is necessary in more severe cases.

Unified View

More recently, Raimondi (1994) has proposed a general definition and classification of hydrocephalus derived from an understanding of the mechanical effects of hydrocephalus on the brain. It is traditional in the neurosurgical literature to separate the various types of hydrocephalus on the basis of presumptions about etiology and different causes of increased intracranial presence and the flow of CSF (McCullough, 1990). Raimondi's model suggests that the effects of increased intracranial pressure and changes in the flow and accumulation of CSF represent different stages in the development of hydrocephalus. In contrast to traditional views of hydrocephalus based on the pressure effects of accumulated CSF, hydrocephalus is viewed more simply as a product of the accumulation of CSF, independent of pressure effects. In this view, hydrocephalus is not a single disease entity or syndrome; rather, it is a common endpoint of a series of pathological events involving a variety of etiological factors, which include congenital malformations, tumors, infectious diseases, and other disorders.

From this unified view, hydrocephalus is classified as (1) intraparenchymal, representing the development of pathological increases in the intracranial volume of CSF, which accumulates inside the parenchyma of the brain; or (2) extraparenchymal, reflecting fluid accumulation in the subarachnoid spaces, cisterns, or ventricles. Intraparenchymal hydrocephalus represents the effects of cerebral edema in association with certain metabolic disorders. Extraparenchymal hydrocephalus is further subclassified as (a) subarachnoid, (b) cisternal, and (c) intraventricular. Classification depends on the stage of CSF shifts—that is, from effects of cerebral edema (accumulation within the parenchyma) to accumulations within the subarachnoid spaces (initial stages of communicating hydrocephalus). Subsequent flow may lead to accumulations in the cisterns and ultimately within the ventricles, the latter representing the significant ventricular dilation and pressure effects on the brain associated with the need for shunting. Both AS and hydrocephalus secondary to Chiari malformations produce extraparenchymal hydrocephalus, representing obstruction within the ventricular system. Communicating forms of hydrocephalus secondary to IVH result because of the obstruction in the subarachnoid spaces that blocks the flow of CSF as it leaves the fourth ventricle to enter the subarachnoid areas. In children with postnatal brain insults, such as meningitis and subarachnoid hemorrhages from CNS trauma, hydrocephalus is also conceptualized as extraparenchymal. Within all these etiologies, further subclassification depends on the stage of fluid accumulation.

Effects on the Brain

Whenever significant hydrocephalus occurs, there are major consequences for the development of the brain (Del Bigio, 1993). Hydrocephalus can stretch and even destroy the corpus callosum; it often leads to hypoplasia, in which all corpus callosum structures are present but thinned. Other white matter tracts can be affected by hydrocephalus, particularly projection fibers near the midline, which connect the hemispheres to the diencephalon and more caudal regions. Vision problems can result from damage to the optic tracts. Longer-term consequences include disruption of the process of myelination, with reductions in thickness of the cortical mantel, reduced overall brain mass, and selective thinning of posterior brain regions. In addition, many children who develop hydrocephalus have other cerebral insults (e.g., anoxia) or other congenital malformations (e.g., agenesis of the corpus callosum).

To illustrate, Figure 8.1 provides a midsagittal view from a magnetic resonance imaging (MRI) scan of a normal child (upper left panel) and a child with AS (upper right panel). The lower panels provide images from the same plane in a child with SB meningomyelocele (lower left) and a child with prematurity/IVH and hydrocephalus (lower right). All three children with hydrocephalus were approximately 8 years of age and were shunted. The scan of the child with AS shows that congenital partial agenesis of the corpus callosum is present, along with dilation of the third ventricle. Other brain anomalies are not readily apparent. In contrast, the scan of the child with SB meningomyelocele (lower left) shows partial agenesis of the corpus callosum, dilation of the third ventricle, and major changes in the cerebellum and hindbrain. Less apparent is the interdigitation of the cortex that often occurs in children with SB. Finally, the slice for the premature child shows very severe hydrocephalus, with an area of periventricular leukomalacia (PVL) represented by the dark shading in the region of the third ventricle. PVL is thought to be the result of deep cystic changes in the periventricular white matter secondary to anoxia, and may be thrombotic in nature (Volpe, 1989).

In addition to the effects of hydrocephalus and other congenital malformations, these children often have associated motor problems, demonstrate ocular–motor disturbances such as strabismus, and may develop seizures. They receive various treatments, usually shunts and/or medication to control and regulate the flow of CSF. Parents of a child with hydrocephalus face a lifetime of monitoring the child's condition, with recurrent concerns about possible relapse, shunt dysfunction, and the need for additional surgeries. Understanding the development of the child with hydrocephalus involves an understanding of the pathophysiological features of the brain injury, as well as a knowledge of the disorder itself, its treatment, and the effects of the disorder on the child's ability to interact within the environment.

NEUROBEHAVIORAL OUTCOMES

Overview

Fletcher and Levin (1988) provided an extensive review of the literature on the intellectual, neuropsychological, and behavioral characteristics of

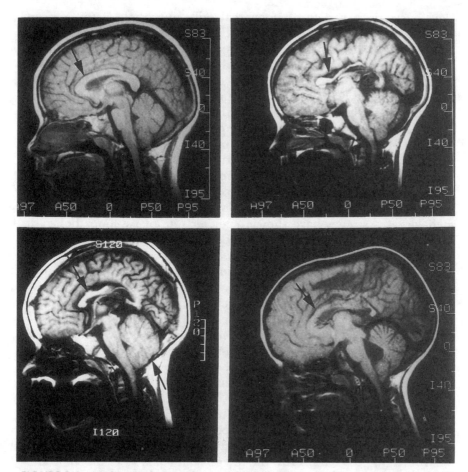

FIGURE 8.1. Midsagittal views from magnetic resonance imaging of a normal child (upper left panel) and children with aqueductal stenosis and shunted hydrocephalus (upper right panel); spina bifida meningomyelocele and shunted hydrocephalus (lower left panel); and prematurity/intraventricular hemorrhage and shunted hydrocephalus (lower right panel). All three cases show abnormalities of the corpus callosum and ventricular dilation. The child with spina bifida also shows a Chiari II malformation, while the child with prematurity also shows periventricular leukomalacia.

children with hydrocephalus. Since that time, the review has been updated (Fletcher, Levin, & Butler, 1995). Additional reviews have been published by Wills (1993), Baron, Fennell, and Voeller (1995), and Dennis (in press).

This literature suggests characteristics consistent with descriptions of the Nonverbal Learning Disabilities (NLD) syndrome (Rourke, 1989). To summarize, hydrocephalus per se is clearly associated with significant deficiencies in a variety of nonverbal skills, including motor, perceptual–motor, and visual–spatial skills. Comparisons of psychometric intelligence test scores invariably show significantly lower scores on performance-based measures than on verbal measures (Dennis et al., 1981; Fletcher, Francis, et al., 1992). Some aspects of language ability may be relatively preserved (e.g., semantic language), but children with hydrocephalus have significant problems with language at the level of discourse (Dennis, Hendrick, Hoffman, & Humphreys, 1987; Dennis, Jacennik, & Barnes, 1994). The few studies of memory, attention, and executive functions have shown inconsistent findings in children with hydrocephalus. Academically, decoding skills appear intact, but problems with writing, math computation, and reading comprehension have been described (Barnes & Dennis, 1992; Wills, Holmbeck, Dillon, & McLone, 1990). Behaviorally, studies have shown a higher rate of psychopathology in children with hydrocephalus (Donders, Rourke, & Canady, 1992; Fletcher, Brookshire, et al., 1995), but only Fletcher, Brookshire, et al. (1995) have produced evidence relating behavior problems to the presence of hydrocephalus.

This summary shows that many children with hydrocephalus show neurobehavioral characteristics of the NLD syndrome (Rourke, 1989). However, much of the literature on children with hydrocephalus is characterized by small and poorly characterized samples and by an absence of appropriate comparison groups. There is excessive reliance on studies of children with SB, with insufficient attention to the presence and severity of hydrocephalus in these children. Many studies do not even identify which children with SB are shunted. In addition, studies have often not been constructed in a manner that permits comparisons across ability domains. Finally, many studies rely on history as opposed to concurrent neuroimaging to characterize the integrity of a child's CNS. Some children with SB will show arrested hydrocephalus that has not been identified because the children have been asymptomatic.

To address the neurobehavioral characteristics of hydrocephalus in relation to the NLD syndrome, we now summarize findings from a large sample of children with hydrocephalus and related medical conditions. The presentation is similar to that of Rourke (1989). The chapter concludes with a discussion of the relationship of these findings to neuroimaging and other indices of the CNS, and more generally to the NLD syndrome.

Sample

The cohort at this point consists of 187 children who were 5 to 14 years of age at recruitment. Children were selected from one of four etiological groups: AS ($n = 17$), SB ($n = 64$), prematurity ($n = 61$), and achondroplasia (n = 16), a form of dwarfism associated with hydrocephalus. In addition, neurologically normal children (n = 29)were recruited. Children with severe psychiatric disorders (infantile autism, psychosis), a history of abuse or other neurological problems not related to hydrocephalus (e.g., stroke), or cerebral palsy of sufficient severity that the children were severely spastic or had no hand use were excluded. In addition, the children (but not the parents) had to be fluent in English.

The sample was 52% female. About 70% of the sample was European-American, with 15% Latin-American, 12% African-American, and 3% Asian-American or Native American. The socioeconomic levels were fairly evenly stratified across the 5 levels of the Hollingshead and Redlich (1958) scale. None of these sociodemographic differences significantly differentiated the etiology groups, but there was a tendency toward more females and Latin-Americans in the SB group. This is consistent with the epidemiology of SB (Wishell, Tuttle, Northam, & Simonds, 1990).

The original intent was to have contrast groups of children with and without hydrocephalus in the SB, prematurity, and achondroplasia groups. Children with AS almost always require shunting, so comparison with the normal group was originally planned. However, concurrent MRI revealed few children in the SB and achondroplasia groups without arrested hydrocephalus. Consequently, children within the etiology groups were subclassified according to the presence of shunted hydrocephalus (n = 75), arrested hydrocephalus (n = 40), and no hydrocephalus (n = 73). Children in the no-hydrocephalus group could have other findings on MRI, mostly mild features of a Chiari I malformation or PVL. Since many children who had arrested and shunted hydrocephalus also had PVL, these children were not retained in order to better establish the effects of hydrocephalus.

For the present chapter, the group with achondroplasia was dropped because of the inability to address the effects of dwarfism and the skeletal abnormalities characteristic of these children. In addition, children with both Verbal IQ and Performance IQ below 70 on the Wechsler Intelligence Scale for Children—Revised (WISC-R) were dropped (n = 6), to avoid problems with examining hypotheses concerning ability discrepancy because of mental deficiency (see Dennis et al., 1981; Fletcher, Francis, et al., 1992). In 20 cases siblings were also studied, so that one sibling was dropped to avoid problems with violations of the assumption of independence for parametric statistical tests (Maxwell & Delaney, 1990). This left a final sample of 145 cases, subdivided as follows: normal (n = 21); AS (arrested n = 1, shunted n = 14); SB (no hydrocephalus n = 12, arrested n = 7, shunted n = 40); and premature (no hydrocephalus n = 22, arrested n = 16, shunted n = 12). With the exception of the single case of AS with arrested hydrocephalus (this child was dropped), the cell sizes are adequate for descriptive purposes.

Each of tese subjects received a comprehensive neuropsychological assessment, neurological exam, and (in all but 24 cases) MRI of the brain. (In these 24 cases, previous scans and history were adequate to document CNS status.) Parents were interviewed to provide history and to complete the Vineland Adaptive Behavior Scales. In addition, parents completed several questionnaires addressing a child's behavioral adjustment and various family/environmental influences on development. Later in this chapter, selected results of these assessments are summarized in relation to the NLD syndrome.

Findings

Tactile-Perceptual Skills

The tactile-proprioceptive abilities of the children were not assessed in this study. Several previous studies of children with SB and hydrocephalus (presumably shunted) have shown lower scores on tests of finger agnosia and graphesthesia (Grimm, 1976), tests of tactile matching (Miller & Sethi, 1971), and the Tactual Performance Test of the Halstead–Reitan Neuropsychological Test Battery (Grimm, 1976). However, Zeiner and Prigatano (1982) were not able to replicate the tactile-matching findings. Although these studies did not control for IQ levels and did not adequately specify the nature and severity of the hydrocephalus, they are consistent with the NLD model. Neurologically, problems with sensory functions are common in children with hydrocephalus, particularly those with SB.

Motor and Psychomotor Skills

Problems with motor skills broadly characterize children with hydrocephalus. Children in our study received several tests of psychomotor ability. For example, Figure 8.2 illustrates results for the dominant and nondominant hands of the Grooved Pegboard. It is apparent that all three groups with shunted hydrocephalus showed significant bilateral impairment, relative to children with arrested hydrocephalus and with no hydrocephalus. The children with arrested hydrocephalus (both those with SB and those with prematurity) also showed poorer fine motor skills relative to the no-hydrocephalus group.

The neurological examination showed abnormalities in fine motor coordination in 74% of children with shunted hydrocephalus, 30% of children with arrested hydrocephalus, and 25% of children with no hydrocephalus. Gross motor problems with the lower extremities are extremely common in children with SB meningomyelocele because of the spinal lesion. For example, the rate of gait abnormalities was high in the shunted

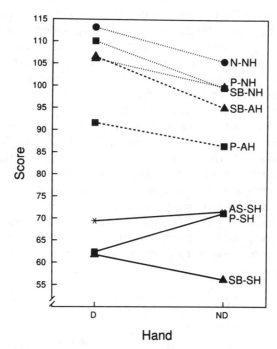

FIGURE 8.2. Grooved Pegboard Test performance ($M = 100$, $SD = 15$) on the dominant (D) and nondominant (ND) hands for children with spina bifida (SB), prematurity (P), or aqueductal stenosis (AS) who had shunted hydrocephalus (SH); children with SB or P who had arrested hydrocephalus (AH); and children with SB or P, or normal children (N), who had no hydrocephalus (NH).

SB group (92%) and the arrested group with SB (83%). However, the shunted groups with prematurity and AS also had a higher percentage of gait abnormalities (prematurity = 44%; AS = 36%) than did the arrested group with prematurity (6%) and the no-hydrocephalus groups (prematurity = 12%; SB = 33%; normal = 0%). There is a broad array of additional literature demonstrating problems with psychomotor skills, hand function, and other motor-based functions in children with hydrocephalus (see Baron et al., 1995; Fletcher & Levin, 1988; Wills, 1993). These findings in the motor system are important, because the NLD model is predicated in part on the role of early motor-based deficiencies, which clearly characterize children with hydrocephalus (Rourke, 1989).

Visual–Spatial–Organizational Abilities

Numerous studies attest to the frequently observed problems with visual–spatial processing characteristic of children with hydrocephalus (see

Fletcher & Levin, 1988; Wills, 1993). It is important to recognize that these deficiencies occur in the context of better development of certain language skills. The clearest examples occur in the numerous comparisons of Verbal and Performance IQ test scores in children with hydrocephalus. The largest studies found lower Performance than Verbal scores across a range of hydrocephalus etiologies (Dennis et al., 1981; Fletcher, Francis, et al., 1992; Raimondi & Soare, 1974; Soare & Raimondi, 1977; Shurtleff, Foltz, & Loesen, 1973). In the present sample, each of the three etiology groups with shunted hydrocephalus showed significantly lower Performance than verbal scores on the McCarthy Scales of Children's Abilities (see Figure 8.3; McCarthy, 1972) and the WISC-R (see Figure 8.4). There was a tendency for the shunted group with AS to score higher on both scales and show more discrepancy than the shunted groups with SB and prematurity. The least discrepant shunted group was the group with SB. In the arrested and no-hydrocephalus groups, scores were not significantly discrepant and were clearly in the average range.

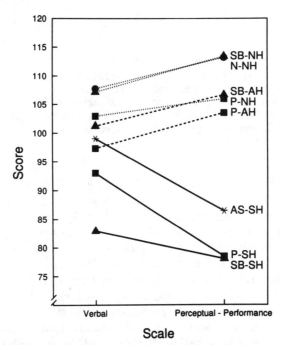

FIGURE 8.3. Performance ($M = 100$, $SD = 15$) on the Verbal and Perceptual–Performance scales of the McCarthy Scales of Children's Abilities for children with spina bifida (SB), prematurity (P), or aqueductal stenosis (AS) who had shunted hydrocephalus (SH); children with SB or P who had arrested hydrocephalus (AH); and children with SB or P, or normal children (N), who had no hydrocephalus (NH).

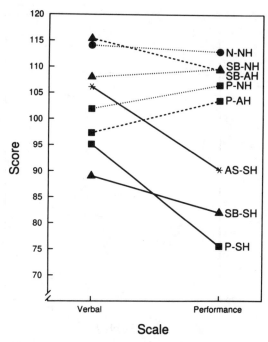

FIGURE 8.4. Performance ($M = 100, SD = 15$) on the Verbal and Performance scales of the Wechsler Intelligence Scale for Children—Revised (WISC-R) for children with spina bifida (SB), prematurity (P), or aqueductal stenosis (AS) who had shunted hydrocephalus (SH); children with SB or P who had arrested hydrocephalus (AH); and children with SB or P, or normal children (N), who had no hydrocephalus.

The visual–spatial problems of these children were quite significant. Since many of the tests used to assess visual–spatial skills in children with hydrocephalus have a motor component, it is tempting to propose that the motor component of these tasks explains the deficiencies observed in children with hydrocephalus. However, a comparison of motor-based and motor-free spatial tasks shows significant impairment in children with shunted hydrocephalus. This is clearly apparent in Figure 8.5, which compares the performance of children with shunted hydrocephalus, arrested hydrocephalus, and no hydrocephalus (collapsed across etiologies) on the Beery Test of Visual–Motor Integration (Beery, 1982) and the Judgement of Line Orientation Test (Lindgren & Benton, 1980). The former test requires graphomotor skills (copying), whereas the latter is motor-free and does not require graphomotor ability. Roughly equivalent levels of impairment are apparent for the three groups, with the shunted group obtaining significantly lower scores on both measures.

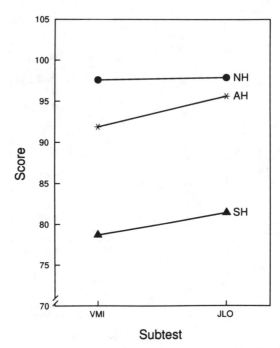

FIGURE 8.5. Performance (M = 100, SD = 15) on the Berry Test of Visual–Motor Integration (VMI; motor-based) and the Judgement of Line Orientation Test (JLO; motor-free) for children had shunted hydrocephalus (SH), arrested hydrocephalus (AH), or no hydrocephalus (NH).

The possibility of spared areas of visual–spatial functioning was also explored in this cohort. Table 8.1 shows that the overall Perceptual Quotient on the Test of Visual-Perceptual Skills (Gardner, 1988) was significantly lower in the shunted groups than in the arrested and no-hydrocephalus groups. Figure 8.6 summarizes performance on the seven subtests of the Test of Visual-Perceptual Skills (Gardner, 1988) for chil-

TABLE 8.1. Means and Standard Deviations by Group for the Perceptual Quotient of the Test of Visual-Perceptual Skills

	Shunted hyd.			Arrested hyd.		No hyd.		
	AS	SB	P	SB	P	SB	P	N
n	12	32	6	5	15	9	17	17
M	83.6	84.0	85.0	100.2	96.3	106.6	101.6	110.6
SD	24.4	17.2	24.4	12.9	19.9	11.7	19.6	13.6

Note. AS, aqueductal stenosis; SB, spina bifida; P, prematurity; N, normal comparison group; hyd., hydrocephalus.

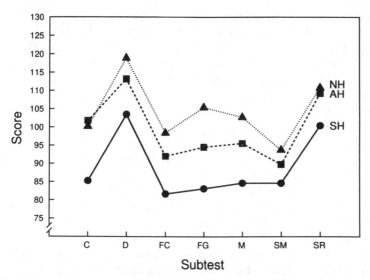

FIGURE 8.6. Performance ($M = 100$, $SD = 15$) on the subtests of the Test of Visual-Perceptual Skills for children who had shunted hydrocephalus (SH), arrested hydrocephalus (AH), or no hydrocephalus (NH). Subtest abbreviations: C, Visual Closure; D, Visual Discrimination; FC, Visual Form Constancy; FG, Visual Figure–Ground; M, Visual Memory; SM, Visual Sequential Memory; SR, Visual Spatial Relationships.

dren with shunted, arrested, and no hydrocephalus. There was a clear tendency for the children with shunted hydrocephalus to score lower than the other groups on all subtests. However, the differences were smaller for simple matching-to-sample (Discrimination) and form-matching (Spatial Relations) subtests. The differences were larger for complex subtests involving form consistency, figure–ground relationships, and spatial memory. As Thompson et al. (1991) showed, visual–spatial processing problems are more apparent on more complex tasks. Figure 8.6 indicates that there was some relative sparing on more simple tasks, but the children with shunted hydrocephalus had lower scores even on these less complex tasks.

Language

The language functioning of children with hydrocephalus was reviewed by Fletcher and Levin (1988), Dennis et al. (1987), and Wills (1993). It has been common to conclude that language is an area of strength in children with hydrocephalus. However, it has also been noted that the speech of children with hydrocephalus has other unusual features. The notion that children with SB have a speech disorder known as "cocktail party syndrome" is well known (Tew, 1979). This syndrome represents the ability to produce fluent expressive language that is tangential and irrelevant to the context of the conversation. Stereotypic phrases and the use of vocabulary above the apparent mental level of the child are also characteristics. Indeed, descriptions of cocktail party speech are somewhat similar to the characteristics of discourse in children with Williams syndrome (see Chapter 6, this volume).

In addition to the studies and overall review by Tew (1979), Dennis and associates have completed the most extensive research on the language of children with hydrocephalus. Dennis et al. (1987) noted that cocktail party syndrome is actually a collection of different language characteristics that make speech atypical in some, but not all, children with hydrocephalus. They suggested that an understanding of this syndrome required studies of the discourse characteristics of children with hydrocephalus.

The discourse characteristics of children with hydrocephalus were thoroughly investigated by Dennis and Barnes (1993) and Dennis et al. (1994). Using a story-retelling format, Dennis et al. (1994) studied the narrative content of the discourse of 49 children with early-onset hydrocephalus and 51 age-matched controls 6 to 15 years of age. They showed that children with hydrocephalus produced oral language that was less coherent and less cohesive than that of controls. Children with hydrocephalus also communicated less of the actual content of the story. In addition, their narrations included more ambiguous material and more content that was implausible or difficult to interpret. Finally, the children with hydrocephalus were more verbose and convoluted in producing narrations. Dennis et al. (1994) interpreted these difficulties as problems with the *usage* of language (i.e., pragmatics), suggesting that the deficits were cognitively derived because the *textual* components of the discourse was impaired. In contrast, the *social* component was preserved because the interpersonal part of the narrations was intact.

The problem with discourse, as well as the relative strengths on the types of semantic language tasks measured by IQ tests, is consistent with the NLD syndrome. Dennis et al. (1987) also suggested that other structural components of language were preserved in children with hydrocephalus. In an earlier study, we (Brookshire et al., 1993) found more pervasive language deficits in children with hydrocephalus than described by Dennis et al. (1987). Figure 8.7 plots scores on four language tests for the normal children and the three groups of children with shunted hydrocephalus in the present sample. The language tests were selected to address phonological awareness skills (the Auditory Analysis Test; Rosner & Simon, 1971), word retrieval under timed conditions for letters (word fluency) and categories (verbal fluency), and automaticity (the Rapid Automatized Naming Test; Denckla & Rudel, 1974). The groups

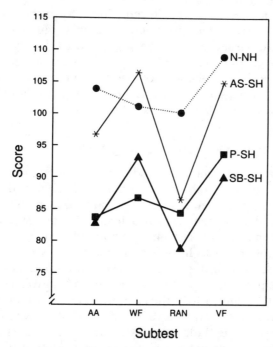

FIGURE 8.7. Performance ($M = 100$, $SD = 15$) on the Auditory Analysis (AA), Word Fluency (WF), Rapid Automatized Naming (RAN), and Verbal Fluency (VF) tests for children who had spina bifida and shunted hydrocephalus (SB-SH), prematurity and shunted hydrocephalus (P-SH), or aqueductal stenosis and shunted hydrocephalus (AS-SH), and normal children (N-NH).

with SB and prematurity scored well below the normal children and the group with AS on the measure of phonological awareness and both retrieval tasks. The group with AS had some difficulty on the Rapid Automized Naming Test, implying problems with automaticity, since this group's performance on the two word retrieval tasks was in the average range. Data for the other no-hydrocephalus groups and for the groups with arrested hydrocephalus were not plotted; they were generally in the average range.

As the plots of IQ tests scores show (see Figures 8.3 and 8.4), language is better developed but not fully preserved in children with hydrocephalus. The strengths and weaknesses are certainly consistent with the NLD model. The weaknesses apparent in the hydrocephalic groups with SB and prematurity may well reflect the influence of the other cerebral malformations and insults characteristic of many such children, which may lead to impairment of left-hemisphere systems. The automaticity deficits in the group with AS may reflect the corpus callosum defects characteristic of 80% of such children. To perform the Rapid Automatized Naming Test, visual information (pictures) must be attached to a name. Since the visual information presented to the right hemisphere must cross the corpus callosum to access the naming centers of the left hemisphere, the partial agenesis of the callosum characteristic of many of these children may be highly relevant for explaining their poor performance on the Rapid Automatized Naming Test.

Attention, Memory, and Problem-Solving Skills

The areas of attention, memory, and problem-solving skills are virtually unstudied in children with hydrocephalus. Fletcher and Levin (1988) and Wills (1993) reviewed studies suggesting that many children with hydrocephalus have attentional problems. Memory studies have produced results that are at best mixed. No studies of concept-formation and problem-solving skills have been reported.

The children in this sample reviewed several tests of verbal and nonverbal memory skills, including verbal and nonverbal selective reminding tests (Fletcher, 1985), the Continuous Recognition Memory Test (Hannay, Levin, & Grossman, 1979), and the Story Recall and Design Memory subtests of the Wide Range Assessment of Memory and Learning (WRAML). Results are not presented in detail, except to note that we (Fletcher, Francis, et al., 1992) previously reported significant deficiencies on both the verbal and nonverbal selective reminding tests. The shunted, arrested, and no-hydrocephalus groups in this cohort did not show large differences on the Continuous Recognition Memory Test. Lower performance was apparent on the Story Recall subtest of the WRAML for the group with shunted hydrocephalus, but this deficit was largely in immediate recall and not in delayed recall. It also was primarily apparent in the shunted groups with SB and prematurity. Given the discourse problems of children with hydrocephalus (Dennis et al., 1994), and these findings of poorer language skills in shunted children with SB and prematurity, such findings may stem from deficiencies in language as opposed to memory. The fact that children with shunted hydrocephalus showed much greater impairment on the Design Memory subtests of the WRAML, but largely in the immediate recall component and not the one for delayed recall, may reflect motor-based problems in these children.

We (Fletcher et al., 1994) administered tests commonly interpreted in terms of problem-solving skills (Tower of London, Wisconsin Card Sorting Test), selective attention (Stroop test), and focused attention (verbal and nonverbal cancellation tests). These results are summarized for the children with shunted, arrested, and no hydrocephalus.

The Tower of London (Shallice, 1982) is a currently popular measure of what are broadly defined as "executive functions" (Pennington,

1994). The task requires a child to transfer beads from an initial position to a goal position in three, four, or five moves. The three groups did not differ significantly in mean initial planning time, mean solution time, number of broken rules, and number of trials to criterion. However, the group with shunted hydrocephalus solved fewer problems, largely on more complex trials, and was less likely to solve the problem on the first trial. It is interesting that the major finding was simply that fewer problems were correctly solved, and that the groups did not appear to differ on the indices commonly associated with planning and the formation of mental representations underlying problem-solving skills.

The Wisconsin Card Sorting Test is a widely used measure of concept-formation and problem-solving abilities. It has also been interpreted as a measure of the ability to shift attention. On this task, the children with shunted and arrested hydrocephalus completed significantly fewer categories. However, the groups did not differ in the ability to maintain set or the number of perseverative errors. As with the Tower of London, fewer problems were solved, but the basis for this finding is not clear.

The Stroop test measures naming speed for colors and words; it includes an interference condition, in which the child is required to read a color name that conflicts with the color of the word. The group with shunted hydrocephalus had slower speeds for all these conditions than did the groups with arrested and no hydrocephalus. However, the interference effect was not significant. This finding suggests that children with shunted hydrocephalus are slower on any naming test that requires cross-modal processing, and it is consistent with the data for the Rapid Automized Naming test (see Figure 8.7).

The cancellation task requires children to search a page for either target letters or shapes among a variety of distractors; the search task stimuli are either randomly arranged or laid out in rows. Hence, this task allows evaluation of focused attentional skills for verbal and nonverbal information and for effects of random versus organized structure. These results are summarized in Figure 8.8. There was a significant group × stimulus interaction (see Figure 8.8). For both the random and the organized conditions, the group with shunted hydrocephalus had relatively poorer performance on the verbal than on the nonverbal task. All groups found the nonverbal and random tasks more difficult than the verbal and organized tasks. The greater difference on the verbal task is surprising, but the nonverbal task was difficult for all groups and may have minimized the motor requirements of the nonverbal task relative to the verbal task.

These results show that children with shunted hydrocephalus are deficient on tasks that require problem-solving skills. However, many of these results can be interpreted in terms of problems with attention systems mediated by posterior (white matter) regions of the brain. In

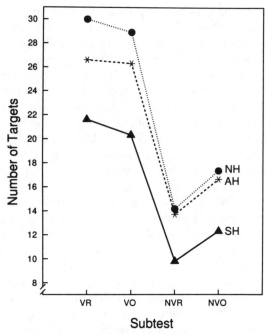

FIGURE 8.8. Number of correctly identified targets on verbal (V) and nonverbal (NV) visual cancellation tasks presented in random (R) and organized (O) formats for children who had shunted hydrocephalus (SH), arrested hydrocephalus (AH), or no hydrocephalus (NH).

this respect, the focused attention task yielded the largest group differences. The Stroop Test seemed to reflect problems with automaticity that may be mediated by corpus callosum pathology. The deficiencies on the Tower of London did not seem mediated by traditional indices of problem-solving ability. Rather, children with shunted hydrocephalus solved fewer problems on the Tower of London and achieved fewer categories on the Wisconsin Card Sorting Test. In addition, the Tower of London showed that children with shunted hydrocephalus were less likely to solve a problem on the first trial. This may reflect problems with focusing and orienting to the task, as opposed to problems with working memory.

Academic Skills

The literature suggests that children with hydrocephalus have preservation of word-decoding skills, but may have problems with reading comprehension, writing, and math computations (Fletcher & Levin, 1988;

Barnes & Dennis, 1992; Wills, 1993). Table 8.2 presents results of an assessment of academic achievement for the present cohort, showing that the shunted groups with SB and prematurity did tend to score below the other groups on the measure of reading decoding skills (Basic Reading), which is a composite measure involving recognitive of real words and nonsense words (Woodcock & Johnson, 1989). The group with AS was clearly in the average range on this measure and on the Spelling subtest from the Wide Range Achievement Test—Revised (WRAT-R; Jastak & Wilkinson, 1984). In contrast, the AS group was markedly discrepant in arithmetic ability. The other two shunted groups (and the two prematurity groups) were also discrepant on the WRAT-R Arithmetic subtest relative to reading decoding. Only the shunted groups with SB and prematurity showed lower scores on the Passing Comprehension measure from the Woodcock–Johnson. The AS group scored in the Average range.

This *pattern* of results is largely consistent with predictions for the NLD model. The shunted groups with SB and prematurity appeared to

TABLE 8.2. Means and Standard Deviations for the Woodcock–Johnson Psycho-Educational Test Battery (Basic Reading, Passage Comprehension) and Wide Range Achievement Test—Revised (WRAT-R; Spelling, Arithmetic) by Group

	Shunted hyd.			Arrested hyd.		No hyd.		
	AS	SB	P	SB	P	SB	P	N
n	13	37	10	7	15	9	20	18
			Woodcock–Johnson					
Basic Reading								
M	104.8	90.9	90.5	117.0	96.9	108.2	102.2	106.4
SD	23.1	19.3	17.7	22.4	12.4	17.9	15.9	15.7
Passage Comprehension								
M	104.8	92.5	93.6	125.1	104.3	109.8	108.2	111.4
SD	22.3	23.0	25.5	19.3	14.1	17.4	17.3	14.9
			WRAT-R					
Spelling								
M	96.0	87.9	85.1	111.1	88.2	98.1	92.6	99.7
SD	26.8	21.5	22.4	25.8	13.2	15.3	15.3	18.4
Arithmetic								
M	85.9	80.4	80.4	95.9	83.2	92.4	91.1	96.9
SD	20.6	15.1	20.2	18.0	13.8	16.6	12.5	11.5

Note. AS, aqueductal stenosis; SB, spina bifida; P, prematurity; N, normal comparison group; hyd., hydrocephalus.

be more impaired on language-related academic tasks, but these groups also had other cerebral anomalies.

Psychosocial Adjustment

Several studies have concluded that hydrocephalus per se is not associated with difficulties in behavioral adjustment (e.g., Donders et al., 1992). More recently, we (Fletcher, Brookshire, et al., 1995) evaluated the behavioral adjustment of children in the present cohort in the 5- to 7-year age range. Group average scores on the Internalizing and Externalizing scales of the Child Behavior Checklist (CBCL; Achenbach, 1991) were not significantly different. However, children with hydrocephalus were more likely to obtain elevations consistent with at least mild behavior disorders. Categorical modeling methods showed that hydrocephalus and its treatment, gender (being male), and several family variables predicted the emergence of a behavior disorder.

In a series of studies summarized by Landry, Jordan, and Fletcher (1994), observational methods were used to characterize the mastery motivation and goal-directed behavior of children with SB, most of whom had hydrocephalus. Children with SB showed reductions in goal-related behaviors and the ability to direct their own behavior. In addition, the perceived competence of these children was lower. However, differences in perceived self-competence, along with intellectual and socioeconomic variables, did not explain the reductions in goal-related and self-directed behaviors. Nonverbal cognitive and motor problems seemed more related to the latter behaviors. These findings are interesting because they are similar to some of the language findings by Dennis et al. (1994), as well as to expectations from the NLD model.

The parents of children in the present cohort completed the Personality Inventory for Children—Revised (PIC-R; Lachar, 1982) and the CBCL. The results for the four broad-based factor scales of the PIC-R and the Internalizing and Externalizing scales of the CBCL are presented in Table 8.3. For both measures, scale elevations above 64 are regarded as mildly abnormal. With the exception of the high elevations for the Cognitive Development factor (Factor IV) of the PIC-R for the three shunted groups, and for the shunted group with prematurity on Factor III, these averages were well within the average range. Children with shunted hydrocephalus were more likely to obtain T scores ≥ 64, but the overall rate was only slightly higher than that for the contrast groups.

To summarize, we (Fletcher, Brookshire, et al., 1995) showed that hydrocephalus and its treatment was related to the emergence of behavior problems in an assessment of psychosocial adjustment of this cohort when younger. However, family and sociodemographic variables were also important predictors. The PIC-R and CBCL scores were generally

TABLE 8.3. Means and Standard Deviations for the Broad-Based Factor Scales (I–IV) of the Personality Inventory for Children—Revised (PIC-R), and the Internalizing and Externalizing Scales of the Child Behavior Checklist (CBCL)

	Shunted hyd.			Arrested hyd.		No hyd.		
	AS	SB	P	SB	P	SB	P	N
n	12	37	12	7	12	10	16	18
			PIC-R[a]					
I								
M	52.5	50.2	55.8	48.6	55.3	50.5	55.4	53.9
SD	8.6	8.3	11.0	11.8	16.2	13.4	13.8	11.8
II								
M	52.1	54.1	63.2	55.6	57.0	49.3	48.3	50.1
SD	10.3	9.4	14.2	8.4	14.5	11.0	7.2	13.0
III								
M	54.6	58.8	66.8	55.3	56.2	57.7	56.0	58.1
SD	15.2	13.9	19.8	13.7	12.4	15.8	10.8	13.6
IV								
M	64.8	74.4	80.9	51.4	61.4	47.0	53.0	50.9
SD	20.0	20.5	18.9	8.5	12.7	9.1	12.2	11.1
			CBCL					
Internalizing								
M	53.4	55.2	61.2	51.0	53.6	53.1	55.1	52.9
SD	12.8	9.1	7.6	8.3	9.4	11.0	7.3	10.1
Externalizing								
M	54.1	55.8	60.8	51.1	52.6	51.8	56.5	52.7
SD	11.9	8.7	9.7	9.7	10.3	8.9	9.6	9.8

Note. AS, aqueductal stenosis; SB, spina bifida; P, prematurity; N, normal comparison group; hyd., hydrocephalus.
[a] Each scale standardized with $M = 50$ and $SD = 10$.

lower than those reported for children selected for specific arithmetic disabilities and an absence of acquired disorder (Rourke & Fuerst, 1991). There are undoubtedly individual cases that represent the full NLD syndrome in children with hydrocephalus (see the case example presented later in this chapter), but the social component of the NLD model in children with hydrocephalus needs more research.

Neurobehavioral Outcomes and the NLD Model

It is clear that children with hydrocephalus have motor and cognitive characteristics that are consistent with predictions of the NLD model. In addition, children with hydrocephalus have cerebral pathology that clearly involves white matter tracts. This section addresses the issue of whether the behavioral and CNS findings are related. With the advent of contemporary neuroimaging modalities, such studies are now possible.

In an initial study, we (Fletcher, Bohan, et al., 1992) obtained assessments of verbal and nonverbal skills and concurrent MRI in children with shunted hydrocephalus (who had AS or SB), arrested hydrocephalus (who had SB), and normal controls. The cognitive measures included the Verbal and Performance scales from the McCarthy Scales of Children's Abilities and the WISC-R. In addition, neuropsychological measures of verbal and nonverbal skills were arranged into composites. The MRI data were downloaded to a computer for area measurements of the corpus callosum (commissural fibers), internal capsules (projection fibers), and centrum semiovale (association fibers). In addition, the volumes of the lateral ventricles in both hemispheres were measured.

Bivariate correlations between the cognitive measures and the MRI measures revealed that the volume of the lateral ventricles and the cross-sectional areas of the corpus callosum and internal capsules were significantly correlated with measures of both verbal and nonverbal cognitive skills, but that the relationship was stronger for nonverbal skills. There was a positive and robust relationship of nonverbal skills, but not verbal skills, with the size of the corpus callosum. In addition, nonverbal measures correlated with the volume of the right, but not the left lateral ventricle and with the area of the right and left internal capsules. The language tasks correlated with the volume of the left, but not right, lateral ventricle and with the area of the left, but not the right, internal capsule.

The results of this study showed a relationship between the corpus callosum and cognitive skills, as well as relationships between cognitive skills and hydrocephalus-related changes in the lateral ventricles and tracts in the cerebral white matter, supporting the NLD model. These results have been replicated (Fletcher et al., 1993) in a larger sample, with the correlations between corpus callosum and nonverbal cognitive skills continuing to show particular robustness.

Another study examined patterns of myelination in relationship to scores on the Bayley Scales of Infant Development in infants with progressive hydrocephalus (van der Knaap et al., 1991). The children were shunted and received MRI and the Bayley at the time of admission, and 6 weeks and 6 months after admission. Volumes of CSF, white matter, and grey matter were computed. Significant correlations between Bayley scores and extent of myelination (white matter) were observed, but there was no relationship of Bayley scores with CSF and grey matter. These findings, along with other studies, have been interpreted to reflect specific relationships of the degree of myelination and the degree to which cognitive skills develop in children with hydrocephalus (Sobkowiak, 1992).

Several other studies have examined variables that characterize hydrocephalus and its treatment in relation to cognitive skills (reviewed in Fletcher & Levin, 1988; Wills, 1993). Hydrocephalus and its treatment, including shunting and shunt revisions, have effects on cognitive skills. In her review, Wills (1993) suggested that the presence of shunted hydrocephalus reduced intelligence test scores. Complications of hydrocephalus (e.g., association with CNS infection) also reduced cognitive skills. Various results were apparent for the number of shunt revisions, with some studies showing reductions in cognitive skills and some finding no relationships. Severity of hydrocephalus was clearly a factor in the development of cognitive skills.

More recently, Riva et al. (1994) examined several variables characterizing hydrocephalus, brain malformations, and treatment in relation to measures of verbal and nonverbal psychometric intelligence. Weak relationships were apparent for Verbal IQ, but the Performance IQ score was correlated with (1) supratentorial abnormalities, (2) shunting age and shunt type, (3) ocular–motor deficits, and (4) use of anticonvulsant medications. Etiology, site of obstruction, duration of time prior to shunting, number of shunt revisions, and other complications were not related to intelligence test scores.

The varying findings on the relationship of medical variables and cognitive functioning across studies are most likely attributable to variations in the samples. The technology with which hydrocephalic children are treated change, so there is a need to continue the types of monitoring studies reviewed by Wills (1993) and Fletcher and Levin (1988) if we are to understand the consequences of hydrocephalus and its treatment.

CASE EXAMPLE

To further illustrate the relevance of the NLD model for children with hydrocephalus, we have a prototypical case selected for review. This child was evaluated for our study at age of 9 years, 5 months. He was identified with AS very early in his development, and was shunted for hydrocephalus 1 week after birth. He required a revision of the shunt approximately 4 months after birth. Other significant medical history included the need for multiple eye muscle surgeries to correct strabismus beginning at 21 months of age. In addition, this child developed a significant seizure disorder at 15 months, which began as partial complex seizures but evolved into major motor seizures. At times this child's epilepsy was poorly controlled, and he had been in status at least twice. However, the seizures were well controlled on Felbamate at the time of our evaluation.

This child was also grossly hyperactive. He had been treated with a variety of stimulant medications, with efficacy resulting from Cylert. The mother noted that the hyperactivity was present very early in development. For example, at the age of 2 months this child had a period of about 1 week during which he slept (at the mother's estimate) for approximately 2½ hours. At the time of our evaluation, the child was widely viewed as bright. Although he had been in special education classes in the past, he was now mainstreamed with support services. The parents expressed concerns about his motor abilities, math and writing skills, weak social skills, and behavior problems related to his hyperactivity.

A neuropsychological assessment was completed for research purposes. Figure 8.9 summarizes this child's performance on measures described previously in this chapter. A review of this figure shows that

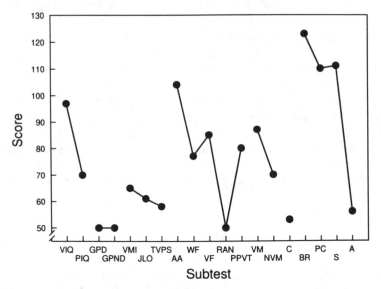

FIGURE 8.9. Neuropsychological profile ($M = 100$, $SD = 15$) for a child with aqueductal stenosis and shunted hydrocephalus who represents a prototype for the Nonverbal Learning Disabilities syndrome. Abbreviations: VIQ, Verbal IQ, WISC-R; PIQ, Performance IQ, WISC-R; GPD, Grooved Pegboard Test, dominant hand; GPND, Grooved Pegboard Test, nondominant hand; VMI, Beery Test of Visual–Motor Integration; JLO, Judgement of Line Orientation Test; TVPS, Test of Visual–Perceptual Skills, overall score; AA, Auditory Analysis Test; WF, Word Fluency; VF, Verbal Fluency; RAN, Rapid Automatized Naming Test; PPVT, Peabody Picture Vocabulary Test—Revised; VM, Verbal Selective Reminding, Consistent Long-Term Retrieval; NVM, Nonverbal Selective Reminding, Consistent Long-Term Retrieval; C, average score on visual cancellation tests; BR, Basic Reading, Woodcock–Johnson; PC, Passage Comprehension, Woodcock–Johnson; S, Spelling, WRAT-R; A, Arithmetic, WRAT-R.

the child had a 27-point discrepancy between WISC-R Verbal IQ and Performance IQ, with the Performance score much lower and the Verbal score clearly in the average range. Severe fine motor coordination problems were apparent for both hands on the Grooved Pegboard Test. In addition, the child showed extremely poor performance on the Beery Test of Visual–Motor Integration and the Judgement of Line Orientation Test, and obtained a Perceptual Quotient on the Test of Visual-Perceptual Skills of 58. In the language area, the child was quite proficient on the Auditory Analysis Test (104), but had difficulty on both word fluency (retrieval to letters) and verbal fluency (retrieval to categories). Severe impairment was apparent on the Rapid Automized Naming test. The child had a Peabody Picture Vocabulary Test—Revised standard score of 80. In the memory area, the child had difficulty on both verbal and nonverbal selective reminding tests, but the problem was more apparent for the nonverbal task. The visual cancellation tasks (see Figure 8.8) yielded an average score across different subtests that was severely deficient. Academically, the child showed extremely good development of basic reading skills. He obtained a high average score on the cloze-based Woodcock–Johnson measure of Passage Comprehension, as well as the WRAT-R Spelling test. He was widely viewed as an excellent reader. However, his performance on a measure of math computations was extremely deficient. Psychosocially, this child had poor social skills and was extremely difficult to control when he was not on his medication. The mother noted that he could be "wild."

His response to language samples using a story-retelling format revealed narrations that were often irrelevant to the context of the story. He had a tendency to use elaborate and convoluted vocabulary that contrasted with the standard score on the Peabody Picture Vocabulary Test—Revised (80), as well as with the standard score on the Vocabulary subtest of the WISC-R (7). Indeed, his highest subtest score on the WISC-R was on the Information subtest (18), reflecting this child's extremely good development of rote verbal memory. The mother reported that one of his favorite activities was to read encyclopedias. He was able to give back the information that he read almost for verbatim. His discourse difficulties were readily apparent in the evaluation; for example, he referred to a female examiner as a "bodacious babe." He obtained uniformly high elevations on all four factor scales of the PIC-R. He was also regarded as a child who related much better to adults, who had few friends, and who struggled with peer relationships.

This child clearly epitomized the neuropsychological assets and deficits associated with the NLD syndrome. In addition, he had the social characteristics that are described by Rourke and Fuerst (1991), although he also had a significant externalizing disorder reflected by his severe hyperactivity.

Figure 8.10 presents the midsagittal view from his MRI, which shows significant ventricular dilation associated with the hydrocephalus. In addition, there is clear partial agenesis of the corpus callosum. Particularly noteworthy in this scan is the atrophy of the midline posterior parietal and occipital cortex, which is replaced by a supracerebellar cyst. The image also shows dysplasia of the cerebellum. The attention-deficit/hyperactivity disorder shown by the child may reflect the extension of the fourth ventricle into the locus coeruleus and other areas representing major dopaminergic pathways in the brain.

CONCLUSIONS

When the neuropsychological, psychosocial, and neuropathological characteristics of children with hydrocephalus are examined, it is clear that hydrocephalus represents a prototypical NLD disorder. In this respect, hydrocephalus is certainly a Level 1 manifestation of the NLD syndrome (see Chapter 18 of this volume). This is particularly important, because hydrocephalus is one of the only disorders identified at Level 1 for which

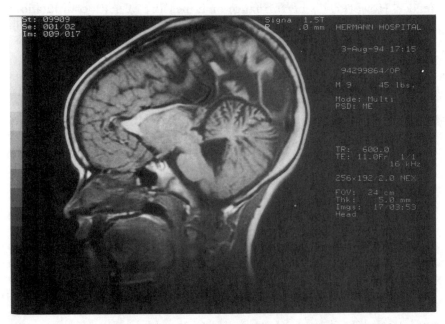

FIGURE 8.10. Midsagittal view from magnetic resonance imaging of a child with aqueductal stenosis and shunted hydrocephalus who represents a prototype for the Nonverbal Learning Disabilities syndrome.

the neurobehavioral characteristics have been thoroughly investigated and initial investigations are occurring that relate these characteristics to neuroimaging studies of the brain. It is clear that early hydrocephalus across all three etiologies is associated with significant changes in the cerebral white matter. In addition, hydrocephalic children with both SB and AS show other congenital alterations of the cerebral white matter, most notably involving the corpus callosum. These changes also seem related to the neuropsychological characteristics of children with hydrocephalus. The only areas where some deviations are observed from the NLD model involve memory and language performance and the psychosocial characteristics.

In terms of memory performance, children with hydrocephalus do show significant problems on various tests of memory and learning. However, this may not represent a manifestation of the memory system; rather, the types of tests that are being employed often require attention and organization abilities. For example, successful execution of the verbal selective reminding task requires a child to develop a strategy for organizing and retrieving the words (Pennington, 1994). In addition, the child must persist in control of the focus of attention across several trials. Problems with either the organizational component or with attentional skills could disrupt performance on these types of tasks. The attention problems of many of these children are clearly apparent and are consistent with predictions from the NLD model.

Some of the language characteristics observed in these children are very consistent with the NLD model, particularly in the area of discourse. However, children with etiologies involving SB and prematurity show deficiencies on other language tests that would not be observed in, for example, children with NLD selected because of specific arithmetic disability. It is likely that the lower language scores depicted in Figure 8.7 reflect the effects of other cerebral insults. For example, there was no control over the presence of PVL in the children selected for this study. In addition, children with prematurity often have significant hypoxic–ischemic encephalopathy, which can have a more general effect on cognition. Children with SB have the Chiari malformation, heterotopias, and other CNS anomalies. The investigation of why ability discrepancies do not emerge in some cases with hydrocephalus is an area that would be fruitful for study.

The area representing the most difficulty for the NLD model in children with hydrocephalus is that of the psychosocial characteristics. The child in the case example presented above would not meet the current diagnostic criteria for Asperger syndrome, but showed a number of similarities in the social area. However, this presentation in our study was quite rare. In addition, we do not see very many children with hydrocephalus who would actually be described as having a "cocktail party syndrome" as defined by Tew (1979). The discourse deficits are readily apparent, but other characteristics of the so-called cocktail party syndrome are not apparent. Many of the children in our study have psychosocial problems that were largely secondary to the effects of poor motor skills, difficulties in school, and other problems associated with generically handicapping conditions. There were certainly exceptions, but full-blown presentations of NLD syndromes that included the internalizing psychosocial component were relatively rare in this sample.

It is important to recognize that this sample differed significantly from other descriptions of children with hydrocephalus in that the children were selected specifically for research and were not part of a clinical population. Many of the children come in only for the research and were not observed to have significant problems in school or with behavior. In our experience, the psychosocial characteristics of children with hydrocephalus do not parallel the consistent forms of psychosocial disturbance observed in children identified with NLD and specific arithmetic disability (Rourke & Fuerst, 1991).

Future directions for research on the NLD syndrome in relationship to hydrocephalus should focus on language and psychosocial characteristics. It would seem particularly important to understand why some children manifest the NLD syndrome to different degrees. It is likely that a variety of factors will be relevant, including the family and social environment in which a child is raised, as well as the influence of other cerebral anomalies in treatment. Nonetheless, the NLD model provides a good framework for capturing the neurobehavioral characteristics of many children with hydrocephalus. Particularly relevant are those studies showing that the nonverbal cognitive deficiencies of these children are related to measurable abnormalities in the cerebral white matter.

REFERENCES

Achenbach, T. M. (1991). *Manual for the Child Behavior Checklist/4–18 and 1991 Profile*. Burlington: University of Vermont, Department of Psychiatry.

Barnes, M. A., & Dennis, M. (1992). Reading in children and adolescents after early onset hydrocephalus and in normally developing age peers: Phonological analysis, word recognition, word comprehension, and passage comprehension skills. *Journal of Pediatric Psychology, 17*, 445–465.

Baron, I. S., Fennell, E., & Voeller, K. (1995). *Pediatric neuropsychology in the medical setting*. New York: Oxford University Press.

Barkovich, A. J. (1990). *Pediatric neuroimaging*. New York: Raven Press.

Beery, K. E. (1982). *Revised administration, scoring, and teaching manual for the Developmental Test of Visual–Motor Integration*. Cleveland, OH: Modern Curriculum Press.

Bohan, T. P., Dominguez, R., Fenstermacher, M., Kramer, L., Fletcher, J. M., Miner, M. E., Beaver, S., & Brookshire, B. (1994). *Diffuse central nervous system anomalies associated with myelomeningocele.* Manuscript submitted for publication.

Brookshire, B. L., Fletcher, J. M., Francis, D. J., Thompson, N., Bohan, T. P., Landry, S. H., Davidson, K. C., & Miner, M. E. (1993). Language functions in children with hydrocephalus. *Journal of Clinical and Experimental Neuropsychology, 15,* 58. (Abstract)

Del Bigio, M. R. (1993). Neuropathological changes caused by hydrocephalus. *Acta Neuropathologica, 85,* 573–585.

Denckla, M. B., & Rudel, R. G. (1974). Rapid "automatized" naming of pictured objects, colors, letters, and numbers by normal children. *Cortex,* 10, 186–202.

Dennis, M. (in press). Hydrocephalus. In J. G. Beaumont & J. Sergent (Eds.), *The Blackwell dictionary of neuropsychology.* Oxford: Blackwell.

Dennis, M., & Barnes, M. A. (1993). Oral discourse after early-onset hydrocephalus: Linguistic ambiguity, figurative language, speech acts, and script-based inferences. *Journal of Pediatric Psychology, 18,* 639–652.

Dennis, M., Fitz, C. R., Netley, C. T., Sugar, J., Derek, C. F., Harwood-Nash, M. B., Hendrick, H. B., Hoffman, H. J., & Humphreys, R. P. (1981). The intelligence of hydrocephalic children. *Archives of Neurology, 38,* 607–715.

Dennis, M., Hendrick, E. B., Hoffman, H. J., & Humphreys, R. P. (1987). The language of hydrocephalic children. *Journal of Clinical and Experimental Neuropsychology, 9,* 593–621.

Dennis, M., Jacennik, B., & Barnes, M. A. (1994). The content of narrative discourse in children and adolescents after early-onset hydrocephalus and in normally-developing age peers. *Brain and Language, 46,* 129–165.

Donders, J., Rourke, B. P., & Canady, A. I. (1992). Behavioral adjustment of children with hydrocephalus and of their parents. *Journal of Child Neurology, 7,* 375–380.

Fletcher, J. M. (1985). Memory for verbal and nonverbal stimuli in learning disability subgroups: Analysis by selective reminding. *Journal of Experimental Child Psychology, 40,* 244–259.

Fletcher, J. M., Bohan, T. P., Brandt, M., Beaver, S. R., Thorstad, K., Brookshire, B. L., Francis, D. J., Davidson, K. C., & Thompson, N. (1993). Relationships of cognitive skills and cerebral white matter in hydrocephalic children. *Journal of Clinical and Experimental Neuropsychology, 15,* 40–41.

Fletcher, J. M., Bohan, T. P., Brandt, M. E., Brookshire, B. L., Beaver, S. R., Francis, D. J., Davidson, K. C., Thompson, N. M., & Miner, M. E. (1992). Cerebral white matter and cognition in hydrocephalic children. *Archives of Neurology, 49,* 818–824.

Fletcher, J. M., Brookshire, B. L., Bohan, T. P., Davidson, K., Brandt, M., Landry, S. H., & Francis, D. J. (1994). *Executive functions in children with early hydrocephalus.* Manuscript submitted for publication.

Fletcher, J. M., Brookshire, B. L., Landry, S. H., Bohan, T. P., Davidson, K. C., Francis, D. J., Thompson, N. M., & Miner, M. E. (1995). Behavioral adjustment of hydrocephalic children: Relationships with etiology, neurological, and family status. *Journal of Pediatric Psychology, 20,* 765–781.

Fletcher, J. M., Francis, D. J., Thompson, N. M., Brookshire, B. L., Bohan, T. P., Landry, S. H., Davidson, K. C., & Miner, M. E. (1992). Verbal and nonverbal skill discrepancies in hydrocephalic children. *Journal of Clinical and Experimental Neuropsychology, 14*, 593–609.

Fletcher, J. M., & Levin, H. S. (1988). Neurobehavioral effects of brain injury in children. In D. Routh (Ed.), *Handbook of pediatric psychology* (pp. 258–296). New York: Guilford Press.

Fletcher, J. M., Levin, H. S., & Butler, I. J. (1995). Neurobehavioral effects of brain injury in children: Hydrocephalus, traumatic brain injury, and cerebral palsy. In M. Roberts (Ed.), *Handbook of pediatric psychology* (2nd ed.). New York: Guilford Press.

Gardner, M. F. (1988). *Test of Visual-Perceptual Skills*. San Francisco: Health.

Grimm, R. (1976). Hand function and tactile perception in a sample of children with myelomeningocele. *American Journal of Occupational Therapy, 30*, 234–240.

Hannay, H. J., Levin, H. S., & Grossman, R. G. (1979). Impaired recognition memory after head injury. *Cortex, 15*, 269–283.

Hollingshead, A. B., & Redlich, F. C. (1958). *Two factor index of social status*. New York: Wiley.

Jastak, S., & Wilkinson, A. (1984). *Wide Range Achievement Test—Revised*. Wilmington, DE: Guidance Associates.

Lachar, D. (1982). *Personality Inventory for Children (PIC): Revised format supplement*. Los Angeles: Western Psychological Services.

Landry, S. H., Jordan, T., & Fletcher, J. M. (1994). Developmental outcomes for children with spina bifida. In M. G. Tramontana & S. R. Hooper (Eds.), *Advances in neuropsychology* (Vol. 2, pp. 85–118). New York: Springer-Verlag.

Lindgren, S. D., & Benton, A. L. (1980). Developmental patterns of visuospatial judgement. *Journal of Pediatric Psychology, 5*, 217–225.

Liptak, G., Bloss, J. W., Briskin, H., Campbell, J. E., Hebert, E. B., & Revell, G. M. (1988). The management of children with spinal dysraphism. *Journal of Child Neurology, 3*, 3–20.

Maxwell, S. E., & Delaney, H. D. (1990). *Designing experiments and analyzing data: A model comparisons approach*. Belmont, CA: Wadsworth.

McCarthy, D. (1972). *McCarthy Scales of Children's Abilities*. New York: Psychological Corporation.

McCullough, D. (1990). Hydrocephalus: Etiology, pathologic effects, diagnosis and natural history. In R. M. Scott (Ed.), *Hydrocephalus* (pp. 180–199). Baltimore: Williams & Wilkins.

Menkes, J. (1985). *Textbook of child neurology* (3rd ed.). Philadelphia: Lea & Febiger.

Miller, E., & Sethi, L. (1971). Tactile matching in children with hydrocephalus. *Neuropediatrica, 3*, 191–194.

Papile, L. A., Burstein, J., Burstein, R., & Koffler, H. (1978). Incidence and evaluation of subependymal and intraventricular hemorrhage: A study of infants with birth weight less than 1,500 gm. *Journal of Pediatrics, 92*, 529–534.

Pennington, B. F. (1994). The working memory function of the prefrontal cortices: Implications for developmental and individual differences in cognition. In M. M. Haith, J. Benson, R. Roberts, & B. F. Pennington (Eds.), *Future-oriented processes in development* (pp. 243–289). Chicago: University of Chicago Press.

Raimondi, A. J. (1994). A unifying theory for the definition and classification of hydrocephalus. *Child's Nervous System, 10,* 2–12.

Raimondi, A. J., & Soare, P. (1974). Intellectual development in shunted hydrocephalic children. *American Journal of Diseases of Children, 127,* 664–671.

Riva, D., Milani, N., Giorgi, C., Pantaleoni, C., Zorzi, C., & Devoti, M. Intelligence outcome in children with shunted hydrocephalus of different etiology. *Child's Nervous System, 10,* 70–73.

Rosner, J., & Simon, P. (1971). The Auditory Analysis Test. *Journal of Learning Disabilities, 8,* 24–37.

Rourke, B. P. (1989). *Nonverbal learning disabilities: The syndrome and the model.* New York: Guilford Press.

Rourke, B. P., & Fuerst, D. R. (1991). *Learning disabilities and psychosocial functioning: A neuropsychological perspective.* New York: Guilford Press.

Shallice, T. (1982). Specific impairments of planning. *Philosophical Transactions of the Royal Society of London, Part B, 298,* 199–209.

Shurtleff, D. B., Foltz, E. L., & Loeser, J. D. (1973). Hydrocephalus: A definition of its progression and relationship to intellectual function, diagnosis, and complications. *American Journal of Diseases of Children, 125,* 688–693.

Soare, P. L., & Raimondi, A. J. (1977). Intellectual and perceptual–motor characteristics of treated myelomeningocele children. *American Journal of Diseases of Children, 131,* 199–204.

Sobkowiak, C. A. (1992). Effect of hydrocephalus on neuronal migration and maturation. *European Journal of Pediatric Surgery, 2,* 7–11.

Tew, B. (1979). The "cocktail party syndrome" in children with hydrocephalus and spina bifida. *British Journal of Disorders of Communication, 14,* 89–101.

Thompson, N. M., Fletcher, J. M., Chapieski, L., Landry, S. H., Miner, M. E., & Bixby, J. (1991). Cognitive and motor abilities in preschool hydrocephalics. *Journal of Clinical and Experimental Neuropsychology, 13,* 245–253.

van der Knaap, M. S., Valk, J., Bakker, C. J., Schoonewaveld, M., Faber, J. A. J., Willemse, J., & Gooskens, R. H. M. (1991). Myelination as an expression of the functional maturity of the brain. *Developmental Medicine and Child Neurology, 33,* 849–857.

Volpe, J. L. (1989). Intraventricular hemorrhage in the premature infant—current concepts: Part I. *Annals of Neurology, 25,* 3–11.

Wechsler, D. (1974). *Wechsler Intelligence Scale for Children—Revised.* New York: Psychological Corporation.

Wills, K. E. (193). Neuropsychological functioning in children with spina bifida and/or hydrocephalus. *Journal of Clinical Child Psychology, 22,* 247–265.

Wills, K. E., Holmbeck, G. N., Dillon, K., & McLone, D. G. (1990). Intelligence and academic achievement in children with meningomyelocele. *Journal of Pediatric Psychology, 15,* 161–176.

Wishell, T. E., Tuttle, D. J., Northam, R. S., & Simonds, G. R. (1990). Major congenital neurologic malformations. *American Journal of Diseases of Children, 144*, 61–67.

Woodcock, R. W., & Johnson, M. B. (1989). *Woodcock–Johnson Psycho-Educational Test Battery—Revised.* Allen, TX: DLM Teaching Resources.

Zeiner, H. K., & Prigatano, G. P. (1982). Information processing deficits in hydrocephalic and letter reversal children. *Neuropsychologia, 20*, 483–492.

9

Sotos Syndrome

Catherine B. Dool
Katy B. Fuerst
Byron P. Rourke

Sotos syndrome, also known as cerebral gigantism, is a rare growth disorder first identified by Sotos and colleagues in 1964. It is marked by rapid growth in early childhood, characteristic facial features, and nonprogressive cognitive impairment (Sotos, Dodge, Muirhead, Crawford, & Talbot, 1964). At present, there is no diagnostic test for this syndrome; therefore, it must be identified on the basis of physical characteristics and developmental history.

In this chapter the clinical features of Sotos syndrome are presented, including findings of accelerated growth, craniofacial features, genetics, neurological and neuroradiological characteristics, and issues concerning differential diagnosis. Research addressing the psychological functioning of children with Sotos syndrome is then examined; following this, a comparison is made between the cognitive profiles of Sotos syndrome and the Nonverbal Learning Disabilities (NLD) syndrome. Finally, the evidence is weighed for the presence of white matter involvement.

CLINICAL MANIFESTATIONS OF SOTOS SYNDROME

Accelerated Growth

The excessive growth in Sotos syndrome begins prenatally. At birth, the babies tend to be very large (above the 90th centile), especially in length (Cole & Hughes, 1990; Ott & Robinson, 1969; Wit et al., 1985). Over the next few years, these children grow at an accelerated rate, so that their height, weight, and bone age are typically 2 to 4 years beyond their chronological age. This growth rate then tends to level off. However, the children remain markedly above average in height (Milunsky, Cowie, & Donoghue, 1967; Ott & Robinson, 1969; Sotos, Cutler, & Dodge, 1977).

Because of the advanced bone age, puberty is usually reached early in relation to chronological age (Dodge, Holmes, & Sotos, 1983; Sotos et al., 1964). As little growth occurs after puberty, children with this syndrome do not generally go on to reach gigantic heights in adulthood. However, they are typically tall, with long arms, large hands, and large feet (Dodge et al., 1983; Ott & Robinson, 1969).

The cause of the excessive growth in Sotos syndrome is still unknown. Endocrine abnormalities, including an excess of growth hormone, have typically not been found. Pancreatic, adrenal, pituitary, gonadal, and thyroid functions are usually normal (Dodge et al., 1983; Ferrier, de Meuron, Korol, & Hauser, 1980).

Craniofacial Features

This accelerated growth also affects craniofacial structures (Motohashi, Pruzansky, & Kawata, 1981). The characteristic facies in Sotos syndrome include a large head (macrocephaly) that is frequently long from front to back (dolichocephaly). The forehead tends to be broad and prominent (bossed); the eyes are widely spaced (hypertelorism); the palpebral fissures slant downward; and the hairline is receding. The jaw may be prominent (prognathism) and the palate highly arched (Dodge et al., 1983; Milunsky et al., 1967). Patients may not present with all the facial characteristics, and some variability has been noted even in the affected members of one family (Halal, 1982). These dysmorphic features also tend to become less obvious with advancing age (Cole & Hughes, 1990). It should be noted that selection factors may be operating here; a patient without the typical dysmorphic facies is not likely to be diagnosed with the syndrome (Ott & Robinson, 1969).

Genetics

Sotos syndrome is thought to be a hereditary disorder, although the mode of transmission has been debated. There is strongest support for autosomal dominant inheritance: Parent-to-child transmission has been documented in a number of families over three generations; males and females appear to be equally involved; and male-to-male transmission has been documented (Dodge et al., 1983; Halal, 1982; Sotos et al., 1977;

Winship, 1985; Zonana et al., 1977). Most of the cases appear to be sporadic. However, since adult cases of Sotos syndrome may go undiagnosed (because of less pronounced dysmorphic facial features and the fact that after puberty bone age is not a useful diagnostic sign), in some "sporadic" cases there may, in fact, be other affected family members (Zonana et al., 1977). The incidence of Sotos syndrome is not known.

Neurological Findings

Findings on neurological examination are usually limited to hypotonia, clumsiness, and some degree of cognitive impairment (Cole & Hughes, 1990; Dodge et al., 1983; Ferrier et al., 1980; Sotos et al., 1964). During infancy, hypotonia is usually present. Motor development (including sitting, crawling, and walking) is often delayed, probably secondary to decreased muscle tone (Cole & Hughes, 1990; Ott & Robinson, 1969). Hypotonia of the oral musculature has also been found; this results in drooling and may contribute to speech problems. Muscle tone and coordination problems have been noted to improve in these children as they get older, although some impairment may persist (Cole & Hughes, 1990).

Neuroradiological Findings

Dilation of the ventricular system is the most common neuroradiological finding in Sotos syndrome; it has been reported in between 69% (Wit et al., 1985) and 91% (Milunsky et al., 1967) of cases. However, increased intracranial pressure, progressive hydrocephalus, and cerebral atrophy have not been reported (Dodge et al., 1983; Poznanski & Stephenson, 1967; Sotos et al., 1964). In some cases, megalencephaly may be present with no ventricular dilation (Hulse, 1981). Midline cava have been reported with some frequency (Barth, Vlasveld, & Valk, 1980; Poznanski & Stephenson, 1967). (As the brain develops it encloses several cavities, or cava. With growth the cava are usually obliterated. In some cases, such as the cavum between the septa pellucida, the cavities may persist in the mature brain as a normal variant of no clinical significance. Other cava are rarely seen in mature brains and are more likely to occur with congenital brain anomalies [Sarnat, 1992]).

Abnormally shaped dorsum sellae were found in one investigation (Poznanski & Stephenson, 1967). Agenesis or dysgenesis of the corpus callosum was found in two patients (Ferrier et al., 1980; Marie et al., 1965, cited in Poznanski & Stephenson, 1967). In some instances cortical sulci, including the sylvian fissure, have been reported to be prominent

(Barth et al., 1980; Hulse, 1981; Wit et al., 1985; Zonana et al., 1977). Barth et al. (1980) reported a case of a 15-day-old infant with a right sylvian abnormality, in which the right frontal, parietal, and temporal opercula had not yet grown to cover the insula, as is usually the case at birth. By 27 months of age, this abnormality had resolved, with complete opercularization occurring.

Electroencephalographic (EEG) abnormalities have been reported in as many as 70% of cases and usually consist of nonspecific abnormalities (Milunsky et al., 1969; Ott & Robinson, 1969). Seizure disorders are less common than EEG abnormalities; when they occur, they have often been associated with febrile episodes (Dodge et al., 1983).

Postmortem Findings

Only one autopsy has been reported to date (Sugarman, Heuser, & Reed, 1977). The brain was found to be large, apparently due to an increase in grey matter. Microgyria were found in the occipital area. Dilation of the ventricles was not found. Histology revealed generalized angular shrinkage of neurons, as well as binucleate neurons in the temporal cortex and basal ganglia. The significance of these findings is not known (Dodge et al., 1983).

Diagnosis

Diagnosis of Sotos syndrome is complicated by a number of factors. First, many of the physical characteristics are not specific to this syndrome (Dodge et al., 1983). Some of these features (such as the facial anomalies), can be minor, and the criteria for identification are rather subjective. It is also clear that as the individual with Sotos syndrome ages, changes in phenotype also occur; however, little is known about Sotos syndrome in adults. It has also become increasingly evident that there is considerable variation in the observed phenotype of this disorder. These factors make diagnosis, especially in mildly affected individuals and/or adolescents and adults, very difficult (Beemer, Veenema, & de Pater, 1986; Cole & Hughes, 1990). Given the variability of expression, it has been increasingly suggested that Sotos syndrome may represent a heterogeneous disorder (Beemer et al., 1986; Cole & Hughes, 1990; Milunsky et al., 1967; Zonana et al., 1977).

Children with Sotos syndrome frequently come to medical attention because of developmental delay and/or their large size. Sotos syndrome must therefore be distinguished from other conditions that can lead to early excessive growth and/or mental retardation. A partial list includes such disorders as Marfan syndrome, adrenogenital syndrome, neurofibromatosis, hydrocephalus, acromegaly, pituitary gigantism, Albright syndrome, Beckwith syndrome, Weaver syndrome, and fragile-X syndrome (Cole & Hughes, 1990; Ott & Robinson, 1969). Depending on the age of presentation and the severity of the disorder, some syndromes, such as the Weaver and fragile-X syndromes, may be difficult to distinguish from Sotos syndrome because of overlap in phenotype (Cole & Hughes, 1990). A differential diagnosis can usually be made on the basis of history, physical findings, biochemical, endocrinological, and chromosomal studies (Cole & Hughes, 1990; Ott & Robinson, 1969).

ETIOLOGY AND PATHOPHYSIOLOGY

As is the case in numerous malformation syndromes, the etiology and pathophysiology of Sotos syndrome have not yet been clearly delineated. However, several authors have suggested that the observed concurrence of cancer and Sotos syndrome may provide valuable clues to the syndrome's etiology. Wit et al. (1985) reported a 7% incidence of solid tumors in patients with Sotos syndrome. However, this number may be exaggerated because of a bias toward reporting two concurrent rare disorders (Cole & Hughes, 1990). Maldonado, Gaynon, and Poznanski (1984) reviewed 132 cases reported before 1981 and found 8 (6%) with tumors. Cohen (1989) reports a more conservative estimate of 3.9% risk. Although there is disagreement over the precise incidence, there is general agreement among many authors that patients with Sotos syndrome, when compared to the general population, are at an increased risk for developing some form of malignancy. Of the tumor types reported, Wilm tumor and hepatocarcinoma have occurred more than once (Cole & Hughes, 1990). Other types have included vaginal, parotid, and neuroectodermal tumors, as well as cavernous hemangiomas, osteochondroma, giant-cell granuloma of the mandible, neuroblastoma (Nance, Neglia, Talwar, & Berry, 1990), and small-cell lung carcinoma (SCLC; Cole, Hughes, Jeffries, Williams, & Arnold, 1992).

In addition to Sotos syndrome (e.g., Wit et al., 1985), tumors have been reported in several other overgrowth syndromes, including congenital hemihypertrophy (Fraumeni, Geiser, & Manning, 1967), Perlman syndrome (Neri, Martini-Neri, Katz, & Opitz, 1984), and Wiedemann–Beckwith syndrome (Kosseff et al., 1976). The Wiedemann–Beckwith and Perlman syndromes are characterized by macrosomia and frequently include Wilms tumor. Neurofibromatosis involves abnormal neural growth regulation with tumors of peripheral neural tissue. Ruvalcaba–Myhre–Smith syndrome is characterized by early macrosomia, hypotonia, ocular signs, and intestinal polyposis. Although the majority of these syndromes appear to be linked with a particular type of tumor, Sotos syndrome has been associated with a variety of solid tumors of ectodermal or mesodermal origin. Of further interest is the increased risk for childhood cancer with high birth weight, as well as with macrosomia of unknown origin (Nance et al., 1990).

The association between somatic overgrowth and cancer has led to the suggestion that both the malformation and the increased risk for tumor formation are caused by a genetic defect that precipitates abnormal organogenesis. Not surprisingly, the involvement of humoral factors has not been substantiated. An endocrine imbalance, for example, would be expected to have generalized effects. On the contrary, localized overgrowth in Sotos syndrome is most extreme in the cranium, while asymmetry is evident in hemihypertrophy (Bale, Drum, Parry, & Mulvihill, 1985). Overgrowth in Wiedemann–Beckwith syndrome may affect most of the body, one side of the body, or select organs or tissues (Kosseff et al., 1976). Kosseff and colleagues have proposed that in syndromes involving overgrowth and malignancies, such as the Wiedemann–Beckwith syndrome, a genetic defect could adversely affect cellular development, differentiation, and function. The resultant anomalies in the formation of organs and tissues could account for the selective overgrowth and malformations, as well as the predisposition for malignancies.

Several authors have postulated specific loci for the gene or genes related to Sotos syndrome. For example, Cole et al. (1992) have reported on a patient with SCLC and Sotos syndrome. The association of these two disorders is significant, because a particular genetic defect that has been identified in SCLC has also been reported in at least one patient with Sotos syndrome. In SCLC, a loss of heterozygosity of markers at chromosome 3p21 has been identified. Schrander-Stumpel, Fryns, and Hamer (1990) reported an apparently balanced 3p/6p translocation (between the short arms of chromosomes 3 and 6), and suggested that one of these two sites, 3p21 or 6p21, may the location of the gene or genes for Sotos syndrome. One of these locations (3p21) is the same as that identified in SCLC. Although there have been reports of chromosomal abnormalities in other locations (e.g., Cole & Hughes, 1990; Tamaki et al., 1989), Cole et al. (1992) argue that the phenotype described by Schrander-Stumpel et al. was "classical," whereas those described by the other authors were merely "Sotos-like" (p. 340).

The proposed pathophysiological mechanisms involved in both Sotos and SCLC involve the loss of a protective gene, suppressor gene, or antioncogene. Cole et al. (1992) have hypothesized that a germline mutation resulting in only one copy of the normal gene may be the cause of the malformations seen in Sotos syndrome. It is possible that this suppressor gene is not specific to SCLC, but has a protective effect against a variety of tumors. This may explain the association of Sotos with many different types of tumors. There has, in fact, been a specific suppressor oncogene (v-erb a) localized to the chromosomal region of 3p21. It is possible that mutations in this region remove the beneficial suppressor effects of this or other oncogenes.

Research into childhood retinoblastoma has yielded evidence for both suppressor and expressor systems in the development of that tumor (Murphree & Benedict, 1984). A diploid pair of suppressor alleles at the chromosomal locus for retinoblastoma has been implicated in tumor formation when chromosome changes in the retinoblast result in homozygosity for the generally inactive allele. An expressor gene or oncogene may also be involved. Murphree and Benedict (1984) suggest that other childhood tumors similar to retinoblastoma, such as Wilms tumor and neuroblastoma, as well as other cancers (including familial renal cell carcinoma and SCLC), may fit the same model of tumorigenesis. Although the possible role of specific genes in the etiology of Sotos and the tumors often associated with it remains obscure, the considerable overlap among Sotos syndrome, other malformation syndromes, and various cancers is striking, and the human genetic and cancer research to date is compelling.

PSYCHOLOGICAL CHARACTERISTICS

Early descriptions of Sotos syndrome listed mental retardation as one of the characteristic symptoms of this disorder. In a review of 80 cases, 83% of the children with Sotos syndrome were described as developmentally retarded (Jaeken, Van der Schueren-Lodeweyckx, & Eeckels, 1972). Other studies with smaller samples have differed in the percentage of children classified as mentally retarded; the figures have varied from 33% (Rutter & Cole, 1991) to 73% (Varley & Crnic, 1984). The levels of impairment ranged from mild to profound retardation.

Continued research into this disorder has shown that the cognitive profiles of children with Sotos syndrome may vary greatly. Although many children do appear to have pervasive cognitive deficits consistent with a diagnosis of mental retardation, others present with specific learning disabilities. The tendency in many studies to limit the cognitive assessment to an intelligence test may have meant that some children with a specific language or visual-perceptual deficit were not identified. Also, the results of assessments have often been presented as summary IQ scores. Given a large discrepancy between verbal and performance skills, children with a specific learning disability may have been inappropriately classified as retarded on the basis of their overall IQ scores.

Another difficulty with many studies to date has been the tendency to group children across age ranges. This is problematic because of increasing evidence that at least some children with Sotos syndrome exhibit very different cognitive abilities, depending upon their age (Bale et al., 1985; Bloom et al., 1983; Ott & Robinson, 1969; Rutter & Cole, 1991). Evidence from studies in which children have been followed longitudinally (Bale et al., 1985; Bloom et al., 1983) suggest that with few exceptions, infants and toddlers show evidence of early cognitive, motor, and language delay. Despite what were often significant early delays, a number of children go on to obtain intelligence test scores in the average range. However, even in those instances where the child's intellectual abilities "normalize," there is still evidence of learning disabilities.

It is not clear what proportion of children with Sotos syndrome demonstrate this developmental pattern. In one study of six children who were reassessed after the age of 6 years, four demonstrated this pattern; early in their development there was evidence of motor, language, and cognitive deficits, but over time these children obtained scores on measures of psychometric intelligence that fell within the average range (Bloom et al., 1983). Two of the six children continued to demonstrate impaired intellectual abilities after the age of 6 years. Bale et al. (1985) present the cases of two sisters who exhibited this same course of early developmental delay, with average intelligence test scores evident later in childhood. It is not known whether any features in the early profiles of children with Sotos syndrome may distinguish those who will go on to exhibit specific learning difficulties from those who present with more pervasive cognitive deficits. The variability of cognitive deficits again raises the possibility of various subtypes of Sotos syndrome.

Neuropsychological Findings

In this section, the performances in specific areas of functioning of children with Sotos syndrome are examined. A few cautionary points should be made. Most studies are based upon relatively, or sometimes very, small sample sizes. Often the test results of children with a wide range of IQ scores are presented together, which may mask patterns of findings. Finally, in no study were comprehensive neuropsychological assessments done; this leaves many gaps in our knowledge.

Motor Skills

Children with Sotos syndrome demonstrate significant delays in attaining motor milestones. Psychomotor impairment often persists throughout childhood. These children are frequently described as being clumsy, having poor fine motor coordination, and exhibiting an awkward gait (Bale et al., 1985; Dodge et al., 1977; Jaeken et al., 1972; Milunsky et al., 1967; Ott & Robinson, 1969). When assessed with the Bruininks–Oseretsky Test of Motor Proficiency, a battery of tests examining gross and fine motor abilities, children with Sotos syndrome scored below the mean in all areas (Stewart & Deitz, 1986). Tests of strength, gross motor speed, and agility were performed relatively better than were tests of balance, coordination, and visual–motor control.

Visual–Spatial Skills

Visual-perceptual abilities have not typically been assessed. Some children with Sotos syndrome show a lower Performance IQ than Verbal IQ, but this is not always the case. Indeed, in approximately half of the cases, the opposite pattern of a higher Performance than Verbal IQ was observed, or no significant discrepancy was found (Morrow, Whitman & Accardo, 1990; Ott & Robinson, 1969; Patterson, Bloom, Reese, & Weisskopf, 1978; Varley & Crnic, 1984). Impairment on a visual–spatial drawing task has been noted (Patterson et al., 1978), although the extent to which poor performance is attributable to impaired coordination rather than to impaired visual-perceptual or visual–spatial skills per se is not clear. The use of visual-perceptual tests without a drawing or constructional component would help to clarify this issue.

Problem-Solving Ability

Anecdotal reports suggest that children with Sotos syndrome tend to display concrete thinking (Patterson et al., 1978), are impaired on creative tasks (Rutter & Cole, 1991), and are perseverative in their responding (Patterson et al., 1978).

Language Skills

Infants and toddlers with Sotos syndrome typically exhibit delayed language milestones. Language skills remain impaired over the next few years (ages 3 to 6), although expressive language skills tend to be slightly more impaired than are receptive skills (Bale et al., 1985; Livingood & Borengasser, 1981). At this age, children have been noted to rely more on gestures than on speech to communicate during the assessment (Bloom et al., 1983). It has been suggested that an "oral apraxia" may contribute to the delay in expressive language, because some children's speech has been noted to be marked by articulation difficulties, drooling, and difficulty with chewing (Bale et al., 1985; Livingood & Borengasser, 1991). It is not clear whether these difficulties are attributable to hypotonia rather than to a true apraxia. Voice quality has often been noted to be unusually low and hoarse (Hulse, 1981; Livingood & Borengasser, 1981; Ott & Robinson, 1969).

Bloom et al. (1983) noted that in all of their cases, even in those children with normal Verbal IQs, there were word-finding difficulties and unusually long response times to auditory material; these findings suggest some impairment of auditory processing. Auditory-perceptual abilities, however, have not been formally assessed. Little is known about the verbal attentional and memory skills of these children.

Academic Achievement

Discrepancies exist in the literature regarding the reading skills of children with Sotos syndrome. The results of one study suggested that reading accuracy and reading comprehension skills were, on average, 2 years or more below chronological age (Rutter & Cole, 1991). The results of another study suggested that word identification and reading comprehension skills were average or even advanced for the child's mental and chronological age (Patterson et al., 1978). In all cases, reading comprehension was slightly poorer than word decoding (Patterson et al., 1978; Rutter & Cole, 1991). Arithmetic computation and reasoning have been found to be impaired relative to reading skills (Bloom et al., 1983; Patterson et al., 1978). Frequently these children require special educational programs, either for developmental retardation or for specific learning disabilities (Varley & Crnic, 1984).

Socioemotional/Adaptational Functioning

In addition to their cognitive deficits, children with Sotos syndrome frequently experience difficulties in their socioemotional functioning (Rutter & Cole, 1991; Varley & Crnic, 1984). These children have been reported to have few if any close friends, and typically prefer the company of adults (Rutter & Cole, 1991). They have been noted to be withdrawn, or to have a manner of interacting that tends to lead to isolation. They may be teased or not accepted at school (Varley & Crnic, 1984). They may also encounter difficulties when unrealistic expectations arise because they are perceived as being older than they are, due to their large size (Dodge, Holmes, & Sotos, 1983; Livingood & Borengasser, 1981). This may be compounded by the fact that developmental delays may make even age-appropriate goals difficult for some of these children to attain.

In addition to their poor social functioning, the majority of children with Sotos syndrome have been reported to exhibit some type of behavioral problem (Rutter & Cole, 1991; Varley & Crnic, 1984). These authors found hyperactivity (56–64%) and tempter tantrums (81%) to be common. Some children were noted to be obsessive or to display ritualistic behavior (27–50%) and/or phobias (67%). Many children had sleep problems, typically early-morning awakening (69%). Excessive eating or fluid intake was seen in some children (31% and 56%, respectively), raising questions about hypothalamic involvement. They have also been noted to have very little awareness of danger, which entails that they be closely supervised (56%). Some children have been noted to exhibit precocious or inappropriate sexual behavior (31%). Overall, more children were classified as neurotic (36–44%) than as antisocial (14–25%) on the Rutter Parent and Teacher Scales (Rutter & Cole, 1991). Morrow et al. (1990) describes one case of a child with Sotos syndrome who presented with normal psychometric intelligence and an autistic disorder.

Comparison to Neuropsychological Profile of Children with NLD

Many similarities to the cognitive and psychological profiles of children with the NLD syndrome can be seen in the descriptions of children with Sotos syndrome. Certainly this is the case with respect to their motor skills. Specifically, in both syndromes there are delays in attaining motor milestones, poor psychomotor skills throughout childhood, poor gross motor skills, and clumsiness (Rourke, 1989). However, it is not yet known whether the developmental changes in motor skills of children with Sotos syndrome also parallel those changes seen with development in children with the NLD syndrome. For example, it is not clear whether simple motor skills become a strength by the middle-school years. Nor is it known whether psychomotor skills tend to worsen with age, with the exception of those skills (such as handwriting) that a child is able to practice repeatedly until they become routine (Rourke, 1989).

Impairments in visual skills (including visual perception, attention, memory, and visual–spatial ability), which constitute a hallmark of the NLD syndrome, have been shown to be impaired in some but not all children with Sotos syndrome. Although some children with Sotos syndrome appear to have impairments on drawing and on the Performance subtests of the Wechsler and other scales, this has not been shown to be an invariant pattern.

Formal evaluation of problem-solving and concept-forming ability of children with Sotos syndrome is needed. Certainly, anecdotal reports would suggest that this is an area of deficit, as is the case in the NLD syndrome. Marked difficulties with concept formation, complex problem-solving ability, the appreciation of humor, and cause-and-effect relationships have all been noted in children with the NLD syndrome (Rourke, 1989). These deficits have been found to be more marked in older as compared to younger children with NLD, especially as they enter the period of formal operational thought (Casey, Rourke, & Picard, 1991).

When the language abilities of children with Sotos syndrome and of children with the NLD syndrome are compared, both similarities and differences are noted. Both show early language difficulties, with speech marked by an apparent oral–motor apraxia. Children with NLD typically go on to develop very good auditory-perceptual skills, attention for simple auditory stimuli, and memory for rote verbal material (Rourke, 1989). This has not been demonstrated in the case of children with Sotos syndrome. In one study (Bloom et al., 1983), the slow response style and uneven performance were suggestive of auditory-perceptual problems, and word-finding difficulties were also noted. Children with Sotos syndrome also have not been noted to demonstrate the "cocktail party" chatter often seen in youngsters with NLD (Rourke, 1989).

A hallmark of the NLD syndrome is the discrepancy between Verbal and Performance IQs on the Wechsler scales. Given their excellent auditory perception, attention, and memory, children with NLD are able to develop a large store of rote verbal material and verbal associations, which is reflected on their scores on the Verbal subtests (Rourke, 1989). In Sotos syndrome, the Verbal IQ has not consistently been found to be elevated relative to the Performance IQ.

As a result of their excellent auditory perception, attention, and memory, children with the NLD syndrome tend to develop excellent phonological skills, word recognition, and receptive and associative skills. These skills may develop to extreme degrees. In keeping with their less well-developed conceptual than phonological abilities, reading comprehension appears to be deficient in comparison with their word-decoding skills (Rourke, 1989). Findings in this area in children with Sotos syndrome have been less consistent. One study suggested that some children with Sotos syndrome develop normal to advanced word-decoding and reading comprehension skills (Patterson et al., 1978) A second study found both single-word reading and reading comprehension to be decreased (Rutter & Cole, 1991). However, in each case the pattern of relatively better word-decoding than comprehension skills was found, as has been described in the NLD syndrome.

As in Sotos syndrome, children with the NLD syndrome have been shown to be markedly impaired in arithmetic computation and reasoning. In the NLD syndrome, some difficulties in written arithmetic appear to be attributable to their visual-perceptual and visual–spatial–organizational problems, and poor graphomotor skills. In addition, children with NLD develop poor conceptual understanding of mathematical concepts, and have difficulty generalizing a previously learned concept to novel problems (Strang & Rourke, 1985). It is not clear in Sotos syndrome which primary deficits contribute to the poor arithmetic skills, but these children do indeed have difficulties in this area.

Finally, there are a number of similarities in the socioemotional functioning of children with NLD and those with Sotos syndrome. In both instances, deficient social interaction skills have been noted; the children preferring to interact with adults or younger children, both of whom are probably more tolerant of the affected children's method of relating. Poor social judgment (such as not being aware of dangerous situations or exhibiting inappropriate sexual behavior in public) has been described in both groups of children (Rourke, 1989; Rourke & Fuerst, 1991). Hyperactivity has been noted as common in both instances. Children with NLD, who have been noted to be hyperactive in early grades, often later become quite hypoactive (Rourke, 1989). It is not known whether the same is the case for children with Sotos syndrome as they become older. Psychopathology is commonly seen in both groups of children, with internalized forms, including anxiety, depression, and social withdrawal, being more common than acting-out behavior (Rourke, 1989; Rourke & Fuerst, 1991). Some behaviors frequently noted in Sotos syndrome, including temper tantrums, insomnia, and eating disturbances, have not been commonly reported in the NLD syndrome.

WHITE MATTER INVOLVEMENT

Various brain anomalies have been noted in children with Sotos syndrome. Although a few cases clearly have white matter involvement, such as those with callosal agenesis, the link in most cases is not as clear. As mentioned, megalencephaly, enlarged ventricles, and increases in cerebral sulci have been noted. Typically, with enlarged ventricles secondary to hydrocephalus, the white matter is particularly vulnerable to forces exerted upon it. However, given the absence of increased intracranial pressure in Sotos syndrome, the effect on the white matter is not clear. Sarnat (1992) speculates that the megalencephaly may be related either to an increase in neurons resulting from the failure of embryonic death of neuroblasts, or to late differentiation of the ependyma leading to an increase in mitotic neuroepithelial cells. In the one autopsied brain to date, grey matter abnormalities were noted.

CONCLUSION

To sum up, some interesting similarities in cognitive and psychosocial functioning between children with Sotos syndrome and those with the NLD syndrome have been noted. However, the evidence of white matter involvement is less clear. Given the present state of our knowledge of Sotos syndrome, the parallel between these two disorders must remain descriptive in nature at this time.

A number of avenues of investigation in future research appear to be in order. Given the variability in cognitive abilities (some children with Sotos syndrome having learning difficulties, whereas others may be profoundly retarded), the examination of larger numbers of children for evidence of specific subtypes of Sotos syndrome may be fruitful. This in turn requires the utilization of more complete neuropsychological assessments, to fill the gaps in our present knowledge of the cognitive functioning of these children. Such comprehensive assessment should increase the probability of the identification of primary deficits that may be contributing to problems in complex behaviors, such as arithmetic, problem solving, and social interactions. Finally, the use of more recently developed radiographic techniques (computed tomography and magnetic resonance imaging) is needed. An examination of possible links between radiographic and neuropsychological results would allow for a better test of the white matter hypothesis.

REFERENCES

Bale, A. E., Drum, M. A., Parry, D. M., & Mulvihill, J. J. (1985). Familial Sotos syndrome (cerebral gigantism): Craniofacial and psychological characteristics. *American Journal of Medical Genetics, 20*, 613–624.

Barth, P. G., Vlasveld, L., & Valk, J. (1980). Unilateral delayed opercularization in a case of Sotos syndrome (cerebral gigantism). *Neuroradiology, 20*, 49–52.

Beemer, F. A., Veenema, H., & Pater, J. M. (1986). Cerebral gigantism (Sotos syndrome) in two patients with Fra(X) chromosomes. *American Journal of Medical Genetics, 23*, 221–226.

Bloom, A. S., Reese, A., Hersh, J. H., Podruch, P. E., Weisskopf, B., & Dinno, N. (1983). Cognition in cerebral gigantism: Are the estimates of mental retardation too high? *Journal of Developmental and Behavioral Pediatrics, 4*, 250–252.

Casey, J. E., Rourke, B. P., & Picard, E. M. (1991). Syndrome of nonverbal learning disabilities: Age differences in neuropsychological, academic, and socioemotional functioning. *Development and Psychopathology, 3*, 329–345.

Cohen, M. M. J. (1989). A comprehensive and critical assessment of overgrowth syndromes. In H. Harris & K. Hirschhorn (Eds.), *Advances in human genetics* (Vol. 18, pp. 181–303). New York: Plenum Press.

Cole, T. R. P., & Hughes, H. E. (1990). Sotos syndrome. *Journal of Medical Genetics, 27*, 571–576.

Cole, T. R. P., Hughes, H. E., Jeffries, M. J., Williams, G. T., & Arnold, M. M. (1992). Small cell lung carcinoma in a patient with Sotos syndrome: Are genes at 3p21 involved in both conditions? *Journal of Medical Genetics, 29*, 338–341.

Dodge, P. R., Holmes, S. J., & Sotos, J. F. (1983). Cerebral gigantism. *Developmental Medicine and Child Neurology, 25*, 248–252.

Ferrier, P. E., de Meuron, G., Korol, S., & Hauser, H. (1980). Cerebral gigantism (Sotos syndrome) with juvenile macular degeneration. *Helvetica Paediatrica Acta*, *35*, 97–102.

Fraumeni, J. F., Geiser, C. F., & Manning, M. D. (1967). Wilms tumor and congenital hemihypertrophy: Report of five new cases and a review of the literature. *Pediatrics*, *40*, 886–899.

Halal, F. (1982). Male to male transmission of cerebral gigantism. *American Journal of Medical Genetics*, *12*, 411–419.

Hulse, J. A. (1981). Two children with cerebral gigantism and congenital primary hypothyroidism. *Developmental Medicine and Child Neurology*, *23*, 242–246.

Jaeken, J., Van der Schueren-Lodeweyckx, M., & Eeckels, R. (1972). Cerebral gigantism syndrome: A report of 4 cases and review of the literature. *Zeitschrift für Kinderheilkunde*, *112*, 332–346.

Kosseff, A. L., Herrmann, J., Gilbert, E. F., Visekul, C., Lubinsky, M., & Opitz, J. M. (1976). Studies of malformation syndromes of man: XXIX. The Wiedemann–Beckwith syndrome. *European Journal of Pediatrics*, *123*, 139–166.

Livingood, A. B., & Borengasser, M. A. (1991). Cerebral gigantism in infancy: Implications for psychological and social development. *Child Psychiatry and Human Development*, *12*, 46–53.

Maldonado, V., Gaynon, P. S., & Poznanski, A. K. (1984). Cerebral gigantism associated with Wilm's tumor. *American Journal of Diseases of Children*, *138*, 486–488.

Milunsky, A., Cowie, V. A., & Donoghue, E. C. (1967). Cerebral gigantism in childhood: A report of two cases and a review of the literature. *Pediatrics*, *40*, 395–402.

Morrow, J. D., Whitman, B. Y., & Accardo, P. J. (1990). Autistic disorders in Sotos syndrome: A case report. *European Journal of Pediatrics*, *149*, 567–569.

Motohashi, N., Pruzansky, S., & Kawata, T. (1981). Roentgencephalometric analysis of cerebral gigantism: Report of four patients. *Journal of Craniofacial Genetics and Developmental Biology*, *1*, 73–94.

Murphree, A. L., & Benedict, W. F. (1984). Retinoblastoma: Clues to human oncogenesis. *Science*, *223*, 1028–1033.

Nance, M. A., Neglia, J. P., Talwar, D., & Berry, S. A. (1990). Neuroblastoma in a patient with Sotos syndrome. *Journal of Medical Genetics*, *27*, 130–132.

Neri, G., Martini-Neri, N. E., Katz, B. E., & Opitz, J. M. (1984). The Perlman syndrome: Familial renal dysplasia with Wilms tumor, fetal gigantism, and multiple congenital anomalies. *American Journal of Medical Genetics*, *19*, 195–207.

Ott, J. E., & Robinson, A. (1969). Cerebral gigantism. *American Journal of Diseases of Children*, *117*, 357–368.

Patterson, R., Bloom, A., Reese, A., & Weisskopf, B. (1978). Psychological aspects of cerebral gigantism. *Journal of Pediatric Psychology*, *3*, 6–8.

Poznanski, A. K., & Stephenson, J. M. (1967). Radiographic findings in hypothalamic acceleration of growth associated with cerebral atrophy and mental retardation (cerebral gigantism). *Radiology*, *88*, 446–456.

Rourke, B. P. (1989). *Nonverbal learning disabilities: The syndrome and the model.* New York: Guilford Press.

Rourke, B. P., & Fuerst, D. R. (1991). *Learning disabilities and psychosocial functioning: A neuropsychological perspective.* New York: Guilford Press.

Rutter, S. C., & Cole, T. R. P. (1991). Psychological characteristics of Sotos syndrome. *Developmental Medicine and Child Neurology, 33,* 898–902.

Sarnat, H. B. (1992). *Cerebral dysgenesis: Embryology and clinical expression.* New York: Oxford University Press.

Schrander-Stumpel, C. T. R. M., Fryns, J. P., & Hamer, G. G. (1990). Sotos syndrome and *de novo* balanced autosomal translocation (t(3;6)(p21;21)). *Clinical Genetics, 37,* 226–229.

Sotos, J. F., Cutler, E. A., & Dodge, P. (1977). Cerebral gigantism. *American Journal of Diseases of Children, 131,* 625–627.

Sotos, J. F., Dodge, P. R., Muirhead, D., Crawford, J. D., & Talbot, N. B. (1964). Cerebral gigantism in childhood. *New England Journal of Medicine, 271,* 109–116.

Stewart, K. B., & Deitz, J. C. (1986). Motor development in children with Sotos' cerebral gigantism. *Physical and Occupational Therapy in Pediatrics, 6,* 41–53.

Strang, J. D., & Rourke, B. P. (1985). Arithmetic disability subtypes: The neuropsychological significance of specific arithmetic impairment in childhood. In B. P. Rourke (Ed.), *Neuropsychology of learning disabilities: Essentials of subtype analysis* (pp. 167–186). New York: Guilford Press.

Sugarman, G. I., Heuser, E. T., & Reed, W. B. (1977). A case of cerebral gigantism and hepatocarcinoma. *American Journal of Diseases of Children, 131,* 631–633.

Tamaki, K., Horie, K., Go, T., Okuno, T., Mikawa, H., Hua, Z. Y., & Abe, T. (1989). Sotos syndrome with a balanced reciprocal translocation t(2;12)(q33.3;q15). *Annales de Génétique, 32* (4), 244–246.

Varley, C. K., & Crnic, K. (1984). Emotional, behavioral, and cognitive status of children with cerebral gigantism. *Journal of Developmental and Behavioral Pediatrics, 5,* 132–134.

Winship, I. M. (1985). Sotos syndrome: Autosomal dominant inheritance substantiated. *Clinical Genetics, 28,* 243–246.

Wit, J. M., Beemer, F. A., Barth, P. G., Oorthuys, J. W. E., Dijkstra, P. F., Van den Brande, J. L., & Leschot, N. J. (1985). Cerebral gigantism (Sotos syndrome): Compiled data of 22 cases. *European Journal of Pediatrics, 144,* 131–140.

Zonana, J., Sotos, J. F., Romshe, C. A., Fisher, D. A., Elders, M. J., & Rimoin, D. L. (1977). Dominant inheritance of cerebral gigantism. *Journal of Pediatrics, 91,* 251–256.

10

Congenital Hypothyroidism

Joanne Rovet

Congenital hypothyroidism (CH) is a disorder of newborns that results from insufficient production of thyroid hormone (TH), an essential hormone for early brain development. Because the clinical features of CH appear relatively late in infancy, children with this disorder were diagnosed and treated after the critical period for preventing widespread and irreversible brain damage; as a result, CH was a leading cause of mental retardation (Crome & Stern, 1972). However, with the recent advent of mandatory programs to screen newborns for CH *en masse*, these children are now treated soon after birth without ever evidencing any clinical signs of the disease. Prospective studies demonstrate that newborn screening has definitely been effective in preventing mental retardation, but that subtle residual deficits still may occur in neuromotor, language, and cognitive areas (Rovet, Glorieux, & Heyerdahl, 1987).

Research, primarily on animals, has shown that TH plays a central role in a number of important neurobiological processes. These include cell division and neurogenesis (Shapiro, 1966), axon and dendrite formation (Legrand, 1984), neuronal migration (Potter et al., 1982), synaptogenesis (Nicholson & Altman, 1972), and myelination (Rosman, Malone, Helfenstein, & Kraft, 1972); hence TH is involved in both grey and white matter formation. There are two ways in which this hormone affects white matter production: by controlling the production of glial cells, the procurers of myelin (Lauder & Krebs, 1986); and by regulating two genes that control myelin production, myelin basic protein and myelin-associated glycoprotein (Munoz et al., 1991).

At the time of diagnosis, children with CH identified by screening lack TH to varying degrees. They differ in the time at which hypothyroidism begins, which for many is the last trimester of pregnancy. They also differ in postnatal duration of hypothyroidism, which can be up to 2–3 months; the duration depends on initial severity of hypothyroidism, the time at which treatment is initiated, and initial dose levels. Because the period of TH insufficiency appears to reflect a critical window when certain brain sites urgently need TH for their development, the specific sequelae will reflect the exact points at which the hormone is missing (both pre- and postnatally), as well as the unique developmental schedules of specific sites (Dobbing & Sands, 1973). Studies of children with CH identified by newborn screening show a pattern of deficits suggestive of the syndrome of Nonverbal Learning Disabilities (NLD). Although the severity of impairment is mild relative to that seen in other conditions producing an NLD effect, CH represents a prototypic example of this syndrome. Furthermore, recent studies in neurobiology and molecular biology also support an interpretation involving white matter dysfunction operating within a highly circumscribed point in time.

This chapter reviews the evidence on the role of TH in early brain development and subsequent behavior, which is based both on animal studies and on findings from children with CH. It shows that these children exhibit a neurodevelopmental profile characteristic of the NLD syndrome (to a mild degree), which is manifested in relative weakness only in arithmetic and reading comprehension. Recent findings showing effects of TH on attention and activity levels are also described. These reflect both organizational effects (those that occur at times when specific brain structures critically need TH) and activational effects (those that occur later in development and may signify the role of TH in neurotransmission). Whereas organizational effects appear to be associated with initial disease severity and timing of treatment onset, activational effects are associated with later adequacy of concurrent therapy and circulating hormone levels.

TH PHYSIOLOGY AND PATHOPHYSIOLOGY

The thyroid gland, which is located at the base of the neck, is regulated by a negative feedback system with the hypothalamus, which produces thyrotropin-releasing hormone (TRH), and the pituitary, which produces thyroid-stimulating hormone (TSH; thyrotropin). When TH is lacking, the levels of TRH and TSH are elevated; when TH is present in excess, levels are low or suppressed. In fact, elevations in TSH serve as a diagnostic indicator of hypothyroidism, while the converse is true for hyperthyroidism.

The thyroid gland develops during the second trimester of pregnancy and becomes functional during the third. Prior to this, the fetus depends on the maternal thyroid system; in fact, children of mothers with thyroid abnormalities represent a distinct subgroup at risk for learning disabilities (Man, Jones, Holden, & Mellits, 1971; Interagency Committee on Learning Disabilities, 1987). However, once the child's system comes into effect, there is minimal maternal contribution, although this continues to be an issue of debate (Burrow, Fisher, & Larsen, 1994). Even though levels of maternal TH may be detected in the newborn (Vulsma & DeViljder, 1989), this may not be sufficient to prevent damage in some tissues. For example, about 60% of neonates with CH have significantly delayed skeletal maturity (at or below 36 weeks' gestation), which is correlated with subsequently poorer intellectual outcome (Rovet, Ehrlich, & Sorbara, 1987).

There are actually two thyroid hormones produced by the thyroid gland: triiodothyronine (T_3) and tetraiodothyronine (T_4), also known as thyroxine. Both hormones travel in the bloodstream via binding proteins to different target tissues in the body, which include muscle, adipocyte, lung, kidney, and the central nervous system (CNS). There, they are involved in various processes of growth and metabolism. Although TH is important at any age to maintain body metabolic homeostasis, it is critically important during early development in controlling the manifold maturational events involved in the transformation of the newborn into the mature organism. At the target tissue site, all T_4 is converted to T_3, the active hormone T_3 then enters the cell and binds to a nuclear receptor; this complex activates DNA resulting in a cascade of biochemical events that ultimately produce specific proteins. Two such proteins regulated by TH are tubulin (Francon, Fellous, Lennon, & Nunez, 1977), which forms the cytoskeleton of developing axons and dendrites (Nunez, 1984), and microtubule-associated proteins, which are required for neuronal migration (Fellous, Lennon, Francon, & Nunez, 1979).

In recent years, molecular biologists have identified four TH receptors, three of which are localized in the brain (Bradley, Young, & Weinberger, 1989). "Alpha$_1$" is found almost exclusively in the cerebellum and "beta$_1$" only in the pituitary, whereas "alpha$_2$" is more widespread and found in hippocampus, cortex, and striatum. Recent studies indicate that these receptors also differ temporally in their periods of peak receptivity to TH. For example, alpha$_2$ is most active at a time that corresponds to birth in the human, whereas beta$_1$ has a more protracted period of receptivity (Strait, Schwartz, Perez-Castillo, & Oppenheimer, 1990). Because this signifies unique periods when different brain structures critically need TH, the sequelae of neonatal TH deficiency will vary, depending on the times when TH is missing and the unique developmental schedules of different brain tissues (Dobbing & Sands, 1973).

TH is also known to play a role in modulating neurotransmitter receptor sensitivity (Prange, Wilson, Rabon, & Lipton, 1969). Animal research has shown that receptor sensitivity to CNS catecholamines is decreased in hypothyroidism, leading to a compensatory increase in catechol concentration (Klawans, Goetz, & Weiner, 1974). Further alterations in T_4 level—as, for example, with dose changes—may precipitate a hyper-catecholaminergic state leading to behavioral (Josephson & Mackenzie, 1979) and cognitive (Johnston & Singer, 1982) changes. In the immature laboratory animal, hyperthyroidism has been found to be associated with increased synthesis and utilization of catecholamines and serotonin, as well as with increased motor activity; in the mature animal, neurotransmitter changes are more subtle and have less effect on behavioral activity (Rastogi & Singhal, 1976). In humans, hyperthyroidism is associated with poorer concentration, increased distractibility, and hyperactivity (Alvarez, Gomez, Alvarez, & Navarro, 1983; Wallace & MacCrimmon, 1990). This suggests that TH plays a role in attention and associated cognitive processes (e.g., working memory, learning), and that optimal functioning requires circulating TH levels well within the normal range.

CH: INCIDENCE, TREATMENT, AND SCREENING

CH is a disease characterized by a deficiency in TH production in the neonatal period. By contrast, juvenile or acquired hypothyroidism develops during middle childhood, although there are recent reports indicating onset in infancy (Foley, Abbassi, Copeland, & Draznin, 1994). CH, if untreated within the first few months of life, will lead to mental retardation. Untreated juvenile acquired hypothyroidism, by contrast, is not associated with mental deficiency; however, poorer learning, attention, and school functioning (in either reading or arithmetic areas) may occur following the initiation of L-thyroxine treatment, particularly if the condition is severe and the treatment more aggressive (Rovet, Daneman, & Bailey, 1993).

CH is a relatively common disorder of newborns, with an incidence rate of between 1 in 3000 and 1 in 4000 children (this varies according to racial and ethnic/cultural composition of the population). There is a marked female preponderance, with a male–female ratio of 1:2.5. Primary CH is caused by a defect in the thyroid gland, although in a small number of cases CH will also result from a CNS defect in either the hypothalamus (secondary CH) or pituitary gland (tertiary CH). The major causes of primary CH include an absent gland (athyrosis), the reasons for which are unknown; a gland that is improperly located because of a failure in embryonic migration (ectopia); a small hypoplastic gland (hypoplasia); and a dysfunctional gland, often accompanied by goiter (dyshormonogenesis). Ectopic and hypoplastic conditions, which represent less severe forms of hypothyroidism, account for about 40–45% of cases; athyrosis occurs in about 30–35% and dyshormonogenesis in about 15–20%.

Although children with CH vary considerably in terms of age of prenatal onset of hypothyroidism, it is well established that the earlier in infancy these children are treated, the better the outcome. As a rule, retardation will occur in 75% of children treated after the third month of life (Klein, 1980), whereas IQs will be in the normal range in 75% of such children treated before the third month (Hulse, 1984). However, even children treated immediately after birth may still have selective deficits, particularly in nonverbal visual–spatial skill areas (MacFaul, Dorner, Brett, & Grant, 1978).

The treatment of CH involves daily oral ingestion of L-thyroxine in pill form, for which dosage guidelines are now available (American Academy of Pediatrics, Committee on Genetics, 1987; American Academy of Pediatrics, Section on Endocrinology and Committee on Genetics, 1993). However, the optimal dose levels of L-thyroxine have not been satisfactorily established, particularly since overtreatment can lead to hyperthyroidism, which can also adversely affect neurodevelopment (Daneman & Howard, 1980). My colleagues and I have found that infants with levels of circulating T_4 above the normal range have more difficult temperaments than do those with levels within the normal range (Rovet, Ehrlich, & Sorbara, 1989). Because temperamental difficulty is reflected in elevated scores on scales of arousal and activity levels, this may also reflect enhanced maturation of the adrenal system, as was shown in rats comparably exposed to high TH levels in infancy (Meserve & Leathem, 1974).

Because treatment for children with clinically diagnosed CH was until recently begun past the critical time for preventing mental retardation and massive brain damage (Benda, 1941), they were not a useful model for studying the selective effects of TH on brain development; this accounts for the almost exclusive reliance on animal models in this research (e.g., Eayrs, 1960). One early study by MacFaul et al. (1978) did show differential effects reflecting timing of treatment onset in children with clinically diagnosed CH. In these children, Verbal IQ declined steadily as a function of delay in treatment, whereas Performance IQ, which was below normal from birth, was relatively unaffected by the time of treatment onset. One interpretation of this finding is that the brain regions underlying visual–spatial skills need TH prior to birth, whereas those underlying verbal processing require it postnatally.

In recent years, newborn screening programs for CH, in conjunction with established programs for the neonatal detection of phenylketonuria, have been implemented throughout the developed world. As a result, children with CH are now diagnosed and treated at a very young age, long before symptoms are ever evident. However, because these children still do undergo a period of hypothyroidism, which can begin *in utero* and extend up to the second month of life (when TH levels have normalized), they provide a unique opportunity to observe in humans *selective* effects of TH on cognition, and presumably on the associated underlying cerebral structures. These could not formerly be studied in the children who were clinically diagnosed. Although there are a number of prospective follow-up studies of children with CH detected by newborn screening, ours may be the only one to approach the topic from the perspective of using the findings to achieve a better understanding of TH's effets on the developing brain.

Despite considerable methodological variation among the many follow-up studies of children whose CH was identified through screening, there is remarkable consensus in their findings. The average Full Scale IQ falls in the normal range (94.0 to 105.2; see Rovet, 1990), representing a significant improvement over the children who were clinically diagnosed, whose Full Scale IQ was in the borderline or mentally deficient ranges. The incidence of mental retardation is also substantially reduced and does not appear to deviate from the normal population. The most severely affected children appear to be those with athyrosis, who also have the lowest levels of TH at birth and the most delayed skeletal maturities. However, despite normal IQs, many children identified by screening demonstrate poorer functioning in selective ability areas, such as speech and language (Glorieux, Dussault, Letarte, Guyda, & Morissette, 1983; Gottschalk, Richman, & Lewandowski, 1994; Rovet, 1991), motor skills (Fuggle, Grant, Smith & Murphy, 1991; Rochiccioli et al., 1983), and eye–hand coordination (Murphy, Hulse, Smith, & Grant, 1990). Preliminary findings for school-age children with CH (Glorieux, 1989; New England Congenital Hypothyroidism Collaborative, 1994; Rovet, Ehrlich, Sorbara, & Czuchta, 1990; Toublanc & Rives, 1994) indicate lower levels of achievement, with arithmetic being most problematic.

THE TORONTO CH PROSPECTIVE STUDY

Sample and Methods

In 1981, Robert Ehrlich, a pediatric endocrinologist at the Hospital for Sick Children in Toronto, and I began a prospective study to evaluate outcome in children with CH. These children were just beginning to be identified by local and regional newborn screening programs. Because Toronto was a pioneering city in newborn screening for CH, children with early-treated CH from the Toronto area represented a unique opportunity to study the effects of TH on human cognition and brain function. We recruited into our study the majority of children who were available to us at that time (about 50), and from 1981 to 1986 we obtained a further 60 or so as they were born. In all, we were able to enlist about

95% of the eligible cases diagnosed by screening that were being treated at the Hospital for Sick Children.

The children were assessed annually with age-appropriate psychometric tests until they reached 9 years of age (Phase 1). In Phase 1, children with CH were compared with sibling controls, who were tested regularly but somewhat less frequently. When the children with CH reached the third and sixth grades at school, they were additionally assessed during the spring semester with a comprehensive battery of psychoeducational tasks (Phase 2). Also included were teacher evaluations with standardized questionnaires, and classmates served as controls. As of this writing, Phase 1 is completed (with the exception of one child); Phase 2, particularly for sixth-graders, is still continuing. In 1993 a third phase was begun, which involves detailed physical and neuropsychological evaluations of these children as teenagers. We have been fortunate to have both a high participation rate (about 95% of eligible cases) and a low rate of attrition (1% per annum for Phase 1). In addition, because most children were assessed in Phase 1 on the same day as their annual endocrine appointment, we have available both early TH level values and values throughout childhood, including those concurrent with day of testing. Our approach is not just descriptive, documenting outcome; it also aims to characterize the neurodevelopmental profiles of specific ability domains and to identify the predictors of poorer outcome for various abilities.

Results

Our findings to date show that Full Scale IQ is moderately but significantly lower in the children with CH than in sibling controls, particularly those with an athyrotic etiology (Figure 10.1). The differences appear to increase with age, presumably reflecting the age-related increase in the reliability of IQ tests and in their demands on complex cognitive functions. Elevated scores for all groups in the first 3 years of life are thought to reflect the old norms for the Griffiths test, which was standardized over three decades ago. At age 9, children with CH scored below controls on both Verbal IQ (99.3 vs. 107.4; $p < .01$) and Performance IQ (104.2 vs. 112.0; $p < .05$). They also differed significantly on the Similarities, Vocabulary, Digit Span, Object Assembly, and Coding subtests of the Wechsler Intelligence Scale for Children—Revised (WISC-R; Wechsler, 1974).

Children with CH also show a characteristic neurodevelopmental profile and achievement pattern reminiscent of the NLD syndrome (Rovet, Ehrlich, & Sorbara, 1992). The specific results of our investigations

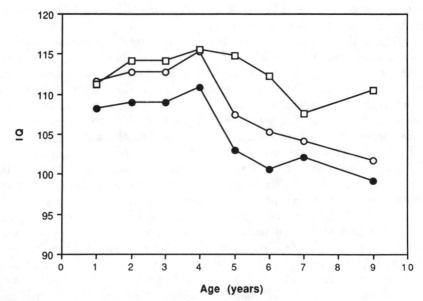

FIGURE 10.1. IQ by age for children with CH and control children. Tests given were the Griffiths Mental Development Scales at 1 to 3 years, the McCarthy Scales of Children's Abilities at 4 and 6 years, the Wechsler Pre-school and Primary Scale of Intelligence (WPPSI) at 5 years, and the Wechsler Intelligence Scale for Children—Revised (WISC-R) at 7 and 9 years. Open circles represent total group with CH; filled circles, athyrotic group only; open squares, controls. Children with CH scored significantly lower than control children at 5 and 9 years; athyrotic children scored significantly lower than controls at 1, 3, 4, 5, 6, and 9 years.

are described below, with the major developmental findings summarized in Figure 10.2.

Motor Skills

According to the protocol for Phase 1, motor skills were assessed regularly until age 6. From 1 to 3 years of age, children were evaluated with the Locomotor scale of the Griffiths tests (Griffiths, 1964, 1970); from 3 through 5 years, with the Motor scale of the McCarthy Scales of Children's Abilities (McCarthy, 1972); and at age 6, with the short form of the Bruininks–Oseretsky Test of Motor Proficiency (Bruininks, 1978), which provides a more detailed assessment of a wide range of fine and gross motor skills. As shown in Figure 10.2A, the total sample of children with CH evidenced initial delays in their motor development (in terms of milestones), but then seemed to catch up. However, when tested with

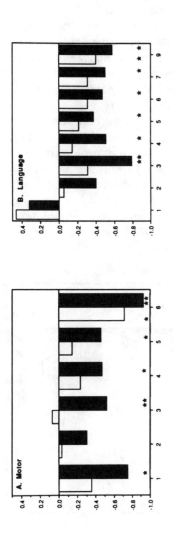

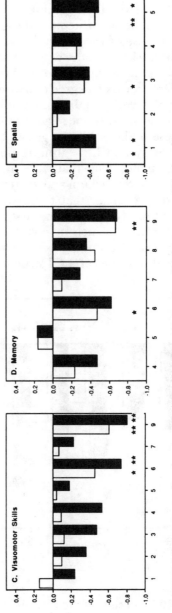

FIGURE 10.2. Neurodevelopmental profiles for (A) motor, (B) language, (C) visual–motor, (D) memory, and (E) spatial abilities in children with CH. Results are expressed as differences from the results for controls, in standard deviation (*SD*) units. Open bars represent total group with CH; filled bars, athyrotic group only, *$p < .05$; **$p < .01$.

the Bruininks at age 6, they showed significantly poorer performance than did controls. Children with athyrosis were affected to a far greater degree than were those with other etiologies, showing significantly poorer motor performance than controls at most ages, and in particular at age 6 when tested with the Bruininks. The results at age 6 indicated a selective deficit on gross motor items and suggested a selective difficulty or weakness in the use of the lower limbs (Figure 10.3). As in the total sample of children with CH, the deficit in children with athyrosis was confined to activities involving the lower limbs. Correlational analyses revealed associations between degree of motor impairment and postnatal duration and initial severity of hypothyroidism; however, prenatal duration of hypothyroidism was not related to level of motor ability.

These findings have suggested to us that different components of the motor system have unique periods of critical sensitivity to TH. Since the motor skills that were most affected in our sample appeared to involve the cerebellum and ventromedial motor systems, we have interpreted this to mean that these structures and pathways are critically dependent on TH during the first month of life. On the other hand, as fine motor skills, which involve the neocerebellum and/or dorsolateral corticospinal (pyramidal) motor system, were unaffected, we have hypothesized that the cerebral structures underlying these skills either are

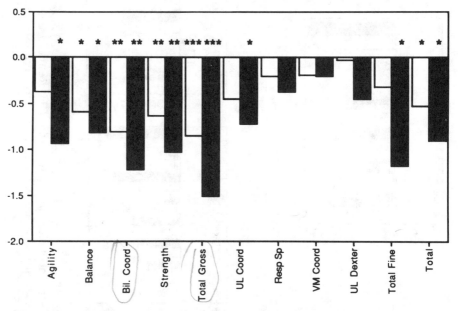

FIGURE 10.3. Results of the Bruininks–Oseretsky Test of Motor Proficiency. Open bars represent total group with CH; filled bars, the athyrotic group. Results are expressed as differences from the results for controls, in *SD* units. *$p < .05$; **$p < .01$; ***$p < .001$.

insensitive to TH or have a different developmental window. Given that children who were diagnosed clinically in the era prior to screening, and who were treated later, had increased spasticity, incoordination, tremor, and clumsiness (Frost & Parkin, 1986; MacFaul et al., 1978; Smith, Blizzard, & Wilkins, 1957), it is likely that TH is indeed necessary, but at a later stage of infancy.

Language

Figure 10.2B shows that for the total sample of children with CH, the global language composite score was lower from age 2 on and was lowest at age 3 years. There appeared to be some improvement after age 3, and then another decline after age 6. For children with athyrosis, impaired language functioning was evident from age 2 onward and was poorest at about 3 years of age. Our clinical experience with these children, suggests that this profile reflects a delay in speech acquisition that is most obvious at about age 3; after this, for some reason, the children seem to show remarkable catch-up. Their later language problems appear to reflect difficulties in processing more complex linguistic structures, as well as poorer verbal reasoning skills.

The Reynell Developmental Language scales (Reynell, 1977) were given annually through age 6. As shown in Figure 10.4, the children's expressive language skills were below those of controls from age 2 on, and were significantly different at 3 years of age. However, children with CH were not clinically delayed, according to the standards of the test. (A standard score of 0 for the test is thought to represent language functions at age level, but the superior performance of controls at certain ages suggests to us that the norms may be outdated.) In the receptive domain, children with CH performed below controls after age 3, and significantly below them at 3 and 4 years. Children with CH also scored lower, but not significantly so, on the Carrow Elicited Language Inventory (Carrow-Woolfolk, 1974) administered at age 7 (69.5% vs. 80.4%). Qualitative analysis of their responses on this test indicated that they made more substitutions and additions than did controls, but that they did not differ in terms of omitted, transposed, or reversed wordings.

Correlations and regressions computed between the language composite and variables reflecting disease and treatment factors indicated that the longer the postnatal duration of hypothyroidism, the poorer the language outcome. This suggests that the cerebral structures underlying speech and language may have a critical period of sensitivity to TH in the postnatal period during the first few months of life.

Auditory Abilities

Auditory discrimination was assessed in our children between 5 and 9 years of age with the Wepman Auditory Discrimination Test (Wepman,

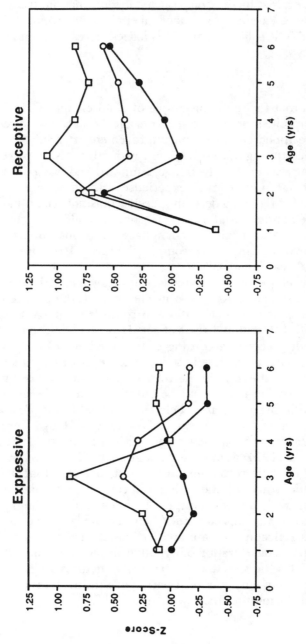

FIGURE 10.4. Results of Reynell Developmental Language Scales. Data are expressed as standard score units based on developmental norms of the test (mean = 0; *SD* = 1). A score of 0 signifies performance at age level; a negative score, below age level for the test; and a positive score, above age level for the test. Open circles represent the total group with CH; filled circles, the athyrotic grop; open squares, controls. Children with CH scored significantly lower than did controls in expressive language at 3 years of age (*p* < .05), and in receptive language at 3 years (*p* < .01) and 4 years (*p* < .05). Athyrotic subjects scored significantly lower than controls in expressive language at 2 years (*p* < .05) and 3 years (*p* < .05), and in receptive language at 3 years of age (*p* < .05).

1958). Our interest in this domain was based on findings in the literature showing that TH plays a role in the development of the ear (Deol, 1976; Meyerhoff, 1979), and that children with CH, despite screening, may be susceptible to mild hearing loss (Francois, Bonfils, Leger, Czernichow, & Narcy, 1994). Our findings indicate that children with CH scored consistently below controls on the Wepman at all ages; however, none of the differences were statistically significant. The averaged score across assessments was 60.2% for children with CH and 66.8% for controls. At age 5, both prenatal and postnatal durations of hypothyroidism significantly predicted ability in this domain. We are currently examining whether children with documented hearing impairment not only perform more poorly on this task, but are the ones contributing to the relationships with prenatal and postnatal factors. These results indicate mild to moderate hearing loss in 17%, which is subsequently associated with poorer reading and spelling but does not affect language (Rovet & Walker, 1995).

Visual–Motor Ability

Although upper-limb and graphomotor skills were not compromised, children with CH performed more poorly than controls at age 6 on a task of design copying (46.3 vs. 66.5%; $p < .01$) using the Beery Developmental Test of Visual–Motor Integration (Beery & Buktenica, 1982). Figure 10.2C shows that at all ages when this domain was assessed, composite scores were lower for the group with CH; however, the differences were only significant at 6 and 9 years. Once again, the effects were stronger and more frequently significant for children with athyrosis than for the group at large. On the Goodenough–Harris Draw-a-Person task (Harris, 1963), administered at age 8, children with CH indicated a trend ($p < .10$) toward lower standard scores (91.2 vs. 99.5).

Visual–Spatial Ability

On tasks in the nonverbal visual–spatial domain, deficits were observed at almost all ages and in all children with CH, regardless of etiology (Figure 10.2E). As mentioned above, children with CH had significantly lower Performance IQ scores at age 9; they differed significantly on Object Assembly (11.3 vs. 13.7; $p < .05$) and Coding (9.0 vs. 10.8; $p < .01$), but not on the Block Design, Picture Completion, or Picture Arrangement subtests.

Memory and Attention

The results for the memory composite are shown in Figure 10.2D. Memory scores are based on the following indices: the McCarthy Memory scale from 4 to 8 years; the Sentences subtest of the Wechsler Preschool and Primary Scale of Intelligence (WPPSI; Wechsler, 1989) at age 5; and the WISC-R Digit Span subtest at 7 and 9 years. At most ages, children with CH performed more poorly than controls, with the differences being significant at 6 and 9 years. There were no effects of etiology of hypothyroidism on performance in this domain, signifying that all groups were equally affected. Correlation analyses indicated that there were no effects of prenatal and initial disease factors on memory, whereas postnatal duration of hypothyroidism and TH levels in both early childhood and later childhood had significant effects. We found a negative association between level of circulating T_4 at 7 and 9 years and concurrent Digit Span performance, particularly on the backward span component (Rovet, Ehrlich, & Donner, 1993).

Comparisons of groups according to type of memory task revealed that children with CH differed most from controls on the Verbal Memory II component of the McCarthy test, which required them to listen to and retell a story. They did not differ on tasks from the McCarthy scales involving visual memory or rote repetition. Poorer WISC-R Digit Span performance, as described above, reflected the backward rather than the forward component, suggesting a problem in working memory. As part of the protocol for Phase 2, sixth-grade children were also assessed with the short form of the Denman Neuropsychological Memory Scale (Denman, 1984). Preliminary findings reveal that the only verbal memory subtest differentiating children with CH from controls was Delayed Recall of Story ($p < .05$). Children with CH performed at the same level as did controls on the Paired-Associate Learning and Immediate Story Recall subtests.

Regression analyses revealed no significant disease-related predictors of memory task performance prior to the age of 9 years; however, at age 9, initial severity of hypothyroidism, initial dose level, and concurrent dose level all accounted for a significant proportion ($p < .001$) of the variance in this domain. At age 8, children who received a higher initial dose of L-thyroxine had higher McCarthy memory scores, whereas children who were concurrently receiving higher dosages of L-thyroxine had lower memory scores. This suggested to us that there may be different mechanisms associated with TH at the newborn and school-age periods (Rovet & Ehrlich, 1995).

Attention was assessed directly with the Freedom from Distractibility (FFD) index of the WISC-R, and indirectly from parent and teacher reports on standardized questionnaires. Children with CH obtained lower FFD scores than controls at 9 years of age (9.6 vs. 11.4; $p < .01$), but not 7 years (10.2 vs. 10.4). Teachers reported greater inattention on the ACTeRS among children with CH than their classmates (centile scores: CH = 47.3, controls = 61.7; $p < .05$), while parents reported more attention problems (T scores: CH = 59.0, controls = 54.4) on the Child

Behavior Checklist (CBCL; Achenbach, 1981) and the Conners (1990) Hyperactivity Index (.60 vs. .20) at age 7. Previous analyses revealed that the strongest predictor of the attention composite at age 7 was concurrent level of circulating T_4. To our surprise, the association was negative, signifying that children with higher TH levels at time of testing were attending less well (Rovet, Ehrlich, & Donner, 1993). More recent analyses have revealed that children with a combination of high T_4 and high TSH had the lowest FFD scores of all children with CH, suggesting to us a direct link between TH and attention (Rovet & Alvarez, 1995a).

Concept Formation and Problem Solving

The domain of concept formation and problem solving has not been adequately studied in our children. Teachers reported that children with CH at the third-grade level did not appear to be working hard or learning as well as classmate controls. At age 5, we found that the children with CH were outscored by controls on the Mazes subtest of the WPPSI. Another study of 6-year-olds with CH revealed no difference between them and controls on the Category Test (New England Congenital Hypothyroidism Collaborative, 1985).

School Achievement

In Phase 1, achievement was assessed at 7, 8, and 9 years of age with the Wide Range Achievement Test—Revised (WRAT-R; Jastak & Wilkinson, 1984) and the Passage Comprehension subtest of the Woodcock Reading Mastery Tests (Woodcock & Johnson, 1987). As shown in Table 10.1, children with CH performed significantly more poorly than controls on the WRAT-R Arithmetic subtest at age 8.

TABLE 10.1. Achievement Test Results for Children with CH and Control Children (Phase 1)

	7 years		8 years		9 years	
	CH	Cont.	CH	Cont.	CH	Cont.
n	93	20	86	15	77	24
WRAT-R (centile)						
Reading	41.7	46.9	42.4	55.9	42.3	46.9
Spelling	39.0	40.9	40.6	42.1	39.2	40.9
Arithmetic	42.4	40.9	33.3	46.5*	42.3	53.0
Woodcock (centile)						
Passage Comprehension	58.2	67.7	54.8	60.2	58.2	67.7

* CH < control, $p < .05$.

When compared to Grade 3 class controls (Phase 2), children with CH again scored significantly lower in Arithmetic ($p < .01$). Results for the Keymath Diagnostic Arithmetic Test (Connelly, Nachtman, & Pritchett, 1981) indicated poorer performance in all domains; these differences were statistically significant for the Division and Numeric Reasoning scales (Table 10.2). Children with CH performed, on average, about one-third of a grade below their current grade level, whereas controls were performing exactly at grade level. Poorer numeric ability was also observed in Phase 1 at age 6 on the McCarthy Quantitative scale (T scores: CH = 51.3, controls = 56.4; $p < .05$). Error analyses of WRAT-R and Keymath responses suggested different types of difficulties for CH versus classmate controls at the grade 3 level (Rovet & Petric, 1995). Children with CH appeared to mix up calculations (e.g., to add instead of subtract within a set of substeps of a problem) or failed to complete

TABLE 10.2. Grade 3 Achievement Test Results for Children with CH and Control Children (Phase 2)

	CH ($n = 51$)	Control ($n = 42$)	t	p
Age (years)	8.81	8.88		
Grade (years)	3.73	3.82		
WRAT-R (centile)				
Reading	41.1	51.1		
Spelling	49.4	38.4	1.79	.07
Arithmetic	36.5	50.7	−2.48	.01
Woodcock (centile)				
Basic Skills Cluster	55.4	55.2	0.03	
Comprehension Cluster	36.9	41.2	−0.78	
Total Reading	48.2	50.8	−0.42	
Gilmore (grade equivalent)				
Accuracy	5.34	5.66	−0.77	
Comprehension	4.44	5.59	−2.37	.05
Keymath (grade equivalent)[a]				
Total	3.38	3.85	−2.20	.03
Fractions	3.34	3.94	−1.79	.07
Geometry and Symbols	3.51	3.87	−1.63	.10
Division	2.44	3.11	−2.84	.005
Reasoning	4.02	4.56	−1.96	.05
Test of Written Language (centile)				
Thematic Maturity	33.7	25.8	1.24	
Vocabulary	30.1	32.1	−0.34	
Syntax	31.3	32.3	−0.14	
Spelling	27.0	27.7	−0.11	
Style	29.8	25.9	0.71	

[a] Only subtests with large differences reported.

problems, whereas controls were more likely than the children with CH to confuse component steps (e.g., to add two columns independently without borrowing).

Children with CH scored below controls ($p < .05$) on the comprehension component of the Gilmore Oral Reading Test (Gilmore & Gilmore, 1968). They did not differ in mechanical reading abilities or written language skills.

Subjects were also assigned to different learning disability (LD) subgroups, according to the Rourke and Strang criteria (Rourke & Strang, 1983) and to a more stringent set of criteria involving lower cutoffs (Rovet, 1993). The results, shown in Figure 10.5, indicate that regardless of the criteria employed, children with CH assigned to an LD subgroup were mostly categorized as arithmetic-disabled, whereas controls were mostly categorized as reading-disabled. There were fewer non-learning-disabled children in the group with CH (Rourke & Strang, 44%; stringent, 67%) than in the control group (Rourke & Strang, 55%; stringent, 75%). Therefore, CH modestly increases the risk of a specific academic LD affecting primarily arithmetic skills.

Social/Adaptive Skills

Children with CH do not seem to exhibit any major social or behavioral problems (Rovet, 1986). However, they were described as having more difficult temperaments at 6 months of age (Rovet, Ehrlich, & Sorbara, 1987). This finding was not replicated at age 8 with the Middle Childhood Temperament Questionnaire (McDevitt & Carey, 1978), which instead showed them to be more predictable and persistent and to have more positive dispositions (Rovet & Alvarez, 1995b). However, they had higher Conduct Problems scores on the Conners and higher Attention Problems scores on the CBCL. Correlation analyses revealed that behavior problems in children with CH were associated with a concurrent biochemical profile suggestive of hyperthyroidism (high T_4, low TSH).

At 8 years of age, children with CH also reported lower total self-esteem than controls on the Piers–Harris Self-Concept Inventory (Piers & Harris, 1969) (total scores: 66.7% vs. 88.6%; $p < .05$).

Brain Function

There are no comprehensive neuroimaging studies on early-treated children with CH, presumably because these children are thought to be developing so well relative to their predecessors. We have performed no such studies. A recent single-case description of an 11-month-old child, who received weekly (vs. daily) dosing with L-thyroxine and was markedly delayed and cretinoid in appearance, revealed delayed myelination on

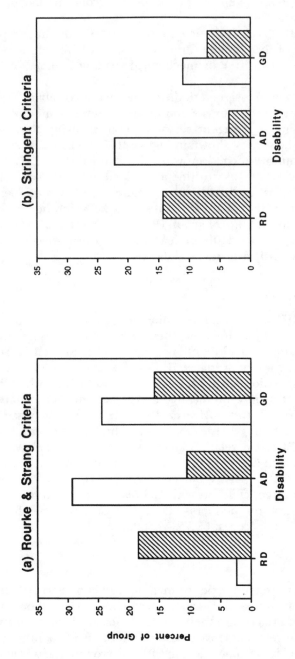

FIGURE 10.5. LD subtypes using (a) Rourke and Strang's (1983) criteria and (b) stringent criteria. The data are represented as percentages of the total group with CH (open bars) and of the control group (hatched bars). RD, reading disability; AD, arithmetic disability; GD, general disability.

magnetic resonance imaging (Rivkees & Hardin, 1994). Autopsy findings obtained shortly thereafter indicated microcephaly, but no focal abnormalities in grey or white matter, cerebellum, or brain stem. Ectopic neurons in deep white matter adjacent to the lining of the cerebellum suggested a migrational defect. However, the authors could not be certain whether this pattern of CNS impairment was attributable to hypothyroidism per se, or to the combined effects of cyclic hyperthyroidism (following supraphysiological dosing) and hypothyroidism (at end of each week), on the developing brain.

A previous study of CNS and peripheral nervous system maturation using electroencephalography indicated focal patterns with slow waves in 3 of 42 cases (7%) (Moschini et al., 1986). Evoked potential testing of these same patients revealed an increased latency of the P2 waveform component for 2-year-olds. Because this was subsequently normalized, these findings may signify an early difficulty in perceptual discrimination that disappeared with time (Moschini et al., 1986).

CH AND THE NLD SYNDROME

Our results are consistent with the NLD syndrome, but indicate a very mild form of the disorder. According to the model described in Chapter 1, children with this syndrome demonstrate a characteristic neurodevelopmental profile with strengths and weaknesses in specific ability areas. The syndrome is believed to arise from certain primary neuropsychological assets and deficits, which lead to a common set of secondary, tertiary, and linguistic features. This hierarchy of features contributes to particular academic disabilities and socioemotional/adaptive characteristics.

The Three Levels

According to the NLD model, primary-level assets include intact simple motor skills, good auditory perception, and rote memory abilities, whereas primary-level deficits include poor tactile and visual perception, as well as difficulty on complex psychomotor tasks and on tasks with novel stimulus configurations. The findings for children with CH are generally consistent with this profile. Our results indicated that children with CH did not differ from controls on auditory discrimination or rote repetition tasks. Assessment of simple motor functions in 6-year-old children with CH by the New England Congenital Hypothyroidism Collaborative (1985), using the Reitan–Indiana test battery, indicated that the children with CH also did not differ from controls on pure motor and simple psychomotor tasks. Although there is no evidence of poorer tactile discrimination in children with CH (New England Congenital Hypothyroidism Collaborative, 1985), they do show early, but not later, difficulties in visual discrimination (Moschini et al., 1986), and have greater difficulty on complex psychomotor tasks (Fuggle et al., 1991; Gottschalk et al., 1994). We found that the motor deficit may be selective for functions involving the lower limbs. Hypotonia and poorer reflexes (Moschini et al., 1986), as well as problems with balance (Fuggle et al., 1991; see above), have also been observed.

At the secondary level, NLD symptoms are said to be manifested in poorer attention to tactile or visual input, whereas attentional deployment for simple repetitive verbal materials (especially if delivered through the auditory modality) is adequate. The only data at present supporting this model are the good forward Digit Span scores of our children on the WISC-R, and the longer visual evoked potential latencies in the P2 wave component of other children with CH (Moschini et al., 1986).

At the tertiary level, it is predicted that rote memory skills will be adequate, whereas difficulties will be observed on tasks of visual or complex verbal recall. Our findings that children with CH did more poorly than controls in their recall of the Denman complex figure and in their story repetition and recall, but not in simple recall tasks, are consistent with the profile at this level. Visual–spatial processing problems, reflecting poorer skills in constructing puzzles, solving mazes, and learning visually presented numerical sequences, also supports the model. Difficulties in visual–spatial and visual-perceptual skills have been observed in the children in our cohort at most ages.

Supplementary Features

According to the NLD model, children will show early delays in speech and language development, rapid subsequent catch-up, excellent phonological processing skills, and a high volume of speech output. Except for speech output, which has not been assessed, the neurobehavioral profile of our children with CH is consistent with the NLD model. In particular, our observation of a marked delay in expressive and receptive language skills at age 3 years with later catch-up is a classic example of the model. When their phonological skills were assessed directly in Grade 3 with the Illinois Test of Psycholinguistic Abilities (Kirk, McCarthy, & Kirk, 1968), no problems were observed in their ability to analyze or blend sounds.

Academically, the NLD model predicts good word-decoding and spelling skills, whereas difficulties in mechanical arithmetic and reading comprehension are expected. We have observed that with the exception of children with hearing impairment, most children with CH did not exhibit any difficulties with mechanical reading or spelling and their written language skills were at par, whereas many evidenced difficulties with mechanical arithmetic from an early age (6 years on the McCarthy), which persisted until at least the third-grade level. Poorer reading comprehension was also observed, particularly on the Gilmore Oral Reading Test, which requires more elaborate responses than does the Woodcock Passage Comprehension subtest (which requires only single-word responses). However, the level of deficit was not remarkable, and, as a group, children with CH performed only about one-third of a grade below expectations and below controls. Continued follow-up of our cohort will determine whether this effect persists with age.

Socioemotional difficulties are expected in the areas of adaptability, social competence, emotional stability, and activity level, according to the NLD model. Although early temperament problems were observed in our children with CH, reflecting increased arousability, major behavior problems have not been observed subsequently. However, the children do appear to be at risk for attentional difficulties, which are directly related to their TH levels at time of testing. Lower self-esteem was also observed at age 8. Social problems are rare in children with CH, and those that occur may be attributable to increased family dysfunction (Heyerdahl, 1987; Illig & Largo, 1987), possibly as a result of a positive screening diagnosis at a vulnerable age (Rovet, 1992).

The Underlying Neurological Mechanism

According to Rourke (1989), cognitive and behavioral manifestations of the NLD syndrome reflect inadequacies in cerebral white matter development, which is necessary to maintain the integrity of the behavioral systems that underlie the NLD model. Although white matter abnormalities are not inconsistent with the neurobiological findings for early thyroid disease, which reveal decreased myelination in hypothyroid animals (Lauder & Krebs, 1986), there is no direct evidence to show such neurological abnormalities in children with CH. Nevertheless, the neurocognitive profiles of children with CH suggest that the lack of TH at a critical stage in early development produces a characteristic set of selective impairments, suggestive of organizational effects of this hormone on the developing brain. Since a recent study by Munoz et al. (1991) shows that the genes for myelin production are regulated by TH, it is not unlikely that the organizational deficits will involve white matter in these children.

Our findings on children with CH also suggest that there may be activational effects of atypical levels of TH at time of testing, which are directly associated with performance on tasks requiring attentional focus and demands on working memory. The relationship appears to be negative, such that poorer performance is associated with higher circulating levels of TH. Recent studies of children with resistance to TH (Hauser et al., 1993) and with attention deficit disorder (Elia, Gulota, Rose, Marin, & Rapaport, 1994) are consistent with these activational effects, showing an effect of high TH levels on activity level and attention.

CONCLUSION

Despite earlier diagnosis and treatment, and IQs in the normal range, children with CH may have subtle residual cognitive impairment that is directly associated with the severity and duration of disease, as well as with TH levels at time of testing. The neurodevelopmental profile and the pattern of impairment are consistent with the NLD model, although the problems are far milder in CH than in most other conditions described in this volume. The role of TH in regulating myelin production supports a white matter interpretation. Additional attentional and memory deficits associated with levels of concurrent TH also suggest an activational basis for some of the cognitive disabilities in these children.

REFERENCES

Achenbach, T. (1981). *Child Behavior Checklist for Ages 4–18*. Burlington: University of Vermont, Department of Psychiatry.

Alvarez, M., Gomez, A., Alvarez, E., & Navarro, D. (1983). Attention disturbance in Graves' disease. *Psychoneuroendocrinology, 8*, 451–454.

American Academy of Pediatrics, Committee on Genetics. (1987). Newborn screening for congenital hypothyroidism: Recommended guidelines. *Pediatrics, 90*, 298–301.

American Academy of Pediatrics, Section on Endocrinology and Committee on Genetics. (1993). Newborn screening for congenital hypothyroidism: Recommended guidelines. *Pediatrics, 91*, 1203–1209.

Beery, K., & Buktenica, N. (1982). *Developmental Test of Visual–Motor Integration*. Cleveland, OH: Modern Curriculum Press.

Benda, C. (1941). *Mongolism and cretinism: A study of the clinical manifestations and the general pathology of pituitary and thyroid deficiency*. London: Heinemann.

Bradley, D., Young, S., & Weinberger, C. (1989). Differential expression of alpha and beta thyroid hormone receptor genes in rat brain and pituitary. *Proceedings of the National Academy of Sciences USA, 80*, 7250–7254.

Bruininks, R. (1978). *Bruininks–Oseretsky Test of Motor Proficiency*. Circle Pines, MN: American Guidance Service.

Burrow, G., Fisher, D., & Larsen, P. (1994). Maternal and fetal thyroid function. *New England Journal of Medicine, 331*, 1072–1078.

Carrow-Woolfolk, E. (1974). *Carrow Elicited Language Inventory.* Allen, TX: DLM Teaching Resources.

Connelly, A., Nachtman, W., & Pritchett, E. (1981). *Keymath Diagnostic Arithmetic Test.* Circle Pines, MN: American Guidance Service.

Conners, K. (1990). *Conners' Rating Scales manual.* Toronto: Multi-Health Systems.

Crome, L., & Stern, J. (1972). *Pathology of mental retardation.* Edinburgh: Churchill Livingstone.

Daneman, D., & Howard, N. (1980). Neonatal thyrotoxicosis: Intellectual impairment and craniosynostosis in later years. *Journal of Pediatrics, 97,* 257–259.

Denman, S. B. (1984). *Denman Neuropsychology Memory Scale.* Charleston, SC: Author.

Deol, M. (1976). The role of thyroxine in the differentiation of the organ of corti. *Acta Otolaryngologica, 81,* 429–435.

Dobbing, J., & Sands, J. (1973). Quantitative growth and development of the human brain. *Archives of Disease in Childhood, 48,* 757–767.

Eayrs, J. (1960). Influence of the thyroid on the central nervous system. *British Medical Bulletin, 16,* 122–127.

Elia, J., Gulota, C., Rose, S., Marin, G., & Rapaport, J. (1994). Thyroid function and attention-deficit hyperactivity disorder. *Journal of the American Academy of Child and Adolescent Psychiatry, 33,* 169–172.

Fellous, A., Lennon, A., Francon, J., & Nunez, J. (1979). Thyroid hormones and neurotubule assembly in vitro during brain development. *European Journal of Biochemistry, 101,* 365–376.

Foley, T., Abbassi, V., Copeland, K., & Draznin, M. (1994). Brief report: Hypothyroidism caused by chronic autoimmune thyroiditis in very young infants. *New England Journal of Medicine, 330,* 466–468.

Francois, M., Bonfils, P., Leger, J., Czernichow, P., & Narcy, P. (1994). Role of congenital hypothyroidism in hearing loss in children. *Journal of Pediatrics, 124,* 444–446.

Francon, J., Fellous, A., Lennon, A.-M., & Nunez, J. (1977). Is thyroxine a regulatory signal for neurotubule assembly during brain development? *Nature, 266,* 188–189.

Frost, G., & Parkin, M. (1986). A comparison between the neurological and intellectual abnormalities in children and adults with congenital hypothyroidism. *European Journal of Pediatrics, 145,* 480–484.

Fuggle, P., Grant, D., Smith, I., & Murphy, G. (1991). Intelligence, motor skills and behavior at 5 years in early-treated congenital hypothyroidism. *European Journal of Pediatrics, 150,* 570–574.

Gilmore, J. V., & Gilmore, E. C. (1968). *Gilmore Oral Reading Test.* New York: Psychological Corporation.

Glorieux, J. (1989). Mental development of patients with congenital hypothyroidism detected by screening: Quebec experience. In F. Delange, D. Fisher, & D. Glinoer (Eds.), *Research in congenital hypothyroidism* (pp. 281–289). New York: Plenum Press.

Glorieux, J., Dussault, J., Letarte, J., Guyda, H., & Morissette, J. (1983). Preliminary results on the mental development of hypothyroid infants detected by the Quebec Screening Program. *Journal of Pediatrics, 102,* 19–22.

Gottschalk, B., Richman, R., & Lewandowski, L. (1994). Subtle speech and motor deficits of children with congenital hypothyroid treated early. *Developmental Medicine and Child Neurology, 36,* 216–220.

Griffiths, R. (1964). *Griffiths Mental Development Scales.* Milton Keynes, England: The Test Agency.

Griffiths, R. (1970). *Griffiths Mental Development Scales.* Milton Keynes, England: The Test Agency.

Harris, D. (1963). *Goodenough–Harris Drawing* Test. New York: Harcourt Brace Jovanovich.

Hauser, P., Zametkin, A., Martinez, P., Vitielo, B., Matochick, J., & Mixson, J. (1993). Attention deficit-hyperactivity disorder in people with generalized resistance to thyroid hormone. *New England Journal of Medicine, 328,* 997–1001.

Heyerdahl, S. (1987). Development of children with congenital hypothyroidism diagnosed by neonatal screening in Norway. In B. Therrell (Ed.), *Advances in neonatal screening* (pp. 81–89). Amsterdam: Elsevier.

Hulse, J. (1984). Outcome for congenital hypothyroidism. *Archives of Disease in Childhood, 59,* 23–30.

Illig, R., & Largo, R. (1987). Mental development of 60 children with congenital hypothyroidism: Prospective follow-up study at one, four and seven years of age. In B. Therrell (Ed.), *Advances in neonatal screening* (pp. 85–89). Amsterdam: Elsevier.

Interagency Committee on Learning Disabilities. (1987). *Learning disabilities: A report to the U.S. Congress.* Washington, DC: U.S. Government Printing Office.

Jastak, S., & Wilkinson, G. (1984). *Wide Range Achievement Test—Revised.* Wilmington, DE: Jastak Associates.

Johnston, M., & Singer, H. (1982). Brain neurotransmitters and neuromodulators in pediatrics. *Pediatrics, 70,* 57–68.

Josephson, A., & Mackenzie, T. (1979). Appearance of manic psychosis following rapid normalization of thyroid status. *American Journal of Psychiatry, 136,* 846–847.

Kirk, S., McCarthy, J., & Kirk, W. (1968). *Illinois Test of Psycholinguistic Abilities.* Urbana: University of Illinois Press.

Klawans, H., Goetz, C., & Weiner, W. (1974). Dopamine receptor site sensitivity in hyperthyroid and hyperthyroid guinea pigs. *Advances in Neurology, 5,* 495–500.

Klein, R. (1980). History of congenital hypothyroidism. In G. Burrow & J. Dussault (Eds.), *Neonatal thyroid screening* (pp. 57–58). New York: Raven Press.

Lauder, J., & Krebs, H. (1986). Do neurotransmitters, neurohumors, and hormones specify critical periods? In W. Greenough & J. Juraska (Eds.), *Developmental neuropsychobiology* (pp. 119–174). New York: Academic Press.

Legrand, J. (1984). Effects of thyroid hormones on central nervous system development. In J. Yanat (ed.), *Neurobehavioral teratology* (pp. 331–363). Amsterdam: Elsevier.

MacFaul, R., Dorner, S., Brett, E., & Grant, D. (1978). Neurological abnormalities in patients treated for hypothyroidism in early life. *Archives of Disease in Childhood, 53,* 611–619.

Man, E., Jones, W., Holden, R., & Mellits, E. (1971). Thyroid function in human pregnancy. *American Journal of Obstetrics and Gynecology, 111*, 905–916.

McCarthy, D. (1972). *McCarthy Scales of Children's Abilities*. New York: Psychological Corporation.

McDevitt, S., & Carey, W. (1978). The measurement of temperament in 3–7 year old children. *Journal of Child Psychology and Psychiatry, 19*, 245–253.

Meserve, L., & Leathem, J. (1974). Neonatal hyperthyroidism and maturation of the rat hypothalamo–hypohyseal–adrenal axis. *Proceedings of the Society for Experimental Biology and Medicine, 147*, 510–512.

Meyerhoff, W. (1979). Hypothyroidism and the ear: Electro-physiological morphological, and chemical considerations. *Laryngoscope, 89* (Suppl. 19), 1–25.

Moschini, L., Costa, P., Marinelli, E., Maggioni, G., Carta, M., Fazzini, C., Diodata, A., Sabini, G., Grandolfo, M., Carta, S., Porro, G., & Paolella, A. (1986). Longitudinal assessment of children with congenital hypothyroidism detected by neonatal screening. *Helvetica Paediatrica Acta, 41*, 415–424.

Munoz, A., Rodriguez-Pena, A., Perez-Castillo, A., Ferreiro, B., Sutcliffe, J., & Bernal, J. (1991). Effects of neonatal hypothyroidism on rat brain gene expression. *Molecular Endocrinology, 5*, 273–280.

Murphy, G., Hulse, J., Smith, I., & Grant, D. (1990). Congenital hypothyroidism: Physiological and psychological factors in early development. *Journal of Child Psychology and Psychiatry, 31*, 711–725.

New England Congenital Hypothyroidism Collaborative. (1985). Neonatal hypothyroidism screening: Status of patients at 6 years of age. *Journal of Pediatrics, 107*, 915–918.

New England Congenital Hypothyroidism Collaborative. (1994). Correlation of cognitive test scores and adequacy of treatment in adolescents with congenital hypothyroidism. *Journal of Pediatrics, 124*, 383–387.

Nicholson, J., & Altman, J. (1972). Synoptogenesis in the rat cerebellum: Effects of early hypo and hyperthyroidism. *Science, 176*, 530–531.

Nunez, J. (1984). Effects of thyroid hormones during brain differentiation. *Molecular and Cellular Endocrinology, 37*, 125–132.

Piers, E., & Harris, D. (1969). *The Piers–Harris Children's Self-Concept Scale*. Los Angeles: Western Psychological Services.

Potter, B., Mano, M., Belling, G., McIntosh, G., Hua, C., Cragg, B., Marshall, J., Wellby, M., & Hetzel, B. (1982). Retarded fetal brain development resulting from severe dietary iodine deficiency in sheep. *Neuropathology and Applied Neurobiology, 8*, 303–313.

Prange, A., Wilson, I., Rabon, A., & Lipton, M. (1969). Enhancement of imipramine antidepressant activity by thyroid hormone. *American Journal of Psychiatry, 126*, 457–469.

Rastogi, R., & Singhal, R. (1976). Influence of neonatal and adult hyperthyroidism on behavior and biosynthetic capacity for norepinephrine, dopamine and 5-hydroxytryptamine in rat brain. *Journal of Pharmacology, 198*, 609–618.

Reynell, J. (1977). *Reynell Developmental Language Scales*. Windsor, England: NFER–Nelson.

Rivkees, S. A., & Hardin, D. S. (1994). Cretinism after weekly dosing with levathyroxine for treatment of congenital hypothyroidism. *Journal of Pediatrics, 125*, 147–149.

Rochiccioli, P., Roge, B., Alexandre, F., Coll, J., Dutau, G., Enjaume, C., & Augier, D. (1983). Résultats du développement psychomoteur des hypothyroidies dépistées a la naissance. *Archives of French Pediatrics, 40,* 537–541.

Rosman, P., Malone, M., Helfenstein, M., & Kraft, E. (1972). The effect of thyroid deficiency on myelination of brain. *Neurology, 22,* 99–106.

Rourke, B. P. (1989). *Nonverbal learning disabilities. The syndrome and the model.* New York: Guilford Press.

Rourke, B. P., & Strang, J. (1983). Subtypes of reading and arithmetic disabilities: A neuropsychological analysis. In M. Rutter (Ed.) *Developmental neuropsychiatry* (pp. 473–486). New York: Guilford Press.

Rovet, J. (1986). A prospective investigation of children with congenital hypothyroidism identified by neonatal thyroid screening in Ontario. *Canadian Journal of Public Health, 77,* 164–173.

Rovet, J. (1990). Neuropsychological outcome and risk factors following neonatal screening for congenital hypothyroidism: A review of 23 cases. *Infant Screening, 14,* 23–27.

Rovet, J. (1991). Does newborn screening increase the risk of the vulnerable child syndrome? In K. Possie (Ed.), *Proceedings of the 8th National Neonatal Screening Symposium and XXI Birth Defects Symposium* (pp. 211–218). Washington, DC: Association of State and Territorial Public Health Laboratory Directors.

Rovet, J. (1993). The psychoeducational characteristics of children with Turner syndrome. *Journal of Learning Disabilities, 26,* 333–341.

Rovet, J., & Alvarez, M. (1995a). *Attentional correlates of atypical thyroid hormone levels in school-age children with congenital hypothyroidism.* Manuscript submitted for publication.

Rovet, J., & Alvarez, M. (1995b). *The relation of thyroid function to attention and behavior in eight-year-old children with congenital hypothyroidism.* Manuscript submitted for publication.

Rovet, J., Daneman, D., & Bailey, J. (1993). Psychologic and psychoeducational consequences of thyroxine therapy for juvenile acquired hypothyroidism. *Journal of Pediatrics, 122,* 543–549.

Rovet, J., & Ehrlich, R. (1995). Long-term effects of L-thyroxine therapy for congenital hypothyroidism. *Journal of Pediatrics, 126,* 380–386.

Rovet, J., Ehrlich, R., & Donner, E. (1993). Long-term neurodevelopmental correlates of treatment adequacy in screened hypothyroid children. *Pediatric Research, 33,* S91.

Rovet, J., Ehrlich, R., & Sorbara, D. (1987). Intellectual outcome in children with fetal hypothyroidism. *Journal of Pediatrics, 110,* 700–704.

Rovet, J., Ehrlich, R., & Sorbara, D. (1989). Effect of thyroid hormone level on temperament in infants with congenital hypothyroidism detected by screening of neonates. *Journal of Pediatrics, 114,* 63–68.

Rovet, J., Ehrlich, R., & Sorbara, D. (1992). Neurodevelopmental outcome in infants and preschool children following newborn screening for congenital hypothyroidism. *Journal of Pediatric Psychology, 17,* 187–213.

Rovet, J., Ehrlich, R., Sorbara, D., & Czuchta, D. (1990). The psychoeducational characteristics of hypothyroid children identified by newborn screening.

In H. B. Bradford, W. H. Hannon, & B. L. Therrell (Eds.), *Proceedings of the 7th National Neonatal Screening Symposium* (pp. 212–215). Washington, DC: Association of State and Territorial Public Health Laboratory Directors.

Rovet, J., Glorieux, J., & Heyerdahl, S. (1987). Summary of presentations and discussion of the psychological follow-up of CH children identified by screening. In B. Therrell (Ed.), *Advances in neonatal screening* (pp. 71–76). Amsterdam: Elsevier.

Rovet, J., & Petric, C. (1995) *Congenital hypothyroidism and arithmetic disabilities*. Manuscript in preparation.

Rovet, J., & Walker, W. (1995). *Long-term sequelae of hearing impairment associated with congenital hypothyroidism*. Manuscript in preparation.

Shapiro, S. (1966). Metabolic and maturational effects of thyroxine in the infant rat. *Endocrinology, 78*, 527–532.

Smith, D., Blizzard, R., & Wilkins, L. (1957). The mental prognosis in hypothyroidism of infancy and childhood. *Pediatrics, 19*, 1011–1022.

Strait, K., Schwartz, H. L., Perez-Castillo, A., & Oppenheimer, J. H. (1990). Relationship of c-erbA mRNA content to tissue triiodothyronine nuclear binding capacity and function in developing and adult rats. *Journal of Biochemistry, 265*, 105–114.

Toublanc, J., & Rives, S. (1994, September 13–17). *Preliminary results of national tests of congenital hypothyroid (CH) children screened at birth*. Poster presented at the Ninth International Neonatal Screening Symposium and Second Meeting of the International Society for Neonatal Screening, Lille, France.

Vulsma, T., & DeVijlder, J. (1989). Maternal–fetal transfer of thyroxine in congenital hypothyroidism due to a total organification defect of thyroid agenesis. *New England Journal of Medicine, 321*, 13–16.

Wallace, J., & MacCrimmon, D. (1990). Hyperthyroidism: Cognitive and emotional factors. In C. Holmes (Ed.), *Psychoneuroendocrinology* (pp. 323–343). New York: Springer-Verlag.

Wechsler, D. (1974). *Wechsler Intelligence Scale for Children—Revised*. New York: Psychological Corporation.

Wechsler, D. (1989). *Wechsler Preschool and Primary Scale of Intelligence*. New York: Psychological Corporation.

Wepman, J. (1958). *Wepman Auditory Discrimination Test*. Los Angeles: Western Psychological Services.

Woodcock, R., & Johnson, M. B. (1987). *Woodcock Reading Mastery Tests—Revised*. Circle Pines, MN: American Guidance Service.

11

Neuropsychological Consequences of Prophylactic Treatment for Acute Lymphocytic Leukemia

Erin M. Picard
Byron P. Rourke

As recently as 1968, fewer than 1% of children diagnosed with acute lymphocytic leukemia (ALL) survived more than a few years. Today, 55–65% of these children are anticipated to achieve long-term disease-free survival. Of the medical innovations responsible for increased survival rates, none has had a greater impact on treatment efficacy than the addition of central nervous system (CNS) prophylaxis. CNS prophylactic treatment was implemented in the 1970s in response to the high CNS relapse rates found to accompany prolonged systemic remissions. The addition of CNS therapy to treatment protocols has been a major factor in improved disease control, and ultimately in survival.

Unfortunately, survival has not been won without cost. Although it is now a standard of practice when treating children with ALL, CNS prophylaxis can have devastating neurological and neuropsychological consequences (Brown & Madan-Swain, 1993; Cousens, Waters, Said, & Stevens, 1988; Fletcher & Copeland, 1988; Gamis & Nesbit, 1991; Johnston, 1985; Kirs & Herman, 1980; Madan-Swain & Brown, 1991; Ochs, 1989; Packer, Meadows, Rorke, Goldwein, & D'Angio, 1987; Poplack & Brouwers, 1988; Williams & Davis, 1986). Almost two decades of research have demonstrated that such effects are most pronounced when treatment involves the administration of high doses of therapeutic radiation and/or methotrexate (MTX), when radiation is directed toward the entire craniospinal axis, and when radiation is administered at younger ages. The medical literature further reveals a potential toxic synergism of chemotherapies and radiation therapies that is dependent upon the sequence of administration of these agents (Balsom et al., 1987; Gamis & Nesbit, 1991; Ochs, 1989). It also has been postulated that treatment-related effects may not be manifested for many years, because of the slow replication of the cellular components of the CNS (Packer et al., 1987).

The potentially deleterious effects of CNS prophylaxis and chemotherapy (especially MTX) have been debated since the early 1970s. Within the medical literature, it is widely acknowledged that pediatric cancer therapy may have a detrimental effect upon the CNS. Unfortunately, the same cannot be said of the literature specific to the area of neuropsychology. Despite almost two decades of research in this field, there is little consensus regarding the implication of CNS pathology for the functional integrity of the brain. The confusion stemming from neuropsychological inquiries is hardly surprising, given that a significant portion of this literature is ill conceived and poorly executed. Although the debate has yet to be resolved, concerns about myriad late treatment-related effects provided the impetus for reform of the standard of CNS prophylactic treatment of children with ALL (Gamis & Nesbit, 1991).

CNS prophylaxis in the 1990s has been altered significantly in response to concerns about neurotoxicity. Developments in cell morphology, cytogenetics, and immunology have enabled researchers to identify subtypes of ALL; each type theoretically carries a different relative risk for relapse, and hence for ultimate prognosis. Consequently, a standard treatment protocol for children with ALL is clearly inappropriate. On the basis of several presenting features at diagnosis, children with ALL are now classified as standard-risk (low-risk) or high-risk patients. With respect to the former, attempts are being made to reduce the potential toxicity associated with treatment without altering the efficacy of treatment (Coccia, Bleyer, Siegel, et al., 1981; McKenna & Baehner, 1991; Miller, 1989; Miller & Miller, 1983). Conversely, more aggressive treatments for those with a greater relative risk of relapse are being assessed. Research has demonstrated that treatment-related toxicity can be minimized among standard-risk patients, with little impact upon treatment efficacy (Gamis & Nesbit, 1991).

In response to evolving treatment protocols, the objectives of neuropsychological research have of necessity changed. Traditional treatment protocols consisting of 2400-cGy cranial or craniospinal irradiation have been replaced by equally effective but less neurotoxic forms of prophylaxis. Consequently, whether or not there are neuropsychological sequelae associated with the use of 2400-cGy irradiation is a moot point. The purposes of this chapter are to clarify the risks associated with CNS therapy among ALL patients; to identify the circumstances under which the effects of treatment may be intensified; and to relate findings in this area to the Nonverbal Learning Disabilities (NLD)/white matter model.

ALL: ITS NATURE AND TREATMENT

Definition and History

The acute leukemias are a subgroup of neoplasms that arise primarily from the hematopoietic system. They are cancers of the blood-forming cells thought to arise in the bone marrow (McKenna & Baehner, 1991). ALL is the predominant form of leukemia occurring during the childhood years. It is a malignant cancer characterized by proliferation of leukocytes and their precursors, accompanied by a reduction in blood platelets and erythrocytes (Johnston, 1985). It was once uniformly fatal; however, as noted earlier, over 50% of children so afflicted are now expected to achieve long-term disease-free survival (Gamis & Nesbit, 1991; McKenna & Baehner, 1991; Miller, 1989; Simone, Aur, Hustu, Versoza, & Pinkel, 1978).

Prior to 1948, death within 3 to 6 months of diagnosis of ALL typically ensued. In 1948, Farber, Diamond, Mercer, Sylvester, and Wolff described a 20% remission induction rate with the use of the folic acid antagonist aminopterin. Although the remissions induced were temporary, Farber et al.'s modest success with aminopterin hailed the beginning of an era of research on chemotherapeutic agents. Over the next decade, the beneficial effects of a number of drugs were demonstrated. Because remissions were short-lived, an era of palliative treatment ensued.

Significant changes in survival rates, however, were not realized until combinations of drugs were implemented in treatment protocols (Gamis & Nesbit, 1991; McKenna & Baehner, 1991; Miller, 1989). By the early 1960s, a treatment strategy had emerged: Effective treatment involved combining drugs in such a manner that leukemic cell kill was maximized while suppressive effects on normal bone-marrow cell proliferation were minimized. Since 1963, the administration of vincristine and prednisone for remission induction has been the standard protocol against which the effects of other chemotherapeutic agents have been compared. With this protocol, 90% of children can be anticipated to enter remission within approximately 4 weeks.

In the era preceding effective systemic control of acute leukemia, CNS leukemia was rare (Gamis & Nesbit, 1991). The base rate occurrence of CNS leukemia was 5% prior to the introduction of combination chemotherapeutic agents in treatment protocols. With prolonged survival, 50–75% of children developed CNS leukemia while apparently still in hematological remission (Evans, Gilbert, & Zandstra, 1970; Gamis & Nesbit, 1991). Proliferation of the disease at this site had not been anticipated. The "CNS as sanctuary" theory was proposed to account for this phenomenon. The unfortunate consequence of this early undetected deposition of leukemic blasts in the leptomeninges was that over 50% of children treated with chemotherapeutic regimens experienced their first relapse in the CNS. CNS relapse, for the most part, signaled the impending onset of a full systemic relapse. The proliferation of leukemic blast cells in the leptomeninges emerged as a major limiting factor for disease control (Price, 1983), because of the high mortality rate associated with CNS relapse. If greater survival rates were to be achieved, it was clear that some form of prophylactic treatment would be necessary.

The use of radiation as a means of preventing leukemic proliferation in the CNS was first investigated by the St. Jude's research center (Aur, Hustu, Versoza, Wood, & Simone, 1973; Aur et al., 1971; Aur, Simone, Hustu, & Versoza, 1972; Hustu, Aur, Versoza, Simone, & Pinkel, 1973; Simone et al., 1978). These researchers demonstrated that a significant number of children could achieve continuous complete remission for up to 5 years if CNS prophylaxis was undertaken early in the course of treatment for ALL. CNS prophylaxis initially consisted of 2400-cGy radiation applied to the entire craniospinal axis. This protocol yielded CNS relapse rates (5%) that approximated the base rate in an untreated population (Aur et al., 1971).

Soon after the addition of prophylactic therapy directed toward the resolution of subclinical foci sequestered within the CNS, reports of late sequelae (neurological, neuropsychological) associated with treatment began to emerge in the literature. Thus began almost two decades of controversy regarding the neurobehavioral consequences of prophylactic treatment. Although this issue is far from resolved, the mere suggestion of potential deleterious effects associated with treatment was sufficient to precipitate a search for alternative forms of prophylactic therapy.

Epidemiology

Neoplasms are the leading cause of death by disease in children under 15 years of age. Malignant disease ranks second only to accidents in mortality rates for this age group. The most frequent types of neoplasms observed in children include the leukemias and brain tumors, which together account for approximately 62% of all pediatric cancers. Although the incidence of cancer varies somewhat according to both race and country, ALL and CNS tumors remain the predominant forms of cancer among children.

Forty-one percent of childhood cancers occur between birth and 4 years of age. In the youngest group, infants below 1 year of age, neuroblastomas replace ALL as the leading form of pediatric malignancy. In the long run, however, the leukemias rank first in mortality rates because of greater survival rates among neuroblastoma patients (Hockenberry, Coody, & Falletta, 1986).

The acute leukemias, the most common form of pediatric cancer, account for 30–45% of all pediatric malignancies (McKenna & Baehner, 1991; Miller, 1989; Miller & Miller, 1983; Neglia & Robison, 1988). Of these, ALL is the predominant form, accounting for 70–90% of all cases. ALL has a peak incidence between the ages of 3 and 5 years. Thereafter, the incidence of this disease declines, but it subsequently rises again during the third decade of life (Neglia & Robison, 1988). It has been speculated that the early peak of childhood ALL may be related to something gone awry during gestation or during the initial development of the immune system (Neglia & Robison, 1988).

The small but significant predominance of ALL in males is consistent across racial and geographic boundaries. Males, being more susceptible to high-risk forms of ALL, have a poorer prognosis for long-term disease-free survival. Consequently, gender is an important prognostic variable (Sather, Miller, Nesbit, Heyn, & Hammond, 1981).

Although the effect of socioeconomic status is less clear (the etiology of this effect may be attributable to race, maternal age, parental education, or occupational exposures), it has been demonstrated to be associated with the incidence of ALL (Neglia & Robison, 1988). ALL has sometimes been referred to as a disease of the middle and upper middle classes. ALL is also 20–30% more common in white children than in black children. Whether this reflects a social class difference or a genuine racial difference is unclear.

The peak age of onset of ALL is not known in many developing nations. A peak age evolved during the early 20th century in North America and Europe at the time of rapid industrialization. The peak age of onset observed in most industrialized nations has led to speculation that environmental exposures associated with industrialization may play a significant role in the etiology of ALL (Neglia & Robison, 1988).

The relationship between seasonal and geographic variations and the incidence of childhood ALL has been examined. Studies of seasonal variations have been inconsistent with respect to the season purportedly associated with increased incidences and the number of peaks identified during any given year. There is some evidence, however, to suggest that the incidence of ALL varies according to geographic regions. Specifically, in the United States, the upper Midwestern states appear to be differentially affected. Given the agricultural nature of these states, it has been speculated that environmental toxins (herbicides, pesticides) may play a role in the etiology of ALL.

Etiology

What is known about the etiology of ALL is the by-product of studies of associations between environmental agents or genetic characteristics and the incidence of the disease. Typically, documentation of these associations has predated an understanding of the biological mechanism responsible. Whether or not a causative relationship is inferred is dependent upon the strength of the association observed, the consistency of the findings across studies, the proper temporal sequence, and the biological plausibility of the relationship (Neglia & Robison, 1988).

The difficulties inherent in establishing a causative relationship cannot be overstated. The latency period of many agents, following which their consequences become manifest, is in most cases too long to enable them to be defined as having a causative role. Although many factors have been implicated in the etiology of ALL, we can only speculate regarding the mechanism or mechanisms by which they cause a malignant transformation. One hypothesis advanced to explain this transformation is the oncogenic hypothesis. This hypothesis states that certain cells carry information for malignant transformation, but that they require activation by an intracellular event such as irradiation, chemical carcinogens, or perhaps even viruses (Lusher & Ravindranath, 1979).

There are a number of variables of potential epidemiological significance in ALL. These include the following: prenatal and perinatal risk factors, irradiation exposure, and viruses. With respect to the first of these, advanced maternal age and poor maternal reproductive history are associated with increased incidences of ALL. It has been speculated that these events implicate a common environmental exposure, an abnormal intrauterine environment, or a genetic predisposition as the biological mechanism responsible for the increased risk (Neglia & Robison, 1988).

Low birth weight has consistently been found to be associated with an increased incidence of ALL, particularly ALL diagnosed at younger ages. Though this is seemingly a robust finding in the epidemiological literature, a biological mechanism has yet to be proposed to account for this association (Neglia & Robison, 1988). Use of oral contraceptives and maternal substance use have also been hypothesized to be associated with an increased risk of ALL. These findings have yet to be confirmed.

Among the environmental influences associated with increased incidences of ALL, ionizing radiation has been the most comprehensively studied (Neglia & Robison, 1988). Prenatal exposure to diagnostic ionizing radiation has repeatedly been shown to be associated with an almost twofold increase in the incidence of ALL. The role of postnatal irradiation in the etiology of ALL has also been the subject of many investigations. The incidence of ALL among those exposed to atomic blasts was up to 20 times that of the normal population among certain age cohorts. Postnatal exposure to therapeutic radiation to treat benign or malignant conditions is likewise associated with an increased risk of ALL. No consistent associations between ALL and the use of diagnostic irradiation postnatally, exposure to electromagnetic fields, or occupational exposure of parents have been demonstrated.

According to McKenna and Baehner (1991), increasing circumstantial evidence implicates viruses in the genesis of ALL. Clustering of cases by season or by geographic location would support a viral etiology. McKenna and Baehner (1991) maintain that the failure to find viral footprints using known technology does not rule out the existence of another subclass of viruses. In all probability, the etiology of ALL will be found to be the result of a complex interaction among genetic, immunological, environmental, and growth-regulating factors.

Increased incidences of ALL have been associated with pre-existing chromosomal abnormalities, such as Down, Bloom, and Fanconi syndromes; this has led to speculation that chromosomal aberrations may be etiologically significant in the genesis of leukemia. Increased incidences of ALL among siblings and identical twins of children diagnosed with this disease further implicate the involvement of genetics in the etiology of ALL. Other abnormalities associated with a predisposition for the development of ALL include the following: (1) ataxia telangiectasia and xeroderma pigmentosum, in which defective repair of DNA occurs; and (2) immunodeficiency disorders (McKenna & Baehner, 1991; Miller, 1989; Neglia & Robison, 1988).

Diagnosis, Classification, and Prognosis

ALL is diagnosed when more than 25–30% of the cells in the bone marrow are lymphoblasts (Baldy, 1986; McKenna & Baehner, 1991; Miller, 1989; Porth, 1990). It is readily established in the child who presents with anemia, thrombocytopenia, hepatosplenomegaly, and lymphoblasts in the peripheral blood and bone marrow (Miller, 1989).

There are multiple ways to characterize the leukemias. The most common classification of ALL—developed in 1976 by a group of French, American, and British hematologists, and thus referred to as the "FAB classification"—is based on distinctive morphological and histochemical characteristics of the immature leukemic blast cell (McKenna & Baehner, 1991; Miller, 1989; Miller & Miller, 1983; Neglia & Robison, 1988). Three prognostically significant subtypes of lymphoblasts are identifiable by means of this classification scheme: L1, L2, and L3. The L1 subtype, the most common, carries the most favorable prognosis for treatment outcome. Somewhat less common, the L2 subtype is claimed by some to carry an intermediate prognosis. The L3 subtype is very uncommon and is reported to carry a poor prognosis. In recent years, the prognostic significance of a distinction between the L1 and L2 subtypes has been questioned. Classification based on cell surface markers (immunology) suggests that these two subtypes are in fact indistinguishable.

In addition to disease characteristics (morphology, immunopheno-type, FAB classification), several presenting features of the child at diagnosis have been found to be important prognostic variables. Included among these are the following: age, white blood count (WBC), race, hemoglobin, sex, hepatosplenomegaly, platelet count, presence of CNS disease, immunoglobulin levels, and time to achieve remission (McKenna & Baehner, 1991; Miller, 1989; Miller & Miller, 1983). Given that many of these variables are interdependent, multivariate techniques have been used to assess the relative contribution of each in predicting outcome. Of the aforementioned variables, age and WBC are perhaps the best predictors of treatment outcome. The single most important predictor of remission and disease-free survival is initial leukocyte count (WBC).

The identification of prognostically important clinical and laboratory features has greatly improved the ability to predict the likelihood of successful treatment at the time of diagnosis (Miller et al., 1980). On the basis of these features, the patient can be determined to be at high, intermediate, or low risk of relapse at the time of diagnosis (Neglia & Robison, 1988); this determination permits treatment to be tailored to individual needs. A standard treatment for all children with ALL is clearly inappropriate. Determining whether treatment-related toxicity can be reduced in standard-risk children without increasing mortality rates or whether intensification of treatment for high-risk children is warranted will be the challenge confronting medical researchers, both now and in the foreseeable future.

Pathophysiology/Pathogenesis

Systemic ALL

To understand the means by which leukemic blasts are disseminated in the blood, one must possess a working knowledge of hematopoiesis—the formation and maturation of blood cells. All normal blood cells are thought to derive from a single pluripotential stem cell (Baldy, 1986; Porth, 1990). This stem cell is capable of differentiating into the progenitors of two cell lineages: the lymphoid and the myeloid progenitors. Considered committed unipotential cells (they differentiate along a single pathway), they give rise to precursors of one of several blood cell types.

ALL is characterized by an uncontrolled proliferation of immature lymphoid-type cells. Being immature and poorly differentiated, they are capable of an increased proliferation and a prolonged lifespan (Porth, 1990). Furthermore, they are unable to perform the functions of mature cells. The leukemic blast cell is simply an immature and mobile type of leukocyte that is disseminated throughout the circulatory system quite rapidly and from the earliest stages of the disease process. With increasing leukemic burden, the blasts gradually replace normal marrow elements and infiltrate many of the organs of the body. Although the basic clonal abnormality does not involve the pluripotential stem cell, the growth and maturation of all normal bone marrow cells are nevertheless affected. There are two critical components to the process by which the leukemic blasts devastate the system: a proliferative syndrome and a bone marrow insufficiency syndrome.

Almost all of the clinical symptoms of ALL are the results of either the replacement of normal bone marrow components or the infiltration of extramedullary sites by leukemic cells (Baldy, 1986; McKenna & Baehner, 1991; Miller, 1989; Porth, 1990). Typically, a child with ALL will present with complaints that reflect the paucity of normal blood cells. Replacement of normal bone marrow elements by leukemic blasts results in anemia, neutropenia, and thrombocytopenia. Thus, a child's presenting complaints may include pallor, excessive fatiguability, and lethargy as a consequence of anemia. Bleeding, including cutaneous bruising, purpura, petechiae, and gingival bleeding, occurs as a result of thrombocytopenia (decreased platelet count). Gastrointestinal and intracranial hemorrhaging are the more severe manifestations of this condition. Granulocytopenia (neutropenia) is the consequence of a compromised immune system that is susceptible to opportunistic infection. Leukemic infiltration of the liver, spleen, or lymph nodes may cause hepatomegaly, splenomegaly, lymphadenopathy, or some combination thereof (Miller, 1989). Bone pain, the result of leukemic infiltration of the cortex and periosteum (McKenna & Baehner, 1991; Miller, 1989), is also a frequent complaint. Sternal pain is almost pathognomonic of the disease.

Leukemia has been referred to as the "great imitator," because of its ability to infiltrate almost any organ of the body and thus present as a number of other common childhood illnesses. The clinical presentation of the child at diagnosis may range from no evidence of disease to extensive organ involvement (McKenna & Baehner, 1991). Onset may be insidious or abrupt, and any or all of the aforementioned symptoms may be in evidence.

CNS (Meningeal) Leukemia

Our current understanding of the pathogenesis of meningeal leukemia indicates that although, in essence, the leukemic cells that infiltrate the CNS are in sanctuary, they are not localized in the parenchyma (as had been envisioned by some). During the early years of CNS prophylaxis, the relative impermeability of the blood–brain barrier to chemotherapeutic agents was said to be responsible for later proliferation of the disease at this site. In fact, leukemic blasts localized within the CNS rarely infiltrate neural tissue directly (Price, 1983).

By definition, prophylactic treatment is treatment for occult CNS disease (Ochs, 1989). All available evidence indicates that subclinical foci of the disease are present within the leptomeninges at the time of hematological diagnosis, or soon thereafter (Price, 1983). Sequestered within the superficial arachnoid by direct perivascular invasion, the leukemic blasts acquire resistance to intravenous (IV) chemotherapeutic agents, thus successfully evading the full thrust of the first line of defense mobilized against them. Without adequate prophylactic treatment, leukemic infiltration of the leptomeninges progresses unchecked and produces characteristic anatomical sequelae and predictable clinical manifestations (Price, 1983).

During the initial stages of CNS leukemia, deeper portions of the arachnoid, the arachnoid trabeculae, and the cerebrospinal fluid (CSF) are free of leukemic blasts (Price, 1983). At this early stage, diagnosis cannot be made by CSF cytology. With increasing leukemic burden and the concomitant destruction of the arachnoid trabeculae, the leukemic blasts are released into the CSF. At this juncture, diagnosis of CNS leukemia by CSF cytology is possible. Of those diagnosed, 90% will have no symptoms of CNS involvement (Price, 1983).

As the leukemic burden increases, the deepest portions of the arachnoid are packed with blasts. Even at this advanced stage, infiltration of the CNS remains extraneural (Price, 1983). In the final stages of CNS leukemia, the resistant pial–glial membrane succumbs to the destructive effects of an expanding cell mass (Price, 1983), thus allowing direct infiltration of neural tissue.

The symptoms of CNS involvement are dependent upon the total leukemic burden and the progression of the disease. The cranial and spinal nerves, which pass through the leptomeninges, are susceptible to the effects of disease within the arachnoid. Cranial nerve palsies result from compression of the vascular supply of the nerves or from direct infiltration of the nerve fibers (Price, 1983). With increasing leukemic burden within the arachnoid, compression of vessels may result in a hypoperfusion encephalopathy. Residual neurological deficits are largely dependent upon the duration and degree of compression of vessels.

Hydrocephalus secondary to the obliteration or compression of the CSF channels was a common finding during the early years of chemotherapy (Price, 1983). The use of the intrathecal (IT) route of administration of chemotherapeutic agents has resulted in decreased incidences of CSF obstruction. Manifestations of increased intracranial pressure (e.g., vomiting, headache, papilledema, and lethargy) may accompany CSF obstruction.

Treatment Principles

The treatment for ALL is now aimed at total eradication of the disease. A child diagnosed with ALL today has a 95% chance of achieving remission, and in excess of a 50% chance of remaining in complete continuous remission for at least 5 years (McKenna & Baehner, 1991; Miller, 1989). This progress can be attributed largely to the use of more effective drugs, the development of better chemotherapeutic regimens, better supportive therapy (e.g., antibiotics), and the addition of CNS prophylactic treatment. Although diagnosis of ALL is made at an early clinical stage, the disease is identified relatively late in its biological growth cycle (Miller, 1989). At this late stage, few doublings may have a dramatic effect on the total cell population. Whereas cure involves total eradication of the leukemic burden, chemotherapeutic agents only kill a constant percentage of leukemic blasts (first-order kinetics). Beacuse a single cell can kill, treatment beyond remission induction is necessary.

In the treatment of ALL, the strategy adopted has been to take advantage of drug combinations that offer the greatest amount of cell kill, yet have the least powerful suppressive effects (McKenna & Baehner, 1991). The goal of treatment is to maximize survival rates while minimizing potential toxicities. For standard-risk ALL children, this involves determining the impact of reducing treatment-related toxicity upon survival rates. Conversely, this involves determining the impact of more aggressive treatments upon survival rates in high-risk ALL children.

There are potentially four phases in the treatment of childhood ALL. These include the following: induction, consolidation or intensification, CNS prophylaxis, and maintenance therapy. During the remission induction phase of treatment, over 90% of children with ALL enter complete remission after 4 weeks of treatment with vincristine and prednisone. Since 1963, this has been the standard combination used for remission induction (McKenna & Baehner, 1991). Although other drugs have been added to this standard protocol over the years, their addition has been found to increase the risk of toxicity without significantly altering remission rates. Recently, Niemeyer et al. (1991) have demonstrated that including IV MTX during the induction phase prolongs the duration of remission. Other agents may be used for those children who fail to achieve remission (fewer than 5% of cells) within the designated period of time. Remission is not akin to total eradication of the leukemic blasts. It simply means that the resolution power of the available instruments is insufficient to detect the small number of cells present.

Following remission, consolidation therapy (also called intensification therapy) may be initiated. The benefits of this phase of therapy have been debated. The rationale behind maintenance therapy has been to reduce the leukemic burden further. This phase of treatment has not been demonstrated to have any beneficial effects in standard-risk patients, but may be of benefit to those patients with a poorer prognosis for continuous complete remission.

CNS prophylaxis was implemented to prevent the development of meningeal leukemia, found in an alarming number of children following the introduction of multiagent chemotherapy. Initially, CNS prophylaxis consisted of the administration of 2400-cGy irradiation to the entire craniospinal axis. Over the years, however, CNS prophylactic treatment protocols have been refined to reduce the toxicity associated with treatment without sacrificing long-term survival. In subsequent comparisons of craniospinal irradiation (2400 cGy) to cranial vault irradiation (2400 cGy), the two regimens were found to be equally effective in preventing CNS relapse. Cranial vault irradiation became the preferred regimen because of the lower incidences of bone marrow suppression and subsequent morbidity associated with its use. Myelosuppression came to be considered a particularly undesirable consequence, given evidence that it may compromise the concomitant use of systemic chemotherapy.

More recently, it has been demonstrated that a reduced dose of cranial irradiation (1800 cGy) is as effective as the conventional dose in preventing CNS relapse in low-risk ALL children (Nesbit et al., 1981). Tubergen et al. (1988) have also found that IT chemotherapy alone is as effective as the latter treatment protocol in preventing CNS relapse in children with low-risk ALL. Conversely, relapse rates are higher among high-risk patients treated with anything but the conventional protocol.

It has been well established that continued therapy prolongs the period of remission (McKenna & Baehner, 1991). Maintenance therapy consists of the administration of multiple drugs at maximally tolerated dosage levels. The agents used during maintenance are often agents that have not been used for remission induction. Furthermore, these agents are reported to have fewer side effects and to be better suited to prolonged usage. The most common drugs used during this phase of therapy include 6-mercaptopurine and MTX (McKenna & Baehner, 1991; Miller, 1989). The addition of other agents provides no clear benefit in terms of disease control, and increases the risk of infection secondary to immunosuppression. With prolonged remissions, a concomitant increase in mortality and morbidity rates because of intercurrent infections has been found. There appears to be no advantage to continuing treatment beyond 3 years (Nesbit, Sather, Robison, Ortega, & Hammond, 1983).

Neurotoxicity Associated with Treatment for ALL

The treatment of childhood ALL involves the administration of multiple agents that may affect the CNS adversely. Although radiation and IT

MTX have often been implicated as the major causes of CNS damage among these children, several other agents administered in treatment protocols potentially neurotoxic. The acute effects of treatment are frequently caused by chemotherapeutic agents. Often transient, they tend to be overshadowed by iatrogenic influences on other systems of rapidly dividing cells (Packer et al., 1987). Although the number and dosage of agents vary considerably across studies (because these studies are part of cooperative research efforts designed to assess the efficacy of certain drugs in combination), the most commonly employed agents include vincristine, prednisone, cytosine arabinoside, daunomocin, 6-mercaptopurine, L-asparaginase, and MTX. Whether a given agent will culminate in acute or delayed effects is determined by such factors as dosage, route of administration, and the use of concomitant radiotherapy (Ochs, 1989).

There is ample evidence to suggest that many of the agents administered during the induction, consolidation, and maintenance phases of treatment have the potential to damage the CNS (Ochs, 1989; Packer et al., 1987). The toxicity of their combined effects merits consideration, particularly in light of a recent trend toward the use of more aggressive systemic therapies. A summary of the acute and delayed neurotoxic effects of several chemotherapeutic agents is presented in Table 11.1. Somnolence, chemical arachnoiditis, transient paraparesis, and leukoencephalopathy are among the acute and subacute neurotoxic effects attributed to methotrexate and irradiation.

Delayed treatment-related effects, ranging from mild neurocognitive impairment to clear evidence of CNS damage, become increasingly evident with the prolonged survival of children with ALL. Although radiotherapy has been incriminated as the causative agent, high-dose infusions of MTX have been found to be equally neurotoxic (Ch'ien et al., 1981; Ochs, 1989; Packer et al., 1987).

Prophylactic CNS treatment has been associated with delayed CNS toxicity, manifested as leukoencephalopathy, neuroendocrine dysfunction, intracranial calcifications, and cerebral atrophy (Bleyer, 1981; Bleyer, Drake, & Chabner, 1973; Crosley, Rorke, Evans, & Nigro, 1978; Glass, Lee, Bruner, & Fields, 1986; Kay et al., 1972; Ochs, 1989; Ochs, Parvey, & Mulhern, 1986; Packer et al., 1987; Peylan-Ramu et al., 1977; Peylan-Ramu, Poplack, Pizzo, Adornato, & DiChiro, 1978; Poplack, 1983; Poplack & Brouwers, 1988; Price, 1983; Price & Birdwell, 1978; Price & Jamieson, 1975a, 1975b; Schriock, Schell, Carter, Hustu, & Ochs, 1991; Skullerud & Halvorsen, 1978). Evidence of such damage has been found among asymptomatic survivors who had received 2400-cGy craniospinal irradiation or 2400-cGy cranial irradiation plus concurrent IT MTX for CNS therapy. By simply changing the temporal sequence of the administration of irradiation and IT MTX, investigators have found higher (IT MTX after) or lower (IT MTX before) rates of CNS pathology.

TABLE 11.1. Neurotoxicity of Chemotherapeutic Agents

Drug	Acute effects	Permanent long-term effects
Methotrexate (intrathecal or intraventricular)	Encephalopathy; meningitis; radiculitis; myelitis; focal brain necrosis	Focal deficits after brain necrosis; leukoencephalopathy[a]; myelitis; neurocognitive deficits[a]; myelitis
Methotrexate (high-dose, intravenous)	Transient encephalopathy; focal cortical deficits; seizures	Leukoencephalopathy[a]; neurocognitive deficits[a]
Methotrexate (intravenous)		Leukoencephalopathy[a]; neurocognitive deficits[a]
Vincristine	Peripheral neuropathy; cranial nerve palsies; seizures	Peripheral neuropathy
L-Asparaginase	Seizures; cerebrovascular accidents; encephalopathy	Residual seizures and focal deficits secondary to cerebrovascular accident
Cis-platinum	Focal brain necrosis (if given intra-arterially); seizures; coma; ototoxicity; peripheral neuropathy	Ototoxicity; peripheral neuropathy; blindness, leukoencephalopathy, focal necrosis after intra-arterial infusion
Cytosine arabinoside (intrathecal or intraventricular)	Radiculitis; myelitis; focal brain necrosis (if intraparenchymal infusion)	Focal deficits after brain necrosis; myelitis
Cytosine arabinoside (high-dose, intravenous)	Encephalopathy; cerebellar ataxia	Cerebellar ataxia
Actinomycin D	Myelitis[a]; focal brain necrosis[a]	Myelitis[a]; focal deficits[a]
5-Fluorouracil	Cerebellar ataxia; extrapyramidal deficits	Cerebellar ataxia; extrapyramidal deficits
BCNU	Focal brain necrosis, blindness after intra-arterial infusion	Focal brain necrosis, blindness, and leukoencephalopathy after intra-arterial infusion
Mechlorethamine	Hemiplegia; coma; seizures, hearing loss, and vestibular loss after intra-arterial infusion	Hearing loss; vestibular dysfunction after intra-arterial infusion
Procarbazine	Somnolence; encephalopathy; peripheral neuropathy	?
Thiotepa (intrathecal)	Weakness; radiculitis	Weakness; radiculitis; myelitis
5-Azacytidine	Weakness (? myopathy); encephalopathy; coma	?
VP16-VM26	Peripheral neuropathy	Peripheral neuropathy

Note. From Packer, Meadows, Rorke, Goldwein, and D'Angio (1987, p. 250). Copyright 1987 by John Wiley & Sons, Inc. Reprinted by permission.

[a] Occurs when used with concomitant radiotherapy.

Although the mechanism underlying the interaction between IT MTX and irradiation is uncertain, IT MTX would appear to have a direct radiosensitizing effect (Bleyer, 1981; Bleyer et al., 1973; Bleyer & Griffin, 1980; Packer et al., 1987). Because radiation alters the integrity of the blood–brain barrier, MTX may diffuse more easily into the parenchyma, and clearance from the brain may be decreased. Lower rates of CNS change have been observed following combination chemoprophylaxis. Among children so treated, calcifications have not been detected.

The pathogenesis of late radiation-induced CNS damage is imprecisely understood. Nevertheless, three hypotheses have been advanced to account for the delayed neuropathological changes detected on neuroimaging. The first of these identifies the capillary endothelial cell as being most susceptible to the effects of radiation, because of its capacity for replication. Damage to these cells is manifested as cell death or endothelial hyperplasia following attempts to replicate. Relatively speaking, the rate of turnover for these cells is rather slow. Consequently, the effects of therapeutic irradiation may be expected to occur over a prolonged period. This hypothesis seems to be the best explanation for the most common form of focal injury secondary to irradiation: mineralizing microangiopathy with dystrophic calcification (Packer et al., 1987).

A second hypothesis advanced to account for radiation-induced injury suggests that the glial cell is differentially susceptible. Damage to the oligodendroglial cells in particular results in transient demyelination and abnormal glial proliferation (Packer et al., 1987). The young child, undergoing a period of active myelinogenesis, may be particularly vulnerable to this type of damage. Leukoencephalopathy may develop secondary to either endothelial (Mildenberger, Beach, McGeer, & Ludgate, 1990) or glial damage. MTX, a folic acid antagonist, can also cause leukoencephalopathy by inhibiting the formation of a lipid that is a major component of myelin (Meadows & Evans, 1976; Packer et al., 1987; Waskerwitz & Fergusson, 1986). More subtle forms of treatment-induced injury, such as alterations of dendritic arborization and synaptogenesis, would not be expected to be detectable by routine light microscopy methods (Packer et al., 1987).

A third and final proposed mechanism of radiation-induced injury maintains that delayed damage results from an allergic response to antigens released from damaged glial cells (Packer et al., 1987). As yet, there is no evidence to support or counter this proposal.

Summary

The past 40 years have yielded major inroads with respect to treatment effectiveness. Currently, over 50% of patients treated for ALL will achieve long-term disease-free survival. As such, this disease has evolved in status over the past several decades from an acute to a chronic condition. Because of the increased survival rates of patients with ALL, we are now confronted with the issues of treatment toxicity, disease chronicity, and the impact of treatment regimens upon the functional integrity of the brain. This last issue forms the basis for the rest of this chapter.

NEUROPSYCHOLOGICAL CONSEQUENCES OF TREATMENT FOR ALL

Delayed treatment-related effects, in the form of varying degrees of neurocognitive impairment, have been reported among long-term survivors of ALL. Since the pioneering paper by Soni, Marten, Pitner, Duenas, and Powazek (1975), more than 60 articles have been published addressing the neuropsychological sequelae of CNS prophylactic treatment in children with ALL. The evidence for neuropsychological impairment is inconsistent, and, unfortunately, many of the studies were poorly executed. In many cases, the conclusions are not warranted, nor can alternative interpretations of the evidence be ruled out. To complicate matters, the direction of this research has changed in response to evolving treatment protocols; the implication of this is that recent research into the neurobehavioral consequences of irradiation/chemotherapy is not necessarily comparable to the pioneering studies in this area.

Since 1986, six reviews of this literature (Brown & Madan-Swain, 1993; Fletcher & Copeland, 1988; Gamis & Nesbit, 1991; Johnston, 1985; Madan- Swain & Brown, 1991; Williams & Davis, 1986) and one meta-analysis (Cousens et al., 1988) have been published. Although the majority of these have concluded that there are neuropsychological sequelae associated with CNS therapy for childhood ALL, there is little consensus among them regarding the nature and severity of impairment and whether or not it can be attributed to therapeutic radiation alone.

Fletcher and Copeland (1988) cautioned that the conclusions drawn from their review of this literature were tentative and merited further research. Nevertheless, their impressions were that CNS prophylaxis (particularly cranial radiation therapy [CRT]) does impair cognitive development; that these effects are most pronounced among those treated at younger ages; and that nonlanguage skills appear to be differentially susceptible to the adverse effects of treatment. By contrast, Williams and Davis (1986) were more inclined to minimize the severity of impairment associated with treatment. They concluded that there are few cognitive differences between leukemic patients and controls. The differences found, moreover, were not felt to be severe. Their sentiment is reminiscent of the statement of Versoza, Aur, Simone, Hustu, and Pinkel (1976) with reference to CNS therapy as being "destitute of prohibitive toxicity" (p. 209). Despite these disclaimers, Williams and Davis (1986) conceded that CNS therapy does appear to have a deleterious effect on cognitive function.

Confronted with contradiction and inconsistency, researchers have seized upon methodological issues as the source of discrepancy. Rare is the article that does not list a host of design flaws. To summarily review methodological issues without discarding studies would seem imprudent; yet it is done. Discarding such studies and controlling for design considerations render the task of reconciling differences among studies, and drawing meaningful conclusions from them, somewhat less daunting. In so doing, one finds a remarkable degree of consistency where once confusion was rife.

For the sake of brevity, methodological issues are not discussed at length here. Suffice it to say that rigorous scrutiny of studies resulted in 23 of them being deemed inadequate, and therefore not retained for the purposes of this discussion (Eiser, 1978; Eiser & Lansdown, 1977; Fallovalita et al., 1987; Gutjahr & Walther, 1981; Inati et al., 1983; McIntosh et al., 1976; Meadows & Evans, 1976; Meadows, Gordon, Littman, Glaser, & Fergusson, 1980; Meadows et al., 1981; Obetz et al., 1979; Paolucci & Rosito, 1983; Pavlovsky et al., 1983; Pfefferbaum-Levine et al., 1984; Poplack, 1983; Rowland et al., 1984; Schuler et al., 1981; Soni et al., 1975; Stehbens, Ford, Kisker, Clarke, & Strayer, 1981; Tamaroff et al., 1982; Tamaroff, Salwen, Miller, Murphy, & Nir, 1984; Versoza et al., 1976; Whitt, Wells, Lauria, Wilhem, & McMillan, 1984).

A further 33 studies were found to be comparatively better designed than those that were discarded outright. Though by no means without flaws of their own, they were deemed adequate (i.e., their limitations were not considered excessive). Some, in fact, were found to be quite well designed. These studies form the foundation upon which we make a renewed attempt to clarify the neuropsychological consequences of prophylactic treatment for childhood ALL (see Table 11.2).

Adverse Effects of Treatment

Of the 33 studies reviewed, 25 found performance decrements in some area. Without exception, the studies that failed to find adverse effects associated with CNS therapy had design variations that would account for the null findings. Berg et al. (1983), Moehle and Berg (1985), Williams et al. (1986), and Copeland, Dowell, Fletcher, Sullivan, et al. (1988) assessed children undergoing treatment. As pointed out by Fletcher and Copeland (1988), the neuropsychological functioning of such children tends not to be compromised. The subjects of Harten et al. (1984) and Trautman et al. (1988), conversely, were assessed at varying points after CNS treatment, thus risking the nullifying effects of combining hetero-geneous samples. The last of these studies, conducted by Ivnik, Colligan, Obetz, and Smithson (1981) and Mulhern, Fairclough, and Ochs (1991), compared the performance of long-term survivors in three CNS treat-ment groups without the benefit of a non-CNS-treated comparison group. It is possible that no form of prophylactic treatment is destitute of toxicity.

Time since Treatment Effects

Studies classified according to time since treatment indicate that the adverse effects of CNS prophylaxis may not be manifested for several years. In-treatment studies, which consist of subjects assessed less than 3 years after CNS therapy, often fail to reveal significant effects associated with treatment. Long-term survivor studies, conversely, almost uniformly reveal adverse sequelae of CNS treatment. With mixed-subject designs, the outcome is variable. Both comparative study designs, whereby newly diagnosed subjects are compared to long-term survivors, and longitudinal designs that extend beyond 3 years after CNS therapy, indicate that adverse sequelae emerge with prolonged survival.

In-Treatment Studies

Of five in-treatment studies reviewed (Berg et al., 1983; Copeland, Dow-ell, Fletcher, Sullivan et al., 1988; Moehle & Berg, 1985; Stehbens, Kisker, & Wilson, 1983; Williams et al., 1986), four indicate that with the excep-tion of an early vincristine-induced peripheral neuropathy, no adverse effects are demonstrated within the first 3 years after CNS treatment. The fifth, a study conducted by Stehbens et al. (1983), found a higher proportion of lower Verbal IQ to Performance IQ scores among patients with ALL. Their failure to replicate this particular finding, and their small sample size, raise the possibility that their results represent a statisti-cal aberration.

The results of the in-treatment studies suggest that if the late effects of treatment are attributable to CNS prophylaxis, then the pathological process must be insidious and progressive. This would appear to lend credence to the hypothesis that the vascular endothelial cell is differen-tially susceptible to the effects of radiation. Fletcher and Copeland (1988) offer an alternative explanation: They suggest that the performance decrements observed in long-term survivors reflect cumulative treat-ment effects.

TABLE 11.2. Adequate Studies of CNS-Treated Children with ALL

Article	Adverse effects	Age at diagnosis	Gender effects	Comparison group(s)	Treatment group(s)	Methodology	Limitations/confounds
Eiser (1980)	Yes	Yes <5 >5	N/A	1. 56 controls matched for age, sex, and SES	1. 2400 CRT + IT MTX (40) 2. Solid tumor (16)	1. R:112 2. LTS study (approx. 56 mos. since dx.); single assessment 3. Multiple *t* tests 4. WISC-R and Burt Reading 5. Treatment groups not compared	• Healthy comparison group • Tests of learning and memory not standardized • Time-since-treatment effect N/A • Coverage
Goff et al. (1980)	Yes	Yes <8 (30) >8 (7)	N/A	1. Newly diagnosed patients (18)	1. 2400 CNSP (9) or 2400 CRT + IT MTX (21)	1. Cross-sectional study 2. Relapse included but dealt with appropriately 3. Comprehensive battery 4. 4.5 to 11 yrs. survival	• No statistics to support age-at-diagnosis effect • No demographic comparisons • CNS therapy, gender, and time-since-treatment effects N/A
Ivnik et al. (1981)	No	No <6 (18) 6+ (15)	N/A		1. IT MTX (8) or IT MTX + IV MTX (6) 2. 2400 CRT + IT MTX (19)	1. R:33 2. LTS study (0.5 to 8 yrs. since treatment) 3. Multiple *t* tests and chi-square 4. Comprehensive battery	• Small *n* • Interaction terms N/A (age at dx. × treatment) • Time-since-treatment and gender effects N/A
Moss et al. (1981)	Yes	Yes <92 mos. (12) >92 mos. (12)	N/A	1. Siblings (24) 2. No-CRT siblings (10)	1. 2400 CRT + IT MTX or IT araC (24) 2. No-CRT ALL Ss (13)	1. P:24 ALL 2. Longitudinal LTS study: baseline (1.5 to 5.8 yrs, mean 3–11); assessed 1 yr. later (at least 1 patient still receiving treatment) 3. Multiple *t* tests 4. IQ and VMI	• Comparison group not well matched • Gender effect N/A • No initial assessment

Study							
Berg et al. (1983)	No, when compared to normative data; yes, when each testing compared (declines overtime)	No <5 (11) >5 (9)	No	1. Normative data	1. 2400 CRT + IT MTX	1. P:20 2. Longitudinal in-treatment design: assessments at average of 0.5, 1.6, and 3.1 yrs. 3. IQ and achievement	• Small *n* • Normative comparisons not appropriate • Interaction terms N/A (dx. × gender) • Brief FU interval • Coverage • Different chemo. protocols
Jannoun (1983)	Yes	Yes	Yes	1. Siblings (67)	1. CNS therapy <3 yrs. (43) 2. CNS therapy 3–6 yrs. (43) 3. CNS therapy 7+ yrs. (43) All patients received 2400 CRT + IT MTX (129)	1. R:129 2. Survivor study (at least 2.5 yrs. since dx.); single assessment 3. All Ss off treatment 4. IQ (British Ability Scales) and behavior 5. WISC-R IQ prorated	• Inappropriate comparison
Moehle et al. (1988)	Yes	Yes	N/A	None	Four groups based on age at dx. (≤5 or >5.1) and age at evaluation (≥13 or <13.1) All patients received 2400 CRT + IT MTX (110)	1. R:110 2. LTS study (mean of 9 mos. to 85 mos. off treatment) 3. Time on therapy and time off therapy controlled for 4. Assessment of language only	• No demographic comparisons • Scores not standardized • Limited to Ss over 9 yrs. of age at assessment • Gender a potential confound • Coverage
Stehbens et al. (1983)	Yes	Yes <8 (9) >8 (7)	N/A	1. 2400 CRT + IT MTX (16) 2. Solid tumor (17): No CNS therapy		1. P:16 2. Longitudinal in-treatment study: assessments at dx. and 1 yr. 3. IQ, achievement, and behavior	• Small *n* • Brief FU interval • No demographics • Gender effect N/A

(continued)

TABLE 11.2. (*Continued*)

Article	Adverse effects	Age at diagnosis	Gender effects	Comparison group(s)	Treatment group(s)	Methodology	Limitations/confounds
Harten et al. (1984)	No	N/A	N/A	1. Nonhematological malignancies (30); 11M/19F	1. <1800 to 2400 CRT + IT MTX (51); 29M/21F	1. R:51 2. Mixed LTS study (1.3 to 12.8 yrs.); single assessment 3. Reliability/validity of assessment tools	• Mixed CNS therapy protocols • Effects of age at dx., gender, and time since treatment N/A • Inappropriate comparison group
Lansky et al. (1984)	Yes	Yes	N/A	1. Healthy sibling controls (9) 2. Matched comparison group (sex, age, and initial IQ) (12)	1. CRT + IT MTX (17) 2. IT MTX only (13) 3. No CNS therapy (16)	1. P:62 2. Mixed longitudinal design: baseline at >1 yrs. post-dx. and assessment again 1 yr. later 3. IQ, BG, WRAT, and school records 4. Regression and discriminant-function analyses 5. Details of CNS treatment protocols not available	• No demographic comparisons • Gender effect N/A • Different diagnostic categories within treatment groups • Basis for combining groups for comparison unclear
Meadows et al. (1984)	Yes	N/A	N/A	None	1. 1800 CRT + IT MTX or IT MTX only	1. P:60 2. Mixed in-treatment and posttreatment longitudinal study: assessments at 1, 2, and 3 yrs. (final at least 3 mos. after D/C of therapy) 3. Abstract 4. Assessment instruments not reported (said to be comprehensive)	• Different diagnostic categories • Brief FU interval • Mixed CNS treatment protocols

302

Study				Controls	Treatment groups	Design/Methods	Limitations
Stehbens & Kisker (1984)	Yes	Yes <8 ≥8	N/A	1. Solid tumor (11)	2. 1800 (2) or 2400 (11) CRT + IT MTX	1. R:24 2. Longitudinal in-treatment design: assessments at 1 mo., 1 yr., and 3 yrs. Three-way ANOVA 3. IQ and achievement	• Gender effect N/A • Limited power for statistical comparisons • Coverage
Copeland et al. (1985)	Yes	Yes <60 mos. >60 mos.	N/A	1. Solid tumor and Hodgkin disease (25)	1. 2400 CRT + IT MTX (25) 2. IT chemo., no CRT (24)	1. R:74 2. LTS study (>5 yrs. disease-free survival) 3. Comprehensive battery	• Different diagnostic categories • Gender effect N/A
Moehle & Berg (1985)	No	No ≤8 8+	N/A	None	1. 2400 CRT + IT MTX (77)	1. P:77 2. In-treatment longitudinal design: assessments at <6 mos. and 1 yr. later 3. IQ and achievement 4. Multiple t tests	• Brief FU interval • Coverage
Williams et al. (1986)	No	No ≤5 >5	N/A	None	1. 2400 CRT + IT MTX (48) 2. IT MTX (30) 3. 1800 CRT + IT MTX (31) 4. Intensive chemo. + delayed CRT (9)	1. P:117 2. In-treatment (CCR 1 yr.); single assessment 3. Comprehensive battery 4. Multiple t tests	• Brief FU interval • Gender effect N/A
Jannoun & Chessells (1987)	Yes	Yes	No	1. Healthy controls matched for age, sex, and SES	1. 2400 CRT + IT MTX (19)	1. P:19 2. Longitudinal LTS study: assessments before radiotherapy and annually thereafter	• Gender effect N/A

(continued)

303

TABLE 11.. (Continued)

Article	Adverse effects	Age at diagnosis	Gender effects	Comparison group(s)	Treatment group(s)	Methodology	Limitations/confounds
Taylor et al. (1987)	Yes	N/A	N/A	1. Healthy siblings (26) matched for age	1. 1800–4800 CRT + IT MTX (26); 12M/14F	1. R:26 2. Mixed design (15–119 mos. since dx.) 3. Comprehensive battery and parent/teacher ratings	• Mixed CNS therapy protocols • Age-at-dx., gender, and time-since-treatment effects N/A
Copeland, Dowell, Fletcher, Bordeaux, et al. (1988)	Yes	N/A	N/A	None	1. ND: IT chemo. (29) 2. ND: no CNS therapy (21) 3. LTS: IT chemo. (24) 4. LTS: IT chemo. + 2400 CRT (25) 5. LTS: no CNS therapy (25)	1. Cross-sectional design (106): ND, evaluated within 3 mos.; LTS, at least 5 yrs. disease-free survival 2. Comprehensive battery	• Different diagnostic categories • Age at dx. N/A • Gender effect N/A
Copeland, Dowell, Fletcher, Sullivan, et al. (1988)	No	N/A	N/A	None	1. CNS therapy and systemic chemo. (19); 15M/4F 2. Systemic chemo., no CNS therapy (19); 9M/10F	1. P:38 2. In-treatment longitudinal design: baseline, and 1 yr. later 3. MANOVA design 4. Comprehensive battery 5. Sample restricted to those 6 yrs. or more at diagnosis	• No demographic comparisons • Brief FU interval • Different diagnostic categories • Groups divided by diagnosis only when significance found
Mulhern et al. (1988)	Yes	No ≤5 >5	N/A	1. Normative data	1. 1800 CRT + IT MTX (20) 2. IT MTX + IV MTX (20)	1. R:40 2. LTS study (>5 yrs. from CNS therapy); single assessment 3. Focus on memory	• Gender effect N/A

Study			Comparison group	Treatment		Methodological notes
Trautman et al. (1988)	No	N/A	1. Normative data	1. 1800 or 2400 CRT	1. R:34 2. Mixed design (9–110 mos. post-dx.) 3. IQ and (PIAT)	• Gender effect N/A • Inappropriate comparison group
Said et al. (1989)	Yes	N/A	1. Healthy siblings (near in age)	1. 2400 CRT	1. R:65/106 2. Mixed survivor study (1 to 13 yrs. since CNS therapy); single assessment 3. ANOVA, multiple regression, and ANCOVA 4. Abbreviated battery	• Coverage
Schlieper et al. (1989)	Yes	N/A	1. Healthy siblings (23)	1. IT MTX ± IV MTX (13); 8F/5M 2. 2400 CRT (16) or 1200 CRT (1) + IT MTX; 8F/9M	1. R:30 ALL 2. LTS study (>4 yrs. from dx.) 3. Comprehensive battery	• Limited power to assess interaction effects • Age-at-dx. effect N/A
Bleyer et al. (1990)	Yes <5 >5	Yes	None	1. 2400 CNSP or 2400 CRT + IT MTX	1. R:70 2. LTS study (3.5 to 10 yrs. after CNS therapy); single assessment 3. IQ only 4. Multiple t tests	• Mixed CNS therapy protocols • Different IQ measures combined
Waber, Gioia, et al. (1990)	Yes	N/A	1. Wilm tumor (15), age and sex matched	1. 2400 CRT + IT MTX	1. R:51 2. LTS study (disease-free 5 to 12 yrs.); single assessment 3. Article intended to identify specific cognitive processes that underlie functional deficits (not to determine degree of impairment)	• Suitability of comparison group

(continued)

TABLE 11.2. (Continued)

Article	Adverse effects	Age at diagnosis	Gender effects	Comparison group(s)	Treatment group(s)	Methodology	Limitations/confounds
Waber, Urion, et al. (1990)	Yes	Yes	Yes	1. Wilm tumor (15), age and sex matched 2. Normative data	1. 2400 CRT + IT MTX	1. R:51 2. LTS study (disease-free 5 to 12 yrs.); single assessment 3. IQ and achievement 4. Impairment index 5. Height/weight	• Suitability of comparison group
Dowell et al. (1991)	Yes	N/A	N/A	None	1. CRT + IT MTX (25) 2. CRT, no IT MTX (11) 3. No CRT, IT MTX (24) 4. No CRT, no IT MTX (25)	1. R:85 2. Purpose of article to evaluate synergism 3. Comprehensive battery	• Different diagnostic categories • Treatment varies • Time-since-treatment effect N/A • Age at dx. not used as covariate
Moore et al. (1991)	Yes	Yes <48 mos. >48 mos. No stats.	N/A	None	1. 2400 CRT + IT MTX (20) 2. 1800 CRT + IT MTX (15)	1. R:35 2. Survivor study 3. IQ, achievement, VMI	• Time since treatment potential confound • Gender effect N/A • Coverage • Limited power to assess interactions
Mulhern et al. (1991)	No	No	Yes	None	1. 2400 CRT + IT MTX (28) 2. 1800 CRT + IT MTX (23) 3. IV MTX + IT MTX (26)	1. R:77 2. LTS study (5 to 11 years after CNS therapy); single assessment 3. Comprehensive battery	• No comparison group or baseline performance

Reference						
Ochs et al. (1991)	Yes	N/A	No	None	1. 1800 CRT + IT MTX (23) 2. Parenteral MTX (26)	1. P:49 2. Longitudinal LTS study: following remission, yearly until D/C therapy, every other year 3. Comprehensive battery
Waber, Bernstein, et al. (1992)	Yes	Yes <36 mos. >36 mos.	Yes	Yes	1. Wilm tumor (15); age and sex matched	1. 2400 CRT + IT MTX	1. R:49 2. LTS study (disease-free survival 5 to 12 yrs.); single assessment 3. Purpose of article to assess relationship of functional outcome to age at CNS therapy and gender; diagnostic profiles
Brown et al. (1992)	Yes	No	N/A	1. Siblings	1. Recently dx. 2. 1 yr. post-dx. 3. Off therapy	1. Cross-sectional design (46)
Waber, Tarbell, et al. (1992)	Yes	N/A	Yes	1. Normative data	1. Grouped according to standard risk (1800) or high risk (2400), MTX (low dose vs. high dose), and gender	1. R:51 2. LTS study (>6 yrs. disease-free) 3. Selected subsets of WISC-R and WRAT 4. Regression model

Note. N/A, not assessed; IT MTX, intrathecal methotrexate; CRT, cranial radiation therapy; CNSP, craniospinal radiation; dx., diagnosis; Ss, subjects; P, prospective; R, retrospective; LTS, long-term survivor; FU, follow-up; CCR, complete continuous remission; SES, socioeconomic status; VMI, measure of visual–motor integration; araC, cytosine arabinoside; IV, intravenous; BG, Bender–Gestalt; WISC-R, Wechsler Intelligence Scale for Children — Revised; WRAT, Wide Range Achievement Test; PIAT, Peabody Individual Achievement Test; ND, newly diagnosed; D/C, discontinuation; ANOVA, analysis of variance; MANOVA, multivariate analysis of variance; ANCOVA, analysis of covariance.

Long-Term Survivor Studies

The results of 19 studies of long-term survivors reviewed are unequivocal: There is unanimous agreement that CNS therapy results in neuropsychological performance decrements. The one exception, a study conducted by Ivnik et al. (1981), compared two treatment protocols without the benefit of a control group, thus accounting for their null findings. The investigations of Eiser (1980), Moss, Nannis, and Poplack (1981), Jannoun (1983), Bleyer et al. (1990), Waber, Urion, et al. (1990), Moore, Kramer, Wara, Halberg, and Ablin (1991), Brown et al. (1992), and Waber, Tarbell, Kahn, Gelber, and Sallan (1992) were restricted to assessing the impact of treatment upon performance on measures of psychometric intelligence, academic achievement, and (less often) visual–motor integration. In the balance of the long-term survivor studies, comprehensive neuropsychological assessments were undertaken (Copeland et al., 1985; Dowell, Copeland, Francis, Fletcher, & Stovall, 1991; Jannoun & Chessells, 1987; Mulhern et al., 1991; Ochs et al., 1991; Schlieper, Esseltine, & Tarshis, 1989). In two of these, assessments were limited to a specific area of functioning (Moehle, Berg, Ch'ien, & Lancaster, 1983; Mulhern, Wasserman, Fairclough, & Ochs, 1988). Specific findings are presented later in the chapter, within the context of a discussion of the nature and severity of impairment associated with CNS treatment.

Mixed Studies

As anticipated, those studies in which the samples of patients were assessed at different points after CNS treatment were divided with respect to their conclusions. Of the five mixed studies identified, three found adverse effects associated with CNS treatment (Lansky et al., 1984; Taylor, Albo, Phebus, Sachs, & Bierl, 1987; Said, Waters, Cousens, & Stevens, 1989), and two reported null findings (Harten et al., 1984; Trautman et al., 1988). Times since treatment in these studies ranged from as little as 9 months post CNS therapy to as much as 13 years after such therapy at assessment.

Comparison Studies

Comparison studies include those that enabled contrasts to be made between newly diagnosed patients and long-term survivors by means of longitudinal or cross-sectional designs. Six such studies were identified (Brown et al., 1992; Copeland, Dowell, Fletcher, Bordeaux, et al., 1988; Goff, Anderson, & Cooper, 1980; Jannoun & Chessells, 1986; Meadows, Massari, & Obringer, 1984; Moss et al., 1981; Stehbens & Kisker, 1984).

These studies reinforce the impression that the neuropsychological functioning of patients assessed within the first few years of treatment is not compromised. Moreover, they indicate that treatment-related deficits emerge with prolonged survival.

Effects of Age at Diagnosis

Of the 23 studies that examined the effects of treatment at different age levels, 16 consistently identified younger children as more susceptible to delayed treatment-related neuropsychological impairment. With one exception (Brown et al., 1992), those studies that failed to find age-at-diagnosis effects had design variations that decreased the likelihood of obtaining significant results. Of these, three did not use a comparison group (Mulhern et al., 1988, 1991; Ochs et al., 1991). In the remaining five, in-treatment (Berg et al., 1983; Moehle & Berg, 1985; Williams et al., 1986) or mixed (Ivnik et al., 1981; Trautman et al., 1988) study designs were used.

Undue confusion regarding what "younger" means has been created by the failure of researchers to reach a consensus regarding appropriate cutoffs. In these studies, the criteria for inclusion in the younger group has been quite variable, ranging from as low as 3 years to as high as 8 years. Some have argued that the development of the nervous system continues through the seventh year, and thus have advocated the use of 8 years as a cutoff (Stehbens et al., 1983). Others have argued that 5 years of age is a more appropriate cutoff, given that a period of rapid cognitive growth occurs between the ages of 5 and 7 years (Copeland et al., 1985). If the purpose of this exercise is to identify whether CNS prophylaxis produces age-related constraints on neurobehavioral development (Waber, Bernstein, Kammerer, Tarbell, & Sallan, 1992), this issue would be addressed best through the assessment of performance across the spectrum of ages in question.

Gender Effects

The relationship between gender and the neuropsychological consequences of CNS therapy has been poorly researched, despite the fact that it was identified as a potentially important variable as early as 1983. Of 10 articles published that assessed the variance in outcome associated with gender, 8 found that females risk being more adversely affected by CNS treatment. Of these, the same sample was used in four publications. When this issue was reconsidered, 6 of 8 studies found females to be at a greater risk for consequent neuropsychological impairment. Additional research would appear warranted to confirm this association.

Treatment Comparisons

Relatively few studies have endeavored to assess the dose–response relationship between radiation and impairment. Given the restricted range of dosages administered within treatment protocols, such an undertaking would probably prove fruitless. Comparisons, however, have been made among several different prophylactic regimens (Bleyer et al., 1990; Copeland et al., 1985; Copeland, Dowell, Fletcher, Sullivan, et al., 1988; Dowell et al., 1991; Ivnik et al., 1981; Moore et al., 1991; Mulhern et al., 1988, 1991; Ochs et al., 1991; Williams et al., 1986).

Among treatment comparisons involving contrasts between IT or IV MTX with or without the concurrent administration of 2400-cGy CRT (Copeland et al., 1985; Copeland, Dowell, Fletcher, Bordeaux, et al., 1988; Dowell et al., 1991; Ivnik et al., 1981; Mulhern et al., 1991; Schlieper et al., 1989), the results have been variable. Copeland et al. (1985), Copeland, Dowell, Fletcher, Bordeaux, et al., 1988, Dowell et al. (1991), and Schlieper et al. (1989) found that children treated with both CRT and IT MTX consistently performed more poorly than did their nonirradiated counterparts. Ivnik et al. (1981), Mulhern et al. (1988, 1991), and Ochs et al. (1991), however, found no performance differences among children treated with IT or IV MTX as compared to those treated with either 2400- or 1800-cGy CRT and the concurrent administration of IT MTX. Furthermore, the investigations of Mulhern and colleagues and of Ochs et al. (1991) suggested that no prophylactic treatment protocol is destitute of toxicity. This finding is echoed by Moore et al. (1991), who found performance discrepancies thought to be due to radiation dosage to be attributable, in fact, to differences in time since treatment between their groups.

The treatment comparison studies of Williams et al. (1986) and Copeland, Dowell, Fletcher, Sullivan, et al. (1988) both made use of in-treatment study designs; null findings would thus be anticipated. Williams et al. (1986) found no early adverse effects associated with any type of CNS treatment. Copeland, Dowell, Fletcher, Sullivan, et al. (1988), by contrast, found both between- and within-group performance differences on measures of fine motor and tactile-perceptual skills during the early stages of treatment. These were attributed to a vincristine-induced peripheral neuropathy.

Comparisons to Other Groups

Included in this section are studies in which the performance of CNS-treated patients with ALL was compared to that of one of the following groups: (1) patients with solid tumors; (2) matched controls or siblings; or (3) normative data.

Patients with Solid Tumors

In five studies, the performance of patients with ALL was compared to that of non-CNS-treated patients with solid tumors. The results of these five studies (Copeland et al., 1985; Harten et al., 1984; Waber, Bernstein, et al., 1992; Waber, Gioia, et al., 1990; Waber, Urion, et al., 1990) consistently found children with ALL to be more severely affected than their counterparts with solid tumors.

Matched Controls or Siblings

Of the eight studies comparing the performance of patients with ALL to that of matched controls or siblings (Brown et al., 1992; Eiser, 1980; Jannoun, 1983; Lansky et al., 1984; Moss et al., 1981; Said et al., 1989; Schlieper et al., 1989; Taylor et al., 1987), the patients were consistently found to perform more poorly. Where more comprehensive assessments were undertaken (Taylor et al., 1987), the group with ALL was found to perform less well than matched siblings on tests of IQ, neuropsychological skills, and academic achievement. Schlieper et al. (1989) found that those patients treated only with IT MTX did not differ from their siblings on any measure.

Normative Data

When the performance of patients with ALL has been compared to normative data, the results have been somewhat more variable. In three of these studies, the performance of the patients fell below normative expectations (Ivnik et al., 1981; Mulhern et al., 1988; Waber, Urion, et al., 1990). In the remaining three studies, the performance of patients as a group did not differ significantly from normative expectations (Berg et al., 1983; Trautman et al., 1988; Waber, Tarbell, et al., 1992); however, two of these used in-treatment or mixed study designs.

The constitution of suitable comparison groups continues to be a point of contention among researchers. Many argue that healthy siblings or matched controls are inappropriate. Most advocate the use of non-CNS-treated patients with solid tumors as a comparison group, to control for the effects of illness and school absence. However, this group may be inappropriate for comparative purposes if socioeconomic status is not taken into consideration. If one refers to the epidemiology of childhood ALL, one finds an increased incidence of this disease among higher socioeconomic levels, as noted earlier in the chapter. Therefore, a bias toward higher levels of premorbid functioning would be anticipated. Comparisons to normative data or to other groups not matched for socioeconomic status would likewise be inappropriate, given that substantial declines in skills and abilities might well result in "normal" performance. The results of studies in which such comparisons have been made must be interpreted with due caution.

Neuropsychological Assets and Deficits Associated with CNS Prophylaxis

That there are adverse sequelae associated with CNS prophylaxis is the least one can conclude from a review of studies assessing the neuropsychological functioning of long-term survivors of childhood ALL. The severity of impairment of skills most often falls within the mild to moderate ranges. The final issue to be resolved concerns the nature of the deficits following treatment.

Only those studies that have assessed long-term survivors of childhood ALL have been retained for the purpose of this section. In-treatment and mixed studies were excluded, because, with few exceptions, the neuropsychological functioning of children undergoing treatment has not been found to be adversely affected. Comparative treatment studies that failed to include a control group are also not considered here. The remaining 14 studies vary in coverage and methodological sophistication. These studies suggest a remarkable degree of consistency between the neuropsychological assets and deficits demonstrated by children having undergone prophylaxis and those displaying the NLD syndrome.

Heretofore lacking in this literature has been a conceptual framework to guide research endeavors. The NLD model (Rourke, 1989) is proposed to bridge this gap. It is a conceptual framework that provides specific hypotheses regarding the constellation of neuropsychological assets and deficits anticipated secondary to white matter damage. This model enables predictions to be made regarding the impact of the amount of white matter destruction and the developmental stage at which the damage occurs, thereby serving to integrate the findings of this literature.

Although the NLD syndrome is manifested most clearly on a developmental basis, it also may be found among groups of children with various forms of neurological disease, disorder, or dysfunction in which significant white matter damage has been sustained. Manifestations of the NLD syndrome in children with neurological disease are hypothesized to occur to the extent that these involve white matter destruction. Conditions that involve generalized or diffuse destruction of white matter would be most likely to result in this syndrome in its entirety. Consequently, to the extent that the damage induced by CNS prophylaxis for treatment of ALL alters the integrity of the white matter, we would expect the neuropsychological assets and deficits exhibited to conform to the NLD syndrome. However, it should be understood that very extensive and severe white matter perturbations would be expected to eventuate in structural deviations so pronounced that the pattern of assets and deficits characteristic of the NLD syndrome would not be discernible.

There is ample evidence to indicate that the white matter of the brain is differentially susceptible to damage following CNS prophylaxis. At least four neuropathologically distinctive forms of delayed CNS toxicity have been identified among long-term survivors of ALL who had received CNS treatment (Poplack & Brouwers, 1988). Three of these are germane to the current discussion: subacute (necrotizing) leukoencephalopathy, mineralizing microangiopathy, and cortical atrophy. Findings consistent with these types of lesions have been found on autopsy and on computed tomography (CT) scans (Ochs, 1989; Ochs et al., 1986; Pedersen & Clausen, 1981; Peylan-Ramu et al., 1977; Peylan-Ramu et al., 1978; Price & Birdwell, 1978; Price & Jamieson, 1975a, 1975b; Riccardi, Brouwers, DiChiro, & Poplack, 1985).

In the first of several CT brain scan studies, Peylan-Ramu et al. (1978) found one or more abnormalities in over 50% of otherwise asymptomatic children 1 month after CNS prophylaxis. A greater or lesser frequency of CT abnormalities has been found, depending upon the sequence of administration of prophylactic agents (Ochs, 1989). Included among the CT abnormalities observed are the following: (1) areas of decreased attenuation coefficient (white matter hypodensity); (2) ventricular dilation; (3) widening of subarachnoid spaces; and (4) intracerebral calcifications (Poplack & Brouwers, 1988). White matter hypodensity, most common in the periventricular areas, reflects demyelination. It is said to be the hallmark of subacute leukoencephalopathy (Poplack & Brouwers, 1988). Cortical atrophy is denoted on CT by ventricular dilation and widening of the subarachnoid spaces. Intracerebral calcifications have been presumed to be mediated by damage to the capillary endothelial cells. Experimental evidence suggests that because of the nature of the vascularization of the brain, this form of damage may also have a more detrimental effect upon white than upon grey matter (Mildenberger et al., 1990).

Significant white matter alteration may occur secondary to treatment with CRT or MTX (Ochs, 1989; Packer et al., 1987). The mechanism of radiation-induced white matter damage, although not precisely known, appears to be related to injury sustained by the capillary endothelial cell (Mildenberger et al., 1990; Packer et al., 1987). MTX, which has been demonstrated to be capable of producing leukoencephalopathy without the use of concomitant radiotherapy (Ochs, 1989; Packer et al., 1987), probably has a more direct effect on glial function.

If the pathophysiology of both CRT and MTX is such that they produce more devastating effects upon the white matter of the brain, what constellation of neuropsychological assets and deficits might we anticipate following CNS treatment for childhood ALL? According to the white matter model, neuropathological conditions that culminate in significant white matter destruction produce a relatively predictable pattern of neuropsychological strengths and weaknesses, which corresponds to that of the NLD syndrome. The following is a review of the evidence to support manifestations (assets and deficits) of the NLD syndrome among long-term survivors of childhood ALL treated with CNS prophylaxis.

Tactile-Perceptual Skills

Tactile-perceptual deficits associated with treatment for ALL may be evidenced early during the course of treatment for childhood ALL; specifically, they appear attributable to a vincristine-induced peripheral neuropathy (Dowell, Copeland, & Judd, 1989). Children exhibiting the NLD syndrome may also demonstrate tactile-perceptual deficits at younger ages, but for much different reasons. In the case of NLD, such deficits usually resolve somewhat as the years pass. Copeland, Dowell, Fletcher, Sullivan, et al. (1988), Copeland et al. (1985), and Dowell et al. (1991) have found that the tactile-perceptual deficits exhibited by those treated for childhood ALL likewise tend to be transient. Among long-term survivors of childhood ALL, treatment-related sensory-perceptual deficits have not been found (Copeland, Dowell, Fletcher, Bordeaux, et al., 1988; Copeland et al., 1985; Mulhern et al., 1991; Schlieper et al., 1989).

Motor and Psychomotor Skills

There is much evidence to suggest that complex psychomotor skills are relatively more impaired among long-term survivors of childhood ALL, as they are in children with the NLD syndrome. Early during the course of treatment for childhood ALL, these children are susceptible to a vincristine-induced peripheral neuropathy that may be disruptive of performance on more complex measures of psychomotor skills (e.g., Grooved Pegboard Test; Copeland, Dowell, Fletcher, Bordeaux, et al., 1988). With prolonged survival, however, performance decrements on complex psychomotor tasks persist, suggesting that impairment is related to CNS prophylactic treatment (Copeland, Dowell, Fletcher, Bordeaux, et al., 1988; Copeland et al., 1985). Whether simple motor skills are adversely affected by CNS prophylaxis is less certain. Although some investigators have found no treatment-related deficits on measures of strength of grip and finger-tapping speed (Goff et al., 1980; Mulhern et al., 1991; Schlieper et al., 1989), others have detected performance decrements on both simple and complex psychomotor tasks (Copeland, Dowell, Fletcher, Bordeaux, et al., 1988; Copeland et al., 1985). Of two studies in which tapping speed was found to be diminished (Copeland, Dowell, Fletcher, Bordeaux, et al., 1988; Copeland et al., 1985), one found this to occur only with the nondominant hand (Copeland et al., 1985). Most investigators, however, found that simple motor skills (finger tapping, grip strength) are impervious to the effects of CNS prophylaxis; this is also typical of children with NLD.

Attention and Memory

Poor attentional capacities (visual and auditory), reflected in weaker performances on selected subtests of the age-appropriate Wechsler scale, have been found among children treated with CNS prophylaxis. Poorest performances have typically been reported on the Arithmetic, Digit Span, and Coding subtests (Copeland et al., 1985; Eiser, 1980; Goff et al., 1980; Waber, Urion, et al., 1990), suggesting that attentional problems may represent an outstanding deficit among these children. Decrements in tactile attention (Mulhern et al., 1991) secondary to CNS prophylaxis have not been observed.

The memory functioning of children treated for ALL has been evaluated by several investigators (Copeland, Dowell, Fletcher, Bordeaux, et al., 1988; Copeland et al., 1985; Jannoun & Chessells, 1987; Mulhern et al., 1988; Schlieper et al., 1989). The consensus among these studies is that both verbal and visual memory may be adversely affected by CNS prophylactic treatment. Mulhern et al. (1988) assessed the memory functioning of 40 patients with ALL, treated with two different prophylactic regimens. No effects of treatment were found on any of the 16 standardized memory measures administered. The entire sample, however, performed more poorly than normative expectations on the Target Test and on 4 of 12 learning efficiency tests (immediate visual and verbal memory). No differences were found on the Memory for Sentences, Visual Auditory Learning, and Number Reversed Tests.

The immediate and delayed visual and verbal memory of 19 patients with ALL who had received 2400-cGy CRT and IT MTX for CNS prophylaxis was assessed by Jannoun and Chessells (1987). Although they found evidence for both verbal and visual memory impairment among their sample, they tended to gloss over this fact in a discussion of their findings. Jannoun and Chessells (1987) suggested that their subjects suffered from a specific auditory–verbal learning deficit. This may have been so. However, the patients also performed more poorly than their siblings on digit span (backward), delayed recall of stories, and the Rey–Osterrieth Complex Figure (copy and delay).

In a cross-sectional study of different treatment regimens undertaken by Copeland, Dowell, Fletcher, Bordeaux, et al. (1988), the verbal and nonverbal memory functioning of both those currently undergoing treatment and long-term survivors were found to be compromised. Investigations conducted by Waber, Tarbell, et al. (1992) and Dowell et al. (1991) confirm the suspicion that the memory impairment secondary to treatment is the product of a complex interaction among the multiple agents used in treatment protocols.

In the only known study to assess performance on a measure involving tactile–spatial memory (memory parameter of the Tactual Performance Test; Goff et al., 1980), children treated for ALL at an older age were found to perform more poorly on this measure than on language-related measures.

The diminished capacity for sustained attention and concentration that is not modality-specific is perhaps the most striking difference between children with ALL and those demonstrating the "developmental" presentation of the NLD syndrome. Although it appears to constitute a generalized deficit, evident from the early stages of treatment, it has most frequently been evaluated and identified in the auditory–verbal realm. There is little conclusive evidence to indicate that such deficits are related to younger age at diagnosis, which would be predicted from the tenets of the NLD model. The impairments in verbal and visual memory demonstrated by children with ALL are the logical outcomes of their heightened distractibility and poor attentional deployment within these modalities. Again, the investigations of Dowell et al. (1991) and Waber, Tarbell, et al. (1992) suggest that the relationship between verbal memory impairment and treatment for childhood ALL is complex. Future research is obviously needed to clarify this relationship.

Psychometric Intelligence

Among children treated for ALL, performance decrements have been found on all three Wechsler summary scales (Copeland, Dowell, Fletcher, Bordeaux, et al., 1988; Copeland et al., 1985; Eiser, 1980; Goff et al., 1980; Moss et al., 1981; Schlieper et al., 1989; Waber, Urion, et al., 1990). Verbal–Performance IQ discrepancies, favoring the former, have been found in just two studies (Jannoun, 1983; Schlieper et al., 1989). Performances on the individual subtests of the Wechsler scales indicate that the most frequently observed pattern of performance has been a clustering of performance inefficiencies on the Arithmetic, Digit Span, and Coding subtests. Nevertheless, depending upon the study examined, evidence can be garnered to support performance decrements on most of the subtests.

In examining the intellectual functioning of children with ALL using the Kaufman Assessment Battery for Children (K-ABC), the Brown et al. (1992) study demonstrates how CNS treatment may affect the patterning of neuropsychological functions. Unlike the aforementioned investigations using the Wechsler scales, Brown et al. (1992) found a selective impairment of certain processing scores on the K-ABC. Specifically, they found children who had received prolonged chemotherapy to be more impaired on tasks associated with the Simultaneous Processing scale than their recently diagnosed or sibling peers. The off-therapy patients performed significantly more poorly than did their siblings on the Triangles and Spatial Memory subtests of the Simultaneous Processing scale. On the Matrix Analogy subtest of this scale, the off-therapy group performed significantly more poorly than did both patients with a recent diagnosis and sibling controls. Brown et al. (1992) present their findings within the context of a discussion of the relative sensitivity of the Wechsler Intelligence Scale for Children—Revised Performance IQ and the K-ABC Simultaneous Processing scale to right hemisphere dysfunction. These authors provide evidence to suggest that Simultaneous Processing scale scores may be more affected by impairment of right hemispheral systems.

Visual–Spatial, Visual-Perceptual, and Visual–Motor Skills

Converging lines of evidence suggest that the visual–spatial–organizational abilities of children who have undergone CNS prophylaxis may be compromised. As part of their comprehensive battery, Copeland, Dowell, Fletcher, Bordeaux, et al. (1988) administered a visual-spatial analysis task to their subjects. Those children who had received CRT as part of their treatment performed significantly more poorly than did their controls on this task. Mulhern et al. (1988) found that their treated subjects performed more poorly on the Target Test, a task in which the subjects are required to reproduce visual–spatial configurations. Brown et al. (1992) found the impairment demonstrated by their off-therapy group with ALL to be spatial–motor in nature. The four tests most adversely affected in their study involved visual stimuli, which required strong spatial and holistic processing skills (Brown et al., 1992). Motor demands were, however, minimal. In seeking to identify the cognitive processes that mediate the performance differentials in intellectual functioning between their children with ALL and controls with solid tumors, Waber, Gioia, et al. (1990) found that the ALL group demonstrated deficits in appreciating the organization inherent in complex visual–spatial material and in alertness. Finally, in a recent study by Butler and Hill (1994), deficits in perceptual localization and susceptibility to perceptual interference were found among children treated with CRT.

Without question, the visual—motor integration skills of children treated for ALL have been found to be deficient. This is borne out by the investigations undertaken by Copeland, Dowell, Fletcher, Bordeaux, et al. (1988), Copeland et al. (1985), Dowell et al. (1991), Moore et al, (1991), and Moss et al. (1981).

Taken together, these studies suggest some impairment in visual—spatial—organizational skills evidenced by children with ALL who have undergone CNS prophylaxis. The deficiencies related to visual memory, outlined earlier, reinforce this impression. Although these abilities may not be compromised to the degree that they are among children with NLD, they nevertheless represent an outstanding deficiency among children treated for ALL. Because the impairment to these skills may be mild, it may not be reflected in global indices such as the Performance IQ.

Concept Formation and Problem Solving

There is a dearth of information available regarding the performance of children with ALL on measures of concept formation and problem solving. Schlieper et al. (1989) found no differences between their CNS-treated group and matched controls on the Wisconsin Card Sorting Test. Goff et al. (1980), by contrast, found that long-term survivors performed more poorly than recently diagnosed children with ALL on the Category Test. Several investigators have found evidence for impairment in nonverbal problem-solving skill, reflected in diminished scores on the Block Design (Copeland, Dowell, Fletcher, Bordeaux, et al., 1988; Copeland et al., 1985; Dowell et al., 1991; Eiser, 1980; Goff et al., 1980; Jannoun, 1983) and Object Assembly (Copeland et al., 1985; Eiser, 1980; Jannoun, 1983; Schlieper et al., 1989) subtests of the age-appropriate Wechsler scales. Also, higher-order cognitive processes are required for success on measures of verbal fluency (categories unspecified) and delayed recall of stories. The performance deficits of children treated for ALL noted on such tests would also be reflective of problems in this class of abilities.

Smatterings of evidence culled from several studies make it difficult to determine conclusively whether the problem-solving and conceptual abilities of long-term survivors of childhood ALL suffer appreciably. Preliminary evidence suggesting that they do is consistent with the NLD syndrome. Nevertheless, future research is needed to determine whether the concept-formation and problem-solving skills of children with ALL constitute a significant area of deficiency, and whether the modality in which such tasks are presented has any bearing on outcome.

Auditory—Verbal and Language-Related Skills

Consistent with the NLD syndrome, the performance of children with ALL on measures of speech and language functioning has been found to be intact, and to represent a relative strength. Performances on such measures as the Rapid Automatized Naming Test, the Peabody Picture Vocabulary Test, and the Token Test have been found to be developed to age-appropriate levels. These results suggest that speech output, receptive vocabulary, and verbal comprehension are adequate.

Verbal assets that characterize the NLD syndrome include excellent phonemic hearing, segmentation, blending, and repetition. These particular skills have not been evaluated among long-term survivors of childhood ALL. Because the development of more complex linguistic skills depends upon the development of these more basic skills, it may be presumed that these skills are intact. Judging by their Wide Range Achievement Test Reading (word recognition) and Spelling scores, which are in the normal range, this would appear to be a safe assumption.

The very well-developed receptive language skills and rote verbal capacities that are defining features of the NLD syndrome have also been demonstrated among children with ALL (Copeland, Dowell, Fletcher, Bordeaux, et al., 1988; Copeland et al., 1985; Jannoun & Chessells, 1987; Moehle et al., 1983). Furthermore, where performance discrepancies have been observed, these have been on more complex language skills (Copeland, Dowell, Fletcher, Bordeaux, et al., 1988; Jannoun & Chessells, 1987).

Academic Achievement

Investigations pertaining to the academic functioning of long-term survivors of ALL are divided with respect to their conclusions (Copeland, Dowell, Fletcher, Bordeaux, et al., 1988; Copeland et al., 1985; Dowell et al., 1991; Eiser, 1980; Goff et al., 1980; Moore et al., 1991; Mulhern et al., 1991; Ochs et al., 1991; Schlieper et al., 1989; Waber, Urion, et al., 1990). A few of these studies did not contain an evaluation of several academic realms. Although four studies suggested that arithmetic achievement may suffer most as a consequence of CNS prophylaxis (Copeland, Dowell, Fletcher, Bordeaux, et al., 1988; Dowell et al., 1991; Mulhern et al., 1991; Ochs et al., 1991), it has yet to be demonstrated conclusively that arithmetic represents an outstanding deficiency in academic achievement among these children, as it is in children with NLD.

The reading comprehension of children having undergone treatment for childhood ALL has been evaluated in just two studies (Schlieper et al., 1989; Waber, Urion, et al., 1990). These too are divided with respect to their conclusions, and consequently the issue merits further research.

Conclusions and Future Directions

Although some issues have yet to be resolved, the very least one can conclude is that CNS prophylaxis has an adverse effect on neuropsychological functioning. Included among the circumstances under which the effects of CNS treatment may be intensified are younger age at diagnosis and, less conclusively, female gender. With respect to the latter of these, the findings of Waber and her colleagues (Waber, Gioia, et al., 1990; Waber, Urion, et al., 1990; Kleinman & Waber, 1992) suggest an interaction between gender and consequent neuropsychological impairment. They maintain that the neuropsychological sequelae of treatment reflect the involvement of at least two processes: one common to CNS-treated patients, and one specific to females so treated. Although this framework is compelling, it must be demonstrated that the gender effect repeatedly reported in their investigations is not a finding peculiar to their sample. Because hormonal influences on manifestations of skills and abilities have been implicated strongly in other conditions (e.g., Turner syndrome; see Chapter 13, this volume) wherein the NLD syndrome appears to be operative, these results raise some intriguing possibilities for theoretical advances. For now, it is clear that future research is needed to clarify the relationship between gender and neuropsychological impairment in children treated for ALL.

With few exceptions, the neuropsychological functioning of those undergoing treatment has not been found to be compromised. Fine motor and tactile-perceptual deficits observed early during the course of treatment have been attributed to a vincristine-induced peripheral neuropathy, and appear to resolve with time.

Unfortunately, however, a trend indicating progressive impairment with prolonged survival is apparent. Neuropathological changes observed on CT have been detected as late as 5 years after CNS therapy (Brouwers & Poplack, 1990; Brouwers, Riccardi, Fedio, & Poplack, 1985; Brouwers, Riccardi, Poplack, & Fedio, 1984; Poplack & Brouwers, 1988). Radiation-induced damage to the vascular endothelial cells would appear to be the principal mechanism to account for late CNS changes.

Although some studies implicate CRT as the source of neuropsychological impairment, the balance of the literature suggests that no treatment regimen is free of toxicity. With the trend toward the use of chemoprophylaxis for treatment, particularly among low-risk candidates, recent investigations have begun to determine the impact of less toxic treatments on neuropsychological outcome (i.e., Brown et al., 1992; Waber, Tarbell, et al., 1992).

Because of their comprehensiveness in terms of coverage, the studies undertaken by Copeland and colleagues (Copeland, Dowell, Fletcher, Bordeaux, et al., 1988; Copeland et al., 1985; Dowell et al., 1991) are perhaps best suited to evaluating the relevance of the NLD model to children treated for childhood ALL. These investigators came to similar conclusions in their studies. They found that their CNS-irradiated group performed significantly more poorly on nonlanguage tasks, including visual–motor integration, arithmetic, coding, spatial memory, and fine motor skills. In their 1988 work, Copeland's group indicated that the pattern of performance demonstrated by their CNS-irradiated treatment group suggests a primary impairment in fine motor, arithmetic, and other nonverbal processing skills.

The results of three other studies that have endeavored to assess the neuropsychological functioning of long-term survivors of childhood ALL in a comprehensive manner found results that support (Butler & Hill, 1994; Goff et al., 1980; Schlieper et al., 1989) and extend (Goff et al., 1980) the findings of Copeland and colleagues. Goff et al. (1980) compared the neuropsychological test performance of newly diagnosed and long-term survivors of childhood ALL treated with CRT. In addition to finding evidence to suggest an impairment in sustained attention and concentration, and heightened distractibility among their long-term survivors, they also reported difficulties on measures of nonverbal problem solving. Schlieper et al. (1989) echoed the results and conclusions of Copeland and colleagues in suggesting that the pattern of specific skill deficits undelying the global decrement found among children treated with radiotherapy occurs in the nonverbal realm. A recent study undertaken by Butler and Hill (1994) provides findings that are consistent with the aforementioned studies, and that indicate that the decreased cognitive efficiency of pediatric cancer patients is reflective of nondominant-hemisphere dysfunction.

The NLD/white matter model provides a framework within which the findings of the literature on the neuropsychological consequences of prophylactic treatment for ALL may be understood. Examining this literature from the perspective of the NLD model reveals that many of the assets and deficits demonstrated by these children are predictable from the tenets of the model. If nothing else, the preceding discussion should have made it abundantly clear that there is a considerable degree of overlap between the assets and deficits demonstrated by children treated for ALL and children who evidence the NLD syndrome.

A relationship between age at diagnosis and neurobehavioral decrement would be predicted from the NLD model, since any skill may be disrupted during its acquisition by white matter damage. Consequently, a spectrum of neuropsychological deficits may be anticipated among those receiving prophylaxis at young ages, and early during the course of their treatment. The possibility that children who receive CNS prophylaxis at earlier developmental levels run a greater risk for consequent neuropsychological impairment is borne out by this research (Bleyer et al., 1990; Copeland et al., 1985; Eiser, 1980; Goff et al., 1980; Jannoun, 1983; Jannoun & Chessells, 1987; Moehle et al., 1983; Moss et al., 1981). The most rigorous of these studies, undertaken by Jannoun (1983), indicated that younger children do indeed risk suffering from a spectrum of delayed neurobehavioral deficits secondary to CNS prophylaxis.

Finally, the psychosocial functioning of children with ALL has infrequently been assessed in conjunction with their neuropsychological abilities. Typically, the questionnaires administered have assessed school absences and difficulties in managing curriculum demands. More detailed personality and behavioral assessments are seldom administered. Given that children with NLD have been found to be at risk for the development of internalized forms of psychopathology (Rourke, 1989; Rourke & Fuerst, 1992), the socioemotional adjustment of children treated for ALL should be more closely scrutinized, particularly in light of the mounting evidence suggesting that the two conditions overlap considerably.

REFERENCES

Aur, R. J. A., Hustu, H. O., Versoza, M. S., Wood, A., & Simone, J. V. (1973). Comparison of two methods of preventing central nervous system leukemia. *Blood, 42,* 349–357.

Aur, R. J. A., Simone, J. V., Hustu, H.O., & Versoza, M. S. (1972). A comparative study of central nervous system irradiation and intensive chemotherapy early in remission of childhood acute lymphocytic leukemia. *Cancer, 29,* 381–391.

Aur, R. J. A., Simone, J. V., Hustu, H. O., Walters, T., Borella, L., Pratt, C., & Pinkel, P. (1971). Central nervous system therapy and combination chemotherapy of childhood lymphocytic leukemia. *Blood, 37,* 272–281.

Baldy, C. M. (1986). The white blood cell. In S. A. Price & L. M. Wilson (Eds.), *Pathophysiology: Clinical concepts of disease processes* (3rd ed., pp. 198–214). New York: McGraw-Hill.

Balsom, B., Bleyer, W. A., Robison, L. L., Heyn, R., Meadows, A., Sitarz, D., Miller, D., Leikin, H., Sather, J., Ortega, J., Nesbit, M., & Hammond, D. (1987). Can intellectual deficits be prevented with pretreatment methotrexate? *Proceedings of the American Society of Clinical Oncology, 6,* 155. (Abstract)

Berg, R. A., Ch'ien, L. T., Bowman, W. P., Ochs, J., Lancaster, W., Goff, J. R., & Anderson, H. R. (1983). The neuropsychological effects of acute lymphocytic leukemia and its treatment—a three year report: Intellectual functioning and academic achievement. *Clinical Neuropsychology, 5*(1), 9–13.

Bleyer, W. A. (1981). Neurologic sequelae of methotrexate and ionizing radiation: A new classification. *Cancer Treatment Report, 65,* 89–98.

Bleyer, W. A., Drake, J. C., & Chabner, B. A. (1973). Neuro-toxicity and elevated cerebrospinal fluid methotrexate concentration in meningeal leukemia. *New England Journal of Medicine, 289,* 770–773.

Bleyer, W. A., Fallavollita, J., Robison, L., Balsom, W., Meadows, A., Heyn, R., Sitarz, A., Ortega, J., Miller, D., Constine, L., Nesbit, M., Sather, H., & Hammond, D. (1990). Influence of age, sex, and concurrent intrathecal methotrexate therapy on intellectual function after cranial irradiation during childhood: A report from the Children's Cancer Study Group. *Pediatric Hematology and Oncology, 7*, 329–338.

Bleyer, W. A., & Griffin, T. W. (1980). White matter necrosis, mineralizing microangiopathy and intellectual abilities in survivors of childhood leukemia. In H. A. Gilbert & A. R. Kagan (Eds.), *Radiation damage to the nervous system* (pp. 155- 173). New York: Raven Press.

Brouwers, P., & Poplack, D. (1990). Memory and learning sequelae in long-term survivors of acute lymphoblastic leukemia: Association with attention deficits. *American Journal of Pediatric Hematology/Oncology, 12*, 174–181.

Brouwers, P., Riccardi, R., Fedio, P., & Poplack, D. G. (1985). Long-term neuropsychologic sequelae of childhood leukemia: Correlation with CT brain scan abnormalities. *Journal of Pediatrics, 106*, 723–728.

Brouwers, P., Riccardi, R., Poplack, D., & Fedio, P. (1984). Attentional deficits in long-term survivors of childhood acute lymphoblastic leukemia (ALL). *Journal of Clinical Neuropsychology, 6*, 325–336.

Brown, R. T., & Madan-Swain, A. (1993). Cognitive, neuropsychological, and academic sequelae in children with leukemia. *Journal of Learning Disabilities, 26*(2), 74–90.

Brown, R. T., Madan-Swain, A., Pais, R., Lambert, R. G., Baldwin, K., Casey, R., Frank, N., Sexson, S. B., Ragab, A., & Kamphaus, R. W. (1992). Cognitive status of children treated with central nervous system prophylactic chemotherapy for acute lymphocytic leukemia. *Archives of Clinical Neuropsychology, 7*, 481–497.

Butler, R. W., & Hill, J. M. (1994, February). *The neuropsychological effects of cranial irradiation, intrathecal methotrexate and systemic methotrexate in childhood cancer.* Paper presented at the meeting of the International Neuropsychological Society, Cincinnati, OH.

Ch'ien, L. T., Aur, R. J. A., Versoza, M. S., Coburn, T. P., Goff, J. R., Hustu, H. O., Price, R. A., Seifert, M. J., & Simone, J. V. (1981). Progression of methotrexate-induced leukoencephalopathy in children with leukemia. *Medical and Pediatric Oncology, 9*, 133–141.

Coccia, P. F., Bleyer, W. A., Siegel, S. E., et al. (1981). Reduced therapy for children with good prognosis acute lymphoblastic leukemia (ALL). *Blood, 58*(Suppl. 1), 137a.

Copeland, D. R., Dowell, R. E., Fletcher, J. M., Bordeaux, J. D., Sullivan, M. P., Jaffe, N., Frankel, L. S., Reid, H. L., & Cangir, A. (1988). Neuropsychological effects of childhood cancer treatment. *Journal of Child Neurology, 3*, 53–62.

Copeland, D. R., Dowell, R. E., Fletcher, J. M., Sullivan, M. P., Jaffe, N., Cangir, A., Frankel, L. S., & Judd, B. W. (1988). Neuropsychological test performance of pediatric cancer patients at diagnosis and one year later. *Journal of Pediatric Psychology, 13*, 183–196.

Copeland, D. R., Fletcher, J. M., Pfefferbaum-Levine, B., Jaffe, M., Ried, H., & Maor, M. (1985). Neuropsychological sequelae of childhood cancer in long-term survivors. *Pediatrics, 75*, 745–753.

Cousens, P., Waters, B., Said, J., & Stevens, M. (1988). Cognitive effects of cranial irradiation in leukemia: A survey and meta-analysis. *Journal of Child Psychology, Psychiatry, and Allied Disciplines, 29*, 839–852.

Crosley, C. J., Rorke, L. B., Evans, A., & Nigro, M. (1978). Central nervous system lesions in childhood leukemia. *Neurology, 28,* 678–685.

Dowell, R. E., Copeland, D. R., Francis, D. J., Fletcher, J. M., & Stovall, M. (1991). Absence of synergistic effects of CNS treatments on neuropsychological test performance among children. *Journal of Clincial Oncology, 9,* 1029–1036.

Dowell, R. E., Copeland, D. R., & Judd, B. W. (1989). Neuro-psychological effects of chemotherapeutic agents. *Developmental Neuropsychology, 5,* 17–24.

Eiser, C. (1978). Intellectual abilities among survivors of childhood leukemia as a function of CNS irradiation. *Archives of Disease in Childhood, 53,* 391–195.

Eiser, C. (1980). Effects of chronic illness on intellectual development. *Archives of Disease in Childhood, 55,* 766–770.

Eiser, C., & Lansdown, R. (1977). Retrospective study of intellectual development in children treated for acute lymphoblastic leukemia. *Archives of Disease in Childhood, 52,* 525–529.

Evans, A. E., Gilbert, E. S., & Zandstra, R. (1970). The increasing incidence of central nervous system leukemia in children. *Cancer, 26,* 404–409.

Fallovalita, J., Bleyer, A., Robison, L., Heyn, R., Meadows, A., Sitarz, A., Ortega, J., Miller, D., Nesbit, M., Sather, H., & Hammond, D. (1987). Intellectual dysfunction after cranial irradiation (CRT) in young children with acute lymphocytic leukemia (ALL): Concurrent intrathecal methotrexate (IT-MTX) is a contributing factor. *Proceedings of the American Society of Clinical Oncology, 6,* 257. (Abstract)

Farber, S., Diamond, L. K., Mercer, R. D., Sylvester, R. F., & Wolff, J. A. (1948). Temporary remission in acute leukemia in children produced by folic acid antagonist 4-aminopteroyl-glutamic acid (aminopterin). *New England Journal of Medicine, 238,* 787–797.

Fletcher, J. M., & Copeland, D. R. (1988). Neurobehavioral effects of central nervous system prophylactic treatment of cancer in children. *Journal of Clinical and Experimental Neuropsychology, 10,* 495–537.

Gamis, A. S., & Nesbit, M. E. (1991). Neuropsychologic (cognitive) disabilities in long-term survivors of childhood cancer. *Pediatrician, 18,* 11–19.

Glass, Y. P., Lee, Y., Bruner, J., & Fields, W. S. (1986). Treatment-related leukoencephalopathy: A study of three cases and literature review. *Medicine, 65*(3), 154–162.

Goff, J. R., Anderson, H. R., & Cooper, P. F. (1980). Distractibility and memory deficits in long-term survivors of acute lymphoblastic leukemia. *Developmental and Behavioral Pediatrics, 1*(4), 158–163.

Gutjahr, P., & Walther, B. (1981). IQ and cognitive function in long-term survivors of childhood acute lymphocytic leukemia. *Lancet, ii,* 1278–1279. (Abstract)

Harten, G., Stephani, U., Henze, G., Langermann, H. J., Riehm, H., & Hanefeld, F. (1984). Slight impairment of psychomotor skills in children after treatment of acute lymphoblastic leukemia. *European Journal of Pediatrics, 142*(3), 189–197.

Hockenberry, M. J., Coody, D. K., & Falletta, J. M. (1986). Introduction to childhood cancer. In M. J. Hockenberry & D. K. Coody (Eds.), *Pediatric oncology and hematology* (pp. 3–13). St. Louis: C.V. Mosby.

Hustu, H. O., Aur, R. J. A., Versoza, M. S., Simone, J. V., & Pinkel, D. (1973). Prevention of central nervous system leukemia by irradiation. *Cancer*, *32*, 585–597.

Inati, A., Sallan, S. E., Cassady, J. R., Hitchcock-Brian, S., Clavell, L. A., Belli, J. A., & Sollee, N. (1983). Efficacy and morbidity of central nervous system "prophylaxis" in childhood acute lymphoblastic leukemia: Eight years' experience with cranial irradiation and intrathecal methotrexate. *Blood*, *61*, 297–303.

Ivnik, R. J., Colligan, R. C., Obetz, S. W., & Smithson, W. A. (1981). Neuropsychologic performance among children in remission from acute lymphocytic leukemia. *Developmental and Behavioral Pediatrics*, *2*(2), 29–34.

Jannoun, L. (1983). Are cognitive and educational development affected by age at which prophylactic therapy is given in acute lymphocytic leukemia? *Archives of Disease in Childhood*, *58*, 953–958.

Jannoun, L., & Chessells, J. M. (1987). Long-term psychological effects of childhood leukemia and its treatment. *Pediatric Hematology and Oncology*, *4*, 293–308.

Johnston, C. W. (1985). Language ability in children treated with central nervous system prophylaxis for acute lymphocytic leukemia. *International Journal of Clinical Neuropsychology*, *7*(1), 25–28.

Kay, H. E. M., Knapton, P. J., O'Sullivan, J. P., Wells, D. G., Harris, R. F., Innes, E. M., Stuart, J., Schwartz, F. C. M., & Thompson, E. N. (1972). Encephalopathy in acute leukemia associated with methotrexate therapy. *Archives of Disease in Childhood*, *47*, 344–348.

Kirs, P. J., & Herman, R. M. (1980). Neuromotor and neuro-psychological manifestations of "total therapy" in children with acute lymphoblastic leukemia. *Cancer Treatment Reviews*, *7*(2), 85–94.

Kleinman, S. N., & Waber, D. P. (1992). Neurodevelopmental bases of spelling acquisition in children treated for acute lymphoblastic leukemia. *Cognitive Neuropsychology*, *9*(5), 403–425.

Lansky, S. B., Cairns, N. V., Lansky, L. L., Cairns, G. F., Stephenson, L., & Garin, G. (1984). Central nervous system prophylaxis: Studies showing impairment in verbal skills and academic achievement. *American Journal of Pediatric Hematology/Oncology*, *6*(2), 183–190.

Lusher, J. M., & Ravindranath, Y. (1979). Acute lymphoid leukemia. In C. Pochedly (Ed.), *Pediatric cancer therapy* (pp. 1–28). Baltimore: University Park Press.

Madan-Swain, A., & Brown, R. T. (1991). Cognitive and psychosocial sequelae for children with acute lymphocytic leukemia and their families. *Clinical Psychology Review*, *11*(3), 267–294.

McIntosh, S., Klatskin, E. H., O'Brien, R. T., Aspnes, G. T., Kammerer, B. L., Snead, C., Kalavsky, S. M., & Pearson, H. A. (1976). Chronic neurologic disturbance in childhood leukemia. *Cancer*, *37*, 853–857.

McKenna, S. M., & Baehner, R. L. (1991). Diagnosis and treatment of childhood acute lymphocytic leukemia. In P. H. Wiernik, G. P. Canellos, R. A. Kyle, & C. A. Schiffer (Eds.), *Neoplastic diseases of the blood* (pp. 231–151). New York: Churchill Livingstone.

Meadows, A. T., & Evans, A. E. (1976). Effects of chemotherapy on the central nervous system: A study of parenteral methotrexate in long-term survivors of leukemia and lymphoma in childhood. *Cancer*, *37*, 1079–1085.

Meadows, A. T., Gordon, J., Littman, P., Glaser, K. M., & Fergusson, J. (1980). Pattern of cognitive dysfunctions in children with acute lymphocytic leukemia (ALL) treated with cranial radiation (RT). *American Society of Clinical Oncology Abstracts, 21*, 386.

Meadows, A. T., Gordon, J., Massari, D. J., Littman, P., Fergusson, J., & Moss, K. (1981). Declines in IQ scores and cognitive dysfunctions in children with acute lymphocytic leukemia treated with cranial irradiation. *Lancet, ii*, 1015–1018.

Meadows, A. T., Massari, D., & Obringer, A. (1984). Cognitive function in children after 1800 rad cranial irradiation (CRT) or periodic intrathecal methotrexate (IT-MTX): A preliminary report. *Proceedings of the American Society of Clinical Oncology, 3*, 71. (Abstract C-278)

Mildenberger, M., Beach, T. G., McGeer, E. G., & Ludgate, C. M. (1990). An animal model of prophylactic cranial irradiation: Histologic effects at acute, early and delayed stages. *International Journal of Radiation, Oncology, Biology and Physiology, 18*, 1051–1060.

Miller, D. R. (1989). Hematologic malignancies: Leukemia and lymphoma. In D. R. Miller, R. L. Baehner, & L. P. Miller (Eds.), *Blood diseases of infancy and childhood* (pp. 604–710). St. Louis: C. V. Mosby..

Miller, D. R., Leikin, S., Albo, V., Vitale, L., Sather, H., Coccia, P., Nesbit, M., Karon, M., & Hammond, D. (1980). Use of prognostic factors in improving the design efficiency of clinical trials in childhood leukemia: Children's Cancer Study Group report. *Cancer Treatment Reports, 64*, 381–392.

Miller, L. P., & Miller, D. R. (1983). Acute lymphoblastic leukemia in children: Current status, controversies, and future perspectives. *CRC Critical Review of Oncology and Hematology, 1*(2), 129–197.

Moehle, K. A., & Berg, R. A. (1985). Academic achievement and intelligence test performance in children with cancer at diagnosis and one year later. *Developmental and Behavioral Pediatrics, 6*, 62–64.

Moehle, K. A., Berg, R. A., Ch'ien, L. T., & Lancaster, W. (1983). Language-related skills in children with acute lymphocytic leukemia. *Developmental and Behavioral Pediatrics, 4*(4), 257–261.

Moore, I. M., Kramer, J. H., Wara, W., Halberg, F., & Ablin, A. R. (1991). Cognitive function in children with leukemia: Effects of radiation dose and time since treatment. *Cancer, 68*, 1913–1917.

Moss, H. A., Nannis, E. D., & Poplack, D. G. (1981). The effects of prophylactic treatment of the central nervous system on the intellectual functioning of children with acute lymphocytic leukemia. *American Journal of Medicine, 71*, 47–52.

Mulhern, R. K., Fairclough, D., & Ochs, J. (1991). A prospective comparison of neuropsychological performance of children surviving leukemia who received 18 Gy, 24 Gy, or no cranial irradiation. *Journal of Clinical Oncology, 9*, 1348–1356.

Mulhern, R. K., Wasserman, A. L., Fairclough, D., & Ochs, J. (1988). Memory function in disease-free survivors of childhood lymphocytic leukemia given CNS prophylaxis with or without 1800 cGy cranial irradiation. *Journal of Clinical Oncology, 6*, 315–320.

Neglia, J. P., & Robison, L. L. (1988). Epidemiology of the childhood acute leukemias. *Pediatric Clinics of North America, 35*, 675–692.

Nesbit, M. E., Sather, H. N., Robison, L. L., Ortega, J. A., & Hammond, G. D. (1983). A randomized study of 3 years versus 5 years of chemotherapy in childhood lymphoblastic leukemia. *Journal of Clinical Oncology, 1,* 308–316.

Nesbit, M. E., Sather, H. N., Robison, L. L., Ortega, J., Littman, P. S., D'Angio, G. J., & Hammond, G. D. (1981). Presymptomatic central nervous system therapy in previously untreated childhood acute lymphoblastic leukemia: Comparison of 1800 rad and 2400 rad: A report from Children's Cancer Study Group. *Lancet, i,* 461–466.

Niemeyer, C. M., Gelber, R. D., Tarbell, N. J., Donnelly, M., Clavell, L. A., Blattner, S. R., Donahue, K., Cohen, H. J., & Sallan, S. E. (1991). Low dose versus high dose methotrexate during remission induction in childhood acute lymphoblastic leukemia (protocol 81–01 update). *Blood, 78,* 2514–2519.

Obetz, S. W., Smithson, W. A., Groover, R. V., Houser, O. W., Klass, D. W., Ivnik, R. J., Colligan, R. C., Gilchrist, G. S., & Burgert, E. O. (1979). Neuropsychologic follow-up study of children with acute lymphocytic leukemia: A preliminary report. *American Journal of Pediatric Hematology/Oncology, 1*(3), 207–213.

Ochs, J. (1989). Neurotoxicity due to central nervous system therapy for childhood leukemia. *American Journal of Pediatric Hematology/Oncology, 11*(1), 93–105.

Ochs, J., Mulhern, R., Fairclough, D., Parvey, L., Whitaker, J., Ch'ien, L., Mauer, A., & Simone, J. (1991). Comparison of neuropsychologic functioning and clinical indicators of neurotoxicity in long-term survivors of childhood leukemia given cranial radiation or parenteral methotrexate: A prospective study. *Journal of Clinical Oncology, 9*(1), 145–151.

Ochs, J., Parvey, L. S., & Mulhern, R. (1986). Prospective study of central nervous system changes in children with acute lymphoblastic leukemia receiving two different methods of central nervous system prophylaxis. *Neurotoxicology, 7*(2), 217–226.

Packer, R. J., Meadows, A. T., Rorke, L. B., Goldwein, J. L., & D'Angio, G. (1987). Long-term sequelae of cancer treatment on the central nervous system in childhood. *Medical and Pediatric Oncology, 15,* 241–253.

Paolucci, G., & Rosito, P. (1983). Adverse sequelae of central nervous system prophylaxis in acute lymphoblastic leukemia. In R. Mastrangelo, D. G. Poplack, & R. Riccardi (Eds.), *Central nervous system leukemia: Prevention and treatment* (pp. 105–112). Boston: Martinus Nijhoff.

Pavlovsky, S., Fisman, N., Arizaga, R., Castano, J., Chamoles, N., Leiguarda, R., & Moreno, R. (1983). Neuropsychological study in patients with ALL: Two different CNS prevention therapies—cranial radiation plus IT methotrexate vs. IT methotrexate alone. *American Journal of Pediatric Hematology/Oncology, 5*(1), 79–86.

Pedersen, H., & Clausen, N. (1981). The development of cerebral CT changes during treatment of acute lymphocytic leukemia in childhood. *Neuroradiology, 22,* 79–84.

Peylan-Ramu, N., Poplack, D. G., Bleir, C. L., Herdt, J. R., Vermess, M., & DiChiro, G. D. (1977). Computer assisted tomography in methotrexate encephalopathy. *Journal of Computer Assisted Tomography*, *1*, 216–221.

Peylan-Ramu, N., Poplack, D. G., Pizzo, P. A., Adornato, B. T., & DiChiro, G. (1978). Abnormal CT scans of the brain in asymptomatic children with acute lymphocytic leukemia after prophylactic treatment of the central nervous system with radiation and intrathecal methotrexate. *New England Journal of Medicine*, *298*, 815–818.

Pfefferbaum-Levine, B., Copeland, D. R., Fletcher, J., Ried, H. L., Jaffe, N., & McKinnon, W. R. (1984). Neuropsychological assessment of long-term survivors of childhood leukemia. *American Journal of Pediatric Hematology/Oncology*, *6*(2), 123–128.

Poplack, D. G. (1983). Evaluation of adverse sequelae of central nervous system prophylaxis in acute lymphoblastic leukemia. In R. Mastrangelo, D. G. Poplack, & R. Riccardi (Eds.), *Central nervous system leukemia: Prevention and treatment* (pp. 95–103). Boston: Martinus Nijhoff.

Poplack, D. G., & Brouwers, P. (1988). Late CNS sequelae in long-term survivors of childhood leukemia. *Anales Españoles de Pediatría*, *29*(Suppl. 34), 19–25.

Porth, C. M. (1990). Disorders of white blood cells and lymphoid tissues. In C. M. Porth (Ed.), *Pathophysiology: Concepts of altered health states* (3rd ed., pp. 218–228). Philadelphia: J. B. Lippincott.

Price, R. A. (1983). The pathology of central nervous system leukemia. In R. Mastrangelo, D. Poplack, & R. Riccardi (Eds.), *Central nervous system leukemia: Prevention and treatment* (pp. 1–10). Boston: Martinus Nijhoff.

Price, R. A., & Birdwell, D. (1978). The central nervous system in childhood leukemia: III. Mineralizing microangiopathy and dystrophic calcifications. *Cancer*, *42*, 717–728.

Price, R. A., & Jamieson, P. A. (1975a). The central nervous system in childhood leukemia. *Cancer*, *35*, 306–317.

Price, R. A., & Jamieson, P. A. (1975b). The central nervous system in childhood leukemia: II. Subacute leuko-encephalopathy. *Cancer*, *35*, 306–318.

Riccardi, R., Brouwers, P., DiChiro, D., & Poplack, D. (1985). Abnormal computed tomography brain scans in children with acute lymphoblastic leukemia: Serial long-term follow-up. *Journal of Clinical Oncology*, *3*, 12–18.

Rourke, B. P. (1989). *Nonverbal learning disabilities: The syndrome and the model.* New York: Guilford Press.

Rourke, B. P., & Fuerst, D. R. (1992). Psychosocial dimensions of learning disability subtypes: Neuropsychological studies in the Windsor Laboratory. *School Psychology Review*, *21*, 360–373.

Rowland, J. H., Glidewell, O. J., Sibley, R. F., Holland, J. C., Tull, R., Berman, A., Brecher, M. L., Harris, M., Gliksman, A. S., Forman, E., Jones, B., Cohen, M. E., Duffner, P. K., & Freeman, A. I. (1984). Effects of different forms of prophylaxis on neuropsychologic function in childhood leukemia. *Journal of Clinical Oncology*, *2*, 1327–1335.

Said, J. A., Waters, B. G., Cousens, P., & Stevens, M. M. (1989). Neuropsychological sequelae of central nervous system prophylaxis in survivors of childhood acute lymphoblastic leukemia. *Journal of Consulting and Clinical Psychology*, *57*(2), 251–256.

Sather, H., Miller, D., Nesbit, M., Heyn, R., & Hammond, D. (1981). Differences in prognosis for boys and girls with acute lymphoblastic leukemia. *Lancet*, *i*, 739–744.

Schlieper, A. E., Esseltine, D. W., & Tarshis, M. A. (1989). Cognitive function in long survivors of childhood acute lymphoblastic leukemia. *Pediatric Hematology and Oncology*, *6*, 1–9.

Schriock, E. A., Schell, M. J., Carter, M., Hustu, O., & Ochs, J. J. (1991). Abnormal growth patterns and adult short stature in 115 long-term survivors of childhood leukemia. *Journal of Clinical Oncology*, *9*, 400–405.

Schuler, D., Bakos, M., Borsi, J., Gascaly, I., Kalmanchey, R., Kardos, G., Koos, R., Nagy, C., Revesz, T., Somlo, P., & Gebauer, E. (1990). Neuropsychologic and CT examinations in leukemic patients surviving 10 or more years. *Medical and Pediatric Oncology*, *18*, 123–125.

Schuler, D., Polcz, A., Revesz, T., Koos, R., Bakos, M., & Gal, N. (1981). Psychological effects of leukemia in children and their prevention. *Medical and Pediatric Oncology*, *9*, 191–194.

Simone, J. V., Aur, R. J. A., Hustu, H. O., Versoza, M. S., & Pinkel, P. (1978). Three to ten years after cessation of therapy in children with leukemia. *Cancer*, *42*, 839–844.

Skullerud, K., & Halvorsen, K. (1978). Encephalomyelopathy following intrathecal methotrexate treatment in a child with leukemia. *Cancer*, *42*, 1211–1214.

Soni, S. S., Marten, G. W., Pitner, S. E., Duenas, D. A., & Powazek, M. (1975). Effects of central nervous system irradiation on neuropsychologic functioning of children with acute lymphocytic leukemia. *New England Journal of Medicine*, *293*, 113–118.

Stehbens, J. A. (1983). A statistical quirk? Reply to Kellerman, Moss, and Siegel. *Journal of Pediatric Psychology*, *8*, 379–381.

Stehbens, J. A., Ford, M. E., Kisker, C. T., Clarke, W. R., & Strayer, F. (1981). WISC-R Verbal/Performance discrepancies in pediatric cancer patients. *Journal of Pediatric Psychology*, *6*(1), 61–68.

Stehbens, J. A., & Kisker, C. T. (1984). Intelligence and achievement testing in childhood cancer: Three years post diagnosis. *Journal of Developmental and Behavioral Pediatrics*, *5*(4), 184–188.

Stehbens, J. A., Kisker, C. T., & Wilson, B. K. (1983). Achievement and intelligence test–retest performance in pediatric cancer patients at diagnosis and one year later. *Journal of Pediatric Psychology*, *8*(1), 47–56.

Tamaroff, M., Miller, D. R., Murphy, M. L., Salwen, R., Ghavimi, F., & Nir, Y. (1982). Immediate and long-term post-therapy neuropsychologic performance in children with acute lymphoblastic leukemia treated without central nervous system radiation. *Journal of Pediatrics*, *101*, 524–529.

Tamaroff, M., Salwen, R., Miller, D. R., Murphy, M. L., & Nir, Y. (1984). Comparison of neuropsychologic performance in children treated for acute lymphoblastic leukemia (ALL) with 1800 rads cranial radiation plus intrathecal methotrexate or intrathecal methotrexate alone. *Proceedings of the American Society of Clinical Oncology*, *3*, 198. (Abstract C-773)

Taylor, H. G., Albo, V. C., Phebus, B. R., Sachs, B. R., & Bierl, P. G. (1987). Postirradiation treatment outcomes for children with acute lymphocytic leukemia: Clarification of risks. *Journal of Pediatric Psychology*, *12*, 395–411.

Trautman, P. D., Erickson, C., Shaffer, D., O'Connor, P. A., Sitarz, A., Correra, A., & Schonfeld, I. S. (1988). Prediction of intellectual deficits in children with acute lymphoblastic leukemia. *Developmental and Behavioral Pediatrics*, *9*(3), 122–128.

Tubergen, D. G., Gilchrist, G. S., Sather, H. N., Coccia, P., Novak, L., O'Brien, R., Waskerwitz, M., & Hammond, D. (1988). Intrathecal methotrexate provides adequate central nervous system therapy in acute lymphoblastic leukemia patients with intermediate risk factors and an age less than ten years. *Proceedings of the American Society of Clinical Oncology*, *7*, 688.

Versoza, M. S., Aur, R. J. A., Simone, J. V., Hustu, H. O., & Pinkel, D. P. (1976). Five years after central nervous system irradiation of children with leukemia. *International Journal of Radiation, Oncology, Biology, and Physiology*, *1*, 209–215.

Waber, D. P., Bernstein, J. H., Kammerer, B. L., Tarbell, N. J., & Sallan, S. E. (1992). Neuropsychological diagnostic profiles of children who received CNS treatment for acute lymphoblastic leukemia: The systemic approach to assessment. *Developmental Neuropsychology*, *8*(1), 1–28.

Waber, D. P., Gioia, G., Paccia, J., Sherman, B., Dinklage, D., Sollee, N., Urion, D. K., Tarbell, N. J., & Sallan, S. E. (1990). Sex differences in cognitive processing in children treated with CNS prophylaxis for acute lymphoblastic leukemia. *Journal of Pediatric Psychology*, *15*(1), 105–122.

Waber, D. P., Tarbell, N. J., Kahn, C. M., Gelber, R. D., & Sallan, S. E. (1992). The relationship of sex and treatment modality to neuropsychological outcome in childhood acute lymphoblastic leukemia. *Journal of Clinical Oncology*, *10*(5), 810–817.

Waber, D. P., Urion, D. K., Tarbell, N. J., Niemeyer, C., Gelber, R., & Sallan, S. E. (1990). Late effects of central nervous system treatment of acute lymphoblastic leukemia in childhood are sex-dependent. *Developmental Medicine and Child Neurology*, *32*, 238–248.

Waskerwitz, M. J., & Fergusson, J. H. (1986). Late effects of cancer treatment in children. In M. J. Hockenberry & D. K. Coody (Eds), *Pediatric oncology and hematology* (pp. 469–492). St Louis: C.V. Mosby.

Whitt, J. K., Wells, R. J., Lauria, M. M., Wilhem, C. I., & McMillan, C. W. (1984). Cranial radiation in childhood acute lymphocytic leukemia. *American Journal of Diseases of Children*, *138*, 730–736.

Williams, J. M., & Davis, K. S. (1986). Central nervous system prophylactic treatment for childhood leukemia: Neuro-psychological outcome studies. *Cancer Treatment Review*, *13*(2), 113–127.

Williams, J. M., Ochs, J., Davis, K. S., Daniel, M., Ragland, R., Mulhern, R. K., & Wasserman, A. (1986). The subacute effects of CNS prophylaxis for acute lymphoblastic leukemia on neuropsychological performance: A comparison of four protocols. *Archives of Clinical Neuropsychology*, *1*, 183–192.

12

Metachromatic Leukodystrophy

Catherine B. Dool
Katy B. Fuerst
Byron P. Rourke

Metachromatic leukodystrophy (MLD) is a genetic disorder caused by a deficiency of arylsulfatase A activity. This enzyme catalyzes the conversion of sulfatides to cerebrosides and sulfate. The deficiency of arylsulfatase A activity in patients with MLD leads to an accumulation of sulfatides in tissues in the body, including both the central nervous system (CNS) and the peripheral nervous system (PNS). This results in a progressive and ultimately fatal neurodegenerative disorder that involves diffuse symmetrical demyelination of the brain, spinal cord, and peripheral nerves (Brett & Lake, 1991).

CLINICAL MANIFESTATIONS OF MLD

MLD exhibits marked clinical heterogeneity, and is divided into different types according to the age at which symptoms develop. Four main types have been described: late infantile, early (or intermediate) juvenile, late juvenile, and adult MLD (Kolodny, 1989; MacFaul, Cavanagh, Lake, Stephens, & Whitfield, 1982). There is, however, some discrepancy in the terminology used and in the age ranges of the different types as defined by different researchers.

Late infantile MLD is the most common form of MLD, making up approximately 44–87% of published cases (Kolodny & Moser, 1982; MacFaul et al., 1982). It typically presents between 1 and 2 years of age. The first signs include an immature gait, delay or deterioration in walking, and strabismus. A progressive loss of motor, social, and linguistic skills is seen, and the disorder eventually leads to coma, generally by age

3. Death usually occurs within 4 years, with a range of 5 months to 8 years reported (MacFaul et al., 1982; Menkes, 1990).

Early juvenile MLD usually manifests itself at approximately 5 years of age in a previously normal child. Motor difficulties, evidenced by tripping and falling, are usually the first symptoms. They may occur alone or in combination with a deterioration in school performance as a result of concentration and memory difficulties and behavioral problems. Death occurs 3 to 17 years later (MacFaul et al., 1982).

Symptoms of late juvenile MLD are typically present by 8 years of age. In this form of the disorder, academic and behavioral problems are usually evident before the motor symptoms. The gait disorder may appear from 6 months to 4 years later, and death occurs from 5 to 11 years after onset (MacFaul et al., 1982).

Adult MLD includes those cases that manifest themselves after age 16, although it can occur later in life. Between one-fifth and one-quarter of all MLD cases are of the adult variety (Kolodny, 1989). When it occurs, it often presents initially as a dementia or as a psychiatric disorder, such as schizophrenia (Alves, Pires, Guimaraes, & Miranda, 1986; Baumann et al., 1991; Fisher, Cope, & Lishman, 1987; Hyde, Ziegler, & Weinberger, 1992; Waltz, Harik, & Kaufman, 1987). In adolescents and adults, some 53% of MLD patients will present with symptoms and/or a diagnosis of psychosis. Delusions, auditory hallucinations, and disorganized cognition are most common (Hyde et al., 1992). The presence of such behavioral disturbance may mask signs of cognitive deterioration (Baumann et al., 1991). Neurological symptoms tend to occur later (often many years later) in the disorder. Because of these factors, patients may be misdiagnosed with schizophrenia, bipolar disorder, Alzheimer disease, Pick disease, or cerebral syphilis (Waltz et al., 1987). Adult MLD tends to have a longer course than infantile or either type of juvenile MLD (Kolodny, 1989).

Approximately 2% of the general population have very low levels of arylsulfatase A activity, but remain asymptomatic (Herz & Bach, 1984). This is referred to as a "pseudodeficiency." It appears that in these cases, there are still sufficient levels of the arylsulfatase A enzyme to metabolize sulfatides normally. Therefore, such individuals remain clinically normal and do not store the excessive amounts of sulfatides that lead to demyelination (Polten et al., 1991; Wenger & Louie, 1991).

GENETICS

MLD is a genetic disorder with autosomal recessive inheritance. Thus, approximately equal numbers of males and females are affected; the parents of patients are carriers of the disorder and often have abnormal levels of arylsulfatase A; and a number of siblings in one family may be affected (Kolodny, 1989). When siblings are affected, the symptoms and time course of the disorder tend to be very similar (Kolodny, 1989), although some exceptions to this have been cited in the literature (Alves et al., 1986; Clarke, Skomorowski, & Chang, 1989). The similarity of clinical course in most siblings has led to the hypothesis that the different forms of MLD may be genetically distinct (Kolodny & Moser, 1982).

Recently, evidence has been generated in support of the hypothesis that genetic heterogeneity may indeed account for the different types of MLD. The gene for arylsulfatase A has been successfully cloned (Kreysing, von Figura, & Gieselmann, 1990), and some of the mutations that cause different types of MLD have been identified (Polten et al., 1991). It was found that all patients homozygous for one allele, labeled allele I, suffered from late infantile MLD. Homozygosity for the second allele, allele A, was associated with either the late juvenile or adult type of MLD. Heterozygosity for both alleles resulted in the intermediate juvenile type of MLD. Thus, the genotype was also associated with the age of onset. Patients homozygous for allele I showed symptoms before 2 years of age. One copy of allele A meant that the onset was delayed until 5.8 years, and homozygosity for allele A meant an average age of onset of 17.3 years. Furthermore, different levels of residual enzyme activity were associated with the different genotypes, with the late infantile form, the most severe type of MLD, demonstrating the lowest amount of residual enzyme activity (Polten et al., 1991). Other studies have failed to find differences in the level of enzyme activity among the different types of MLD (Kolodny, 1989; MacFaul et al., 1982).

INCIDENCE

The incidence of MLD is not known. It has been suggested that the incidence for all types of MLD may be between 1 per 40,000 (Menkes, 1990) and 1 per 130,000 births (Kolodny, 1989). Higher incidences have been reported in certain isolated communities or groups (Kolodny & Moser, 1982). Thus, although MLD is rare, it is one of the more common childhood neurodegenerative diseases (MacFaul et al., 1982). Some adult MLD cases have not been diagnosed until autopsy. It is likely that many other cases with late onset remain undiagnosed because of the presence of solely psychiatric symptoms early in the disorder (Hyde et al., 1992).

DIAGNOSIS

The association of central and peripheral neurological symptoms should raise the possibility of a leukodystrophy (Baumann et al., 1991). When a suspicion of MLD arises, based upon clinical symptoms or family history, the diagnosis can be confirmed through enzymatic assays. A severe reduction or absence of urinary or leukocyte arylsulfatase A activity suggests MLD. Tissue, such as the cells shed in urine, must then be examined for the storage of sulfatides to confirm the diagnosis. This is necessary because people with pseudodeficiency will also show low arylsulfatase A activity levels; however, because they still have sufficient levels of the enzyme to metabolize sulfatides normally, they do not show excessive storage and excretion of sulfatides (Wenger & Louie, 1991). More recently, it has become possible to examine DNA samples for the mutations responsible for MLD and pseudodeficiency (Li, Waye, & Chang, 1992; Polten et al., 1991; Wenger & Louie, 1991).

These laboratory tests have generally replaced the more invasive diagnostic procedures used in the past, such as biopsies of the sural nerve (a sensory nerve in the leg), the skin, or the brain. In MLD, these biopsied tissues will show evidence of metachromatic granules (Hyde et al., 1992; Kolodny & Moser, 1982; Menkes, 1990). The sulfatides in histological preparations form spherical granular masses that stain metachromatically (Kolodny & Moser, 1982)—hence the name of the disorder.

When a diagnosis of MLD is confirmed, the patient's siblings may also be examined for levels of arylsulfatase A activity to determine whether the disorder is present or whether they are carriers (also referred to as "heterozygotes"). Because MLD is an autosomal recessive disorder, the patient's parents will be carriers. MLD heterozygotes typically have reduced levels of arylsulfatase A activity, which fall between the values of patients and those of controls. Activity levels ranging between 19% and 62% of control values have been reported (Kohn, Manowitz, Miller, & Kling, 1988). However, there tends to be some overlap in enzyme values between normal individuals and carriers, and between carriers and those with MLD (Kolodny, 1989).

Prenatal diagnosis is possible by examining the activity of arylsulfatase A in cultured amniotic fluid cells (Wenger & Louie, 1991). Other laboratory tests that may help to confirm the diagnosis of MLD include magnetic resonance imaging (MRI) or computed tomography (CT) scans, nerve conduction studies, electroencephalograms (EEGs), and examination of other organs such as the gallbladder. Typical findings in these studies are reported below.

Neuroimaging

CNS abnormalities are almost invariably found on CT scan or MRI. CT scans typically show diffuse bilateral symmetrical decrease of white matter attenuation in the frontal, parietal, and occipital regions adjacent to the cerebral ventricles. This decreased attenuation of white matter is attributed to loss of myelin and increased water content in structures in those areas of increased sulfatide deposits (Buonnano, Ball, Laster, Moody, & Mclean, 1978; Jayakumar, Aroor, Jha, & Arya, 1989). White matter involvement of the temporal lobes and cerebellum is less commonly seen (Jayakumar et al., 1989).

MRI scans may prove especially useful in studying MLD, because of the high contrast that MRI provides between grey and white matter. It is the most sensitive imaging technique for demonstrating white matter involvement. However, to date, there are only a few reports of MRI findings in individual patients with MLD (Baumann et al., 1991; Klemm & Conzelmann, 1989; Reider-Grosswasser & Bornstein, 1987; Waltz et al., 1987).

MRIs show evidence of demyelination in the same regions in which hypodensities are seen on CT scan, and the white matter abnormalities are sometimes described as more marked on MRI (Klemm & Conzelmann, 1989; Waltz et al., 1987). In one case, whereas the CT scan demonstrated hypodensities in the white matter adjacent to the frontal horns, the MRI revealed more diffuse involvement, with bilateral demyelination throughout the white matter adjacent to the cerebral ventricles (Reider-Grosswasser & Bornstein, 1987). MRI of nine recently reported cases demonstrated widespread demyelination, with anterior regions being most severely involved (Shapiro, Lockman, Knopman, & Krivit, 1994).

Some differences in the results of neuroimaging studies have been found among the various types of MLD. CT abnormalities tend to be evident at an early stage in infantile and juvenile forms of MLD (Buonnano et al., 1978). However, this is not always the case in adult MLD. Some adults may demonstrate less diffuse white matter involvement than is seen with earlier-onset cases, with symmetrical bifrontal or biparietal hypodensities of white matter (Finelli, 1985; Reider-Grosswasser & Bornstein, 1987; Skomer, Stears, & Austin, 1983). In some cases of juvenile MLD, the frontal lobes are reportedly slightly more affected by the demyelination process. It has been suggested that this may be because of the relatively late myelination of the frontal lobes. Those areas of the brain in which myelination occurs early may remain relatively spared from sulfatide accumulation and subsequent demyelination (Schipper & Seidel, 1984). However, as previously mentioned, MRI scans may be necessary to accurately determine the extent of white matter involvement. Ventricular enlargement and cortical atrophy are often seen in adult MLD (Kolodny & Moser, 1982; Waltz et al., 1987), but are minimal or absent in late infantile MLD (Jayakumar et al., 1989; Kolodny & Moser, 1982). Brain stem atrophy is a common finding in late infantile MLD (Jayakumar et al., 1989; Reider-Grosswasser & Bornstein, 1987).

Findings on neuroimaging have not been found to correlate highly with the length of the illness (Boltshauser, Spiess, & Isler, 1978; Jayakumar et al., 1989) or with the clinical severity of the disorder (Dietrich, Vining, Taira, Hall, & Phillipart, 1990).

The diffuse, symmetrical white matter involvement evident on neuroimaging is useful in differentiating MLD from other demyelinating diseases, such as multiple sclerosis, adrenoleukodystrophy, and Schilder disease. In these disorders, asymmetrical, *focal* areas of white matter involvement are more likely than the *diffuse*, symmetrical white matter involvement in MLD (Buonanno et al., 1978; Jayakumar et al., 1989). Neuroimaging may also be helpful in adult cases that present with psychotic symptoms. Although cortical atrophy and ventricular enlargement have been described in schizophrenia, periventricular white matter abnormalities have not been reported and should help to differentiate these disorders (Manowitz, Kling, & Kohn, 1978; Waltz et al., 1987).

Electromyography

Because of the involvement of the PNS in MLD, nerve conduction studies are frequently utilized. Typically, slowed conduction velocities of motor and sensory nerves are found (Baumann et al., 1991; Kolodny & Moser, 1982). Impaired nerve conduction may sometimes be evident before clinical symptoms develop (Clark, Miller, & Vidgoff, 1979). However, in some cases, normal nerve conduction may also be found (MacFaul et al., 1982).

Electroencephalography

Often the EEG is found to be normal in MLD (Jayakumar et al., 1989), especially early in the course of the disease (Blom & Hagberg, 1967; Kolodny & Moser, 1982). As it progresses, diffuse slow-wave activity is seen. In some cases, this slow-wave activity is asymmetrical, and there may be evidence of isolated spikes in both hemispheres. Generalized slow-wave activity is a nonspecific finding, being seen in degenerative, metabolic, or toxic disorders. However, it is indicative of diffuse cerebral dysfunction (Blom & Hagberg, 1967). Seizures, when they occur, tend to be seen only very late in the disorder. This is not surprising, given the general absence of grey matter involvement in early-onset forms (MacFaul et al., 1982).

Cerebrospinal Fluid

In late infantile and early juvenile MLD, cerebrospinal fluid (CSF) protein is typically elevated in the chronic stage of the disease. This protein elevation is not always found in late juvenile or adult MLD (Baumann et al., 1991; Kolodny & Moser, 1982).

Other Organs

Sulfatides accumulate in a number of organs other than the brain. These include the gallbladder, which often shows increasingly abnormal functioning, and the liver and kidneys, which tend to show little impairment despite the evidence of deposits of metachromatic granules. Deposits may also be found in the pancreas, pituitary gland, adrenal cortex, retina, and testes (Kolodny & Moser, 1982).

PATHOLOGY

The pathological processes in MLD consist of the accumulation of metachromatic deposits and demyelination. The demyelination of the CNS and PNS is thought to be caused by this accumulation of sulfatides in the oligodendrocytes and Schwann cells, respectively. These are the cells responsible for the maintenance of myelin. However, the mechanism by which the sulfatide deposits lead to demyelination has been debated. Most evidence supports the view that the accumulation of sulfatide results in the metabolic failure of these cells, and that this in turn triggers demyelination (Kolodny & Moser, 1982; Menkes, 1990).

Arylsulfatase A is the enzyme responsible for catalyzing the conversion of sulfatide to cerebrosides and sulfate. Thus, a deficiency in arylsulfatase A activity in MLD leads to an accumulation of sulfatides in cells that normally synthesize them. The metachromatic granules characteristic of MLD are simply lysosomes that are storing the excess sulfatides. Sulfatides, the sulfate esters of cerebroside, are membrane lipids that are important components of cell membranes, the membranes of organelles within the cell, and the myelin sheath. Sulfatide is most prominent in myelin; its presence elsewhere in the body, such as in other organs, is relatively limited. Thus, the anomaly inherent to MLD has the most devastating effect on nervous system tissues. If sulfatides cannot be broken down, they cannot be converted to cerebrosides, resulting in a decreasing amount of cerebroside in the myelin sheath. This produces an increase in the extracellular negative charge, resulting in physiochemical instability of the myelin sheath (Valk & van der Knaap, 1989).

On examination, the brain shows evidence of a reduction in the amount of central white matter. There is moderate to severe loss of myelin, with reactive gliosis found in areas of demyelination. Some fibers tend to be less involved, including the arcuate fibers, optic radiations, and myelin fibers within the central grey nuclei. An accumulation of metachromatic granules may be found in a variety of structures, including within oligodendrocytes, in the neurons of some cerebellar and brain stem nuclei, and in the grey matter of spinal ganglia. The neurons of the cerebral cortex are usually not involved in late infantile MLD, but more grey matter sulfatide deposits are seen in adult MLD (Kolodny & Moser, 1982). These deposits may be especially common in the frontal lobes (Seidel, Goebel, & Scholz, 1981). The cerebellum typically shows atrophy, with a severe reduction in Purkinje and granule cells, demyelination, gliosis, and marked accumulation of granules (Kolodny & Moser, 1982).

Demyelination is also evident in segmental regions of the peripheral nervous system, with metachromatic granules collecting in the Schwann cells, in endoneural macrophages, and between nerve fibers. The actual number of myelinated fibers may be reduced (Kolodny & Moser, 1982).

TREATMENT

Until recently, there were no effective treatments for MLD. Diet therapy to reduce sulfatide synthesis has been tried unsuccessfully. Drug and enzyme replacement therapies have also failed to produce positive outcomes (Kolodny, 1989).

In the last few years, bone marrow transplantation (BMT) has been used to treat MLD and other lysosomal disorders. This was thought to be a promising treatment because a source of lysosomal enzymes is the bone marrow. However, it was uncertain whether the leukocytes from the bone marrow could pass the blood–brain barrier, penetrate into needed areas of the CNS, and then supply the missing enzyme (Bayever et al., 1985). Four transplants have been reported. Two children with infantile MLD died shortly after transplant (Kolodny, 1989). Preliminary reports of the other two cases suggest that BMT may be beneficial in at least partially halting the progression of this disorder.

Bayever et al. (1985) report the case of an 11-month-old boy with late infantile MLD who received a BMT. Improvement in enzyme activity was immediately evident. Six months after BMT there were leukocytes of bone marrow origin in the patient's CSF, suggesting that penetration of the CNS was possible. The child's development in the 28 months following transplant showed an apparent lack of progression of the disorder in several areas. He acquired developmental milestones in adaptive, social, fine motor, and language skills, but at a slower-than-normal rate. He did not show progress in gross motor skills, perhaps because of continued deterioration in peripheral nerve function. This course contrasts markedly with that of his two siblings with MLD, who at the patient's age were totally incapacitated. It has been repeatedly suggested that the clinical course for siblings tends to be very similar (Kolodny & Moser, 1982). Therefore, this patient's clinical course, in comparison to that of his siblings, suggests that BMT was successful in halting deterioration to some degree in all but his motor skills.

Another patient who underwent a BMT at 4½ years of age has been reported on extensively in the literature (Krivit et al., 1990; Lipton et al., 1986; Shapiro, Lipton, & Krivit, 1992). The patient had an older sister who was diagnosed with MLD at the age of 4 years, was quadriparetic and unable to speak by age 5, and died at age 8. The patient was diagnosed at 8 months of age and showed fairly normal development until age 4, except for mild, slowly progressive motor problems first evident at 17 months of age. By 4½ years of age she showed evidence of hypotonia, hyperreflexia, toe walking, and a mild intention tremor. At age 4 years, 9 months, she received a BMT from a younger unaffected sister. At the time of the most recent report she was 10 years, 9 months of age, and had been followed at regular intervals for some 6 years after transplant.

Following BMT, this patient's arylsulfatase A levels increased from very low levels to normal levels and remained within the normal range over the next 5 years. Although her MRI continued to be abnormal, it showed no evidence of deterioration, and in fact was thought to show some slight improvement. However, there was evidence of continued slow motor deterioration following BMT. At the age of 10 the child required a walker, as well as a keyboard for writing activities. Deterioration was also seen in cognitive abilities over a 3-year period following BMT, but then stabilization occurred. (Her cognitive abilities are discussed in more detail in the next section.) Again, this course was markedly better than that of her affected sibling.

Thus, initial studies have suggested that BMT may be able to halt to some extent the progression of cognitive deficits in this disorder. However, there is little evidence that this procedure is effective in reversing damage that already exists. It is possible that the macrophages are not able to remove previously stored sulfatide (Bayever et al., 1985). Also, as was especially evident in the second case reported above, a period of deterioration of function may occur after transplant. This may reflect a delay in the enzyme reaching the brain and in cell replacement occurring (Shapiro et al., 1992). As the researchers suggest, this makes the timing of transplantation crucial, so that the disease does not progress to the point of severe mental retardation before the enzyme can halt the deterioration. In both cases cited, motor skills showed continued deterioration, raising the possibility that macrophages may be unable to invade the peripheral nerves (Bayever et al., 1985). Given the generally bleak course of MLD, these preliminary attempts at treating the disorder with BMT appear to be promising.

NEUROPSYCHOLOGICAL FINDINGS IN LATE INFANTILE MLD TREATED WITH BMT

There have been few investigations of the cognitive functioning of children with MLD, probably because of the typical course of rapid decline to coma and death. The only detailed neuropsychological study to date has been a report on the second case described above, a child with late infantile MLD who was treated with BMT (Shapiro et al., 1992).

Before BMT, this child's verbal skills were in the high-average range, with a Wechsler Preschool and Primary Scale of Intelligence (WPPSI) Verbal IQ of 116. Her Verbal IQ dropped to 105 1 year after BMT, to 97 at 2 years after BMT, and to 82 at 3 years after BMT, and remained stable thereafter. She did, however, show increases in raw score points on each of the subtests, suggesting that new verbal learning was occurring, but at a decreased rate compared to that of her peers. Performance on a selective reminding test suggested significant difficulty in acquiring new verbal material.

Prior to BMT, the girl's WPPSI Performance IQ was significantly lower than her Verbal IQ. One year after BMT, her Performance PIQ dropped from a score of 95 to 74. This loss was mainly attributable to poorer performance on two subtests with a motor component (Animal House and Geometric Design). Her slowly progressive motor impairments prevented her from completing the Performance subtests at subsequent assessments.

The Kaufman Assessment Battery for Children (K-ABC) was administered several times, beginning approximately 2 years after BMT. Scores on this test were stable, with the Sequential Processing score (high-average range) consistently higher than the Simultaneous Processing score (borderline range). Marked deficits were seen on a spatial memory task and a visual–spatial task similar to Block Design. Immediate recall of sequences of number, words, and hand movements was average to high-average.

The patient learned to read following the BMT. Word decoding and reading comprehension remained stable and in the low-average to average range. Word attack skills were significantly better than was passage comprehension. Arithmetic skills were less well developed than reading skills and were generally in the borderline range.

Nonverbal reasoning skills, as measured by the Raven Colored Progressive Matrices and the Matrix Analogy subtest of the K-ABC, were in the low-average range. The patient had difficulty in word retrieval and expressive vocabulary, but from ages 7 to 10 years of age she showed significant improvement, going from significantly below-average to average levels. She demonstrated slower-than-normal processing speeds.

The child was able to perform normally on a test involving the recognition of simple emotions depicted on faces. She performed more poorly on speeded matching tasks that involved the determination of whether tachistoscopically presented faces were the same or different in terms of affect and identity. Thus, as the speed and visual processing demands of the tasks increased, difficulties were more evident.

School reports suggested that the patient had excellent relationships with her peers. She was in a regular classroom, with withdrawal for her physical and learning problems. This impression of normal socioemotional functioning was also indicated on the Personality Inventory for Children (PIC), completed by the parents when the patient was 10 years of age. There were elevations on the Intellectual Screening and Development scales, but all of the other clinical scales were in the normal range. During the assessment, the child was noted to have normal affect and prosody, with somewhat immature behavior.

There are few childhood disorders that present almost exclusively with white matter involvement. As Shapiro et al. (1992) suggest, this case provides a unique opportunity to examine the effect of documented white matter involvement on cognitive abilities, and in particular to determine whether the pattern of strengths and deficits demonstrated in the Nonverbal Learning Disabilities (NLD) syndrome is present in this case. The following section presents a comparison of this case to the NLD syndrome (Rourke, 1989).

COMPARISON TO THE NLD SYNDROME

Sensory and Perceptual Abilities

As in the NLD syndrome, the child with MLD described above was noted to have difficulty with complex and speeded visual processing. Scores on tasks involving the processing of more simple visual information (e.g., gestalt closure, recognition of facial expressions) were within the low-average to average range. Tactile and auditory processing skills were not reported. Given her generally well-developed language skills, intact auditory processing skills might be inferred.

Motor and Psychomotor Skills

Because of the involvement of the PNS in MLD, motor skills were not assessed in this case, and thus meaningful comparisons to the NLD syndrome cannot be made.

Attention and Memory

This child demonstrated good verbal attention skills, with above-average ability to immediately recall a sequence of digits and words. Her immediate recall of spatial location was very poor. She also showed good recall of a series of hand movements. Although this information was presented through the visual mode, it might be argued that it is readily encoded verbally (e.g., "fist, then palm"), whereas random spatial locations are not easily encoded in this manner. Thus, the child demonstrated the same pattern of attentional skills as is usually seen in the NLD syndrome. Her memory for words on a selective reminding test was very poor. It is not known how she would perform on a less novel verbal memory task, such as repeating naturally spoken language (e.g., sentences of increasing length). Typically, such a task is performed very well in cases of the NLD syndrome.

Visual–Spatial Skills

As in the NLD syndrome, this child had impaired visual–spatial skills, except for a picture arrangement task (K-ABC photo series) that involves some verbal mediation.

Problem Solving and Reasoning

Nonverbal reasoning abilities for this patient were in the low-average to average range, and thus did not show the marked impairment that is usually evident in the NLD syndrome. She was also noted to have a good sense of humor—an area of deficiency in children with the NLD syndrome.

Verbal and Language Skills

On the initial assessments, the child's verbal skills were noted to be well developed in comparison to her nonverbal skills. Deterioration in verbal skills was seen in the 4 years following BMT, but these skills remained relatively better than her visual-perceptual and visual–spatial skills. In terms of speech and language skills, this patient did not show the repetitive, rote, verbose speech that has been described in the NLD syndrome. Nor was she lacking in appropriate affect, prosody, or understanding of speech pragmatics. Her difficulty with word retrieval and expressive vocabulary, evident until about the age of 9, also has not been described in NLD.

Academic Achievement

The child's performance on academic tasks showed a profile similar to that seen in the NLD syndrome. Reading was in the normal range, with passage comprehension significantly poorer than word attack skills. Her word attack or phonemic abilities were not exceptionally well developed, as is seen in the NLD syndrome. Arithmetic skills were poor relative to her reading skills—a hallmark of NLD.

Psychosocial and Adaptive Skills

Children with the NLD syndrome have been noted to lack social competence and interpersonal skills. In later childhood, they may be susceptible to internalized forms of psychopathology, including anxiety, depression, and social withdrawal. These difficulties were clearly not evident in this child. She was reported to have good relationships with her peers, and showed no evidence of socioemotional disturbance on the PIC. Her behavior during the assessment was described as "immature," however.

Summary

In summary, this child would appear to show evidence of a partial NLD syndrome (Shapiro et al., 1992). Although visual-perceptual, visual–spatial, academic, attention, and memory skills were in keeping with the profile seen in NLD, socioemotional functioning, speech and language, and nonverbal reasoning skills did not show the same pattern.

According to Rourke's (1989) NLD model, intact white matter is necessary for the development of left-hemisphere functions, but not for the maintenance of such functions. This child did not show significant clinical evidence of demyelination until the age of 4 years. Although it is not possible to assume that myelin development was entirely normal prior to that point, most of her symptoms were limited to minor motor problems, and she certainly showed well-developed verbal skills. Following evidence of extensive demyelination, her verbal skills remained fairly well developed, albeit not at her previous level. Interestingly, she was also able to learn to read after significant demyelination had occurred.

The NLD model also holds that intact white matter is necessary for the development and maintenance of right-hemisphere functions. The right hemisphere is said to be geared toward intermodal integration, and thus necessary for dealing with novel information-processing demands for which the person has no pre-existing code. This would include such dimensions as nonverbal problem solving, adapting to new social situations, mathematical reasoning and most visual–spatial skills. Thus, even given fairly normal early development, the occurrence of a significant white matter disorder would be expected to disrupt these skills. Because of the inability to generate new descriptive systems, these deficits tend to become more noticeable with age.

In this case, relative impairment was seen in visual–spatial and arithmetic skills. The child did not, however, show impairments in nonverbal problem solving and social interaction skills, and did not fall back on the use of stereotyped and thus inappropriate language in such situations, as would be predicted. However, she was noted to be somewhat immature in her behavior and to be functioning in a fairly protective environment. Shapiro et al. (1992) hypothesize that perhaps white matter integrity is needed for the development but not the maintenance of social skills, as was the case with language. This child had very well-developed social skills by age 4, and these would appear to have been maintained. As the authors suggest, it will be interesting to see whether this child continues to show good psychosocial skills as she faces novel social developmental tasks with puberty.

NEUROPSYCHOLOGICAL FINDINGS IN JUVENILE AND ADULT MLD

Manowitz et al. (1978) reported the case of a brother and sister with MLD who first presented with evidence of impaired visual–spatial skills and nonverbal reasoning abilities relative to language skills. When each of the siblings was in the eighth grade, and before any other signs of MLD were present, testing on the Differential Aptitude Test revealed language skills at or above the 60th centile for the female, and at or above the 75th centile for her brother. These skills were evident on tests of verbal reasoning, spelling, language usage, and clerical speed and accuracy. Performance on tests of visual–spatial relations and abstract reasoning (nonverbal reasoning involving the ability to ascertain relationships among objects, patterns, and designs) was at or below the 35th centile for both siblings. The sister also performed relatively poorly on mechanical reasoning (10th centile) and numerical reasoning (30th centile), while her brother performed somewhat better on these tests (50th and 65th centiles, respectively). It is not known whether this same pattern of relative strengths and weaknesses was present at an earlier age.

This pattern of cognitive abilities was evident 3 and 5 years before psychiatric symptoms first became apparent, and 5 and 18 years before gross neurological symptoms were seen in the sister and brother, respectively.

At the same time as psychiatric symptoms (anxiety, depression, and schizoid behavior) first became evident in the sister, marked deterioration in IQ was seen, with the Performance IQ significantly lower than the Verbal IQ. At the time of diagnosis, the brother had a neuropsychological assessment that included the Halstead–Reitan battery. He initially showed impairment on all tests except for the Speech-Sounds Perception Test and the Aphasia Screening Test. Performance on the Category Test, a measure of nonverbal reasoning, was impaired, with the most difficulty noted on a subtest that required visual–spatial solution. When the brother was reassessed 1½ years later, he showed impaired word fluency and bilateral finger agnosia, in addition to the deficits previously described.

Thus, deficits in visual–spatial relations, nonverbal reasoning, and (at least in one instance) arithmetic skills, in conjunction with preserved language skills, were seen as early indicators of adult MLD. Although a more complete assessment would be needed, these early impairments are also in keeping with a diagnosis of NLD. As the disease progressed in both siblings, cognitive deficits became more widespread, affecting language skills as well.

Several other studies report IQ scores for patients with juvenile or adult MLD. The typical pattern shows a decline in both Verbal and Performance IQs, with markedly lower scores on the Performance subtests (Clarke et al., 1989; Fisher et al., 1987; Manowitz et al., 1978). More detailed assessments of cognitive skills early in the course of the disease would permit a better understanding of the possible differential effect this disorder has on various skills. However, as was previously mentioned, grey matter involvement is frequently seen in MLD cases with later onset. Therefore, compared to cases of childhood MLD, these cases may not provide a particularly good test of the influence of white matter involvement on cognitive abilities.

More recently, Shapiro et al. (1994) have reported the neuropsychological findings for a group of nine patients, including three cases of early juvenile MLD, four cases of late juvenile MLD, and two cases of adult MLD. Although the authors did not present the numerical data, they have described interesting results. Five of the nine patients obtained Wechsler Verbal IQ scores that were greater than their Performance IQ scores by at least 10 points. Arithmetic achievement scores were lower than expected in four of the nine patients, whereas reading skills were normal in seven out of eight patients. Although unimpaired scores on several measures of vocabulary, as well as repetition of sentences and digits, indicated that language skills were intact, the patients obtained severely impaired scores on measures of visual perception and nonverbal reasoning. All patients were impaired on measures of encoding and delayed recall, and visual short-term memory was poor. In addition, all patients demonstrated severe deficits on several variables of a continuous performance attention task. Although verbal fluency scores were normal, all other measures of executive function were impaired. Scores on measures of motor function ranged from low-average to more than four standard deviations below the mean.

In regard to socioemotional functioning, Shapiro et al. (1994) reported that most of their nine subjects demonstrated disinhibition, poor judgment, and socially inappropriate behavior. Although the five oldest patients demonstrated behavior difficulties, none of the patients had manifested affective or psychotic disorders. In addition to their nine cases, Shapiro et al. (1994) analyzed 11 cases from the recent literature and found a high frequency of attentional difficulties, hyperactivity, impulsivity, poor judgment, and emotional lability. Social withdrawal and aggressive behavior were less common; depressed mood, sleeplessness, paranoid behavior, and hallucinations were rare. However, all patients were receiving psychiatric treatment before they were diagnosed as having MLD. Many had also been identified as learning-disabled. MRI findings demonstrated diffuse demyelination, with frontal regions being more severely affected.

Shapiro et al. (1994) concluded that the cognitive–behavioral profile of patients with MLD is in accordance with both white matter disease, as outlined by Rourke (1987), and frontal lobe dysfunction. Neuropsychological deficits consistent with white matter disease or dysfunction in Shapiro et al.'s patients included impaired spatial perception, relative preservation of verbal versus nonverbal skills, and impaired arithmetic skills in the context of comparatively intact reading skills. Behaviorally, these patients with MLD tended toward disinhibition, impulsivity, poor judgment, and social inappropriateness, all of which are characteristics of the NLD syndrome.

NEUROPSYCHOLOGICAL PROFILES OF MLD CARRIERS

Two studies have suggested that the lower arylsulfatase A levels found in MLD carriers may be associated with neuropsychological deficits, especially with deficits on visual–spatial tasks. Preliminary support for this comes from a study that examined enzyme activity and performance on cognitive measures in heterozygotes for various lipisodes (Christomanou, Martinius, Jaffe, Betke, & Forster, 1980). This study included seven members of one family who were carriers of MLD. Control subjects consisted of unaffected family members.

The MLD carriers scored below control subjects on an abbreviated Wechsler IQ test, consisting of the Comprehension, Similarities, Picture Completion, and Block Design subtests. Estimated Full Scale IQ values were 100 and 115 for the MLD carriers and controls, respectively. The MLD carriers made more errors on the Benton Visual Reproduction task, and score differences on the Wechsler Block Design subtest just failed to reach statistical significance. The heterozygotes also performed significantly more slowly on a visual reaction time task. Those with very low arylsulfatase A activity performed more slowly than did the other carriers. Thus, there was some suggestion that visual–spatial–organizational skills, including those with a speed component, may be especially vulnerable to low levels of arylsulfatase A activity.

Further support for this notion comes from a study in which a group of MLD heterozygotes received neuropsychological, neurological, and EEG examinations. Their performance was compared to that of a control group of heterozygotes for Tay–Sachs disease (Kohn et al., 1988). The MLD heterozygotes performed significantly more poorly on neuropsychological tests with a visual–spatial component than did the Tay–Sachs heterozygotes. The visual–spatial tasks utilized included the Kohs Blocks Test, the Benton–Spreen Embedded Figures and Stereognosis Tests, the Trail Making Test, the Category Test, the Tactual Performance Test, and the Halstead Sensory Perceptual exam. Unfortunately, scores on individual tests were not reported. However, 8 of the 10 MLD heterozygotes scored in the impaired range on at least one of the tests, and 7 of these subjects showed deficits on two or more spatial tests. Three out of 10 Tay–Sachs carriers were impaired on at least one visual–spatial task. The two groups did not differ on a series of tests with a language component. No abnormalities on neurological exam or EEG were found.

Kohn et al. (1988) hypothesized that below-normal arylsulfatase A activity results in a buildup of sulfatides, and that this in turn leads to partial demyelination in the CNS. Language skills, being overlearned, may be less susceptible to this disruption. Although this is an interesting hypothesis, the presence of white matter involvement in carriers of MLD has yet to be established, and carriers do not go on to develop clinical symptoms of the disease. However, the possible influence of different levels of enzyme activity on cognitive skills remains an area deserving of more thorough investigation.

CONCLUSION

An overview of MLD, a devastating progressive neurodegenerative disorder, has been presented in this chapter. Until recently, few detailed studies of neuropsychological functioning in MLD had been conducted. Preliminary studies of cognitive functioning in juvenile and adult MLD and in MLD carriers have been presented, and the results are consistent with the NLD syndrome. The results suggest that at least early in the course of juvenile and adult MLD, there is evidence of impaired visual–spatial, nonverbal reasoning, and arithmetic skills, with preserved language. The results of a recent study of nine MLD patients supported these findings, and also found that the psychosocial and behavioral characteristics of these patients were very much like those seen in the NLD syndrome.

Similarly, there is some suggestion that visual–spatial–organizational skills may be disrupted in MLD carriers.

A more detailed longitudinal study of a child with late infantile MLD, treated with BMT, has also been described (Krivit et al., 1990; Lipton et al., 1986; Shapiro et al., 1992). This child demonstrated many, but not all, aspects of the NLD syndrome. These included impaired visual-perceptual and visual–spatial skills compared to rote verbal skills; poor arithmetic skills; relatively better word decoding than reading comprehension; and better verbal than visual attentional and memory skills. However, the marked deficits in socioemotional functioning, impaired nonverbal reasoning skills, and the stereotyped language that are so characteristic of children with NLD were not evident in this case. The relationship of this case to the Rourke (1989) white matter model has been examined. Given the extent of white matter involvement in this disease, similar detailed neuropsychological studies of children with MLD should further our knowledge of the NLD syndrome and the white matter hypothesis.

REFERENCES

Alves, D., Pires, M. M., Guimaraes, A., & Miranda, M. C. (1986). Four cases of late onset metachromatic leukodystrophy manifesting as a schizophrenic disorder: Computer tomographic correlation. *Journal of Neurology, Neurosurgery and Psychiatry, 49*, 1417–1422.

Baumann, N., Masson, M., Carreau, V., Lefevre, M., Herschkowitz, N., & Turpin, J. C. (1991). Adult forms of metachromatic leukodystrophy: Clinical and biochemical approach. *Developmental Neuroscience, 13*, 211–215.

Bayever, E., Ladisch, S., Philippart, M., Brill, N., Nuwer, M., Sparkes, R. S., & Feig, S. A. (1985). Bone-marrow transplantation for metachromatic leucodystrophy. *Lancet, ii*, 471–473.

Blom, S., & Hagberg, B. (1967). EEG findings in late infantile metachromatic and globoid cell leucodystrophy. *Electroencephalography and Clinical Neurophysiology, 22*, 253–259.

Boltshauser, E., Spiess, H., & Isler, W. (1978). Computed tomography in neurodegenerative disorders in childhood. *Neuroradiology, 16*, 838–842.

Brett, E. M., & Lake, B. D. (1991). Progressive metabolic brain diseases. In E. M. Brett (Ed.), *Pediatric neurology* (2nd ed., pp. 141–200). New York: Churchill Livingstone.

Buonanno, F. S., Ball, M. R., Laster, W., Moody, D. M., & Mclean, W. T. (1978). Computed tomography in late-infantile metachromatic leukodystrophy. *Annals of Neurology, 4*, 43–46.

Christomanou, H., Martinius, J., Jaffe, S., Betke, K., & Forster, C. (1980). Biochemical, psychometric, and neuropsychological studies in heterozygotes for various lipidoses. *Human Genetics, 55*, 103–110.

Clark, J. R., Miller, R. G., & Vidgoff, J. M. (1979). Juvenile-onset metachromatic leukodystrophy: Biochemical and electrophysiologic studies. *Neurology, 29*, 346–353.

Clarke, J. T. R., Skomorowski, M. A., & Chang, P. L. (1989). Marked clinical difference between two sibs affected with juvenile metachromatic leukodystrophy. *American Journal of Medical Genetics, 33*, 10–13.

Dietrich, R. B., Vining, E. P., Taira, R. K., Hall, R. R., & Phillipart, M. (1990). Myelin disorders of childhood: Correlation of MR findings and severity of neurological impairment. *Journal of Computer Assisted Tomography, 14*, 693–698.

Finelli, P. F. (1985). Metachromatic leukodystrophy manifesting as a schizophrenic disorder: Computer tomographic correlation. *Annals of Neurology, 18*, 94–95.

Fisher, N. R., Cope, S. J., & Lishman, W. A. (1987). Metachromatic leukodystrophy: Conduct disorder progressing to dementia. *Journal of Neurology, Neurosurgery and Psychiatry, 50*, 488–510.

Herz, B., & Bach G. (1984). Arylsulfatase A in pseudodeficiency. *Human Genetics, 66*, 147–150.

Hyde, T. M., Ziegler, J. C. & Weinberger, D. R. (1992). Psychiatric disturbances in metachromatic leukodystrophy: Insights into the neurobiology of psychosis. *Archives of Neurology, 49*, 401–406.

Jayakumar, P. N., Aroor, S. R., Jha, R. K., & Arya, B. Y. T. (1989). Computed tomography (CT) in late infantile metachromatic leucodystrophy. *Acta Neurologica Scandinavica, 79*, 23–26.

Klemm, E., & Conzelmann, E. (1989). Adult-onset metachromatic leukodystrophy presenting without psychiatric symptoms. *Journal of Neurology, 236*, 427–429.

Kohn, H., Manowitz, P., Miller, M., & Kling, A. (1988). Neuropsychological deficits in obligatory heterozygotes for metachromatic leukodystrophy. *Human Genetics, 79*, 8–12.

Kolodny, E. H. (1989). Metachromatic leukodystrophy and multiple sulfatase deficiency: Sulfatide lipidosis. In C. R. Scriver, A. L. Beaudet, W. S. Sly, & D. Valle (Eds.), *The metabolic basis of inherited disease* (6th ed., Vol. 2, pp. 1721–1750). New York: McGraw-Hill.

Kolodny, E. H., & Moser, H. W. (1982). Sulfatide lipidosis: Metachromatic leukodystrophy. In J. B. Stanbury, J. B. Wyngarden, D. S. Fredrickson, J. L. Goldstein, & M. S. Brown (Eds.), *The metabolic basis of inherited disease* (5th ed., pp. 881–905). New York: McGraw-Hill.

Kreysing, J., von Figura, K., & Gieselmann V. (1990). The structure of the arylsulfatase A gene. *European Journal of Biochemistry, 191*, 627–631.

Krivit, W., Shapiro, E., Kennedy, W., Lipton, M., Lockman, L., Smith, S., Summers, C. G., Wenger, D. A., Tsai, M. Y., Ramsy, N. K. C., Kersey, J. H., Yao, J. K., & Kaye, E. (1990). Treatment of late infantile metachromatic leukodystrophy by bone marrow transplantation. *New England Journal of Medicine, 322*, 28–32.

Li, Z. G., Waye, J. S., & Chang, P. L. (1992). Diagnosis of arylsulfatase A deficiency. *American Journal of Medical Genetics, 43*, 976–982.

Lipton, M., Lockman, L. A., Ramsay, N .K. C., Kersey, J. H., Jacobson, R. I., & Krivit, W. (1986). Bone marrow transplantation in metachromatic leukodystrophy. *Birth Defects, 22*, 57–68.

MacFaul, R., Cavanagh, N., Lake, B. D., Stephens, R., & Whitfield, A. E. (1982). Metachromatic leucodystrophy: Review of 38 cases. *Archives of Diseases in Childhood, 57*, 168–175.

Manowitz, P., Kling, A., & Kohn, H. (1978). Clinical course of adult metachromatic leukodystrophy presenting as schizophrenia. *Journal of Nervous and Mental Disease, 166*, 500–506.

Menkes, J. H. (1990). *Textbook of child neurology* (4th ed.). Philadelphia: Lea & Febiger.

Polten, A., Fluharty, A. L., Fluharty, C. B., Kappler, J., von Figura, K., & Gieselmann, V. (1991). Molecular basis of different forms of metachromatic leukodystrophy. *New England Journal of Medicine, 324*, 18–22.

Reider-Grosswasser, I., & Bornstein, N. (1987). CT and MRI in late-onset metachromatic leukodystrophy. *Acta Neurologica Scandinavica, 75*, 64–69.

Rourke, B. P. (1987). Syndrome of nonverbal learning disabilities: The final common pathway of white-matter disease/dysfunction. *The Clinical Neuropsychologist, 1*, 209–234.

Rourke, B. P. (1989). *Nonverbal learning disabilities: The syndrome and the model.* New York: Guilford Press.

Schipper, H. I., & Seidel, D. (1984). Computed tomography in late-onset metachromatic leucodystrophy. *Neuroradiology, 26*, 39–44.

Seidel, D., Goebel, H. H., & Scholz, W. (1981). Late onset metachromatic leucodystrophy: Diagnostic problems elucidated by a case report. *Journal of Neurology, 226*, 119–124.

Shapiro, E. G., Lipton, M. E., & Krivit, W. (1992). White matter dysfunction and its neuropsychological correlates: A longitudinal study of a case of metachromatic leukodystrophy treated with bone marrow transplant. *Journal of Clinical and Experimental Neuropsychology, 14*, 610–624.

Shapiro, E. G., Lockman, L. A., Knopman, D., & Krivit, W. (1994). Characteristics of the dementia in late-onset metachromatic leukodystrophy. *Neurology, 44*, 662–665.

Skomer, C., Stears, J., & Austin, J. (1983). Metachromatic leukodystrophy (MLD): Adult MLD with focal lesions by computed tomography. *Archives of Neurology, 40*, 354–355.

Valk, J., & van der Knaap, M. S. (1989). *Magnetic resonance of myelin, myelination, and myelin disorders.* Berlin: Springer-Verlag.

Waltz, G., Harik, S. I., & Kaufman, B. (1987). Adult metachromatic leukodystrophy: Value of computed tomographic scanning and magnetic resonance imaging of the brain. *Archives of Neurology, 44*, 225–227.

Wenger, D. A., & Louie, E. (1991). Pseudodeficiencies of arylsulfatase A and galactocerebrosidase activities. *Developmental Neuroscience, 13*, 216–221.

13

Turner Syndrome

Joanne Rovet

Turner syndrome (TS) is a genetic disorder affecting only females. In the majority of cases, it is caused by a loss of all or part of the second X chromosome. The physical phenotype includes a number of characteristic features, the most common of which are short stature, sexual infantilism, mild skeletal abnormalities, and a defect in lymphatic clearance. Although considerable variability exists as to type and severity of presentation of stigmata, almost all individuals with TS are very short, and the majority are infertile.

There are also characteristic behavioral features associated with TS. These include outstanding difficulties in visual–spatial cognition, a weakness in working memory, difficulties at school in mathematics, and social/behavioral problems. In many ways, with TS may be considered a prototype of the syndrome of Nonverbal Learning Disabilities (NLD; Rourke, 1989); however, recent evidence involving neuroimaging techniques suggests that the neuroanatomical basis of the TS psychological profile does not conform completely to a white matter interpretation.

This chapter reviews current findings on the physical, behavioral, and neuropsychological characteristics of TS. The features not only of classic cases, but also of some of the variants, are described. In addition, the genetic literature is reviewed to provide an explanation for some of the heterogeneity, with particular emphasis on recent molecular genetic studies aimed at identifying specific genes for TS. The findings from studies using different neuropsychological approaches are also compared, in order to identify common themes as well as inconsistencies; explanations for the inconsistencies based on procedural/methodological differences among studies are offered. A model is presented that combines both organizational and activational components of neurological development and functioning. It is argued that whereas atypical neuro-

maturational features in TS are a product of the abnormal sex chromosome complement, difficulties with attention, memory, and executive
functioning presenting in adolescence may reflect abnormal levels of
specific hormones—in particular, the lack of estrogen—during a critical
window of development.

PHYSICAL CHARACTERISTICS

TS affects between 1 in 2000 (Nielsen, Nyborg, & Dahl, 1977) and 1 in
5000 (Hook & Warburton, 1983) females; it is similarly represented
among different ethnic and racial groups. TS is caused by the loss of a
single X chromosome, a structural abnormality or rearrangement of one
or both X chromosomes, or mosaicism involving both a normal and an
abnormal cell line. Whereas the single-X or 45X0 condition and some of
the structural abnormalities occur during gamete production prior to
fertilization, and can be maternal or paternal in origin, mosaicism takes
place after fertilization of the ovum. Although most conditions involve
the X chromosome, there is in a small percentage of cases an abnormality
involving a Y chromosome, even though the phenotype is clearly female.
For almost all individuals, TS occurs *de novo*; however, a few inherited
forms have been described (Leichtman et al., 1978).

The physical phenotype of TS is characterized by a generalized
growth defect, ovarian failure, and the variable presence of certain somatic features. Growth failure can begin *in utero*, since newborns with
TS tend to be small for date (approximately 3 cm shorter than normal
children) (Giovannelli & Balestrazzi, 1995). Although there is near-normal growth during infancy and very early childhood, a considerable loss
in height tends to occur between 3 and 12 years of age; the final adult
height averages about 4 feet, 9 inches (Ranke, 1992), depending on
country of origin (Ranke, 1995). Studies of the effects of biosynthetic
growth hormone on children with TS are well underway in a number of
countries, although there is considerable variability as to final outcome
(Neely, 1995; Rongen-Westerlaken et al., 1992; Rosenfeld et al., 1988;
Van Vliet & Collu, 1993).

Ovarian failure occurs because of a massive loss of oocytes *in utero*
and after birth, which results in streak or dysgenetic ovaries. Although
ovarian dysgenesis is a normal process in all females, for some unknown
reason it is highly accelerated in individuals with TS (Singh & Carr,
1966). This results in a lack of secondary sexual development during
adolescence (which can be easily rectified with exogenous hormone replacement) and, for the vast majority of women with TS, in infertility.

With modern advances in assisted reproduction, a few women with TS have now given birth to normal children.

The somatic abnormalities include skeletal deformities, such as an unusual carrying angle of the elbows (cubitus valgus), short fourth meta-carpals, short neck, and spinal deformities. In addition, individuals with TS may also have atypical facies, including micrognathia, a reduced size of the facial skeleton (Weiss, Loevy, Saunders, Pruzansky, & Rosenthal, 1982), and a high-arched palate that can produce feeding difficulties during infancy (Mathisen, Reilly, & Skuse, 1992; Skuse, Percy, Reilly, & Stevenson, 1995). Abnormalities of the facial bone structures are thought to be associated with an elevated incidence of ear infections and resultant hearing loss. Another common abnormality is a basic defect in the lymphatic clearance system, associated with increased risk of aortic coarctation (Lippe, 1982), ptosis, a high dermal ridge count, neck webbing, and a low-set hairline and ears. Individuals with TS may also have nail dysplasia and multiple pigmented nevi (Simpson, 1975).

Except for short stature and infertility, individuals with TS vary considerably in the presentation of the other physical features (Simpson, 1975). As a rule, but not always, more severe presentation occurs if the entire X chromosome is missing (Ross, 1990). The presence of a Y chromosome increases the risk of ambiguous or incompletely developed male genitalia (Ebbin, Howell, & Wilson, 1980) and of gonadoblastoma.

The genetic phenomenon known as X inactivation (Lyon, 1962) signifies that for the vast majority of genes on the X chromosome, only one of the two X copies is expressed—hence the greater number of similarities than differences between females with TS and normal females. However, there are now known to be several sites on the X (or Y) chromosomes that escape X inactivation. These are presumably the sources of somatic (and psychological) features of TS; indeed, current thinking holds that there may be five such sites contributing to the phenotype (Page, 1995). Since an individual with TS has one instead of two copies of these particular genes, she will have reduced expression of the associated proteins (Zinn, Page, & Fisher, 1993). It is thought that the decreased production of these proteins is what contributes to the TS-like stigmata. Variability among persons with TS may be explained in terms of which of the five genes there is only a single copy for, as well as other endocrine and environmental factors (Ross, 1990). One such gene has now been identified and mapped onto the proximal long arm of the X chromosome. Its protein product, RPS4X (Fisher et al., 1990), is essential for normal cellular functioning (Watanabe, Zinn, Page, & Nishimoto, 1993), and is thought in reduced dosage (as in the single-X condition) to contribute to the lymphatic clearance problem causing edema, coarctation of the aorta, neck webbing, and so forth.

BEHAVIORAL FEATURES

Intelligence

In addition to the physical stigmata of TS there are a number of associated behavioral features. Numerous studies, based primarily on adult women with TS, have reported a reduction in global IQ (e.g., Grumbach, Van Wyck, & Wilkens, 1955; Haddad & Wilkens, 1959), but no apparent increase in mental subnormality (Sybert, Reed, & Hall, 1980). In a review of 19 studies in the literature describing the findings from 226 cases of TS, I observed a mean IQ of 94.6, in contrast to 103.9 for controls (Rovet, 1990). Lower IQs were typically associated with a selective impairment in the nonverbal visual–spatial processing components of intelligence testing (Garron, 1977; Shaffer, 1962), which accounted for about a 12-point difference between the Verbal and Performance IQ, favoring the Verbal IQ (Rovet, 1990).

Specific Cognitive Disabilities

Studies have shown that individuals with TS do more poorly on a variety of visual–spatial cognitive tasks, which include the following: design copying (Waber, 1979); directional sense (Alexander, Walker, & Money, 1964); extrapersonal space perception (Alexander & Money, 1966); mazes (Nielsen et al., 1977); mental rotation (Rovet & Netley, 1982); part–whole perception (Silbert, Wolff, & Lilienthal, 1977); rod and frame (Nyborg, 1990); spatial reasoning (Money & Alexander, 1966); visual discrimination (Silbert et al., 1977); visual memory (Shaffer, 1962); visual sequencing (Robinson et al., 1986); and visual–motor integration (Lewandowski, Costenbader, & Richman, 1985). Although one investigator has suggested that individuals with TS appear to exhibit "space–form blindness" (Money, 1963), in their everyday lives they do drive cars and navigate themselves adequately in their environments. They also demonstrate competence in such activities as using new equipment; assembling objects from parts; arranging objects in a balanced and spatially efficient manner; and interpreting graphs, charts, and diagrams. However, they indicate greater-than-usual difficulty "picturing the outcome of a construction project" (Downey et al., 1991).

Whereas the receptive language skills of girls with TS are intact (Rovet & Netley, 1982), those with high arched palates and/or hearing loss may have early speech and language difficulties (Robinson et al., 1986). Similarly, problems in early motor development and subsequent clumsiness are also described. Difficulties with executive functioning have been reported in the areas of fluency, planning, and flexibility (Waber,

1976), as have problems with short-term memory (Berch, 1995), attention (Williams, Richman, & Yarbrough, 1991), temporal analysis, and auditory sequencing (Silbert et al., 1977).

Behavior Problems

Children with TS tend to be more hyperactive than normal (Rovet, 1986; Sonis, Levine-Ross, & Blue, 1983), whereas adults may be phlegmatic with low levels of arousal (Money & Mittenthal, 1970). Nevertheless, there is considerable variability among adults with TS, including excellent adjustment and adaptation (Pavlidis, McCauley, & Sybert, in press). Although behavior problems reflecting poor social skills (McCauley, 1990; Rovet & Ireland, 1994), shyness, poor peer relations, and low self-esteem (Rovet, 1992) have been reported in children and adolescents with TS, adults are not at increased risk for severe psychopathology but may be prone to mild depression (McCauley, 1990).

Lindsay Ireland and I have recently characterized the behavioral phenotype in a large unselected sample of children with TS. This appeared to involve an increased propensity for immature behavior, clinging, and a preference for children younger than themselves (Rovet & Ireland, 1994). They were also more restless and hyperactive than normal. Considerable variability was noted, however, with poorer social competence being linked to shorter stature and behavior problems to specific karyotypes.

Academic Difficulties

School-related difficulties in children with TS may reflect problems with mathematics, primarily mechanical arithmetic (Rovet, 1993). These appear to increase the likelihood of grade retention and the need for special education services. Children with TS are excellent and avid readers, and do not generally indicate difficulties on either word identification or passage comprehension reading tasks. Spelling and written language skills are not affected, although parents frequently describe problems with completing tasks and with written work.

Subtyping subjects with TS into different learning disability groups based on Rourke and Strang's (1983) criteria has indicated that 55% of these subjects have a learning disability, compared with 26% of controls (Rovet, 1993). In TS, this always involved an arithmetic disability, alone, or in combination with reading problems. They never had a reading disability alone unlike controls, who were more evenly distributed across the various subtype groupings. Although problems were observed in all arithmetic processing domains, geometry appeared to be less severely affected than computational arithmetic skills (Rovet, 1992).

In a recent study from our laboratory (Rovet, Szekely, & Hockenberry, 1994), error analyses were conducted on the responses of girls with TS and controls to selected items of the Wide Range Achievement Test—Revised (WRAT-R; Jastak & Wilkinson, 1984) and the Keymath Diagnostic Arithmetic Test (Connelly, Nachtman, & Pritchett, 1981). This analysis was based on the McCloskey, Caramazza, and Basili (1985) model for delineating the dysfunctional cognitive mechanisms in acalculic patients after brain damage, as well as Temple's (1989, 1991) procedures for analyzing arithmetic errors in children with dyscalculia. In these analyses, items were subdivided into number-processing or computational domains, with the latter reflecting fact retrieval or procedural knowledge processes.

For the WRAT-R, 45 subjects with TS were compared with 92 age-matched female controls. Results revealed that the group with TS attempted significantly fewer fact retrieval and procedural knowledge problems, and that they obtained fewer correct solutions on the items they completed, particularly for addition and division problems. On the Keymath, given to 10 of the subjects with TS and 37 of the controls, the results indicated that the group with TS scored significantly below controls in all domains except geometry and symbols. Both groups showed perfect understanding of numbers and operational symbols, and did not differ in either the number of fact or procedure items attempted or the number of fact problems correct. However, the group with TS made significantly more errors in the procedure domain, which occurred primarily for addition and subtraction problems; multiplication and division were equally difficult for both groups. Qualitative analysis of their errors revealed that girls with TS were more likely to confuse component steps and less likely to complete or separate intermediate steps than controls, who were more likely to compute wrong calculations.

Correlational analyses showed that subjects with TS relied more on verbal abilities for arithmetic processing than did controls. For the subjects with TS, visual–spatial ability was correlated with the retrieval of simple multidigit addition facts, as well as with procedural skills in subtraction, multiplication, and division domains; this suggests that a common mechanism may be affecting both visual–spatial task performance (e.g., Block Design on the Wechsler tests) and the carrying out of sequential steps in arithmetic problems. Since the breakdown in procedure problems took place in computing a number of different sequential components, the mechanism underlying the arithmetic difficulty may reflect a basic defect in working memory: As the demands on memory increased, so did basic difficulty.

Correlations between Phenotype and Behavior

As with the physical features, there exists considerable heterogeneity in the behavioral features of individuals with TS (Temple & Carney, 1993; Rovet, 1992). For example, in one study 50% of subjects had significant visual–spatial impairments, whereas 10–20% exhibited superior nonverbal ability compared to their verbal skills (Pennington et al., 1985). Similarly, there are also some children with TS who demonstrate very good figure copying (Rovet, 1992), arithmetic skills (Rovet et al., 1994), and social skills (Rovet & Ireland, 1994).

Several studies have examined the influence of specific karyotype on ability or behavior. As a rule, less cognitive and behavioral deviance is observed in children with a mosaic karyotype than in those with a pure 45X0 chromosomal constitution (Bender, Linden, & Robinson, 1990; Rovet & Ireland, 1994; Swillen et al., 1993; Temple & Carney, 1993); the presence of Y-chromosome material is also associated with a weakness in visual–spatial ability (Ebbin et al., 1980). In our study of the behavioral phenotype, we found that children with chromosomal deletions or with the presence of a Y-chromosome line had the highest behavior problem scores, whereas those with mosaicism were not unlike controls (Rovet & Ireland, 1994).

Studies have also examined the influence of different phenotypic features on psychometric intelligence (Garron, 1977; Money & Granoff, 1965). Their findings have failed to indicate any significant correlations between specific phenotypic characteristics and psychometric intelligence, although lower IQ was associated with the presence of more than three classic stigmata (Garron, 1977). Unfortunately, because these studies did not use a systematic approach to classify physical stigmata (e.g., skeletal growth, gonadal, lymphatic), a real effect may have been missed.

Summary

TS is associated with a wide range of behavioral characteristics. These include difficulties on tasks of visual–spatial processing, executive functioning, memory, attention, and arithmetic. Their arithmetic problems appear to involve a deficit distinct from their visual–spatial impairment; this reflects increased difficulty with the stepwise, componential aspects of procedural problems, as well as poorer fact retrieval during timed testing. A more basic problem involving working memory has been implicated as the core deficit.

Young girls with TS have also been observed to be prone to attentional and social problems, as well as hyperactivity. These features do not persist into adulthood, when the women become more introverted and passive than usual. However it is very important to note that despite consistencies in the behavioral profile, there is also considerable variability among individuals as to severity of presentation, with some not being affected at all. Future research should be directed toward identifing the factors predicting such variability, including the role of the family (Bender, Linden, & Robinson, 1987).

NEUROLOGICAL/NEUROPSYCHOLOGICAL CHARACTERISTICS

An increasing number of studies using a variety of different techniques have been attempting to describe the neuroanatomical basis of the underlying cognitive deficits in TS. The findings suggest no consistency as to either lateralizing or localizing effects (Rovet, 1990). Studies based solely on neuropsychological test batteries indicate variable findings, ranging from a focal right parietal dysfunction (Money, 1973) and more extensive posterior right-hemisphere dysfunction (McGlone, 1985) to dysfunction involving the entire right hemisphere (Silbert et al., 1977) or the parietal and frontal regions of both hemispheres (Waber, 1979). Although this research is limited by relatively small sample sizes, the evidence suggests more diffuse involvement than was originally (Money, 1973) expected.

Neuropathology

The evidence based on three cases with TS autopsied to date suggests considerable heterogeneity. In one case, a neuronal migration defect was found (Kolb & Heaton, 1975). In another case, neurodevelopmental changes were localized to the posterior right hemisphere (Reske-Nielsen, Christensen, & Nielsen, 1982). The third woman showed neither brain pathology nor previous history of cognitive impairment (Reske-Nielsen et al., 1982).

Cerebral Lateralization

Hemispheric laterality testing, which requires subjects to attend and respond to competing stimuli presented unilaterally to each cerebral hemisphere, provides an indirect marker of brain organization and specialization for different types of stimulus information. The results obtained from such tasks given to individuals with TS show that their brain organization is atypical relative to controls. However, considerable variability exists across studies, and there is no consensus as to source of impairment.

Subjects with TS exhibited decreased left-hemisphere specialization for verbal processing (Netley & Rovet, 1982), decreased right-hemisphere specialization in nonverbal processing (McGlone, 1985), or both (Rovet, 1990). In these studies, cognitive impairment correlated only modestly with atypical hemispheric lateralization (Netley & Rovet, 1982).

Electrophysiological Findings

Although electroencephalographic studies have shown atypical recordings in many subjects with TS (Poenaru, Stanesco, Poenaru, & Stoian, 1970; Tsuboi & Nielsen, 1976), no single problem has as yet been identified, and considerable variability exists both among individuals and across studies (see Rovet, 1990, for a review). A recent study (Portellano-Perez, Bouthelier, & Asensio-Monge, 1994) has shown that for girls with TS, the specific brain structures involved in doing certain cognitive activities may differ from those of controls. For example, reading involved the right hemisphere to a greater degree in girls with TS, whereas arithmetic activated the left parietal lobe in controls but not girls with TS. This suggests that certain neuronal systems may have become specialized differently during development in girls with TS versus normal females.

Two studies have used event-related potential (ERP) paradigms with individuals with TS. When given an auditory ERP paradigm to probe tones, TS subjects produced a profile suggestive of less adequate processing of ongoing irrelevant or competing information by the right hemisphere (Shucard, Shucard, Clopper, & Schachter, 1992). Johnson and Ross (1994) gave adolescents with TS (none treated with hormones) and controls an auditory "oddball" task and a task of visual discrimination (right- vs. left-hand discrimination) while ERPs were simultaneously recorded. Subjects with TS demonstrated two cognitive deficits: one suggestive of a congenital abnormality (from birth) and the other of a maturational problem (during adolescence). Regarding the congenital or "organizational" abnormality, girls with TS did not differ from controls in the ERP components signifying sensory processing, but they did differ in the response execution components of the ERP waveform (Johnson, Rohrbaugh, & Ross, 1993). Regarding the maturational or "activational" component, girls with TS failed to show the normally occurring changes in the O-wave component of the ERP waveform; these changes occur in midpuberty and reflect stimulus orientation and the ability to change contexts. Older subjects with TS appeared to remain hyperoriented, as was typical of controls prior to puberty but not after.

Johnson and Ross (1994) also studied ERP components in one subject with TS who had normal endogenous estrogen levels. Her performance was found to be remarkably similar to that of normal females. In contrast, these researchers also noted that the administration of estrogen therapy to individuals with TS during late adolescence failed to normalize the immature O-wave response. They have proposed that there is a critical period for estrogen exposure, without which this normal adolescent maturation of selective brain systems fails to occur.

Neuroimaging Techniques

At least four studies have now employed brain imaging techniques in girls with TS. Clark, Klonoff, and Hayden (1990), using position emission tomography (PET) scans, described reduced glucose utilization in the parietal and occipital lobes of five women with TS. Reiss et al. (1993) performed magnetic resonance imagining (MRI) scans on a pair of 10-year-old twins discordant for TS. Comprehensive physical and neurocognitive evaluations revealed that the twin with TS was significantly shorter and more delayed in her pubertal development than her sister, and that she also had mild physical TS stigmata; that the affected TS twin did more poorly on tasks of visual–spatial abilities, attention, and executive functioning; and that she was more hyperactive, with greater-than-usual difficulty in reading comprehension but not in math. MRI scans revealed that for the twin with TS, grey matter volume was significantly reduced in the left parietal perisylvian and right prefrontal regions, whereas cerebrospinal fluid was increased in the right posterior parieto-occipital area. The child with TS also had a reversal of left-greater-than-right asymmetry in ventricular volumes; increased volumes of the cisterna magna and fourth ventricle; and decreased sizes of the cerebellar vermis, pons, and medulla. The sisters were remarkably similar in their white matter volumes, which were not unusual. Ross, Reiss, Freund, Roeltgen, and Cutler (1993) compared MRI scans in 8 girls with TS (aged 8 to 14 years) and 13 age-matched female controls. Preliminary evidence based only on assessment of subcortical nuclei and ventricular volumes indicated that the children with TS had increased bilateral ventricular volumes, which were also more variable. These authors attributed the increased volumes to a generalized process operating during neurodevelopment, which could adversely affect subsequent white matter and grey matter formation, as well to specific effects influencing genetic endocrine and environmental factors.

A fourth study obtained MRI scans from nine 30-year-old women with a pure 45X0 karyotype and nine with a mosaic 45X0 karyotype, as well as 19 healthy controls (Murphy et al., 1993). Compared to controls, women with TS had significantly smaller MRI-measured volumes in the hippocampus, caudate, lenticular and thalamic nuclei, and parieto-occipital brain matter on both sides; these volumes were greater on the right than on the left side. They did not differ from controls in frontal, temporal, or cerebellar regions. Women with TS mosaicism had values intermediate between those of the women with pure 45X0 and controls for all affected sites. They also differed significantly from the women with pure 45X0 in their hippocampal volumes—a finding suggesting that this site may be sensitive to gene dosage effects, in contrast to the other sites, which may reflect a more generalized effect of the abnormal X-chromosome complement. These researchers specifically attributed their results to the role of the X chromosome in the development and aging of grey matter in the striatum, diencephalon, and cerebral hemispheres.

Summary

These findings suggest that neuroanatomical abnormalities may be associated with TS, and that the severity of these reflects how much of the X chromosome is missing and which sites on the X chromosome are affected. Although there appear to be neurodevelopmental modifications (which are presumed to be genetically modulated), functional differences may be associated with hormonal abnormalities (Ross et al., 1993). The only study to deal with both organizational and activational components of dysfunction is that by Johnson and Ross (1994). They used the ERP paradigm, in which two distinct abnormalities were identified: one that was congenital in nature, and another that was activationally or functionally based. Current imaging studies suggest that grey matter may be affected to a greater degree than white matter, although the findings are more diffuse than originally predicted.

TS AND THE NLD SYNDROME

The present review of behavioral and neuropsychological research studies of TS has provided considerable, but not complete, support for the NLD model. According to this model, children with the NLD syndrome demonstrate a characteristic profile of assets and deficits as presented in detail in Chapter 1. The syndrome is believed to arise from certain primary neuropsychological assets and deficits, which in turn lead to secondary, tertiary, and linguistic assets and deficits. Particular academic and socioemotional/ adaptive characteristics are attributed to this hierarchy of features.

The Three Levels

Primary-level assets in children with the NLD syndrome reflect intact simple motor skills, as well as good auditory-perceptual and rote memory capabilities. On the other hand, primary-level deficits reflect poor tactile and visual perception, as well as difficulty with complex psychomotor tasks and novel stimulus configurations. Studies of children with TS are generally consistent with this profile. With respect to assets, for example, they are reported to have well-developed auditory perception (Kolb & Heaton, 1975), pattern analysis (Silbert et al., 1977), right–left discrimination (Serra, Pizzamiglio, Boari, & Spera, 1978), finger tapping (Waber, 1979), and two-point tactile perception (McGlone, 1985). Regarding their deficits, they do more poorly on tasks of motor coordination (McGlone, 1985), balance, dexterity, and psychomotor coordination (Lewandowski et al., 1985), as well as perceptual awareness of their bodies in space (Robinson et al., 1986). They also have difficulty with novel stimulus configurations (Silbert et al., 1977). According to McGlone (1985), low scores by subjects with TS on many of the tasks she gave appeared to be secondary to poorer coordination.

At the secondary level, the NLD model predicts that persons so afflicted will be able to deploy attention adequately for simple repetitive verbal materials, especially if information is delivered through the auditory modality. By contrast, attention to tactile or visual input is predicted to be poor, particularly if the stimuli are complex or novel. The findings for individuals with TS also support the model at this level. They show adequate deployment of attention for simple repetitive verbal material (Johnson & Ross, 1994; McGlone, 1985; Rovet & Netley, 1982), whereas on a more involved computerized task of visual sustained attention, they performed very much like children with documented attentional difficulties (Williams et al., 1991). Robinson et al. (1986) reported that 56% of their sample had a diagnosable attentional problem reflecting an inability to remain focused, increased distractibility, and poorer concentration. The NLD model also predicts that at this level, the disparity between attentional capacities for repetitive versus novel stimuli increases with age, as has been observed by Johnson and Ross (1994). Furthermore, it hypothesizes that since there is little physical exploration of any kind in children with the NLD syndrome, the tendency toward sedentary and physically limited modes of functioning increases with age; this is also frequently reported for individuals with TS. However, in the case of TS this is generally attributed to increased social isolation, loneliness, and withdrawal during adolescence, as a result of short stature and sexual infantilism (McCauley, 1994).

The expected pattern of assets and deficits at the tertiary level is also observed in individuals with TS. They demonstrate well-developed rote memory (Berch, 1995; McGlone, 1985; Williams et al., 1991), but show difficulties on tasks of visual memory (Pennington et al., 1985; Shaffer, 1962; Waber, 1979) or complex verbal recall (Pennington et al., 1985); there is no information on tactile memory skills in this population. Consistent with the model, individuals with TS also do more poorly on concept-forming and problem-solving tasks (Pennington et al., 1985), and, of course, have outstanding difficulties in visual–spatial processing (Gordon & Galatzer, 1980; Lewandowski et al., 1985; McGlone, 1985; Rovet & Netley, 1982).

Supplementary Features

The NLD model also predicts characteristic strengths and weaknesses in the language domain, including early delays in speech and language, rapid catch-up, excellent phonological processing, and a high volume of speech output. In TS, Robinson et al. (1986) described adequate receptive and expressive language, with the exception of their understanding of grammatical relations, which was below normal. They also have difficulties with word fluency (Money & Alexander, 1966) and auditory sequencing (Silbert et al., 1977), but not with general verbal ability (Serra et al., 1978; Waber, 1979) or specific understanding of grammatical relations (Rovet & Netley, 1982). Excessive chattiness is a frequent behavioral complaint of parents (Rovet & Ireland, 1994).

Academically, according to the NLD model, word-decoding and spelling skills should be spared, whereas outstanding difficulties in mechanical arithmetic and reading comprehension should be observed. Although the evidence for reading decoding, spelling, and arithmetic in TS clearly supports the model (Rovet, 1993; Rovet et al., 1994), the findings on reading comprehension are less consistent. We observed that comprehension was adequate among children with TS (Rovet et al., 1994), whereas Portellano-Perez et al., (1994) reported that reading comprehension was problematic in older individuals.

In the socioemotional realm, deficits are expected in adaptability, social competence, emotional stability, and activity level. Indeed, poor social competence and increased activity levels have been found to be characteristic of the TS behavioral phenotype (McCauley, 1992; Rovet & Ireland, 1994), although girls with TS are not less adaptable (Rovet, 1986) or more emotionally unstable (McCauley, Ito, & Kay, 1986). Rather, their difficulties primarily reflect low self-esteem (Rovet, 1994) and problems with attention/hyperactivity and social skills (McCauley, 1994; Rovet & Ireland, 1994).

The Underlying Neurological Mechanism

According to Rourke (1989), the cognitive and behavioral manifestations of the NLD model are reflections of inadequate cerebral white matter

development, with the integrity of the white matter system being necessary for the development and maintenance of those behavioral systems
affected by the NLD syndrome. Although studies of the behavioral characteristics of children with circumscribed brain damage and learning
disabilities support this model (Dool, Stelmack, & Rourke, 1993), the
evidence on individuals with TS is not in complete agreement.

Recent findings using PET and MRI techniques with children (Reiss
et al, 1993; Ross et al., 1993) and adults (Murphy et al., 1993) with TS
indicate that grey matter is affected to a greater degree than white matter;
this is attributed to an early neurodevelopmental abnormality. However,
as these studies used static and not active procedures (such as functional
MRI), it is still uncertain whether the brains of individuals with TS might
appear abnormal when specific cognitive processes are called upon. Until
such technology is available for use with this population, at best we can
conclude that females with TS fit the NLD model almost perfectly in terms
of their behavior, whereas the evidence on white matter dysfunction is
still inconclusive.

Alternatively, altered grey matter development may produce white
matter perturbations (e.g., as a result of fewer glial cells), with the result
that white matter is very subtly affected in this population. This cannot
be observed with current imaging methodologies. It is also possible that
the reduced grey matter volumes seen on MRI are the indirect result of
decreased myelination (B. P. Rourke, personal communication, July
1994); this may be resolved once newer neuroimaging technologies can
be used in this population. Indeed, the neuropsychological testing evidence signifying diffuse involvement supports the white matter interpretation and may be borne out in the future.

Until then, however, a more parsimonious interpretation, based on
the research by Johnson and Ross (1994), is that there are at least two
defects. One is organizational in nature, and presumably reflects the
genetic component; the other is purported to be "activational," reflecting
hormonal insufficiencies (Johnson, 1994). At the organizational level,
the lack of an X chromosome contributes to differences in neurodevelopment and specialization; this is thought to occur prior to birth. As a
result, there appear to be neuronal migration defects (Kolb & Heaton,
1975), which may produce structural relationships and patterns of connectivity differing from those usually observed in females without a sex
chromosome anomaly. It is thought that this may contribute to the basic-
level deficits proposed in the NLD model, and, directly or indirectly, to
those at other levels (e.g., visual–spatial and number processing). On
the other hand, the lack of puberty during the adolescent period appears
to contribute to a further functional defect. This is thought to be activational in origin (Johnson, 1994) and perpetuates an immature pattern
of orienting to stimuli, which may be associated with some of the deficits
in executive social and functioning observed among girls with TS.

Alternatively, it is conceivable that these "activational" defects may actually reflect late-occurring organizational processes, which presumably involve the myelination that occurs during puberty in those structures with protracted development, such as the frontal lobes and reticular formation (Yakovlev & Lecours, 1967). Support for this interpretation is that the deficits are neither phasic nor neurotransmitter-related, as is typical of activational processes. Further evidence to determine whether the abilities of girls with TS vary during the monthly cycle, as found in normal females (Hampson & Kimura, 1992), is needed.

CONCLUSION

In conclusion, the behavioral findings on individuals with TS strongly support the NLD syndrome model. Although the MRI evidence to date suggests an absence of white matter involvement in the condition, ERP studies indicate that there are brain abnormalities suggestive of inadequate white matter formation, which may be attributable to a lack of estrogen during a critical window of pubertal development. However, as these findings cannot adequately explain the early cognitive and arithmetic problems exhibited by younger children with TS, it is unlikely that their NLD-like profile can be attributable entirely to inadequate white matter formation. It is expected that the primary neurological basis of the TS deficit, as well as secondary manifestations, will be discovered within the next decade as newer neuroimaging technologies become available for use in this population, and as interest in the syndrome is maintained at both scientific (Broman & Grafman, 1994) and clinical (Rovet & Holland, 1995) levels.

REFERENCES

Alexander, D., & Money, J. (1966). Turner's syndrome and Gerstmann's syndrome: Neuropsychologic comparisons. *Neuropsychologia, 4*, 265–273.

Alexander, D., Walker, H., & Money, J. (1964). Studies in direction sense. *Archives of General Psychiatry, 10*, 337–339.

Bender, B., Linden, M., & Robinson, A. (1987). Environment and developmental risk in children with sex chromosome abnormalities. *Journal of the American Academy of Child Psychiatry, 26*, 499–503.

Bender, B., Linden, M., & Robinson, A. (1990). SCA: In search of developmental patterns. In D. Berch & B. Bender (Eds.), *Sex chromosome abnormalities and human behavior: Psychological studies* (pp. 20–37). Boulder, CO: Westview Press.

Berch, D. (1995). Memory. In J. Rovet & F. J. Holland (Eds.), *Turner syndrome across the lifespan*. Book in preparation.

Broman, S., & Grafman, J. (Eds.). (1994). *Atypical cognitive deficits in developmental disorders: Implications for brain function*. Hillsdale, NJ: Erlbaum.

Clark, C., Klonoff, H., & Hayden, M. (1990). Regional cerebral glucose metabolism in Turner syndrome. *Canadian Journal of Neurological Sciences, 17,* 140–144.

Connelly, A., Nachtman, W., & Pritchett, E. (1981). *Keymath Diagnostic Arithmetic Test.* Circle Pines, MN: American Guidance Service.

Dool, C. B., Stelmack, R., & Rourke, B. P. (1993). Event-related potentials in children with learning disabilities. *Journal of Clinical Child Psychology, 22*(3), 387–398.

Downey, J., Elkin, E., Ehrhardt, E., Meyer-Bahlburg, A., Bell, H., & Akira, J. (1991). Cognitive ability and everyday functioning in women with Turner syndrome. *Journal of Learning Disabilities, 24,* 32–39.

Ebbin, A., Howell, V., & Wilson, M. (1980). Deficits in space–form perception in patients with sex chromosome mosaicism (45,X/46,XY). *Developmental Medicine and Child Neurology, 22,* 352–361.

Fisher, E., Beer-Romano, P., Brown, L., Ridley, A., McNeil, J., Lawrence, J., Willard, H., Bieber, F., & Page, D. (1990). Homologous ribosomal protein genes on the human X and Y chromosomes: Escape from X inactivation and possible implications for Turner syndrome. *Cell, 63,* 1205–1218.

Garron, D. (1977). Intelligence among persons with Turner's syndrome. *Behavior Genetics, 7,* 105–127.

Giovannelli, G., & Balestrazzi, P. (1995). Phenotypic characteristics of Turner syndrome. In J. Rovet & F. J. Holland (Eds.), *Turner syndrome across the lifespan.* Book in preparation.

Gordon, H., & Galatzer, A. (1980). Cerebral organization in patients with gonadal dysgenesis. *Psychoneuroendocrinology, 5,* 235–244.

Grumbach, C., Van Wyck, J., & Wilkens, L. (1955). Chromosomal sex in gonadal dysgenesis relationship to male pseudohermaphroditism and theories of human sex differentiation. *Journal of Clinical Endocrinology, 15,* 1161–1193.

Haddad, H., & Wilkens, L. (1959). Congenital abnormalities associated with gonadal aplasia: Review of 55 cases. *Pediatrics, 23,* 885–902.

Hampson, E., & Kimura, D. (1992). Sex differences and hormonal influences on cognitive function in humans. In J. Becker, S. Breedlove, & D. Crews (Eds.), *Behavioral endocrinology* (pp. 357–398). Cambridge, MA: MIT Press.

Hook, E., & Warburton, D. (1983). The distribution of chromosomal genotypes associated with Turner's syndrome: Live birth prevalence rates and evidence for diminished fetal mortality and severity in genotypes associated with structural X abnormalities or mosaicism. *Human Genetics, 64,* 24–27.

Jastak, S., & Wilkinson, G. (1984). *Wide Range Achievement Test—Revised.* Wilmington, DE: Jastak Associates.

Johnson, R. (1995). Event-related potential indications of altered brain development in Turner syndrome. In J. Rovet & F. J. Holland (Eds.), *Turner syndrome across the lifespan.* Book in preparation.

Johnson, R., Rohrbaugh, J. & Ross, J. (1993). Altered brain development in Turner's syndrome. *Neurology, 43,* 801–808.

Johnson, R., & Ross, J. (1994). Event-related potential indications of altered brain development in Turner syndrome. In S. Broman & J. Grafman (Eds.), *Atypical cognitive deficits in developmental disorders: Implications for brain function* (pp. 217–242). Hillsdale, NJ: Erlbaum.

Kolb, J., & Heaton, R. (1975). Lateralized neurologic deficits and psychopathology in a Turner syndrome patient. *Archives of General Psychiatry, 32*, 1198–1200.

Leichtman, D., Schmickel, R., Gelehrtner, T., Judd, W., Woodbury, M., & Meilinger, K. (1978). Familial Turner syndrome. *Annals of Internal Medicine, 89*, 473–476.

Lewandowski, L., Costenbader, V., & Richman, R. (1985). Neuropsychological aspects of Turner syndrome. *International Journal of Neuropsychology, 1*, 144–147.

Lippe, B. (1982). Primary ovarian failure. In S. Kaplan (Ed.), *Clinical pediatric and adolescent endocrinology* (pp. 269–299). Philadelphia: W. B. Saunders.

Lyon, M. (1962). Sex chromatin and gene action in the mammalian X-chromosome. *American Journal of Human Genetics, 14*, 135.

Mathisen, B., Reilly, S., & Skuse, D. (1992). Oral–motor dysfunction and feeding disorders of infants with Turner syndrome. *Developmental Medicine and Child Neurology, 34*, 141–149.

McCauley, E. (1990). Psychosocial and emotional aspects of Turner syndrome. In D. Berch & B. Bender (Eds.), *Sex chromosome abnormalities and human behavior: Psychological studies* (pp. 78–100). Boulder, CO: Westview Press.

McCauley, E. (1992). Educational concerns at school age and puberty. In A. Longas & C. Basterra (Eds.), *Second International Turner Contact Group Meeting: Proceedings of the meeting held in Zaragoza, Spain, September 25–28* (pp. 207–210). Salamanca, Spain: Tesitex.

McCauley, E. (1995). Social adaptation: Teens. In J. Rovet & F. J. Holland (Eds.), *Turner syndrome across the lifespan.* Book in preparation.

McCauley, E., Ito, J., & Kay, T. (1986). Psychosocial functioning in girls with Turner's syndrome and short stature: Social skills, behavior problems, and self concept. *Journal of the American Academy of Child Psychiatry, 25*, 105–112.

McCloskey, M., Caramazza, A., & Basili, A. (1985). Cognitive mechanisms in number processing and calculation: Evidence from dyscalculia. *Brain and Cognition, 4*, 171–196.

McGlone, J. (1985). Can spatial deficits in Turner's syndrome be explained by focal CNS dysfunction or atypical speech lateralization? *Journal of Clinical and Experimental Neuropsychology, 7*, 375–394.

Money, J. (1963). Cytogenetic and psychosexual incongruities with a note on space-form blindness. *American Journal of Psychiatry, 119*, 820–827.

Money, J. (1973). Turner's syndrome and parietal lobe functions. *Cortex, 9*, 385–393.

Money, J., & Alexander, D. (1966). Turner's syndrome: Further demonstration of the presence of specific cognitive deficiencies. *Journal of Medical Genetics, 3*, 47–48.

Money, J., & Granoff, D. (1965). IQ and the somatic stigmata of Turner's syndrome. *American Journal of Mental Deficiency, 70*, 69–77.

Money, J. & Mittenthal, S. (1970). Lack of personality pathology in Turner's syndrome: Relations to cytogenetics, hormones and physique. *Behavior Genetics, 1*, 43–56.

Murphy, D., DeCarli, C., Daly, E., Haxby, J., Allen, G., White, B., McIntosh, A., Powell, C., Horwitz, B., Rapoport, S., & Schapiro, M. (1993). X-chromosome effects on female brain: A magnetic resonance imaging study of Turner's syndrome. *Lancet, 342,* 1197–1200.

Neely, E. K. (1995). Results of growth hormone studies. In J. Rovet & F. J. Holland (Eds.), *Turner syndrome across the lifespan.* Book in preparation.

Netley, C., & Rovet, J. (1982). Atypical hemispheric lateralization in Turner syndrome subjects. *Cortex, 18,* 377–384.

Nielsen, J., Nyborg, H., & Dahl, G. (1977). Turner's syndrome: A psychiatric–psychological study of 45 women with Turner's syndrome, compared with their sisters and women with normal karyotypes, growth retardation, and primary amenorrhea. *Acta Jutlandica, 45,* (Medicine Series 21), 190.

Nyborg, H. (1990). Sex hormones, brain development, and spatio-perceptual strategies in Turner syndrome. In D. Berch & B. Bender (Eds.), *Sex chromosome abnormalities and human behavior: Psychological studies* (pp. 100–129). Boulder, CO: Westview Press.

Page, D. (1995). The molecular basis of Turner syndrome: Searching the X (and Y) chromosomes for the critical genes. In J. Rovet & F. J. Holland (Eds.), *Turner syndrome across the lifespan.* Book in preparation.

Pavlidis, K., McCauley, E., & Sybert, V. (in press). Psychosocial and sexual functioning in women with Turner syndrome. *Clinical Genetics.*

Pennington, B., Heaton, R., Karzmrak, P., Pendleton, M., Lehman, R., & Shucard, D. (1985). The neuropsychological phenotype in Turner syndrome. *Cortex, 21,* 391–404.

Poenaru, S., Stanesco, V., Poenaru, L., & Stoian, D. (1970). EEG dans le syndrome de Turner. *Acta Neurologica Belgica, 70,* 509–522.

Portellano-Perez, J., Bouthelier, R., & Asensio-Monge, I. (1995). New neurophysiological and neuropsychological contributions about Turner syndrome. In J. Rovet & F. J. Holland (Eds.), *Turner syndrome across the lifespan.* Book in preparation.

Ranke, M. (1992). Growth in Turner syndrome and possibilities for treatment. In A. Longas & C. Basterra (Eds.), *Second International Turner Contact Group Meeting: Proceedings of the meeting held in Zaragoza, Spain, September 25–28* (pp. 45–62). Salamanca, Spain: Tesitex.

Ranke, M. (1995). Growth and prediction of growth in Turner syndrome. In J. Rovet & F. J. Holland (Eds.), *Turner syndrome across the lifespan.* Book in preparation.

Reiss, A., Freund, L., Plotnick, L., Baumgardner, T., Green, K., Sozer, A., Reader, M., Boehm, C., & Denckla, M. (1993). The effects of X monosomy on brain development: Monozygotic twins discordant for Turner's syndrome. *Annals of Neurology, 34,* 95–107.

Reske-Nielsen, E., Christensen, A., & Nielsen, J. (1982). A neuropathological and neuropsychological study of Turner's syndrome. *Cortex, 18,* 181–190.

Robinson, A., Bender, B., Borelli, J., Puck, M., Salbenblatt, J., & Winter, J. (1986). Sex chromosomal aneuploidy: Prospective and longitudinal studies. In S. Ratcliffe & N. Paul (Eds.), *Prospective studies on children with sex chromosome aneuploidy* (pp. 23–73). New York: Alan R. Liss.

Rongen-Westerlaken, C., Wit, J., De Muinck Keizer-Schrama, S., Otten, B., Oostdijk, W., Delemarre-van der Waal, H., Gons, M., Bot, A., & Van den Brande,

J. (1992). Growth hormone treatment in Turner syndrome accelerates growth and skeletal maturation. *European Journal of Pediatrics, 151*, 477–481.

Rosenfeld, R., Hintz, R., Johanson, A., Sherman, B., Brasel, J., Burnstein, S., Chernausek, S., Compton, S., Frane, J., Gotlin, R., Kintze, J., Lippe, B., Mahoney, P., Moore, W., New, M., Saenger, P., & Sybert, V. (1988). Three year results of a randomized prospective trial of methionyl human growth hormone and oxandrolone in Turner syndrome. *Journal of Pediatrics, 113*, 393–400.

Ross, J. L. (1990). Disorders of the sex chromosomes: Medical overview. In C. S. Holmes (ED.) *Psychoneuroendocrinology: Brain, behavior, and hormonal interactions* (pp. 127–137). New York: Springer-Verlag.

Ross, J. L., Reiss, A. L., Freund, L., Roeltgen, D., & Cutler, G. B., Jr. (1993). Neurocognitive function and brain imaging in Turner syndrome: Preliminary results. *Hormone Research, 39*, 65–69

Rourke, B. P. (1989). *Nonverbal learning disabilities: The syndrome and the model.* New York, Guilford Press.

Rourke, B. P., & Strang, J. (1983). Subtypes of reading and arithmetic disabilities: A neuropsychological analysis. In M. Rutter (Ed.), *Developmental neuropsychiatry* (pp. 473–488). New York: Guilford Press.

Rovet, J. (1986). Processing deficits in 45,X females. Paper presented at the meeting of the American Association for the Advancement of Science, Philadelphia.

Rovet, J. (1990). The cognitive and neuropsychological characteristics of children with Turner syndrome. In D. Berch & B. Bender (Eds.), *Sex chromosome abnormalities and human behavior: Psychological studies* (pp. 38–77). Boulder, CO: Westview Press.

Rovet, J. (1992). Neurocognitive and school learning characteristics of children with Turner's syndrome. In A. Longas & C. Basterra (Eds.), *Second International Turner Contact Group Meeting: Proceedings of the meeting held in Zaragoza, Spain, September 25–28* (pp. 239–254). Salamanca, Spain: Tesitex.

Rovet, J. (1993). The psychoeducational characteristics of children with Turner syndrome. *Journal of Learning Disabilities, 26*, 333–341.

Rovet, J. (1994). School outcome in Turner syndrome. In B. Stabler, & L. Underwood (Eds), *Growth stature, and adaptation* (pp 165–180). Chapel Hill: University of North Carolina Press.

Rovet, J., & Holland, F.J. (Eds.). (1995). *Turner syndrome across the lifespan.* Book in preparation.

Rovet, J., & Ireland, L. (1994). The behavioral phenotype of children with Turner syndrome. *Journal of Pediatric Psychology, 19*, 779–790.

Rovet, J., & Netley, C., (1982). Processing deficits in Turner's syndrome. *Developmental Psychology, 18*, 77–94.

Rovet, J., Szekely, C., & Hockenberry, M. (1994). Specific arithmetic deficits in children with Turner syndrome. *Journal of Clinical and Experimental Neuropsychology, 16*, 820–839.

Serra, A., Pizzamiglio, L., Boari, A., & Spera, S. (1978). A comparative study of cognitive traits in human sex chromosome aneuploids and sterile and fertile euploids. *Behavior Genetics, 8*, 144–154.

Shaffer, J. (1962). A specific cognitive deficit observed in gonadal aplasia (Turner's syndrome). *Journal of Clinical Psychology, 18*, 403–406.

Shucard, D. W., Shucard, J. L., Clopper, R. J., & Schachter, M. (1992) Electrophysiological and neuropsychological indices of cognitive processing deficits in Turner syndrome. *Developmental Neuropsychology, 8*, 299–323.

Silbert, A., Wolff, P., & Lilienthal, J. (1977). Spatial and temporal processing in patients with Turner's syndrome. *Behavior Genetics, 7*, 11–21.

Simpson, J. (1975). Gonadal dysgenesis and abnormalities of the human sex chromosomes: Current status of phenotypic–karotypic correlations. *Birth Defects: Original Article Series, 11*, 23–55.

Singh, R., & Carr, H. (1966). The anatomy and histology of human embryos and fetuses. *Anatomy Research, 155*, 369–384.

Skuse, D., Percy, E., Reilly, S., & Stevenson, J. (1995). Behavioural and feeding characteristics of infants with Turner syndrome. In J. Rovet & F. J. Holland (Eds.), *Turner syndrome across the lifespan.* Book in preparation.

Sonis, W., Levine-Ross, J., & Blue, J. (1983). *Hyperactivity in Turner's syndrome.* Paper presented at the meeting of the American Academy of Child Psychiatry, San Francisco.

Swillen, A., Fryns, J., Kleczkowska, A., Massa, G., Vanderschueren-Lodeweyckx, M., & Van Den Berghe, H. (1993). Intelligence, behaviour and psychosocial development in Turner syndrome. *Genetic Counseling, 4*, 7–18.

Sybert, V., Reed, S., & Hall, J. (1980). *Mental retardation in the Turner syndrome.* Paper presented at the 31st annual meeting of the American Society for Human Genetics, New York.

Temple, C. (1989). Digit dyslexia: A category-specific disorder in developmental dyscalculia. *Cognitive Neuropsychology, 6*, 93–116.

Temple, C. (1991). Procedural dyscalculia and number fact dyscalculia: Double dissociation in developmental dyscalculia. *Cognitive Neuropsychology, 8*, 155–176.

Temple, C., & Carney, R. (1993). Intellectual functioning of children with Turner syndrome: A comparison of behavioural phenotypes. *Developmental Medicine and Child Neurology, 35*, 691–698.

Tsuboi, T., & Nielsen, J. (1976). Electroencephalographic examination of 50 women with Turner's syndrome. *Acta Neurologica Scandinavica, 54*, 359–365.

Van Vliet, G., & Collu, R. (1993). Treatment of Turner syndrome with growth hormone. *Journal of Pediatrics, 122*, 671.

Waber, D. (1979). Neuropsychological aspects of Turner syndrome. *Developmental Medicine and Child Neurology, 21*, 58–70.

Watanabe, M., Zinn, A., Page, D., & Nishimoto, T. (1993). Functional equivalence of human X- and Y-linked isoforms of ribosomal protein S4, consistent with a role in Turner syndrome. *Nature Genetics, 4*, 268–274.

Weiss, E., Loevy, H., Saunders, A., Pruzansky, S., & Rosenthal, I. (1982). Monozygotic twins discordant for Ullrich–Turner syndrome. *American Journal of Medical Genetics, 13*, 389–399.

Williams, J., Richman, L., & Yarbrough, D. (1991). A comparison of memory and attention in Turner syndrome and learning disability. *Journal of Pediatric Psychology, 16*, 585–593.

Yakovlev, P., & Lecours, A. (1967). The myelogenetic cycles of regional matura-
     tion of the brain. In A. Minkowski (Ed.), *Regional development of the brain
     in early life* (pp. 3–69). Oxford: Blackwell Scientific.
Zinn, A., Page, D., & Fisher, E. (1993). Turner syndrome: The case of the missing
     sex chromosome. *Trends in Genetics, 9,* 90–93.

14

Fetal Alcohol Syndrome

Audrey Don
Byron P. Rourke

Fetal alcohol syndrome (FAS) is a dysgenic disorder caused by the teratogenic effects of alcohol on the developing fetus. Children with FAS have characteristic facies, growth retardation, and central nervous system (CNS) effects, which often include mental retardation or other impairments in cognitive functioning (Sokol & Clarren, 1989).

HISTORY

Although references throughout history testify to alcohol's ability to intoxicate and cause harm, few involve drinking during pregnancy. The first extensive historical references to alcohol's teratogenic effects come from 18th-century England. At that time, during England's "gin epidemic," maternal alcohol abuse was identified as harmful to the fetus (Abel, 1984; Rosett & Weiner, 1984). The College of Physicians cautioned that consumption of gin during pregnancy resulted in "weak, feeble, and distempered children" (Report to Parliament, 1736, quoted in Abel, 1984, p. 11).

Recognition of alcohol's teratogenic effects seemed to disappear during the 19th century and the first half of the 20th century. Poor nurture was thought to explain the increased mortality and behavioral problems observed in children of alcoholic mothers (Abel, 1984; Rosett & Weiner, 1984).

It was not until the second half of the 20th century that FAS was identified. It was at this time that the impact of alcohol on the developing fetus was once again recognized by the medical profession. In 1968, Lemoine, Harousseau, Borteyru, and Menuet published a study of 127 children born to alcoholic parents. These children were found to exhibit a recognizable pattern of developmental delay and morphological anomalies that identified them as children of alcoholics. The 1968 study was published in France and did not receive widespread attention until Jones and Smith, working independently in the United States, recognized the same clinically distinct pattern of major and minor anomalies and named it "fetal alcohol syndrome" (Jones & Smith, 1973; Jones, Smith, Ulleland, & Streissguth, 1973).

IDENTIFICATION OF FAS

As noted above, FAS is diagnosed according to the presence of (1) characteristic facies, (2) growth retardation, and (3) CNS dysfunction. Signs of abnormality in each of these three areas are necessary to establish the diagnosis of FAS (Sokol & Clarren, 1989). In addition, a history of maternal alcohol use during pregnancy should be available to corroborate the diagnosis (Caruso & ten Bensel, 1993).

The characteristic facies include short palpebral fissures, microcephaly, flattened philtrum, thin upper lip, and flattened maxilla. The presence of a single feature is not significant, but several in combination are diagnostic (Rosett & Weiner, 1984).

Growth deficiency is usually of prenatal onset and continues postnatally. Typically, the child is below the 10th centile for height and weight, with weight being more negatively affected than height (Rosett & Weiner, 1984; Sokol & Clarren, 1989). In other words, affected children are small and thin. In some cases, postnatal growth retardation may not be apparent for 1 to 2 years after birth (Rosett & Weiner, 1984).

CNS involvement is characterized by neurological, developmental, and behavioral and/or intellectual abnormalities that may include microcephaly, tremulousness, motor problems, developmental delays, hyperactivity, intellectual deficits, and learning disabilities (Burd & Martsolf, 1989; Rosett & Weiner, 1984; Sokol & Clarren, 1989).

ALCOHOL TERATOGENESIS AND FAS

Alcohol's effects on the fetus differ, depending on the timing, dose, length of exposure, and individual maternal and fetal characteristics. The effects of alcohol (technically, ethanol) toxicity on the fetus range from mild, with CNS manifestations such as learning disabilities and/or distractibility predominating, to most severe, resulting in fetal death (Rosett & Weiner, 1984). FAS occurs toward the severe end of the spectrum, and develops most commonly in infants of chronically alcoholic women.

Although the diagnosis of FAS is based on the presence of the aforementioned characteristics, alcohol-affected children without characteristic facies may also demonstrate severe cognitive deficits (Caruso & ten Bensel, 1993; Clarren & Smith, 1978; Jones et al., 1973; Little, Snell, Rosenfeld, Gilstrap, & Gant, 1990). Overall, significantly higher rates of perinatal death and prematurity occur in the offspring of alcoholic women. About one-third of the infants born to these women exhibit the full syndrome (Adams & Victor, 1989; Caruso & ten Bensel, 1993; Clarren & Smith, 1978; Jones et al., 1973; Little et al., 1990).

A diverse range of additional abnormalities has been reported in association with FAS. Currently, it is unknown how many of these defects are related to alcohol teratogenesis and how many may be coincidental. Controlled prenatal ethanol exposure, available in animal studies, has established a causal link between prenatal alcohol exposure and a wide range of birth defects and behavioral abnormalities similar to those noted in many children (with and without FAS) born to alcoholic women (Driscoll, Streissguth, & Riley, 1990; Goodlett & West, 1992; Riley, Barron, & Hannigan, 1986). However, a causal link between prenatal alcohol exposure and symptoms associated with, but not diagnostic of, FAS in humans has not been widely accepted by the medical profession (Caruso & ten Bensel, 1993; Burd & Martsolf, 1989; Sokol & Clarren, 1989).

Because of the range of effects of alcohol teratogenesis, the diagnosis of FAS necessarily represents an artificial distinction between individuals affected severely enough to be diagnosed with FAS and those who are apparently less affected. Although similar criteria for the diagnosis of FAS are generally used in Europe, a system of levels, indicative of the severity of manifestations, is used in some countries (e.g., France). In such countries, the diagnosis of FAS may include individuals who do not meet the North American criteria for FAS (Burd & Martsolf, 1989; Lemoine & Lemoine, 1992).

The terms "possible fetal alcohol effects" or "fetal alcohol effects" (both abbreviated FAE), and "alcohol-related birth defects" (ARBD), have been used by clinicians and researchers to categorize birth defects that are not diagnostic of FAS but are thought to be caused by prenatal alcohol exposure (Streissguth, 1990; Abel, 1984; Rosett & Weiner, 1984; Streissguth & LaDue, 1987; Sokol & Clarren, 1989). However, a lack of consensus about the definition and application of these terms to human subjects has limited research. At this time, FAS remains the diagnosable focus of human studies.

ASSOCIATED SYMPTOMATOLOGY

Many associated, though not diagnostic, facial and anatomical anomalies have been reported in patients with FAS. Facial aberrations include the following: epicanthal folds, underdeveloped chin, cleft palate, short up-turned nose, and a flat nasal bridge (described in younger children). Additional anatomical anomalies include cardiac defects (particularly atrial septal defect), dislocation of the hips, flexion deformities of the finger, a limited range of motion of other joints, scoliosis (especially in adolescents), anomalous external genitalia, and capillary hemangiomata (Caruso & ten Bensel, 1993; Jones & Smith, 1973; Jones et al., 1973). Associated neuroanatomical abnormalities include hydrocephaly, neuro-glial meningeal heterotopies, cortical neuronal disorganization, agenesis of the corpus callosum, cerebellar and brain stem abnormalities, and (rarely), neural tube defects (Caruso & ten Bensel, 1993; Clarren, Ells-worth, Sumi, Streissguth, & Smith, 1978; Clarren & Smith, 1978; Galofre, 1987; Schenker et al., 1990).

    Associated CNS dysfunction in infants is noted in the forms of hyper-acusis, irritability, poor suck, and (less often), seizure disorders (Adams & Victor, 1989, Caruso & ten Bensel, 1993; Clarren & Smith, 1978; Jones et al., 1973). In older children, mild alterations in cerebellar function and hypotonicity have been reported (Clarren & Smith, 1978; Marcus, 1987). However, findings from neurological examinations of FAS pa-tients have rarely been reported—either because few affected children exhibit distinct neurological abnormalities, or because the cognitive defi-cits are so predominant that they receive greater attention.

    In a clinical sample of nine children with FAS, Marcus (1987) re-ported that five displayed abnormal neurological findings, whereas the remaining four had normal neurological exams. The symptoms common to the five affected children included kinetic tremor and axial ataxia. Three of the children were dysarthric and displayed dysdiadochokinesis. In one, tendon reflexes were generally decreased. Three of these five children were diagnosed with attention deficit disorder; two were men-tally retarded; and one had epilepsy. The clinical findings from the five affected patients suggest cerebellar dysfunction and diffuse cortical dam-age. Although all children diagnosed with FAS exhibit CNS effects, char-acteristic facial dysmorphology, and growth retardation, the result of Marcus's (1987) neurological examination of these nine FAS patients illustrates the variability that occurs in the manifestations of the syndrome.

DIFFERENTIAL DIAGNOSIS

Clarren and Smith (1978) reported a superficial resemblance to the de Lange syndrome in a few severely affected children with FAS. In addi-tion, two children with extensive prenatal alcohol exposure were reported to resemble patients with Noonan syndrome (Hall & Orenstein, 1974).

The DiGeorge syndrome has also been mentioned in relationship to FAS. Amman, Wara, Cowan, Barrett, and Stiehm (1982) reported four cases of DiGeorge syndrome in infants born to alcoholic mothers. Facial abnormalities and CNS deficits are noted in both syndromes, and a causal link between maternal alcoholism and DiGeorge syndrome was suggested. Common to each of these disorders are patterns of developmental malformation. Generally, however, the FAS phenotype is distinct and is not often confused with other syndromes of developmental malformation.

NEUROPATHOLOGY

The neuropathology associated with FAS occurs as a result of disrupted development of potentially normal neuronal tissue by alcohol teratogenesis, rather than as a result of degeneration of existing tissue. Three possible mechanisms have been postulated for alcohol's teratogenic effects on the fetus. Alcohol (or acetaldehyde) is hypothesized (1) to impair placental–fetal blood flow, resulting in transient hypoxia to the fetus; (2) to derange prostaglandin balance; and/or (3) to have a direct effect upon such cellular processes as protein synthesis, membrane composition, and cell–cell interaction (Schenker et al., 1990).

Malnutrition has been suggested as a possible contributing factor (alcoholics tend to suffer from malnutrition); however, its effects are not considered primary. Children born to severely malnourished women during World War II "were small and often premature, but these infants did not show the pattern of malformations that characterizes the fetal alcohol syndrome" (Adams & Victor, 1989, p. 884).

Although the exact mechanisms by which alcohol exerts its teratogenetic effects are unknown, the means by which alcohol reaches the fetus is known. Once ingested, alcohol is soluble in water and fat; it readily diffuses across cell membranes, included those of the placenta. In the womb, fetal alcohol levels are usually comparable to maternal levels (Abel, 1984). In the fetus, alcohol is absorbed by all tissues. Highest concentrations of alcohol appear in the liver, pancreas, kidney, lung, thymus, heart, and brain (Abel, 1984).

> In the brain, alcohol tends to concentrate more in grey matter, which has greater water content than white matter. In the telencephalon, the areas of highest concentrations are the visual cortex, hippocampus, caudate nucleus, and putamen. The cerebellum, dentate, fastigal nucleus and lateral denticulate also attain relative high concentrations. (Abel, 1984, p. 38)

Given this information, it would appear logical to look for specific neuroanatomical changes in the above-mentioned areas. However, the effects of alcohol teratogenesis are extremely time- and dose-dependent. An organ is most vulnerable to toxic insult during its period of greatest growth and development. This has been demonstrated experimentally in animals for a number of toxins (Light, Serbus, & Santiago, 1989). On the basis of this model, alcohol may be expected to affect the developing fetus differently over the course of prenatal development. The fact that FAS occurs in the children of chronically alcoholic women suggests that FAS reflects an accumulation of pathologies that develop throughout gestation. As alcoholics follow varied patterns of drinking, the manifestations of FAS are expected to vary, and do in each case. Although all individuals diagnosed with FAS show facial dysmorphology, growth retardation, and CNS effects, the extent, severity, and variety of associated deficits differ widely across affected individuals.

Knowledge of the neuroanatomical changes associated with FAS has developed through limited human studies (based on a few autopsy and magnetic resonance imaging [MRI] case reports) and through animal models of FAS. Animal models of FAS have been produced in rats, beagles, swine, nonhuman primates, and other animals. Affected animals show similar facial dysmorphology, growth retardation, and CNS effects (Clarren et al., 1990; Dexter, Tumbleson, Decker, & Middleton, 1980; Driscoll et al., 1990; Ellis & Pick, 1980; Riley, 1990).

Animal Studies: Neuroanatomy

Animal studies provide a model of FAS in controlled experimental situations. The evidence of reliable anatomical, neurological, and behavioral defects apparent in animals exposed prenatally to alcohol provides sound evidence of alcohol's teratogenic properties. In animal studies, widespread neuroanatomical and neurochemical changes are reported. Differential vulnerability of cells to the effects of alcohol is noted. This section and the next one provide a sampling of the neuropathological findings from animal research.

Dexter et al. (1980) found microcephaly, anencephaly, cranial bone hypoplasia, and microphthalmia on gross inspection of miniature swine exposed prenatally to levels of alcohol that resulted in facial dysmorphology similar to that found in FAS.

On a more microscopic level, with a focus on the cerebellum, Pierce, Goodlett, and West (1989) reported that Purkinje cells in the cerebellum were most notably reduced in rats exposed prenatally to ethanol. In addition, cerebellar granule cells were significantly reduced in the granular layer, but not in the external granular layer. The lobules in the cerebellum were also affected differentially, with lobule 1 being most affected. Similar changes in human cases may explain the hypotonicity, axial ataxia, kinetic tremor, and poor coordination reported in children with FAS (Clarren & Smith, 1978; Marcus, 1987).

In another study, reduction in mossy fiber zinc was found in the hippocampus of rats subjected to moderate prenatal alcohol exposure that did not result in growth retardation (Savage, Montano, Paxton, & Kasarskis, 1989). The behavioral consequences of mossy fiber zinc reduction in fetal alcohol rats are not currently understood (Savage et al., 1989). However, experimentally induced depletion of whole-hippo-campal zinc through zinc-deficient diets causes impairments in long-term potentiation and learning. Learning disabilities are commonly reported in children with FAS and may be a result of alcohol-induced hippocampal damage (Burd & Martsolf, 1989; Driscoll et al., 1990; Rosett & Weiner, 1984; Sokol & Clarren, 1989).

Delayed myelinization and thinned myelin in the rat optic nerve were found in rats exposed prenatally and postnatally (third-trimester equivalency) to ethanol (Phillips, Krueger, & Rydquist, 1991). These findings are of special interest in relationship to the white matter model of Nonverbal Learning Disabilities (NLD).

Under electron-microscopic examination, neurons of nonhuman primates exposed prenatally to alcohol were found to display mitochon-drial abnormalities and changes in the distribution of organelles. It is unclear which functional effects are associated with these cellular changes (Clarren et al., 1990).

The range of abnormalities that has been discovered in association with alcohol teratogenesis is astonishing. On a macroscopic level, reduced brain size is the most common finding, although gross structural alter-ations have been reported. On a microscopic level, widespread cellular changes have been reported (Clarren et al., 1990; Dexter et al., 1980). In almost all areas investigated, aberrations have been found. Unfortu-nately, many more studies are needed before a comprehensive picture of the neuroanatomical changes associated with prenatal alcohol expo-sure can be catalogued. It is also important to examine alcohol-induced neurochemical changes, as brain functioning is determined by both struc-ture and chemistry.

Animal Studies: Neurochemistry

Information on neurochemical abnormalities has been obtained almost exclusively through animal studies. Species, ethanol dose, timing of dose, and outcome examinations vary considerably from experiment to experi-ment. Endocrinological studies, with a few exceptions, are notably lack-ing. In a rare exception, Gottesfeld and Silverman (1987) reported that prenatal alcohol exposure in rats was associated with early hypothyroid-ism that was restored to euthyroidism by postnatal day 14.

Greater attention has been given to the effects of prenatal alcohol exposure on brain neurotransmitters. Despite inconsistencies in method-ology and results, Druse (1992) reported that some conclusions about effects on neurotransmitters could be drawn.

Of the neurotransmitters, serotonin and dopamine have received the greatest attention. Serotonergic neurons, found in the raphe nuclei in the brain stem, mature relatively early and influence the development and maturation of target tissues. Rats receiving doses of alcohol that produce effects similar to FAS display considerable decreases (50%) in whole-brain serotonin concentrations. The decreases are most marked in the motor cortex.

There are conflicting findings on the effects of ethanol on whole-brain concentrations of dopamine. In her review of animal studies, Druse (1992) concluded that exposure to higher ethanol doses results in dopa-mine or dopamine receptor deficiency in the hypothalamus, in striatum, and possibly in the frontal cortex. However, transient increases in dopa-mine concentrations have been found at some dose schedules (Clarren et al., 1990).

Studies of norepinephrine, acetylcholine, and gamma-aminobutyric acid in fetal alcohol-affected animals also show changes. Most often, decreased concentrations of these neurotransmitters are found in specific areas of the brain (Clarren et al., 1990; Druse, 1992).

In the investigations to date, chemical changes that are likely to affect brain functioning have been reported in almost all areas investigated. In neuroanatomical studies, widespread changes in brain structure, primarily at the microscopic level, are reported. Unfortunately, each study necessarily focuses on limited aspects of brain structure and chemistry. Much more research, investigating a wider range of brain structure and chemistry, is needed before definitive conclusions about the most salient and important changes associated with alcohol terato-genesis can be drawn.

Because of the wide range of effects of ethanol teratogenesis, it is difficult to determine which neurobehavioral manifestations are pro-duced by which neuroanatomical or neurochemical changes. Changes in specific structures (e.g., the hippocampus and cerebellum) may be re-flected in particular symptoms such as learning disabilities and motor problems. Given the widespread neuroantomical and neurochemical changes, many clinical manifestations of FAS appear to result from the interaction of many dysfunctional systems.

Animal studies provide important clues to understanding FAS. How-ever, human studies (e.g., MRI and autopsy studies) are needed to dis-cover how alcohol teratogenesis specifically affects the human brain.

Human Studies: Neuropathology

Autopsy case reports of infants, stillborn or surviving only a few months (e.g., Clarren et al., 1978; Galofre, 1987), provide a sampling of the neuropathological changes found in human cases. Generally, the characteristics associated with FAS are compatible with life. In the autopsy reports, the development of the affected infant was severely compromised as a result of alcohol toxicity and/or poor nurture by the alcoholic mothers in the perinatal period. Thus, these infants are likely to reflect the severe end of the spectrum of alcohol's toxicity to the fetus. Less severe, but similar, neuropathology is thought to occur in children and adults with FAS.

In autopsy studies, Clarren et al. (1978) found similar malformations in the brains of four infants of alcoholic mothers. All brains showed malformations caused by failure or interruption of neuronal and glial migrations; however, the location of the malformations varied from subject to subject. Leptomeningeal, neuroglial heterotopias (sheets of aberrant neural and glial tissue that cover parts of the brain surface) were found in three subjects. Extensive brain disorganization, as a result of errors of neuronal and glial migration, was found in two of these cases. In one case, widespread cortical, nuclear, and white matter dysplasia was found. Cerebellar and brain stem anomalies produced hydrocephalus in two cases and had no discernible effect on head size in another.

Interestingly, only two of the four patients exhibited the facial dysmorphology required to meet diagnostic criteria for FAS. The fact that severe brain malformations and fetal death occurred as a result of prenatal alcohol exposure in infants who did not meet diagnostic criteria for FAS suggests that several possibly independent factors are important in the development of brain pathology and facial dysmorphology.

In 1987, Galofre reported on an autopsy of a 4-month-old infant with FAS. Neuropathological abnormalities in this patient included microcephaly, uncovered rostral region of the insula, glial meningeal heterotopies, disordered arrangement of cortical neurons, and cortical cerebellar displasies and heterotopies. Similar morphological changes have been reported in the brains of other children affected with FAS (Clarren et al., 1990).

In addition, abnormalities of the dendritic spines were found, similar to those reported in a number of human diseases in which low intellectual performance is the most common clinical sign (e.g., Down syndrome). Galofre (1987) has suggested that the abnormalities of the dendritic spines, if typically present in the brains of children with FAS, may be a morphological substrate for mental retardation.

Human Studies: Radiology and Electroencephalography

Recently, Mattson et al. (1992), Knight et al. (1993), and Loock, Conry, and Clark (1993) reported the results of MRI, electroencephalographic

(EEG), and positron emission tomography (PET) scan studies of individuals with FAS, and provided glimpses of the neuroanatomical effects in living children.

Mattson et al. (1992) reported on the results of MRI scans and EEG studies of two mentally retarded boys with FAS. Reduced volumes of the cerebrum, cerebellum, caudate, lenticular nucleus, cortical grey matter, diencephalon, corpus callosum (in one case, agenesis of the corpus callosum), and cerebral ventricles, as well as abnormal neuronal migration, were found. The EEGs for both boys were moderately abnormal; however, no asymmetry or focal abnormalities were found.

In a preliminary report of the results of MRIs of high-functioning children with FAS (IQ > 70), Knight et al. (1993) found no abnormalities of the size or position of the ventricles, no focal areas of abnormal increased signal intensity intracranially, and no midline shift or mass effect, with the single exception of marked hypoplasia of the pituitary gland in one child with FAS.

Loock et al. (1993) combined MRI and PET scanning in a case study of a 16-year-old female with FAS. From the MRI, the structural integrity of the brain appeared normal. However, the findings of the PET scan suggested abnormalities of caudate and cortical glucose metabolism. The mean rate of cortical glucose metabolism was two standard deviations above normal, while the relative caudate values were significantly below normal.

This study suggests that even when the brain of an individual with FAS appears normal on an MRI, metabolic abnormalities may occur. Autopsy and animal studies point to additional brain abnormalities that cannot be imaged through MRI.

Both animal and human studies have demonstrated varied microscopic changes in cell migration, cell densities, cell development, function, neurochemistry, and organization in the brain affected by fetal alcohol. On a more macroscopic level, the most common finding is reduced brain growth without structural abnormalities, although varied structural abnormalities, such as agenesis of the corpus callosum, cerebellar and brain stem disorganization, hydrocephaly, and leptomeningeal heterotopias, have been found. The observed changes reflect disruptions occurring over the course of gestation and neonatal development.

DEVELOPMENTAL ASPECTS OF FAS PATHOLOGY

Although the pathology associated with FAS varies across affected individuals, developmental characteristics of the fetus allow a probable dating of the different effects associated with prenatal alcohol exposure.

The characteristic facial features that occur with FAS point to disruption in development occurring during the first trimester of human gestation, when major organs are formed (Ellis & Pick, 1980). During this time, alcohol may affect the cell membrane and alter cell migration, which in turn would be expected to alter embryonic organization of tissue. The structural malformations of the cerebral cortex, corpus callosum, and anterior commissure that Clarren (1986) and Mattson et al. (1992) found are most likely to have occurred during this period.

During the second trimester, physical growth and brain development are most at risk. According to Clarren, (1986), the neuroglial heterotopias and cortical dysgenesis that he found on autopsy of alcohol-affected fetuses are most likely to have occurred during this period of development.

During the third trimester, the brain undergoes its most rapid growth and neurophysiologic organization. Secondary and tertiary sulci develop during the last few months before birth (CIBA-Geigy, 1974). Clarren (1986) found cerebral destruction of white matter occurring in some of the autopsies that he performed on FAS infants. This is indicative of damage occurring during this period. One of the most common findings, reflecting third-trimester effects of alcohol teratogenesis, is a reduction in brain growth that is dose-dependent (Pierce et al., 1989). In addition, postmortem examinations of animals exposed to alcohol during their period of rapid brain growth show abnormal glial migration, indicating possible abnormalities of oligodendroglial cells and delayed myelin development (Light et al., 1989).

During the first year of life, an intense period of myelinization occurs within the brain. Alcohol inhibits lactation in high concentrations, but at lower doses it diffuses into the mother's milk and reaches the infant. Results of animal studies suggest that alcohol exposure at this stage leads to reduction of selected neuronal populations in the brain. Myelinization is also delayed, and myelin accumulation is reduced (Lancaster, Phillips, Patsalos, & Wiggens, 1984; Pierce et al., 1989). Severity of white matter destruction is dose dependent. Partial mitigation of this effect was found when animals received nutritional supplementation (Lancaster et al., 1984).

EPIDEMIOLOGY

FAS affects children without regard for sex, nationality, or race. Since Lemoine et al.'s 1968 description of children affected by maternal alcohol abuse, FAS has been reported in many countries around the world (Abel, 1984). Studies in Roubaix, France; Seattle, Washington; and Goteborg, Sweden yielded a prevalence rate of approximately 1 in 750 live births

(Dehaene et al., 1981; Hanson, Streissguth, & Smith, 1978; Olegard et al., 1979, cited in Streissguth & LaDue, 1987).

Prevalence varies as a function of the rate of maternal alcohol abuse. Incidence of FAS on some Native reservations in North America has been reported to be as high as 1 in 99 births. And on those same reservations, the incidence of FAE has been estimated at 1 out of every 49 births (Sokol, Miller, & Reed, 1980; Streissguth, 1990). Current worldwide frequency of FAS is estimated at 1.9 per 1000 live births. On the basis of this estimate, Abel and Sokol (1987) suggested that FAS is the leading recognized disorder in which mental retardation occurs.

The true prevalence of FAS is likely to be higher. There are several reasons for this. First, the diagnosis is just over 20 years old, and many primary physicians are still inadequately informed about the diagnosis. Second, drinking during pregnancy is rarely assessed, so that the potential for FAS in the developing fetus cannot be evaluated. Third, poor prenatal care is often reported among mothers of FAS infants, so that these mothers are less available for evaluation of their gestational drinking patterns (Caruso & ten Bensel, 1993). And fourth, even when drinking is assessed, the information may not be considered in diagnosing associated problems in the resulting children (Little & Streissguth, 1981).

In a study of the records of more than 28,000 deliveries of women in Dallas County, Texas from September 1977 to December 1980, Little et al. (1990) found information regarding alcohol use for only 5602 of these cases. Of these, 38 women reported a history of alcohol abuse during pregnancy. Although physical features consistent with FAS were described in the medical records of 5 of the resultant children, a diagnosis of FAS, FAE, or ARBD did not appear in any of the medical records.

Lastly, developmental characteristics add to the probability of a lower estimate of FAS prevalence. The best time to recognize FAS is probably during early childhood, rather than at birth. During early childhood, the characteristic facies, growth retardation, and CNS effects are most distinct (Rosett, 1980; Sokol & Clarren, 1989; Streissguth, 1990). However, pediatricians are rarely schooled in diagnosing FAS, and information concerning the maternal prenatal alcohol consumption behavior is often lacking; thus, the probability of FAS is again often overlooked. This is especially true because most children with FAS are raised by someone other than their natural mothers, because of the mothers' alcoholism and resultant inability to care for the children (Abel, 1984; Burd & Martsolf, 1989; Rosett & Weiner, 1984; Streissguth et al., 1991).

All children born to women who abuse alcohol are at risk. However, not all infants born to severely alcoholic women develop FAS. Increased maternal age, one or more previous pregnancies, already having an FAS- or FAE-affected child, and longer duration of heavy alcohol abuse have been suggested as contributing factors (Sokol et al., 1980; Streissguth &

LaDue, 1987). However, in a study of pregnant teens, Cornelius et al. (1993) found that the resultant infants were more negatively affected by prenatal alcohol exposure than were the resultant infants from two comparison samples of adults reporting greater amounts of alcohol consumption during pregnancy. In addition, teratogenic effects appeared to depend on both maternal and fetal genetic characteristics. Dizygotic twins of alcoholic mothers have been observed to be differentially affected: Mental retardation is sometimes seen in one twin and not the other (Streissguth & LaDue, 1987).

As long as women abuse alcohol during pregnancy, FAS will continue to occur. The fact that FAS occurs as a result of a known, avoidable cause argues strongly for efforts directed toward prevention. The preventability of FAS is both its greatest tragedy and its greatest hope.

TREATMENT

By the time FAS is diagnosed, developmental changes are irreversible, and treatment is necessarily palliative. The most common childhood treatment is Ritalin, prescribed to reduce the hyperactivity associated with FAS. Differing degrees of success are noted with this medication. Remedial education and a supportive structured environment are also used to help the child grow intellectually and socially and gain behavioral control (Caruso & ten Bensel, 1993; Guinta & Streissguth, 1988; LaDue, Streissguth, & Randels, 1992).

PREVENTION

Although no current treatments are available to cure or to lessen the impact of prenatal alcohol exposure, animal research and clinical studies have provided suggestions for mitigation of the effects of such exposure. Interestingly, aspirin may mitigate the effects of alcohol's exposure on the fetus. A proposed mechanism of alcohol pathogenesis is deranged prostaglandin balance. Alcohol has been shown to influence prostaglandin activity, and it has been hypothesized that this influence increases prostaglandin activity. Because aspirin inhibits prostaglandin synthesis, it may help prevent some of the defects associated with alcohol teratogenesis (Schenker et al., 1990).

Little research has been carried out to test this hypothesis, but aspirin does appear to have a protective effect if given before ethanol ingestion in animals. When it is given after alcohol ingestion, protective effects are not noted (Schenker et al., 1990). In a recent prospective clinical study, Martier, Sokol, and Ager (1993) assessed aspirin use in conjunction with prenatal alcohol intake (they controlled for effects of smoking, other drugs, maternal risk, and demographics), and found that aspirin use was associated with a decreased negative impact for prenatal alcohol exposure.

Vitamin and trace metal deficiencies in alcoholics may also contribute to the effects of alcohol teratogenesis. Providing supplements of these vitamins and trace metals or minerals to pregnant drinking mothers may also reduce the effects of ethanol on the fetus. Of the vitamin deficiencies seen in alcoholics, folate deficiency is the most common. However, folate supplementation did not lessen the effects of prenatal exposure in a rat model of FAS (Schenker et al., 1990).

Zinc deficiency has also been noted. And zinc deficiencies are thought to cause fetal malformations similar to those caused by ethanol. In a study of zinc-deficient pregnant women, zinc supplementation seemed beneficial for the infant. However, these women were not alcoholic, and it remains to be seen whether zinc supplementation would prove helpful for the fetuses of alcoholic women (Schenker et al., 1990).

Gottesfeld and Silverman (1987) reported on the reversal of developmental delays associated with prenatal alcohol exposure in rats that were treated with thyroid hormone (triiodothyronine, or T_3). They found that exposure to alcohol *in utero* was associated with early hypothyroidism that was restored to euthyroidism by postnatal day 14. Treatment with T_3 served to reverse the ethanol-induced delay in appearance of dental eruption and eye opening in the resultant rat pups. However, alcohol-induced delay in reaching other milestones, such as the righting reflex and acoustic startle response, did not respond to T_3. The role of thyroid dysfunction in alcohol teratogenicity is poorly understood and the results from the Gottesfeld and Silverman (1987) study suggest a fascinating direction for further research.

Currently, the only treatment to eliminate FAS is prevention. Education about the effects of alcohol on the fetus is one tool in working toward this goal. Another is social nonacceptance of alcohol ingestion during pregnancy. These tools proved effective in one Aleut village. With the development of a social culture that did not accept drunken behavior, and that educated and treated individuals who drank excessively, a marked decline in the incidence of FAS occurred (Streissguth, 1990).

DEVELOPMENTAL EFFECTS ON THE EXPRESSION OF FAS

From infancy through adulthood, FAS-affected individuals are handicapped by their abnormal morphogenesis as they adapt to the world. Despite wide variability of outcome, FAS-affected individuals manifest a general pattern of deficits that evolves in expression with development and changes in environmental demands. The following sections describe the general pattern of development observed in FAS-affected individuals.

Infancy and Early Childhood

At birth, infants with FAS have been reported to suck and sleep poorly, and to be irritable and hyperactive, although these manifestations may be missed or absent. Most often, weak reflexes and increased startle have been noted (Adams & Victor, 1989; Sokol & Clarren, 1989; Streissguth, 1990). These initial symptoms may be manifestations of retarded prenatal development, CNS deficiencies, and/or withdrawal from alcohol.

The infancy and early childhood of individuals with FAS is characterized by developmental delays, poor appetite, sleep disturbances, delayed or poorly articulated speech, hyperactivity, and motor problems. Motor problems are manifested as tremors, motor incoordination, weak grasp, difficulty with eye–hand coordination, and slowed motor performance (Barr, Streissguth, Darby, & Sampson, 1990; Rosett & Weiner, 1984; Streissguth, 1990; Streissguth & LaDue, 1987).

Because these children are very small, developmental delays are often overlooked. In addition, FAS-affected infants are usually described as socially adapted. They have a notable lack of stranger anxiety, which may be mistakenly interpreted as an indication of social advancement, and they are fearless in new social situations. Developmental delays in the smaller-than-average infant, in conjunction with seemingly normal or advanced social skills, often falsely lead the pediatrician and caregiver to expect the child to outgrow his or her delays.

However, during the preschool years, the early fearlessness and lack of stranger anxiety evolve into an extreme lack of caution that is prominent and problematic. Hyperactivity continues and becomes the most frequently noted behavioral problem. Motor problems remain, and developmental and speech delays are not outgrown (Streissguth & LaDue, 1987). In addition, chronic serous otitis media, probably secondary to eustachian tube dysfunction associated with maxillary hypoplasia, is a common problem in children with FAS. Episodes of serous otitis media may cause intermittent hearing loss and/or lead to permanent hearing loss that further interferes with normal language development (Streissguth, Clarren, & Jones, 1985).

Elementary School Years

When the child with FAS enters school, additional demands on the child may make deficits more evident. Hyperactivity persists into the early grade school years, and attentional problems may become more problematic. Along with poor attention, reaction times are slowed, and deficits in response inhibition and habituation are apparent (Streissguth, Landesman-Dwyer, Martin, & Smith, 1980; Streissguth, 1986). These problems alone are enough to cause academic difficulties in affected individuals.

Moreover, intellectual deficits, including mental retardation, are common with FAS and are often recognized when the affected individual enters school. In clinical studies, approximately half of affected children are mentally retarded (IQ < 70) (Jones, Smith, & Streissguth, 1974; LaDue et al., 1992; Lemoine & Lemoine, 1992; Streissguth et al., 1991). Although intellectual deficiency is common, it does not explain the attentional and impulse control problems; in FAS-affected children with normal IQs, the CNS effects of the syndrome are most often manifested in conspicuous attentional deficits, hyperactivity, and persistent learning problems.

Specific learning difficulties in arithmetic are especially prominent, reflecting difficulties with abstract concepts. Writing and other graphomotor skills are often acquired with difficulty, as a result of fine motor coordination problems, which in turn may slow learning in the early grades. Memory problems are also noted during the grade-school years (Streissguth, 1990).

After initial difficulties, reading and spelling may be mastered. The children often seem to be doing better in reading and spelling than would be predicted on the basis of their Full Scale IQs. However, as these children get older, reading comprehension is found to be poor in comparison to word-recognition. Sight reading and spelling tend to stand out, in later years as their strongest academic skills. Arithmetic difficulties are especially noted when multiplication is introduced (Streissguth & LaDue, 1987).

Social difficulties, often overlooked during early childhood, become more apparent during the elementary school years. The child with FAS is easily influenced by others and does not appear to be able to predict or understand the consequences of his or her actions or their effects on others. Despite difficulty in understanding social rules and expectations, these children are often seen as friendly, perhaps overfriendly, and in need of constant interaction with others (Abel, 1984; Rosett & Weiner, 1984; Streissguth & LaDue, 1987). Despite their poor language and social skills, children with FAS are noted for their prolific verbalization, which resembles the hyperverbal speech patterns or "cocktail party syndrome" seen in other developmental disorders. In addition, because the children are hyperactive and lack impulse control, they do not appear physically or mentally slow, as do children with Down syndrome. Because of this, and their engaging manner, they continue to be seen as more capable than is actually the case (Burd & Martsolf, 1989; Guinta & Streissguth, 1988).

Adolescence and Early Adulthood

Because the diagnosis of FAS is only a little over 20 years old, few studies of older adolescents and adult patients with FAS have been carried out. Two major longitudinal studies have been reported: one by Streissguth et el. (1991), and the other by Lemoine and Lemoine (1992).

The Streissguth et al. (1991) study represents the first systematic follow-up study of adolescent and adult manifestations of FAS and FAE. Physical characteristics; intellectual, academic, and adaptive functioning; and family environment were assessed in 61 individuals with FAS ($n = 43$) and FAE ($n = 18$). Because of the limitations inherent in clinical studies, full information was not always available on all patients.

In a 1992 paper, the France-based team of Lemoine and Lemoine reported on the long-term outcome for 105 individuals identified with FAS and FAE. Many of these individuals were originally described by Lemoine et al. in the 1968 study that first identified FAS. Individuals were classified according to three levels of diagnosis: severe FAS, light FAS, and without dysmorphology. Physical characteristics and intellectual, academic, vocational, and adaptive functioning were assessed.

These two studies reveal that the physical characteristics of FAS become less noticeable with maturity, whereas cognitive deficits persist and have an increasingly negative impact on the lives of the affected individuals (Lemoine & Lemoine, 1992; Streissguth et al, 1991). The specific findings of these and other, shorter-term studies are as follows.

The child with FAS may catch up in height and/or weight during the growth spurt occurring with puberty, although short stature remains common. Males tend to remain thin, while females tend to become heavy during puberty (Church & Gerkin, 1988; Lemoine & Lemoine, 1992; Streissguth et al., 1991). By the end of puberty, facial features may change with growth of the chin, nose, and midface, so that the face appears normalized and the dysmorphic features are less apparent (Lemoine & Lemoine, 1992; Streissguth et al., 1991). However, imbalance in the growth of the midface and mandible may lead to dental misalignments that require braces (Rosett & Weiner, 1984; Streissguth et al., 1985; Streissguth, 1990).

Hyperactivity tends to disappear by adolescence, but attentional, learning, and memory problems persist. In addition, judgment and adaptive behavior appear severely compromised (Lemoine & Lemoine, 1992; Streissguth, 1990; Streissguth et al., 1991). Repeated academic and social failure produce low self-esteem and motivation, and depression may result. Because of lack of social skills, continued lack of judgment, and suggestibility, these individuals are open to being exploited by "friends." Indiscriminate sexual activity and drinking, as well as criminal behavior, were reported in some adolescents with FAS (Lemoine & Lemoine, 1992; Streissguth et al., 1991; Streissguth & LaDue, 1987).

In adulthood, adaptive problems lead to difficulties in vocational placement and independent living. Arithmetic difficulties make money management problematic. When the affected adult is retarded, he or she often does not fit into programs designed for "typical" adults with mental retardation or Down syndrome, because of a relatively higher activity level and a greater number of behavioral problems. In the Streissguth et al. (1991) study, mentally retarded adolescents and adults with FAS exhibited two to four times more behavioral problems, as measured by the Maladaptive Behavior scale of the Vineland Adaptive Behavior Scales (VABS), than were noted in a comparable study of adolescents with Down syndrome (Harris, 1988).

Nonretarded FAS adults also have difficulty with vocational placement and independent living. Although these individuals may be able to perform adequately in school (except in arithmetic), they do not seem able to respond with sufficient flexibility in vocational and social situations (Lemoine & Lemoine, 1992; Streissguth et al., 1991; Streissguth & LaDue, 1987).

VARIABILITY AND SEVERITY OF FAS

Considerations

Just as alcohol's effects on the fetus differ, depending on the timing, dose, length of exposure, and maternal and fetal characteristics, manifestations of FAS also vary. Although all individuals diagnosed with FAS demonstrate symptomatology in the three areas of CNS effects, characteristic facial dysmorphology, and growth retardation, the severity of manifestations within each area varies widely.

The wide variability in expression of FAS points to a difficulty in diagnosis that arises because of the etiology of the syndrome. Teratogens, including alcohol, typically have a range of teratogenicity. Both animal studies and the results of human autopsy studies demonstrate that serious brain malformations can occur as a result of alcohol teratogenesis in the absence of facial dysmorphology. Findings of such brain malformations in animals and humans who do not fulfil the criteria for FAS suggests that FAS is too limited a diagnosis for the classification of all individuals suffering from severe effects of prenatal alcohol exposure.

In the United States, Burd and Martsolf (1989) have argued for a broader definition of FAS and for the elimination of the ill-defined FAE classification. In France, the diagnosis includes levels of severity, so that individuals diagnosed with FAS in that country may display a greater range of symptomatology than do those diagnosed in the United States and Canada (Burd & Martsolf, 1989; Lemoine & Lemoine, 1992). Research on the range and severity of alcohol teratogenicity in humans is limited by the artificial dichotomy created by the diagnostic classification of FAS. The following discussion of the variability of the syndrome is based primarily on research occurring in North America, although results from Lemoine and Lemoine's (1992) longitudinal study in France have also been incorporated.

Findings

One common finding is that the extent of craniofacial abnormalities is directly related to the degree of growth deficiency and intellectual deficit. In other words, children who exhibit the greatest degree of facial dysmorphology are most likely to be smallest and most negatively affected from a cognitive standpoint as well.

Another general finding is the occurrence of a positive dose–response curve in animal studies. This suggests that the severity of maternal alcoholism is positively correlated with the extent of fetal impairment (Streissguth et al., 1985; Streissguth et al., 1991).

Overall, the range of effects of FAS occurs within a normal distribution. In a follow-up study of 61 adolescents and adults with FAS (70% of the sample) and FAE, Streissguth et al. (1991) reported a normal distribution for such characteristics as height, head circumference, and IQ among FAS-affected individuals. However, the distribution was shifted downward—approximately two standard deviations (2 SD) below the mean—from that in the normal population. Lesser but similar shifts were found for the FAE sample.

For example, whereas the average head circumference for the FAS patients was 1.86 SD below the mean, 28% of the sample had normal head sizes. Height was more affected, as only 16% of the FAS patients were within 1 SD of the mean for height. IQ scores were also normally distributed, but shifted approximately 2 SD below average. The average Full Scale IQ of the FAS patients was 66, with scores ranging from 20 to 105. The results of this study are in agreement with those of other investigations, although one FAS patient with a Full Scale IQ of 118 has been reported (e.g., Clarren & Smith, 1978; Don, Kerns, Mateer, & Streissguth, 1994; Jones et al., 1974; Lemoine & Lemoine, 1992; Streissguth et al., 1991).

Although growth, head size, and Full Scale IQ were shifted approximately 2 *SD* below the norm, not all areas of cognitive functioning were equally affected. For example, Verbal IQ was more negatively affected than Performance IQ, which was, on average, 10 points higher than Verbal IQ.

In addition, Streissguth et al. (1991) reported that arithmetic deficits were the most characteristic learning disabilities. The average sight reading, spelling, and arithmetic grade levels of the sample (mean age = 17), as measured on the Wide Range Achievement Test—Revised (WRAT-R), were fourth grade, third grade, and second grade, respectively. Within the sample, considerable variability in academic functioning was noted. Several teenagers had age-appropriate sight reading and spelling skills, whereas some adults were functionally illiterate (Streissguth et al., 1991). These findings have been replicated in additional clinical samples (e.g., Clarren & Smith, 1978; Jones et al., 1974; Lemoine & Lemoine, 1992).

Very few studies have formally assessed adaptive functioning. In the Streissguth et al. (1991) study, mean adaptive levels, as measured by the VABS, were very low—age 9 equivalent for daily living skills, and age 6 equivalent for socialization skills. A few patients scored at age-appropriate levels in daily living skills, but none scored at age-appropriate levels for socialization skills (Streissguth et al., 1991). Patients with FAS thus perform within a range of adaptive functioning extending from near-average to extremely deficient.

Clinically, these patients appear to experience emotional decompensation as they mature, and do not adapt to the demands of maturity. This is especially true of the higher-functioning individuals (IQ > 80) who are aware of their deficits. They exhibit increased levels of depression, anger, antisocial behavior, and substance abuse during adolescence, and appear at risk for psychiatric disturbances (LaDue et al., 1992; Lemoine & Lemoine, 1992; Streissguth et al., 1991).

Although most individuals with FAS fall along the continuum described above, atypical cases have been reported. Nanson (1992) reported on six children who fulfilled criteria for both FAS and autism. In contrast to the overly talkative and overly intrusive characteristic of children with FAS, children with autism are characterized by extreme social withdrawal. Current research in autism is focused on the neurobiological aspects of the disorder. Because the incidences of dysmorphic features, mental retardation, and CNS deficits are increased in the autistic population, some similarities in etiology may occur in autism and FAS. Currently, it is unknown whether the concurrence of FAS and autism in these six individuals is coincidental or linked (Nanson, 1992).

In more typical cases of FAS, cognitive and behavioral deficits persisted as the most profound and significant consequences of FAS (Lemoine & Lemoine, 1992; Streissguth et al., 1991). Lemoine and Lemoine

(1992) noted behavior disorders and conspicuous instability "in every case" (p. 226), while Streissguth et al. (1991) reported that "maladaptive behaviors present the greatest challenge to treatment" in the long-term outcome of FAS patients (p. 1967).

The results of the Streissguth et al. (1991) study and the Lemoine and Lemoine (1992) study are important and point out the devastating long-term effects of FAS. However, the sample populations were clinically obtained, and as such may have been biased. In addition, many FAS-affected children grow up in environments that are unstable, largely because of their mothers' alcoholism (Streissguth et al., 1991). This lack of stability is likely to have a negative impact on the children's development. The children's own difficulties in adaptation may also have a negative effect upon their upbringing. Further research is needed to clarify the role of postnatal environments on the variability of outcome of FAS-affected individuals.

NEUROPSYCHOLOGICAL LITERATURE

Results from neuropsychological evaluations of FAS patients can provide information about a broad range of assets and deficits exhibited by FAS-affected individuals. In particular, this information may be used to provide insight into the cognitive and behavioral difficulties exhibited by individuals with FAS, and to create a detailed base of information from which to design treatment and intervention programs. Unfortunately, to date, few neuropsychological investigations of individuals with FAS have been published. Most studies of the cognitive functioning of individuals with FAS have been limited to measures of IQ and academic achievement (Streissguth, 1992).

To gain a greater understanding of the cognitive deficits associated with FAS, a few studies have included specific neuropsychological tests thought to be sensitive to the effects of alcohol teratogenesis (Carmichael Olson, Feldman, Streissguth, & Gonzales, 1994; Conry, 1990; Don et al., 1994; Gray & Streissguth, 1990; Kodituwakku et al., 1992; Mattson et al., 1992; Mattson, Sadoff, Delis, Jones, & Riley, 1993; Nanson & Hiscock, 1990). A brief review of these studies is presented in this section.

Carmichael Olson et al. (1994) compared the performance of 12 adolescents and young adults with FAS to a sample of 175 adolescents with minimal or no prenatal alcohol exposure. Seven of the group with FAS had IQ scores within the average range (86–118), and five had scores in the borderline range (70–80). Various measures of attention, memory, and executive functioning were used. These included Wechsler's Digits (forward) and the Seashore Rhythm Test as measures of auditory attention and working memory. A continuous-performance test using degraded visual stimuli was used as a measure of complex visual attention. The Stepping Stone Maze was used as a measure of visual–spatial memory. The Stepping Stone Maze (based on Milner's test of hippocampal function) requires a trial-and-error approach and memory for correct moves to find the targeted path through a spatial maze. Wechsler's Digit Span (backward) and the Wisconsin Card Sorting Test (WCST) were used as measures of executive functioning.

Most of the FAS-affected individuals performed more poorly on measures of auditory and visual–spatial attention and memory. In addition, the group with FAS performed more poorly on measures of executive functioning and demonstrated a greater number of impulsive responses on a measure of sustained attention using degraded visual stimuli. It is important to note that despite the overall group performance, no single profile characterized all patients in the group with FAS.

Don et al. (1994) compared the performance of 16 nonretarded (IQ range = 70–118) subjects with FAS to normative data on a variety of neuropsychological measures. On a measure of simple sustained auditory attention, requiring subjects to listen to a series of digits and press a buzzer when a specific number was heard, all subjects performed within 1 SD of the mean. However, when demands for mental processing were included in the auditory attention tasks (e.g., requiring subjects to press a buzzer when the number presented was one less than the preceding number), all subjects performed extremely poorly in comparison to the normative sample.

On the California Verbal Learning Test (CLVT), deficits in word acquisition were found in all subjects. However, as would be predicted, subjects with IQs in the borderline range performed more poorly than did subjects with IQs in the average range. For subjects with average IQ, retention of learned information was normal, whereas poor retention was noted in subjects with borderline IQs. Over half of the subjects, regardless of IQ level, demonstrated excessive intrusions on cued recall and/or a greater-than-expected number of perseverations in comparison to the number of unique designs created on a nonverbal fluency task.

The results of this study suggest that an overall deficit in cognitive functioning is not a sufficient explanation for deficits seen in patients with FAS. In addition, the scattered exhibition of excessive cued-recall intrusions and perseverations suggests that different patterns of neuropsychological performance may be found in subgroups of individuals with FAS. In addition, although the mean Performance IQ was greater than the mean Verbal IQ in both groups, the difference between Verbal IQ and Performance IQ in the average-IQ group with FAS was less (5 points) than in the borderline group (10 points).

Gray and Streissguth (1990) compared seven adult patients with FAS or FAE to seven controls matched for age and sex on measures of memory and receptive language. The Stepping Stone Maze was found to be the most sensitive measure for distinguishing between the groups. The Seashore Rhythm Test, the Wechsler Memory Scale, and the Peabody Picture Vocabulary Test—Revised (PPVT-R) also discriminated between the two groups. Interestingly, the Memory for Faces Test did not discriminate between the groups. The alcohol-affected group demonstrated deficits on measures of receptive vocabulary, visual–spatial memory, and auditory attention and memory.

Unfortunately, information regarding psychometric intelligence for the two groups was not reported. It would be very interesting if lowered scores group on the Wechsler Memory Scale were to occur for subjectswith FAS and controls matched for IQ.

Kodituwakku et al. (1992) compared 10 alcohol-affected children with 10 controls matched for age and sex. The alcohol-affected children's performance was comparable to that of the controls on measures of memory (the Design Memory and Story Memory subtests of the Wide Range Assessment of Memory and Learning) and receptive vocabulary (PPVT-R), but were significantly more impaired on measures of fluid intelligence (Raven's Progressive Matrices) and planning (a modified Tower of Hanoi puzzle). In addition, the group with FAS made significantly more perseverative errors and achieved fewer categories on the WCST. Similarities in receptive language (standard scores of 99 and 87 for the control and alcohol-affected groups, respectively) rendered the specific cognitive deficits of the alcohol-exposed group even more notable.

Mattson et al. (1992) compared the performance on the CVLT of two mentally retarded teenage boys with FAS to that of controls matched for chronological age and mental age. Compared to age-matched controls, the subjects with FAS exhibited impaired immediate and delayed recall, excessive perseveration and intrusions, poor discrimination, and an increase in false-positive errors on recognition. When the performance of the subjects with FAS was compared to that of normal 5-year-old males (mental-age equivalent), relative deficits were found in excessive intrusions, poor recognition, and increased false-positive responses on recognition.

Mattson et al. (1993) reported on a comparison study of 14 children with prenatal alcohol exposure and 14 normal controls matched for age and sex. A free-recall task using large letter shapes (global stimuli) constructed from an arrangement of smaller letters (local stimuli) was employed to assess hierarchical processing of visual information. The alcohol-affected groups showed deficits in recall and reproduction of local but not global features. In contrast, deficits in recall and reproduction of global but not local features were found in a study of children with Williams syndrome (see Chapter 6, this volume).

Nanson and Hiscock (1990) compared 20 alcohol-affected children to equal numbers of children with attention deficit disorder (ADD) and normal controls on measures of psychometric intelligence and attention. The groups with FAS and ADD made significantly more impulsive errors on visual attention tasks (continuous-performance tasks) than did the normal controls. However, on measures of reaction time, the performance of the group with FAS was significantly slower than the equivalent performance of the group with ADD and the normal controls. In addition, the alcohol-affected children were significantly more impaired on measures of psychometric intelligence (mean IQ = 78 for alcohol-affected children, 107 for children with ADD).

Conry (1990) compared a group of 19 alcohol-affected individuals (13 with FAS, 6 with FAE) with controls matched for age (mean = 12.6 years) and sex from the same Native group in Canada. Conry reported on the results of measures of sensorimotor function (e.g., grip strength, finger tapping, finger localization, reaction time), receptive and expressive language (PPVT-R and Expressive One Word Picture Vocabulary Test), and psychometric intelligence (the age-appropriate Wechsler test). Significant deficits were found on measures of grip strength, motor speed/precision, and reaction time with the nondominant hand. No differences were found for finger localization and reaction time with the dominant hand.

Significant deficits of receptive vocabulary and expressive vocabulary were noted in the group with FAS; these paralleled the same group's deficit in Verbal IQ. Interestingly, Conry (1990) reported a relatively greater deficit in Performance IQ than in Verbal IQ for the group with FAE in comparison to the group with FAS when both were compared to the control group.

These studies suggest that a pattern of deficits on measures of auditory and visual attention and memory, and on measures of executive functioning (noted in perseverations, intrusions, and poor performance on the WCST), may be found in FAS-affected subjects. Because of the small number of subjects in each FAS study, within-group variability, differences in ages of the subjects, and the generally lower IQ of the alcohol-affected groups, one cannot determine a general overall pattern of neuropsychological performance, nor can the relationship of any pattern of assets and deficits to psychometric intelligence be determined.

Unfortunately, in each of these studies, measures were chosen for their presumed sensitivity to deficits that occur with FAS. Thus, a full picture of the range of assets and deficits that may be present in patients with FAS has not been obtained. Comprehensive neuropsychological studies of FAS patients are required to provide resolutions to these concerns.

NEUROPSYCHOLOGICAL ASSESSMENT FINDINGS FOR FAS: A COMPARISON WITH THE NLD SYNDROME

Although full neuropsychological assessments of FAS-affected individuals are not available, inferences of probable findings are possible. Findings from the studies reviewed above are used here to formulate, where possible, probable results of a neuropsychological examination (based on an expanded Halstead–Reitan Battery) of a child with FAS. The hypothetical results are compared to the results of a prototypical neuropsychological study of a child with the NLD syndrome (Rourke, 1989).

Basic Sensory-Perceptual Measures: Tactile, Visual, and Auditory Modalities

In the areas of basic tactile- and visual-perceptual ability, too little information is available for conclusions to be drawn. Basic auditory perception is likely to be good, because there are reports of hyperacusis in infants with FAS. This is comparable to results expected in a neuropsychological examination of a child with NLD. However, otitis media, which is common during the early childhood of FAS-affected individuals, may cause impairments in auditory perception.

Lateral Dominance Examination: Motor and Psychomotor Tests

Poor coordination and motor slowness are commonly reported in children with FAS. In addition, some evidence for greater deficits in strength, coordination, speed, and reaction time on the left side has been found (Conry, 1990). This is typical of the level and pattern of deficits reported in children with NLD.

Measures of Attention: Tactile, Visual, and Auditory Modalities

In the area of tactile attention, too little information is available to permit us to speculate on the results of neuropsychological testing.

On measures of simple sustained auditory attention, the individual with FAS is likely to do well. On measures of simple sustained visual attention, such as those of a continuous performance test, the individual with FAS is likely to perform rather poorly and to engage in impulsive responses. The individual with NLD is expected to demonstrate a similar pattern of poorer visual attention than auditory attention. However, because tests of auditory and visual attention are not equivalent in terms of difficulty and complexity, it is not possible to conclude that visual attention is poorer than auditory attention in individuals with FAS.

Attentional difficulties are a very characteristic feature reported in children with FAS. When complexity is added to measures of both auditory and visual attention, the FAS-affected individual is likely to do poorly in both areas. The difficulties with attention appear basic, underlying both the visual and auditory attention deficits, rather than modality-specific. These findings appear to differ from the robust differential findings for visual and auditory attention in NLD. In NLD, auditory attention is good, while visual attention is poor. However, in the typical NLD presentation, auditory attention declines when novel and/or complex stimuli are involved. It would be necessary to determine the level of novelty and/or complexity of the auditory stimuli used in studies of children with FAS in order to make the necessary comparisons. These dimensions of novelty and complexity are difficult to discern in the studies of attention reviewed above.

Measures of Memory: Tactile, Visual, and Auditory Modalities

In the area of tactile memory, again, too little information is available to permit us to speculate about the FAS-affected individual's performance. Deficits in visual–spatial and auditory memory have often been reported in individuals with FAS and would be expected in neuropsychological testing. Whether these deficits are correlated with generally lowered psychometric intelligence is unknown. However, there are indications of differentially affected functioning, in that visual memory appears more negatively affected than is auditory memory (Carmichael Olson et al., 1994; Don et al., 1994). This is somewhat similar to NLD, although the contrast between auditory and visual–spatial memory is not as clearly differentiated. In NLD, rote auditory memory is an asset and is much stronger than is the notably poor visual–spatial memory.

Wechsler Performance Subtests

Subtest scores have not often been reported in studies of the intellectual functioning of individuals with FAS. Generally, Performance IQ is higher than Verbal IQ, and visual–spatial skills are reported to be stronger than verbal skills. This stands in contrast to the lower Performance IQ than Verbal IQ found in children with NLD. However, the degree of disparity may vary as a function of IQ. In the studies by Don et al. (1994) and

Conry (1990), a relatively greater deficit in Performance than in Verbal IQ was reported for a group with FAS and higher (average) IQ and for a higher-IQ group with FAE, respectively. If such findings were replicated in larger groups, this would suggest relatively more similarity between individuals with NLD and individuals with FAS and/or FAE and higher IQ than between those with NLD and lower-IQ individuals with FAS.

Additional Visual–Spatial Measures

On measures of complex visual–spatial tasks, the performance of both FAS- and NLD-affected individuals is very poor.

Measures of Problem Solving, Concept Formation, Hypothesis Testing

Problem solving and concept formation, like attention, are very characteristic areas of deficit for individuals with FAS. Although hypothesis-testing measures (e.g., the WCST) have only rarely been mentioned in the literature on FAS, it is probable that extremely poor performance in this area would be generally found. Difficulties with problem-solving skills have been reported in both retarded and nonretarded individuals with FAS. In addition, scores on measures of fluid intelligence would be expected to be much poorer than would those on measures of crystallized intelligence. Findings in this area would be expected to parallel those for individuals with NLD.

Wechsler Verbal Subtests

As noted previously, and in contrast to children with NLD, children with FAS generally score lower in Verbal IQ than in Performance IQ. Low scores are most often noted in Arithmetic and Digit Span, reflecting poor attention (characteristic of FAS) and poor arithmetic skills (characteristic of both FAS and NLD).

Additional Auditory–Verbal/Linguistic Measures

Both children with FAS and those with NLD would be expected to perform more poorly when challenged by complexity and/or novelty in auditory/linguistic measures.

Academic Achievement Measures

Interestingly, both children with FAS and those with NLD show a pattern on the WRAT-R of better performances in sight (single-word) reading and spelling than in arithmetic. In addition, both groups are better at single-word reading than at reading comprehension. However, the discrepancy between sight reading and spelling on the one hand and arithmetic on the other tends to be less dramatic in FAS. This seems to occur because overall academic achievement is lower.

Measures of Personality, Psychosocial Skills, and Adaptive Abilities

Personality, psychosocial skills, and adaptive abilities develop along generally parallel paths in NLD and FAS. During early childhood, children with either syndrome are seen as more capable than they really are because of superficially well-developed language skills (NLD and FAS) and a social orientation (FAS). However, as the demands of the environment increase, the FAS- and NLD-affected individuals' poor social skills and poor adaptation become apparent. Individuals with either syndrome demonstrate a tendency toward emotional problems in adolescence and later life. However, poorer adaptive abilities and more externalizing disorders are likely to occur in individuals with FAS. At the same time, the results of some recent studies have suggested that children who exhibit important elements of the NLD pattern continue to exhibit "externalizing" forms of psychological disturbance (Fuerst & Rourke, 1995). More longitudinal studies are necessary to further delineate the developmental manifestations of NLD and FAS.

Summary of Neuropsychological Findings and Comparison to NLD

Both individuals affected by FAS and individuals with NLD demonstrate an overall pattern of compromised adaptation that appears to be a result of compromised brain functioning. In FAS, the brain's development is marred throughout gestation. In a generalized overview, this results in deficits in motor skills, impairment in attentional processes, and a general depression in cognitive functioning. Moreover, suggestions of a relatively greater impairment in visual–spatial memory and in fluid intelligence have been made (Carmichael Olson et al., 1994; Kodituwakku et al., 1992).

The resulting deficits in motor skills, coordination, visual–spatial skills, problem solving, and life adjustment resemble the characteristic deficits that occur in NLD. However, two major factors discriminate between NLD and FAS. First, most FAS-affected individuals lack the assets in auditory attention and rote verbal skills seen in individuals with NLD. Second, most FAS-affected individuals display prominent attentional difficulties in both visual and auditory modalities that are not found in individuals with NLD.

Interestingly, the developmental manifestations of FAS and NLD share many similarities. In either syndrome, children may display hyperactive behavior in early years that diminishes in late childhood and adolescence. Because of the NLD-affected child's well-developed rote verbal skills, and because of the FAS-affected child's orientation toward people and superficially developed verbal skills, both appear in early childhood to be capable of functioning better than is actually the case. In addition, children with either FAS or NLD show poor adaptation to novelty. As most FAS- or NLD-affected individuals mature, difficulties with adaptation become more apparent and emotional problems may occur as a result. More externalized problem behaviors are reported in children with FAS than in those with NLD, although the extent of externalized and internalized pathology in either disorder has not been extensively documented.

RELATIONSHIP OF FAS TO THE WHITE MATTER MODEL OF NLD

The NLD syndrome is hypothesized to occur when white matter required for intermodal integration is destroyed or rendered dysfunctional. In addition, a sufficiently intact substrate for the development of language is required. White matter damage or dysfunction occurring after natural language has developed and become automatized is likely to result in NLD. White matter damage or destruction that occurs before language development and that spares the left-hemisphere association fibers is also likely to result in NLD. However, significant disruption of left-hemisphere association fibers occurring before language has developed would be expected to interfere with language development. In such cases, both NLD *and* language impairment would be expected to occur. The timing of white matter disturbance is crucial for the explication of NLD (Rourke, 1989).

In FAS, alcohol damages the developing brain throughout gestation. Because alcohol is absorbed more readily by the grey matter in the brain, grey matter may be more susceptible to damage. Disruption of early neuronal and glial cell migration and organization is characteristically reported in experimental animal models of FAS. Thus, FAS is likely to be characterized by more generalized brain dysfunction than is seen in the typical NLD presentation.

In individuals with FAS, damage that later results in white matter dysfunction may occur early in gestation if the substrates for white matter do not develop properly. For example, if the neurons for the corpus callosum are not laid down properly, agenesis of the corpus callosum may occur. In the reported cases of callosal agenesis in FAS, it appears that much more than the corpus callosum of the developing brain is compromised, and that the resulting individual is so severely affected that deficits such as mental retardation occur in addition to NLD.

Callosal agenesis or hypoplasia may also occur as a result of white matter damage or dysfunction occurring late in gestation and/or during the first year of life. In children with FAS, such damage may occur through exposure to alcohol during the last trimester of pregnancy and during lactation. Children who have suffered the greatest prenatal exposure to alcohol during the last trimester and through breast feeding would be expected to be most similar to children with NLD, because white matter development is particularly vulnerable to disruption during that period. However, in FAS, the characteristic facies points to substantial damage occurring during the first trimester of pregnancy, while other manifestations point to an accumulation of damage occurring throughout gestation.

General attentional deficits, lowered psychometric intelligence, and language deficits occur in FAS, in addition to the more characteristic deficits occurring with NLD. Deficits typically shared by FAS- and NLD-affected individuals include the following: specific mechanical difficulties with arithmetic learning; visual–spatial processing and memory deficits; poor problem solving; difficulty in dealing with novel material; poor social skills; and poor general adaptation. Although NLD and FAS share many of the same deficits, the deficits found in FAS appear to reflect both white matter dysfunction and more generalized brain dysfunction than the primary white matter dysfunction that occurs in NLD. Because of the probable generalized brain dysfunction in addition to probable white matter damage, one would expect to see the deficits but not the assets associated with NLD and deficits characteristic of more widespread (grey matter) brain dysfunction.

Fairly broad individual differences are exhibited by children who have experienced prenatal alcohol exposure resulting in FAS. In some affected individuals, psychometric intelligence is average, and more specific deficits (e.g., attentional problems, especially when requirements for planning and mental flexibility are added; poor arithmetic skills; and difficulty with novelty and mental flexibility) have been reported. In addition, there is some evidence, still in need of replication, that for some average-IQ FAS-affected individuals, the difference between Perform-ance and Verbal IQs in favor of Performance IQ is less than in mentally retarded FAS-affected individuals. It seems possible that a subset of rela-tively high-functioning individuals with FAS would exhibit symptoms of NLD without additional symptomatology.

Children without characteristic facies and with significant alcohol exposure during the last trimester and lactation would be more likely to exhibit the NLD pattern. These individuals would best be diagnosed with FAE or ARBD, which unfortunately are not commonly accepted classifications. Inquiry into the timing of possible prenatal alcohol expo-sure in children who exhibit the developmental manifestation typical of the NLD pattern, and who may in addition display more general atten-tional problems, would help to generate a better understanding of devel-opmental aspects of the etiology of NLD.

There is much evidence to suggest that FAS- and FAE-affected chil-dren have white matter disturbances. However, the extent to which the white matter perturbations in FAS are related to white matter manifesta-tions of NLD is unknown. Investigations into the white matter distur-bances in FAS and their relationship to the behavioral manifestations of NLD should prove to be a fruitful avenue of research.

REFERENCES

Abel, E. L. (1984). *Fetal alcohol syndrome and fetal alcohol effects*. New York: Plen-um Press.

Abel, E. L., & Sokol, R. J. (1987). Incidence of fetal alcohol syndrome and economic impact of FAS-related anomalies. *Journal of the American Medical Association, 245*, 2436–2439.

Adams, R. D., & Victor, M. (1989). *Principles of neurology* (4th ed.). Toronto: McGraw-Hill.

Amman, A. J., Wara, D. W., Cowan, M. J., Barrett, D. J., & Stiehm, E. R. (1982). The DiGeorge syndrome and the fetal alcohol syndrome. *American Journal of Diseases of Children, 136*, 906–908.

Barr, H. M., Streissguth, A. P., Darby, B. L., & Sampson (1990). Prenatal exposure to alcohol, caffeine, tobacco, and aspirin: Effects on fine and gross motor performance in 4-year-old children. *Developmental Psychology, 26*(3), 339–348.

Burd, L., & Martsolf, J. T. (1989). Fetal alcohol syndrome: Diagnosis and syndro-mal variability. *Physiology and Behavior, 46*(1), 39–43.

Carmichael Olson, H., Feldman, J. J., Streissguth, A. P., & Gonzales, R. D. (1994). *Neuropsychological deficits and life adjustment in adolescents and young adults with fetal alcohol syndrome: A comparison to normative data* (Tech. Rep. No. 93-17). Seattle: University of Washington, Pregnancy and Health Study.

Caruso, K., & ten Bensel, R. (1993). Fetal alcohol syndrome and fetal alcohol effects: The University of Minnesota experience. *Minnesota Medicine, 76*, 25–29.

Church, M. W., & Gerkin, D. P. (1988). Hearing disorders in children with fetal alcohol syndrome: Findings from case reports. *Pediatrics*, *82*(2), 147–154.

CIBA-Geigy. (1974). Development of the nervous system: A logical approach to neuroanatomy. *Clinical Symposia*, *26*, 1–32.

Clarren, S. K. (1986). Neuropathology in fetal alcohol syndrome. In J. R. West (Ed.), *Alcohol and brain development* (pp. 158–166). New York: Oxford University Press.

Clarren, S. K., Astley, S. J., Bowden, D. M., Lai, H., Milam, A. H., Rudeen, P. K., & Shoemaker, W. J. (1990). Neuroanatomic and neurochemical abnormalities in non-human primate infants exposed to weekly doses of ethanol during gestation. *Alcoholism: Clinical and Experimental Research*, *14*, 674–683.

Clarren, S. K., Ellsworth, C. A., Sumi, M., Streissguth, A. P., & Smith, D. W. (1978). Brain malformations related to prenatal exposure to ethanol. *Journal of Pediatrics*, *92*(1), 64- 67.

Clarren, S. K., & Smith, D. W. (1978). The fetal alcohol syndrome. *New England Journal of Medicine*, *298*(19), 1063–1067.

Conry, J. (1990). Neuropsychological deficits in fetal alcohol syndrome and fetal alcohol effects. *Alcoholism: Clinical and Experimental Research*, *14*, 650–655.

Cornelius, M. D., Day, N. L., Cornelius, J. R., Geva, D., Taylor, P. M., & Richardson, G. A. (1993). Drinking patterns and correlates of drinking among pregnant teenagers. *Alcoholism: Clinical and Experimental Research*, *17*(2), 290–294.

Dehaene, P., Crepin, G., Delahousse, G., Querleu, D., Walbaum, R., Titran, M., & Samaille-Villette, P. (1981). Aspects épidemiologiques du syndrome d'alcoolisme foetal: 45 observations en 3 ans [Epidemiological aspects of the fetal alcohol syndrome: 45 observations in 3 years]. *La Nouvelle Presse Médicale*, *6*, 2639–2643.

Dexter, J. D., Tumbleson, M. E., Decker, J. D., & Middleton, C. C. (1980). Fetal alcohol syndrome in Sinclair (s-1) miniature swine. *Alcoholism: Clinical and Experimental Research*, *4*, 145–151.

Don, A., Kerns, K., Mateer, C. A., & Streissguth, A. P. (1994). *Cognitive deficits in non-retarded adults with fetal alcohol syndrome*. Manuscript submitted for publication.

Driscoll, C. D., Streissguth, A. P., & Riley, E. P. (1990). Prenatal alcohol exposure: Comparability of effects in humans and animal models. *Neurotoxicology and Teratology*, *12*, 231–237.

Druse, M. F. (1992). Effects of *in utero* exposure on the development of neurotransmitter systems. In M. W. Miller (Ed.), *Development of the central nervous system: Effects of alcohol and opiates* (pp. 139–165). Toronto: Wiley.

Ellis, F. W., & Pick, F. R. (1980). An animal model of the fetal alcohol syndrome in beagles. *Alcoholism: Clinical and Experimental Research*, *4*, 123–134.

Fuerst, D., & Rourke, B. P. (1995). Psychosocial functioning in children with learning disabilities at three age levels. *Child Neuropsychology*, *1*.

Galofre, F. E. (1987). Dendritic spine anomalies in fetal alcohol syndrome. *Neuropediatrics*, *18*, 161–163.

Goodlett, C. R., & West, J. R. (1992). Fetal alcohol effects: Rat model of alcohol exposure during the brain growth spurt. In I. S. Zagon & T. A. Slotkin

(Eds.), *Maternal substance abuse and the developing nervous system* (pp. 45–75). San Diego: Academic Press.

Gottesfeld, Z., & Silverman, P. B. (1990). Developmental delays associated with prenatal alcohol exposure are reversed by thyroid hormone treatment. *Neuroscience Letters, 109*, 42–47.

Gray, J. K., & Streissguth, A. P. (1990). Memory deficits and life adjustment in adults with fetal alcohol syndrome: A case control study. *Alcoholism: Clinical and Experimental Research, 14*, 294.

Guinta, C. T., & Streissguth, A. P. (1988). Patients with fetal alcohol syndrome and their caretakers, *Social Casework: The Journal of Contemporary Social Work, 69*(7), 453–459.

Hall, B. D., & Orenstein, W. A. (1974). Noonan's phenotype in an offspring of an alcoholic mother. *Lancet, ii*, 680–681.

Hanson, J. W., Streissguth, A. P., & Smith, D. W. (1978). The effects of moderate alcohol consumption during pregnancy on fetal growth and morphogenesis. *Journal of Pediatrics, 92*(3), 457–460.

Harris, J. C. (1988). Psychological adaptation and psychiatric disorders in adolescents and young adults with Down syndrome. In S.M. Pueschel (Ed.), *The young person with Down syndrome: Transition from adolescence to adulthood* (pp. 35–51). Baltimore: Paul H. Brookes.

Jones, K. L., & Smith, D. W. (1973). Recognition of the fetal alcohol syndrome in early infancy. *Lancet, ii*, 999–1001.

Jones, K. L., Smith, D. W., & Streissguth, A. P. (1974). Outcome in offspring of chronic alcoholic women. *Lancet, ii*, 1076–1078.

Jones, K. L., Smith, D. W., Ulleland, C. N., & Streissguth, A. P. (1973). Pattern of malformation in offspring of chronic alcoholic mothers. *Lancet, i*, 1267–1271.

Knight, J. E., Kodituwakku, P. W., Orrison, W. W., Lewine, J. D., Maclin, E. L., Weathersby, E. K., Cutler, S. K., McClain, C. H., Handmaker, N.S., & Handmaker, S. D. (1993). Magnetic resonance imaging in high-functioning children with fetal alcohol syndrome who exhibit specific neuropsychological deficits. *Alcoholism: Clinical and Experimental Research, 17*, 485.

Kodituwakku, P. W., Handmaker, N. S., Cutler, S. K., Weathersby, E. K., Handmaker, S. D., & Aase, J. M. (1992). Specific impairments of self regulation in FAS/FAE: A pilot study. *Alcoholism: Clinical and Experimental Research, 16*, 158.

LaDue, R. A., Streissguth, A. P., & Randels, S. P. (1992). Clinical considerations pertaining to adolescents and adults with fetal alcohol syndrome. In R. A. LaDue, A. P. Streissguth, & S. P. Randels (Eds.), *Perinatal substance abuse: Research findings and clinical implications* (pp. 104–131). Baltimore: Johns Hopkins University Press.

Lancaster, F. E., Phillips, S. M., Patsalos, P. N., & Wiggens, R. C. (1984). Brain myelination in the offspring of ethanol-treated rats: *In utero* versus lactational exposure by crossfostering offspring of control, pairfed and ethanol treated dams. *Brain Research, 309*, 209–216.

Lemoine, P., Harousseau, H., Borteyru, J. P., & Menuet, J. C. (1968). Les enfants de parents alcooliques: Anomalies observées à propos de 127 cas [Children of alcoholic parents: Abnormalities observed in 127 cases]. *Ouest Médical*

(Paris), *21*, 476–482. (Available in English from the National Clearinghouse for Alcohol Information, P.O. Box 2345, Rockville, MD 20852.)

Lemoine, P., & Lemoine, P. H. (1992). Avenir des enfants de mères alcooliques (étude de 105 cas retrouvés à l'âge adulte) et quelques constatations d'intérêt phophylactique [Outcome in the offspring of alcoholic mothers (a study of 105 cases in adulthood) and considerations with a view to prophylaxis]. *Annales de Pédiatrie* (Paris), *39*(4), 226–236.

Light, K. E., Serbus, D. C., & Santiago, M. (1989). Exposure of rats to ethanol from postnatal days 4 to 8: Alteration of cholinergic neurochemistry in the cerebral cortex and corpus striatum at day 20. *Alcoholism: Clinical and Experimental Research*, *13*, 29–35.

Little, B. B., Snell, L. M., Rosenfeld, C. R., Gilstrap, L. C., & Gant, N. F. (1990). Failure to recognize fetal alcohol syndrome in newborn infants. *American Journal of Diseases of Children*, *144*, 1142–1146.

Little, R. E., & Streissguth, A. P. (1981). Effects of alcohol on the fetus: Impact and prevention. *Canadian Medical Association Journal*, *125*, 159–164.

Loock, C. A., Conry, J. L., & Clark, C. M. (1993). Disregulation of caudate/cortical metabolism in FAS: A case study. *Alcoholism: Clinical and Experimental Research*, *17*(2), 485.

Marcus, J. C. (1987). Neurological findings in the fetal alcohol syndrome. *Neuropediatrics*, *18*, 158–160.

Martier, S. S., Sokol, R. J., & Ager, J. W. (1993). Aspirin may lessen the impact of alcohol on fetal deficit: A human study. *Alcoholism: Clinical and Experimental Research*, *17*, 456.

Mattson, S. N., Riley, E. P., Jernigan, R. L., Ehlers, C. L., Delis, D. C., Jones, K. J., Stern, C., Johnson, K. A., Hesselink, J. R., & Bellugi, U. (1992). Fetal alcohol syndrome: A case report of neuropsychological, MRI, and EEG assessment of two children. *Alcoholism: Clinical and Experimental Research*, *16*,(5), 1001–1003.

Mattson, S. N., Sadoff, L. J., Delis, D. C., Jones, K. L., & Riley, E. P. (1993). Global and local processing of hierarchical visual stimuli in children with prenatal exposure to alcohol. *Alcoholism: Clinical and Experimental Research*, *17*, 456.

Nanson, J. L. (1992). Autism in fetal alcohol syndrome: A report of six cases. *Alcoholism: Clinical and Experimental Research*, *16*(3), 558–565.

Nanson, J. L., & Hiscock, M. (1990). Attention deficits in children exposed to alcohol prenatally. *Alcoholism: Clinical and Experimental Research*, *14*(5), 656–661.

Phillips, D. E., Krueger, S. K., & Rydquist, J. E. (1991). Short- and long-term effects of combined pre- and postnatal ethanol exposure (three trimester equivalency) on the development of myelin and axons in rat optic nerve. *International Journal of Developmental Neuroscience*, *9*, 631–647.

Pierce, D. R., Goodlett, G. R., & West, J. R. (1989). Differential neuronal loss following early postnatal alcohol exposure. *Teratology*, *40*, 113–126.

Riley, E. P. (1990). The long-term behavioral effects of prenatal alcohol exposure in rats. *Alcoholism: Clinical and Experimental Research*, *14*(5), 670–673,

Riley, E. P., Baron, S., & Hannigan, J. H. (1986). Response inhibition deficits following prenatal alcohol exposure: A comparison to the effects of hippocampal lesions in rats. In J. R. West (Ed.), *Alcohol and brain development* (pp. 71–105). New York: Oxford University Press.

Rosett, H. L. (1980). A clinical perspective of the fetal alcohol syndrome. *Alcoholism: Clinical and Experimental Research, 4,* 119–122.

Rosett, H. L., & Weiner, L. (1984). *Alcohol and the fetus: A clinical perspective.* New York: Oxford University Press.

Rourke, B. P. (1989). *Nonverbal learning disabilities: The syndrome and the model.* New York: Guilford Press.

Savage, D. D., Montano, C. Y., Paxton, L. L., & Kasarskis, E. J. (1989). Prenatal ethanol exposure decreases hippocampal mossy fiber zinc in 45 day-old rats. *Alcoholism: Clinical and Experimental Research, 13,* 588–593.

Schenker, S., Becker, H. C., Randall, C. L., Phillips, D. K., Baskin, G. S., & Henderson, G. I. (1990). Fetal alcohol syndrome: Current status of pathogenesis. *Alcoholism: Clinical and Experimental Research, 14,* 635–647.

Sokol, R. J., & Clarren, S. K. (1989). Guidelines for use of terminology describing the import of prenatal alcohol on the offspring. *Alcoholism: Clinical and Experimental Research, 13,* 146–151.

Sokol, R. J., Miller, S. I., & Reed, G. (1980). Alcohol abuse during pregnancy: An epidemiologic study. *Alcoholism: Clinical and Experimental Research, 4*(2), 135–145.

Streissguth, A. P. (1986). The behavioral teratology of alcohol: Performance, behavioral, and intellectual deficits in prenatally exposed children. In J. R. West (Ed.), *Alcohol and brain development* (pp. 3–44). New York: Oxford University Press.

Streissguth, A. P. (1990). Today I visited an Aleut village: Observations on preventing fetal alcohol syndrome. *The IHS Primary Care Provider, 15,* 125–127.

Streissguth, A. P. (1992). Fetal alcohol syndrome and fetal alcohol effects: A clinical perspective of later developmental consequences. In I. S. Zagon & T. A. Slotkin (Eds.), *Maternal substance abuse and the developing nervous system* (pp. 5–25). San Diego: Academic Press.

Streissguth, A. P., Aase, J. M., Clarren, S. K., Randels, S. P., LaDue, R. A., & Smith, D. F. (1991). Fetal alcohol syndrome in adolescents and adults. *Journal of the American Medical Association, 265*(15), 1961–1967.

Streissguth, A. P., Clarren, S. K., & Jones, K. L. (1985). Natural history of the fetal alcohol syndrome: A ten-year follow-up of eleven patients. *Lancet, ii,* 85–92.

Streissguth, A. P., & LaDue, R. A. (1987). Fetal alcohol: Teratogenic causes of developmental disabilities. In S. R. Schroder (Ed.), *Toxic substances and mental retardation: neurobehavioral toxicology and teratology* (pp. 1–32). Washington, DC: American Association on Mental Deficiency.

Streissguth, A. P., Landesman-Dwyer, S., Martin, J. C., & Smith, D. W. (1980). Teratogenic effects of alcohol in humans and laboratory animals. *Science, 209,* 353–361.

15

Multiple Sclerosis

Roberta F. White
Maxine Krengel

NEUROLOGY OF MULTIPLE SCLEROSIS

Multiple sclerosis (MS) is a demyelinating disorder—that is, a disease in which the myelin sheaths of nerve fibers are damaged, producing lesions called demyelinating plaques.

Findings on Medical Examination

In the early stages, symptoms of MS can be transient and difficult to confirm on physical examination. Patients with MS may show no abnormalities if they are between exacerbations or in the early stages of the illness. Common early symptoms of MS often include weakness in one or more limbs (50% of patients) and partial or total loss of vision lasting several hours or days (25% of patients). In addition, symptoms may include transient episodes of numbness, ataxia, diplopia, vertigo, seizures, deafness, facial paralysis, unformed auditory hallucinations, aphasia, urinary frequency, incontinence, and affective changes. Other common symptoms include fatigue (Krupp, LaRocca, Muir-Nash, & Steinberg, 1989) and sensitivity to heat (Accornero, DeVito, Rotunno, Perugino, & Manfredi, 1989; Nelson & McDowell, 1959).

During exacerbations, after the occurrence of multiple exacerbations, or in continuously progressive stages of the illness, symptoms include nystagmus, limb weakness or numbness, ataxia, gait disorder, incoordination, urinary frequency, and emotional and cognitive changes. Symptoms that occur later in the disease process include hemiparesis, tremor, chorea, diplopia, blindness, field cuts, seizures, incontinence, dizziness, difficulty with balance, dysarthria, dysphasia, dysphagia, and affective changes.

It should be noted that diagnosis of MS requires evidence of two separate lesions in the central nervous system (CNS), supported by clinical examination and laboratory data. Diagnostic criteria, which are used for both clinical and research purposes, have been developed (Poser et al., 1983).

Laboratory Studies

A wide variety of methods can be used to assist in the diagnosis of MS. These include studies of cerebrospinal fluid (CSF), magnetic resonance imaging (MRI), electroencephalography (EEG), and computer tomography (CT).

Studies of CSF

CSF studies are, according to Adams and Victor (1985), highly diagnostic of MS: Virtually all patients with MS show some abnormality in CSF. About 40% of patients show oligoclonal bands. Other CSF abnormalities seen in MS include plecytosis and elevated protein.

Neurophysiological and Neuroimaging Findings

Studies employing MRI and CT often reveal MS lesion sites, although MRI is more sensitive to MS changes than is CT. CT is often useful in detecting ventricular size and cerebral atrophy; the latter occurs in 40% of patients with MS, according to Rao et al. (1985). In fact, it has been speculated that the degree of atrophy may be an important indicator of the amount of cognitive decline.

EEG abnormalities in MS are characterized by focal or diffuse slowing. However, such changes are not specific to MS alone.

Visual, auditory, and tactile evoked potentials are often abnormal in MS, as are the results of blink reflex and critical flicker fusion studies.

Neuropathology

At autopsy, MS lesions, which are typically distributed relatively randomly in the cerebral hemispheres, brain stem, spinal cord, and cerebellar peduncles, are typically grayish-pink in color and are sharply delineated. Plaques often occur in the optic nerves and chiasm, as well as in optic tracts and radiations. In the cortex, high proportions of MS plaques are found in periventricular white matter (PVWM). Cortical lesions are characerized by myelin destruction, but nerve cells usually remain intact (Adams & Victor, 1985).

It is thought that MS lesions develop episodically during exacerbations of the illness, and that a great deal of demyelination may occur with each exacerbation. There has been evidence to suggest that in some cases remyelination may occur, with associated diminution in lesion sizes observed on MRI of lesions in individual patients (Costantino, Black, Carr, Nicholson, & Noseworthy, 1986).

EPIDEMIOLOGY AND GENETICS

It has been suggested that there may be an environmental factor in the development of MS (Kurtzke, 1965). For instance, it has been found that the prevalence of MS is lower in equatorial areas, whereas the prevalence is highest in the northern United States and Europe. It has been noted that people who move from high-risk latitudes to low-risk latitudes carry with them some of the risk from their place of origin, at least if emigration occurs after the age of 15 (Vella, 1984).

There is also evidence to suggest that there may be a genetic component to susceptibility to MS. For instance, first-degree relatives of a patient with MS have a risk of MS that is 5 to 15 times higher than the risk in the general population; the highest risk is among siblings (Kurtzke, 1965). Twin studies suggest that MS affects both twins more frequently in monozygotic than in dizygotic twin dyads. Genetic studies suggest that MS development is based on multigenetic influences rather than on single-gene transmission (Ebers, 1983).

Most likely there is a combined genetic and environmental cause of MS. This notion receives support from the evidence that there are racial differences in the prevalence of MS, which are nonetheless affected by latitude of habitation. Blacks in the United States, for example, have lower rates of MS than whites, but blacks living in the northern United States are more likely to develop MS than are blacks living in the South (Kurtzke, Beebe, & Norman, 1979). In addition, Ebers (1983) has reported that siblings who develop MS tend to do so in the same calendar year, not at the same age; this suggests not only a genetic but an environmental influence.

The mechanism of the proposed environmental influence on development of MS has received much discussion. It has been argued that viral infections encountered early in life produce an autoimmune response later in life, which in turn triggers the demyelinating exacerbations of MS (Raymond, 1986). Recently, Kurtzke, Hyllested, and Heltberg (1993) have temporally related a series of "epidemics" of MS in the Faroe

Islands to the occupation of the islands by British troops from 1941 to 1944. MS had not existed in the Faroes prior to 1943, but since then four epidemics have occurred. Kurtzke et al. attribute clinical MS in the Faroes to an infectious agent affecting many persons, a small portion of whom develop MS.

TREATMENT

Drug Treatment

There is no known treatment that will cure or reverse the progression of MS. Although there are some experimental treatments of MS aimed at treating immune system dysfunction, MS in exacerbation is usually treated symptomatically with adrenocorticotropic hormone (ACTH), a pituitary hormone that stimulates the adrenal glands, or with prednisone. Other drug treatments include psychopharmacological intervention to treat the affective or personality changes that may accompany MS.

Psychotherapy

Patients with MS often need assistance in accepting and learning to adjust to the cognitive and behavioral changes associated with the disorder. Patients who have experienced affective changes often need assistance in adjusting to these changes. When affective symptoms are related to exacerbations, it is helpful to learn to associate these symptoms with the disease process. A patient's intellectual comprehension that hallucinations or other symptoms are caused by CNS dysfunction is often reassuring.

Family therapy or education may also be helpful. For example, family members may need to learn how to deal with the consequences of a chronic illness. For example, a patient may become dependent on his or her family for physical care needs. Also, the family members need to deal with grief over functional loss of the affected family member and fear of losing the affected member through death. In addition, family members may need to adjust to the patient's disease-related mood swings, changes in energy level, and variability in cognitive integrity. At times, problems arise because personality changes occur early in the illness, prior to diagnosis.

In later stages, social workers are often useful in helping patients and family members acquire resources for dealing with the disease, such as respite care. Vocational counseling may also be necessary if the patient is unable to return to his or her previous place of employment following motor or cognitive losses.

Other therapeutic interventions include speech therapy (for patients with motor, speech, or aphasic symptoms), occupational therapy (if a patient is unable to carry out activities of daily living), and physical therapy (for patients with hemiparesis, spasticity, or gait disturbance). Cognitive remediation may assist a patient in learning how to control attentional lapses.

DEVELOPMENTAL EFFECTS ON EXPRESSION OF DISORDER

The disease affects young and middle-aged adults. The mean age of symptom onset is between 29 and 33 years (Matthews, Acheson, Batchelor, & Weller, 1985).

CLASSIC LITERATURE ON BEHAVIORAL FINDINGS

There is a large body of literature on the cognitive, affective, and personality correlates of MS. However, it is difficult to compare results from individual studies because MS has most often been treated as a unitary disorder. As we have seen, lesions can manifest themselves in several parts of the CNS; it may be more appropriate to think of the disease as one with several subtypes of neuropsychological dysfunction, defined by the sites and quantity of focal lesions in individual cases.

One way of classifying MS, as a "subcortical" disorder (Albert, 1978; Rao, 1986, 1990), acknowledges both the neuropathology of MS (i.e., it attacks subcortical structures most commonly) and the particular pattern of neuropsychological deficits seen in MS. This pattern of deficits resembles those seen in other subcortical disorders, such as Huntington disease and Parkinson disease. Common neuropsychological deficits include impairments in visual–spatial processing, problems with effortful memory tasks involving retrieval, and impaired executive system functioning in the context of relatively preserved linguistic aspects of verbal functioning. However, the subcortical characterization does not apply to the entire constellation of symptoms. Dysnomia may occur once there are sufficient numbers of white matter lesions in the dominant hemisphere, and specific subgroups of patients may exhibit aphasic symptoms if they develop areas of demyelination in the white matter of subcortical speech zones.

Specific research studies have examined the relationship between cognitive dysfunction and a number of MS-related variables, including disability ratings (Fink & Houser, 1966; Marsh, 1980) and duration of illness (Ivnik, 1978; Rao et al., 1985; van den Burg, van Zomeren, Minderhoud, Prange, & Meijer, 1987). Two interesting studies agree that simple screening measures such as the Mini-Mental State Exam and clinical examinations underestimate cognitive deficits (DePaulo, Folstein, & Fordon, 1980; Heaton, Nelson, Thompson, Burks, & Franklin, 1985).

Cognitive correlates of MS subtypes have also been studied. Patients with "relapsing–remitting" (characterized by discrete focal lesions) and "chronic/progressive" (characterized by many diffusely represented lesions) MS have been compared. At least three studies of this type have been completed, one reporting no differences between chronic/progressive and relapsing–remitting patients on a rather restricted battery of tests (Raymond, Stern, Authelet, & Penny, 1987). Two other groups of investigators found that the chronic/progressive patients tended to be significantly more impaired than relapsing–remitting patients on a wide variety of tasks (Beatty, Goodkin, Monson, & Beatty, 1989; Heaton et al., 1985). Beatty and coworkers concluded that differences between the groups in disease duration, severity of disability, and disease course could not be ruled out as causes of greater cognitive decline in the chronic/progressive group, but that the differences could not be explained on the basis of age. These subtypes, although somewhat unreliable (Goodkin, Hertgaard, & Rudnick, 1989), may constitute a first step in the attempt to examine neuropathological issues.

NEUROPSYCHOLOGICAL ASSESSMENT

Test Selection

The following basic battery of neuropsychological tests has been found to be useful for making clinical diagnoses. The battery includes tests that are frequently sensitive to MS, that are usually insensitive to MS, or that are sensitive to MS only with specific lesion sites. Asterisked tests have been shown to be particularly sensitive to MS in prior research and in our clinical experience. This battery is similar to that recommended by Peyser, Rao, LaRocca, and Kaplan (1990) for clinical studies.

Wechsler Adult Intelligence Scale—Revised (WAIS-R; Wechsler, 1981)
  *Performance subtests
  *Digit Span, Arithmetic
  *Similarities, Comprehension
  *Other WAIS-R subtests
*Wechsler Memory Scale (WMS; Wechsler, 1945)
*Wisconsin Card Sorting Test (WCST; Heaton, 1981)
*Trail Making Test (Reitan, 1958)
*Controlled Word Association Test (Spreen & Beton, 1969)

Boston Naming Test (usually sensitive only in later stages) (Kaplan, Goodglass, & Weintraub, 1983)

*Writing sample (Goodglass & Kaplan, 1983a)

Reading Comprehension subtest, Boston Diagnostic Aphasia Examination (Goodglass & Kaplan, 1983b)

*Boston Visuospatial Quantitative Battery: drawings, maps, clocks (Goodglass & Kaplan, 1983b)

Hooper Visual Organization Test (Hooper, 1958)

*Finger Tapping Test (Halstead, 1947)

*Grip Strength Test (Reitan & Davison, 1974)

*Delayed Recognition Span Test (Moss, Albert, Butters, & Payne, 1986)

Albert's Famous Faces Test (Albert, Butters, & Levin, 1979)

*Minnesota Multiphasic Personality Inventory-2 (MMPI-2; Hathaway & McKinley, 1989)

*Profile of Mood States (McNair, Lorr, & Droppleman, 1971)

Visual analogue depression scale (Aitken, 1969)

Other tests that may be useful include the following:

Peabody Picture Vocabulary Test—Revised (for estimating premorbid IQ in patients without evidence of spatial hemi-inattention) (Dunn & Dunn, 1981)

*Category Test (Reitan & Davison, 1974)

*Raven's Progressive Matrices (Raven, 1958)

*Paced Auditory Serial Addition Test (PASAT; Gronwall & Sampson, 1974)

*Continuous-performance test

*Cancellation tasks (Weintraub & Mesulam, 1988)

Repeated motor programs (Luria, 1982)

Luria Three-Step (Luria, 1982)

*Tactual Performance Test (Halstead, 1947)

California Verbal Learning Test (CVLT; Delis, Kramer, Kaplan, & Ober, 1987)

*Rey–Osterrieth Complex Figure (Osterrieth, 1946)

*Brown–Peterson Interference Memory Tasks (Peterson, 1966)

*Buschke Selective Reminding Test (Buschke & Fuld, 1974)

*Fatigue Severity Scale (Krupp et al., 1989; a measure of fatigue symptomatology)

Typical Neuropsychological Assessment Findings

Basic Sensory-Perceptual Measures

We do not know of any empirical studies that have found deficits in basic tactile- or auditory-perceptual functions in the early stages of MS.

Because of the most typical lesion sites, deficits in visual processing are often apparent early in the disease.

Lateral Dominance Examination: Motor and Psychomotor Tests

Most investigators agree that motor deficits occur in MS. Given the multiplicity of lesion sites that may produce motor loss, such as the cerebral hemispheres, spinal cord, and cerebellum (sites that are often affected), it is not surprising that motor deficits are seen even early in the disease process.

Motor deficits are commonly seen during neuropsychological testing in handwriting samples, in which writing is often large, irregular, or poorly formed (secondary to poor graphomotor control), or in drawings. For example one patient's drawing of a daisy (Figure 15.1) is notable for impaired fine manual motor control. In addition, impaired performance on simple motor tasks, such as the Grip Strength or Finger Tapping Tests, may be seen. Behaviorally, MS patients may show frank tremor of, more rarely, chorea.

Measures of Attention/Executive Functions

Auditory

Research findings regarding attention deficits for auditorily presented material in MS are inconsistent. Although there have been reports

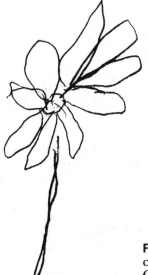

FIGURE 15.1. Fine manual motor control deficit when drawing a daisy (Boston Visuospatial Quantitative Battery).

of impaired Digit Span in performance patients with MS as compared to normal controls (Diers & Brown, 1950; Fink & Houser, 1966; Hirschenfang & Benton, 1966), other investigators have reported no attentional problems in MS (van den Burg et al., 1987) on the WAIS-R Digit Span (Litvan, Grafman, Vendrell, & Martinez, 1988), or on other tasks such as a continuous-performance test (Raymond et al., 1987; Raymond, Authelet, Stern, & Penny, 1989). It appears that when patients with MS are tested for limits, their performances drop off. For example, in one study, PASAT performance was impaired at the two highest speeds (Litvan et al., 1988).

In our clinical experience, attention and executive system dysfunction are frequently prominent in patients with MS, even in early stages of the illness. During exacerbations, even simple attention may be highly affected, and a patient may even be confused. Deficits are noted on tests such as WAIS-R Digit Span (backward) and the PASAT—tests that require complex cognitive tracking. This is particularly true of patients with mild white matter disease, though impairments even in simple attention occur in patients with many white matter lesions or with brain stem involvement.

Visual

Impairments in visual sequencing and complex visual attention are also common in patients with MS. For example, simple tracking and sequencing as measured by the Trail Making Test, Part A are typically intact early in the disease, though alternating sequences (Trail Making Test, Part B and recurrent series writing) may be difficult for a patient with even limited white matter pathology.

Patients may be pulled to the stimulus figure when copying visual stimuli. For example, a patient with relapsing–remitting MS, when asked to copy the pattern "mnmnmn" across the page, copied the sequence unusually close to the original stimulus (Figure 15.2). In addition, he

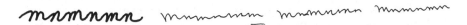

FIGURE 15.2. Example of perseveration when completing recurrent series writing in a 45-year-old patient with MS.

perseverated one "m" on the first segment with both his right and his left hand.

Perseverative contamination is also fairly common in patients with MS. For example, when one female patient with relapsing—remitting MS was asked to draw a cube, she drew a figure similar to the one that she drew previously for delayed recall of the WMS design (Figure 15.3).

Tests of Memory

Memory deficits are often seen in patients with MS (e.g., Beatty, Goodkin, Monson, Beatty, & Hertsgaard, 1988; Carroll, Gates, & Roldan, 1984; Rao, Leo, & St. Aubin-Fanbert, 1989; Vowels, 1979). Rao, Hammeke, McQuillen, Khatri, and Lloyd (1984) found that approximately 20% of a group with chronic/progressive MS were severely impaired on memory tests, whereas 43% were mildly impaired and 36% were indistinguishable from a group of normal control subjects. Specific types of memory deficits vary widely among patients, depending upon the underlying neuropathology of lesion sites in individual patients. In general, memory deficits may be the result of poor attention, impaired encoding or slowed acquisition, decreased spontaneous retrieval, or impaired recognition. In our experience, patients with MS show patterns of poor attention, slowed acquisition, and limited spontaneous recall of new information in the context of relatively intact recognition memory, with little or no forgetting over time. In addition, they are generally better at verbal than at visual—spatial memory tasks, because of the extra burden of perceptual processing on memory in patients for whom such processing is problematic. A review of common neuropsychological findings on tests of verbal, visual—spatial, and retrograde memory is now presented.

Verbal Memory

The performance of patients with MS on verbal memory tasks may be affected by poor attention and inefficient encoding, in addition to slowed information processing. For example, patients may have difficulty learning material without repeated exposure. Because of poor attention

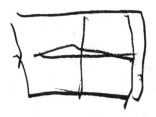

FIGURE 15.3. Perseverative contamination of elements from previously drawn figures and objects in a patient with MS.

and impaired cognitive flexibility, patients may be unable to develop strategies necessary to encode and retrieve newly learned material. Moreover, patients may be unable to work with effort in a situation in which they are presented with an interference task, and rapid forgetting rates may be seen with tasks that are dependent on the ability to learn in the context of divided attention, such as the Brown–Peterson tasks (Beatty et al., 1988).

A 58-year-old right-handed male patient with relapsing–remitting MS showed the typical dissociation between recall and recognition memory on the CVLT. Across five learning trials he showed the following learning curve from a list of 16: 4, 5, 5, 4, 8. Delayed free recall was 3, and cued recall was 5. However, recognition memory testing on long delay showed 15 of 16 hits and no false alarms. This same patient performance as follows on the Logical Memory subtest of the WMS:

Immediate recall: 15 details total.
Delayed recall: 0 details total.
Multiple choice: 16 of 20.

Visual–Spatial Memory

Patients with MS may also have impaired visual–spatial processing, which can affect the ability to learn and remember information that is presented visually. Patients again have an especially difficult time with tasks requiring effort, such as copying and recalling the outer form and inner details of a complex figure. The Rey–Osterrieth Complex Figure can yield some information on *functional* ability to complete effortful memory tasks requiring free recall, but it is often difficult for patients with MS, given their frequent visual–spatial and motor deficits. For example, a 49-year-old male with chronic/progressive MS was unable to maintain the outer form of the Rey–Osterrieth Complex Figure for immediate recall. He simplified the outer configuration and perseverated inner details (Figure 15.4).

In our experience, the Visual Reproduction subtest of the WMS is also quite sensitive to MS. Drawings are often notable for loss of details and perseveration.

Retrograde Memory

Patients with MS (at least in the early to moderate stages) usually show intact retrograde memory for personal and public information. However, they may show some unevenness in retrieval of information such as names on formal testing (this can be assisted for the patients by phonemic cuing), and they may show reduced knowledge of public

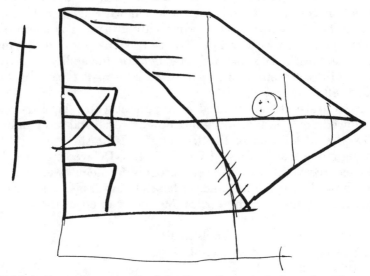

FIGURE 15.4. Immediate recall of the Rey–Osterrieth Complex Figure in a 49-year-old patient with MS.

information and events occurring during exacerbations or following pronounced disability secondary to their illness.

Wechsler Performance Subtests

Patients with MS frequently score relatively poorly on WAIS-R visual–spatial Performance subtests (Diers & Brown, 1950; Heaton et al., 1985); this reflects the multiplicity of MS sites that may produce impaired performance on visual–spatial tasks (e.g., optic nerves, white matter, and cerebellum). Examples of difficulties that these patients often have on the Performance subtests of the WAIS-R include the following: rotation of block designs or pieces of puzzles, "pull" to the red aspects of the Block Design stimuli, and poor visual–spatial planning or impaired sequencing. Lastly, motor slowing may hinder patients on the timed visual–spatial tasks.

Other Measures of Visual–Spatial Abilities

In addition to deficits on the WAIS-R subtests, deficits on the Halstead–Reitan visual–motor tasks have been shown by patients with MS (Beatty & Grange, 1977; Goldstein & Shelly, 1974; Heaton et al., 1985; Ivnik, 1978; Ross & Reitan, 1955). In addition, critical flicker fusion abnormalities have been identified (Ross & Reitan, 1955; Titcombe & Willison, 1961).

Qualitative findings from visual–spatial tests in patients with MS include typical "subcortical" kinds of constructional deficits, including perseveration of parts of drawings on spontaneous or copy constructions (Figure 15.5). In addition, patients with focal cortical lesions or large subcortical lesions may show focal visual–spatial deficits, such as hemi-inattention (parietal), inability to represent perspective (frontal), or loss of appreciation of outer configurations (temporal, parietal), as in the example of a drawing of a cube provided in Figure 15.6.

Measures of Abstract Reasoning

Cognitive flexibility may be affected relatively early in the disease process, producing difficulties on such tasks as the WCST. Specifically, patients with MS often show *qualitative* evidence of frontal system dysfunction; that is, they may perseverate prior sets or have difficulty in generating all of the categorical sets. For example, one of our patients who was diagnosed with MS 5 years prior to testing was unable to get into set or maintain categorical sets on the WCST. She was only able to complete 3 sorts in 168 trials because she continued to perseverate the prior set. In addition, although she was able to verbalize the rules of the test, she lost set on two occasions.

Heaton et al. (1985) reported impaired performance on the Hal-stead–Reitan Category Test in patients with chronic/progressive but not relapsing–remitting MS. Similarly, Peyser, Edwards, Poser, and Filskov (1980) reported that 50% of the patients with MS in their sample had abnormal performance (i.e., error scores greater than 50) on the Category Test. On a reasoning test using blocks, Parsons, Stewart, and Aren-berg (1957) reported impaired abstraction in patients with MS even when other possible sources of error, such as attention, were controlled for.

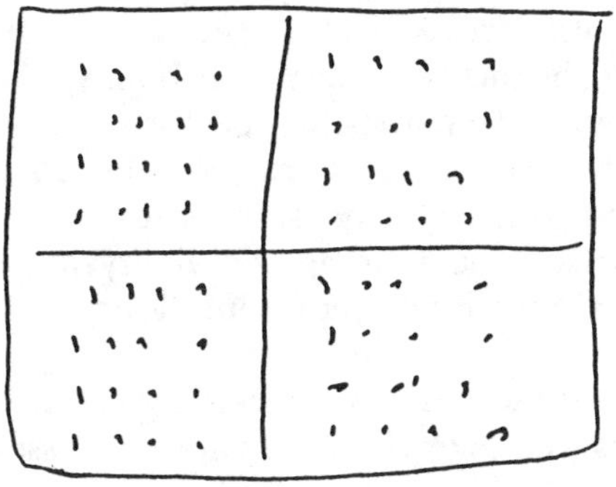

FIGURE 15.5. Perseveration in a drawing from the WMS Visual Reproductions subtest.

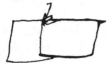

FIGURE 15.6. Examples of loss of outer form in this copy of a cube in a patient with MS.

Perseverative contamination of prior responses into later responses is also common on the Verbal subtests of the WAIS-R (see below). For example, one patient seen shortly after an exacerbation showed such a response on the Vocabulary subtest of the WAIS-R. After having defined "penny" and "winter," she defined "repair" as "having money for winter." Similarly, a patient may be stimulus-bound when completing verbal reasoning tests, may confuse metaphors when interpreting proverbs, or may lose sight of the abstract interpretation of proverbs or metaphorical expressions. For example, when one patient was asked, "What does this saying mean: 'One swallow does not make a summer'?", she replied as follows: "The weather varies from time to time, and you cannot count on anything at any time."

Wechsler Verbal Subtests

In general, the WAIS-R protocols of patients with MS reveal relatively intact verbal skills in the context of relatively impaired visual–spatial skills. When deficits are found on verbal tasks, they are most likely to be the results of impaired abstract reasoning, slowed mental processing, or impaired attention.

Some researchers (Fink & Houser, 1966) have reported impaired performance on the WAIS-R Similarities and Comprehension subtests in patients with MS, compared to normal controls. However, other researchers have reported normal performance on the WAIS-R Verbal reasoning subtests in patients with MS (Diers & Brown, 1950; Jambor, 1969; Litvan et al., 1988). Goldstein and Shelly (1974) found that patients with MS performed similarly to other brain-damaged patients and neuropsychiatric patients on the WAIS-R Similarities and Comprehension subtests. As stated previously, impaired abstract reasoning, which may occur relatively early in the disease process, affects patients' performance on these two subtests. Another WAIS-R subtest that can be affected by loss of abstract set is Vocabulary, in which patients sometimes become concrete in their definitions, while still maintaining the ability to use the words in conversation and retaining inner representations of the words' meaning.

Performance on the Arithmetic subtest may be marred by impaired attention and poor concentration, as well as by slowed mental processing speed. Fund of academic information remains relatively intact, except for occasional problems in retrieving exact information.

Other Measures of Verbal and Language Skills

Goldstein and Shelly (1974) reported intact verbal skills in their samples of patients with MS, compared to neurological and neuropsychiatric controls. However, several investigators have described verbal and language deficits in these patients. For example, deficits have been reported on tests of naming (Caine, Bamford, Schiffer, Shoulson, & Levy, 1986; Jambor, 1969), reading (Jambor, 1969), and verbal fluency (Beatty et al., 1989; Heaton et al., 1985).

The inconsistencies in research findings on verbal dysfunction in MS may reflect the variability of MS lesion sites in the samples used by different investigators. However, there were also differences in the control groups used in these studies. The comparisons made by Goldstein and Shelly (1974) of patients with MS to other patient groups likely to show cognitive loss (neurological patients, neuropsychiatric patients) would be expected to produce fewer effects than would comparisons to normal control subjects. Because MS can have extensive effects on subcortical white matter and cortex, it is reasonable to conclude that some patients will exhibit naming deficits and other symptoms of language loss.

Clinical observation has revealed that patients with MS are often dysarthric (presumably secondary to cerebellar pathology). They are also frequently impaired in verbal fluency, as measured by controlled word association techniques. Dysfluency of this type can be seen in patients with cerebellar, brain stem, cerebral, and white matter involvement. We saw a 36-year-old woman with relapsing–remitting MS of 2 to 3 years' duration who exhibited relatively normal performance on the FAS test at her first testing, at which time there was minimal white matter pathology on MRI. One year later, with increased white matter pathology reported on MRI, her performance on the Controlled Word Association Test dropped considerably. Confrontation naming on the Boston Naming Test was normal at both testings (59 of 60), though mild paraphasia was observed.

In our experience, naming is not usually affected early in the disease unless the patient has a focal left-hemisphere area of demyelination. However, a dysnomia often develops as the disease progresses and as the number and volume of white matter lesions in the left hemisphere increase. This naming deficit is characterized by word retrieval problems and circumlocutions.

As stated previously, patients with MS may also have problems with graphomotor control, and written letters are often poorly formed. In addition, errors in monitoring and perseveration may be seen in the writing of these patients.

Academic Achievement

Reading in patients with MS may be adversely affected by visual-perceptual deficits secondary to optic nerve damage (producing decreased visual acuity and scotoma, nystagmus, or diplopia). In addition, retention of material read may be impaired because of poor encoding secondary to decreased attention. In our experience, the linguistic aspects of reading comprehension are usually well retained unless there is focal left-cortical or extensive left-hemisphere white matter damage. Likewise, comprehension of conversation and repetition are usually intact.

Behavior and Personality

Psychiatric symptoms often predate the existence of cognitive changes. For example, in some cases, depression or other affective symptoms can be the first sign of the disease (Goodstein & Farrell, 1977), with fatigue being the most common symptom. We know of cases in which patients have been hospitalized for psychiatric reasons while physical symptoms, such as incontinence and parasthesias, go unnoticed. The most common psychiatric diagnoses are affective disorders (including depression, euphoria, and bipolar disorders), hysterical symptoms, and psychosis.

RELATIONSHIP TO THE WHITE MATTER MODEL

MS is a white matter disease, and therefore it affects the same cerebral structures as those implicated in the Nonverbal Learning Disabilities (NLD)/white matter model. However, the pathology is much more severe and extensive in the amount of tissue involved. In addition, the NLD model is better fitted to data for children, whose behavioral and cognitive features are *developmentally* affected by underlying pathology. This is a different situation from that seen in adults, in whom MS pathology alters well-established behavioral patterns.

In its broad outlines, MS fits the NLD model (Rourke, 1989; Harnadek & Rourke, 1994) very well. In both MS and the developmental NLD syndrome, the clinician observes deficits in perceptual, motor, visual–spatial, executive, reasoning, and affective functions. The similarities and differences in the particular behaviors observed in children and adults with developmental NLD and MS are quite interesting.

In regard to perceptual processing, patients with MS often have primary visual-perceptual deficits resulting from lesions of the CNS structures mediating visual perception (i.e., the optic chiasm). Such deficits may also be seen when significant lesions occur in posterior portions of the brain. Motor incoordination is very common in MS and can be multiply determined: It may result from white matter lesions or from spinal cord and cerebellar involvement. In our experience, motor deficits are nearly universal in MS patients, and white matter is the most common site of neuropathological damage.

Significant visual–spatial processing problems are seen in most patients diagnosed with MS. Though cerebellar involvement may contribute in some cases, white matter pathology appears to be the usual determinant of visual–spatial–organizational deficit.

Difficulties in problem solving, concept formation, flexible interpretation of incoming information, effective planning, insight, use of effective strategies, and other aspects of executive functioning have been described as a hallmark of NLD syndrome. These are seen in MS, though they appear to be less severe and pervasive in MS than in developmental disorders, and they have a less devastating effect on social interactions. Patients with MS can show remarkable difficulties in planning, and a subset are described as bland and nonreactive to the severity of their illness.

As in NLD, rote verbal skills are generally well retained in MS unless there is focal left-hemisphere damage involving cortical grey areas or until there are large numbers of white matter lesions in the left hemisphere, at which time naming and other basic verbal abilities may be affected. Verbal information that has been held in memory store for a long time is generally retrievable; however, the ability to learn and retrieve new verbal information can be problematic. As in NLD, learning visual–spatial information is more difficult than learning verbal information.

Though patients with MS who have word-finding difficulty (producing circumlocutory speech) or hypomanic affect (with associated press of speech) can be highly verbose, speech is not usually of the "cocktail party" variety seen in children with NLD. Speech prosody is also apparently better retained in patients with MS than in persons with developmentally based NLD.

Although mechanical problems with arithmetic are described in the NLD model, these are generally not seen in patients with MS unless there is extensive left posterior involvement or a developmental history of arithmetic problems. When difficulties arise on arithmetic tests in patients with MS, these are usually secondary to inattention, deficits in cognitive tracking, or visual-perceptual problems.

Deficits in social perception, judgment, and interaction are prominent in NLD but variable in MS. There is no question that there is often a decline in social interaction in MS, and such patients are often

abandoned by spouses. These outcomes appear to be multiply determined; their causes seem to include primary personality changes, as well
as the chronicity of the disease, physical deterioration, and socioeconomic
losses. Patients with MS do develop primary affective disorders such as
those described in the NLD model. These can include major depression,
dysthymic disorders, manic states, and bipolar/cycling disorders in some
patients. Interestingly, the pre-eminent affective tone common to most
patients with MS is a pervasive feeling of fatigue. Perhaps the differences
in social/affective outcomes of patients with MS versus patients with
developmental NLD reflect the former patients' experience of change in
CNS function, rather than the effects of a static condition seen in some
developmental disorders.

In sum, MS can be viewed as an "NLD+ syndrome," with many
features in common with developmental NLD but also some differences.
The differences can probably be attributed to the following:

- Developmental stage of brain structure and function at the time
  that pathological abnormalities begin to occur and express themselves in behavior.
- Existence of neuropathological abnormalities outside of the white
  matter in MS.
- Existence of focal lesions (cortical and subcortical) in MS, with
  associated focal functional abnormalities.
- Progressive nature of MS, which can result in widespread deficits
  in later stages of the disease.

VARIABILITY AND SEVERITY OF DISORDER MANIFESTATIONS

As stated earlier in this chapter, the variability and severity of symptoms
differ widely among patients with MS, depending upon the sites of lesions. In addition to the variability of symptoms, the course of MS also
differs widely among patients. Often an initial symptom occurs with a
long latency before other symptoms appear. Generally, as the disease
progresses, the periods of remission become shorter. The general relapse
rate is about 0.3 to 0.4 exacerbations per year, although this can vary
widely. McAlpine and Compston (1952) reported the following relapse
rates for a sample of patients with MS: 1 year (30%); 2 years (50%); 5
to 9 years (10%); 10 to 30 years (10%). Although there is little agreement
about the events that may precipitate an exacerbation, some investigators
claim that pregnancy may be associated with relapse (Schapira,
Poskanzer, Newell, & Miller, 1966; McAlpine, Lumsden, & Acheson,
1972), and others believe that there is a temporal relationship between
viral infections and subsequent exacerbations of MS (Sibley, Bamford,
& Clark, 1985).

On the basis of clinical course, MS in individual patients is sometimes classified as belonging to one of three types: acute MS, which is rapidly progressive; relapsing–remitting MS, which is characterized by periods of exacerbation followed by recovery; and chronic progressive MS, in which the patient gradually deteriorates. These categories, however, are not completely reliable (Goodkin et al., 1989).

As the disease progresses, patients tend to enter a period of deterioration, which Adams and Victor (1985) attribute to the cumulative number of CNS lesions acquired. Duration of MS is extremely variable: The *average* duration of the disease is over 30 years, but some patients live only a few months after initial symptoms present themselves.

DIFFERENTIAL DIAGNOSTIC CONSIDERATIONS

For the neuropsychologist, it is important to recognize that if MS lesions occur outside of the cerebral parts of the CNS, patients may show no cognitive dysfunction. Also, as stated previously, in early stages or after mild exacerbations cognitive recovery may occur, and no cognitive deficits will be seen on neuropsychological evaluation. Even when neuropsychological deficits are observed, they may be mild or may be evident qualitatively but not quantitatively. Therefore, it is essential to attend to subtle findings on neuropsychological exam. Finally, diagnosis of MS in its early stages can be a tricky endeavor, ultimately involving the integration of multiple test findings—the results of neurological examination and neuroimaging studies, as well as of neuropsychological testing. The neuropsychologist may render an opinion on the pattern of neuropsychological test results: Are they typical for MS, and, if so, where are the lesions likely to be located? Such an opinion is more likely to be accurate when test results are positive and typical than when results are negative. In the latter situation, making a conservative statement that findings typical for MS were not seen (without claiming that the patient does not have MS) is often the most prudent course.

MS patients are most typically misdiagnosed as having psychiatric illnesses, other disorders involving subcortical structures (e.g., Parkinson disease), toxicant-induced encephalopathy, and early dementia of the Alzheimer type or leukoaraiosis.

CASE EXAMPLE

Initial Evaluation

Background

Ms. C. was a right-handed woman with a bachelor's degree who had relapsing–remitting MS and was seen twice for neuropsychological assessment. She was initially referred by her neurologist after neurological examination raised the question of MS versus a degenerative cerebellar disease. Ms. C.'s physical symptoms at the time of her initial testing included difficulties with her balance and numbness on her right side. Her history was notable for hypomania, for which she was hospitalized just prior to her first evaluation. At the time of this first testing, medications included lithium.

Ms. C. was friendly and cooperative with testing. Her mood seemed almost euphoric, and she did not appear to be upset by the fact that she might have MS. She worked very slowly on tasks, and at times she had trouble persisting with tasks requiring fine motor coordination.

Test Results

Initial neuropsychological testing revealed Ms. C.'s IQ to be in the average range, though her premorbid IQ was estimated to be in the bright-normal range on the basis of her performance on Vocabulary (age scaled score = 12). Performance on verbal tasks was significantly better than performance on nonverbal tasks because of motor slowing on the latter tasks. Psychomotor speed was in the borderline range.

On tests of attention and executive function, Ms. C. was slow on tests of mental control, and she made errors when completing a verbal imagery test. She perseverated and lost set when completing recurrent series writing of "mn" with the left hand, and she needed verbal cues when performing a motor sequencing test.

Acquisition of verbal material was intact, although Ms. C. was somewhat susceptible to interference. She also had poor retrieval of nonverbal material. Mild deficits in visual organization were apparent, and motor slowing marred her performances on timed visual–spatial tasks.

Perseveration and disinhibition were apparent on tests requiring problem solving and the ability to plan ahead. Performance on verbal and language testing was mostly within expected levels, although word list generation was notable for perseveration. A writing sample revealed mild tremor.

Second Testing

Background

Ms. C. was seen again for testing 3 years, 5 months later. At that time, she was continuing to have difficulties with her balance. In addition, she was suffering from urinary incontinence and parasthesias in both hands. She had recently been diagnosed with diminished peripheral vision and loss of depth perception, and she noted that she suffered from diplopia when she was tired. Her MS appeared to be equally troubling in cold and warm weather.

During this test session, Ms. C. was friendly and cooperative with testing, but her affect was relatively flat. She often interrupted the examiner, and her performances were marred by restlessness and disinhibition, such as inserting comments into timed tasks.

Test Results

Ms. C.'s overall intellectual functioning was in the average range, but slightly below her level of functioning at initial evaluation. Motor testing revealed significantly slowed left-sided motor speed, and left-sided tremor was noted on writing tasks. Simple attention for auditorily presented material was variable, and she made occasional perseverative errors on executive system tasks.

Ms. C. was able to learn and remember verbal material; however, on this second testing, she confabulated and confused details. In addition, she was unable to retrieve nonverbal material after delays. Set loss marred her performance on a test of visual integration, and she also had difficulty identifying subtle nuances in stimuli on the WAIS-R Picture Arrangement subtest. Ms. C.'s drawings revealed perseveration and inattention to the left side of space.

Problem solving was impaired because of a tendency to lose set repeatedly. Verbal tasks were characterized by verbosity and concreteness. At this test session, Ms. C. had difficulty with word definitions because of underelaboration. She was circumlocutory when answering reasoning questions, and she had difficulty organizing her thoughts when interpreting proverbs. Her performance on a verbal test of abstract reasoning also revealed a tendency to be stimulus-bound. Perseveration affected her performance on a test of word list generation, but her performances on naming and academic achievement tests were unimpaired.

Ms. C.'s MMPI-2 profile showed reports of unusual experiences, as well as restlessness and possible agitation.

Neuropsychological testing showed a tendency to lose set, occasional perseveration, sequencing errors, and a tendency to be stimulus-bound. Motor slowing and tremulousness were also observed, with left-hand motor weakness. She had difficulty with visual organization and integration. Affect was suggestive of denial and restlessness. This profile of neuropsychological deficits is typical of the pattern seen with widespread, diffuse white matter lesions in MS. This case is an interesting demonstration of multifocal progression of cognitive change over time. At the second testing, increased problems with cognitive efficiency were evident;

this finding is typical of those seen in patients with multiple white matter lesions.

Comments

This case illustrates several features of the NLD model. At initial evaluation, the patient showed impaired motor speed, visual imagery, problem solving, and planning. In addition, she showed more difficulty in manual motor dexterity and processing with the left hand than the right hand. At her second evaluation, other features emerged, including loss of behavioral control and verbosity of speech.

REFERENCES

Accornero, N., DeVito, G., Rotunno, A., Perugino, U., & Manfredi, M. (1989). Critical fusion frequency in multiple sclerosis during mild induced hyperthermia. *Acta Neurologica Scandinavica, 79*, 510–514.

Adams, R. D., & Victor, M. (1985). Multiple sclerosis and allied demyelinative diseases. In R. D. Adams & M. Victor (Eds.), *Principles of neurology* (3rd ed., pp. 699–717). New York: McGraw-Hill.

Aitken, R. C. (1969). Measurement of feelings using visual analogue scales. *Proceedings of the Royal Society of Medicine, 62*, 17–24.

Albert, M. L. (1978). Subcortical dementia. In R. Katzman, R. D. Terry, & K. L. Bick (Eds.), *Aging: Vol. 7. Alzheimer's disease, senile dementia and related disorders* (pp. 173–180). New York: Raven Press.

Albert, M. S., Butters, N., & Levin, J. (1979). Temporal gradients in the retrograde amnesia of patients with alcoholic Korsakoff disease. *Archives of Neurology, 36*, 211–216.

Beatty, P. A., & Gange, J. J. (1977). Neuropsychological aspects of multiple sclerosis. *Journal of Nervous and Mental Disease, 164*, 42–50.

Beatty, W. W., Goodkin, D. E., Monson, N., & Beatty, P. A. (1989). Cognitive disturbances in patients with relapsing remitting multiple sclerosis. *Archives of Neurology, 46*, 1113–1119.

Beatty, W. W., Goodkin, D. E., Monson, N., Beatty, P. A., & Hertsgaard, D. (1988). Anterograde and retrograde amnesia in patients with chronic progressive multiple sclerosis. *Archives of Neurology, 45*, 611–619.

Buschke, J., & Fuld, P. A. (1974). Evaluating storage, retention, and retrieval in disordered memory and learning. *Neurology, 11*, 1019–1025.

Caine, E. D., Bamford, H. A., Schiffer, R. B., Shoulson, I., & Levy, S. (1986). A controlled neuropsychological comparison of Huntington's disease and multiple sclerosis. *Archives of Neurology, 43*, 249–254.

Carroll, M., Gates, R., & Roldan, F. (1984). Memory impairment in multiple sclerosis. *Neuropsychologia, 22*, 297–302.

Costantino, A., Black, S. E., Carr, T., Nicholson, R. L., & Noseworthy, J. H. (1986). Dorsal midbrain syndrome in multiple sclerosis with magnetic resonance imaging correlation. *Canadian Journal of Neurological Science, 13,* 62–65.

Delis, D., Kramer, J. H., Kaplan, E., & Ober, B. A. (1987). *California Verbal Learning Test manual.* New York: Psychological Corporation.

DePaulo, J. R., Folstein, M. F., & Fordon, B. (1980). Psychiatric screening on a neurological ward. *Psychological Medicine, 10,* 125–132.

Diers, W. C., & Brown, C. C. (1950). Psychometric patterns associated with multiple sclerosis. *Archives of Neurology and Psychiatry, 63,* 760–765.

Dunn, L. M., & Dunn, L. M. (1981). *Peabody Picture Vocabulary Test—Revised: Manual.* Circle Pines, MN: American Guidance Service.

Ebers, G. C. (1983). Genetic factors in multiple sclerosis. *Neurologic Clinics, 1,* 645–654.

Fink, S. L., & Houser, H. B. (1966). An investigation of physical and intellectual changes in multiple sclerosis. *Archives of Physical Medicine and Rehabilitation, 47,* 56–61.

Goldstein, G., & Shelly, C. H. (1974). Neuropsychological diagnosis of multiple sclerosis in a neuropsychiatric setting. *Journal of Nervous and Mental Disease, 158,* 280–290.

Goodglass, H. C., & Kaplan, E. (1983a). *The assessment of aphasia and related disorders* (2nd ed.). Philadelphia: Lea & Febiger.

Goodglass, H. G., & Kaplan, E. (1983b). *Boston Diagnostic Aphasia Examination* (2nd ed.). Philadelphia: Lea & Febiger.

Goodkin, D. E., Hertsgaard, D., & Rudick, R. A. (1989). Exacerbation rates and adherence to disease type in a prospectively followed population with multiple sclerosis. *Archives of Neurology, 46,* 1107–1112.

Goodstein, R. K., & Ferrell, R. B. (1977). Multiple sclerosis presenting as a depressive illness. *Diseases of the Nervous System, 38,* 127–131.

Gronwall, D. M., & Sampson, H. (1974). *The psychological effects of concussion.* Auckland, New Zealand: Auckland University Press.

Halstead, W. C. (1947). *Brain and intelligence.* Chicago: University of Chicago Press.

Harnadek, C. S., & Rourke, B. P. (1994). Principal identifying features of the syndrome of nonverbal learning disabilities in children. *Journal of Learning Disabilities, 27,* 144–154.

Hathaway, S. R., & McKinley, J. C. (1989). *Minnesota Multiphasic Personality Inventory-2.* Minneapolis: University of Minnesota Press.

Heaton, R. K. (1981). *Wisconsin Card Sorting Test manual.* Odessa, FL: Psychological Assessment Resources.

Heaton, R. K., Nelson, L. M., Thompson, D. S., Burks, J. S., & Franklin, G. M. (1985). Neuropsychological findings in relapsing–remitting and chronic–progressive multiple sclerosis. *Journal of Consulting and Clinical Psychology, 53,* 103–110.

Hirschenfang, S., & Benton, J. G. (1966). Note on intellectual changes in multiple sclerosis. *Perceptual and Motor Skills, 22,* 786.

Hooper, H. E. (1958). *The Hooper Visual Organization Test manual.* Los Angeles: Western Psychological Services.

Ivnik, R. J. (1978). Neuropsychological test performance as a function of the duration of MS-related symptomatology. *Journal of Clinical Psychiatry, 39,* 304–312.

Jambor, K. L. (1969). Cognitive functioning in multiple sclerosis. *British Journal of Psychiatry*, 115, 765–775.

Kaplan, E., Goodglass, H., & Weintraub, S. (1983). *The Boston Naming Test*. Philadelphia: Lea & Febiger.

Krupp, L. B., LaRocca, N. G., Muir-Nash, J., & Steinberg, A. D. (1989). The Fatigue Severity Scale: Application to patients with multiple sclerosis and systemic lupus erythematosus. *Archives of Neurology*, 46, 1121–1123.

Kurtzke, J. F. (1965). Familial incidence and geography in multiple sclerosis. *Acta Neurologica Scandinavica*, 41, 127–139.

Kurtzke, J. F., Beebe, G. W., & Norman, J. E. (1979). Epidemiology of multiple sclerosis in U.S. veterans: I. Race, sex and geographic distribution. *Neurology*, 29, 1228–1235.

Kurtzke, J. F., Hyllested, K., & Heltberg, A. (1993). Multiple sclerosis in the Faroe Islands. In C. A. Molgaard (Ed.), *Neuroepidemiology: Theory and method* (pp. 23–50). New York: Academic Press.

Litvan, I., Graftman, J., Vendrell, P., & Martinez, J. M. (1988). Slowed information processing in multiple sclerosis. *Archives of Neurology*, 45, 281–285.

Luria, A. R. (1982). *Higher cortical functions in man* (2nd ed.). New York: Basic Books.

Marsh, G. G. (1980). Disability and intellectual function in multiple sclerosis patients. *Journal of Nervous and Mental Disease*, 168, 758–762.

Matthews, W. B., Acheson, E. D., Batchelor, J. R., & Weller, R. O. (1985). *McAlpine's multiple sclerosis*. New York: Churchill Livingstone.

McAlpine, D. M., & Compston, N. (1952). Some aspects of the natural history of disseminated sclerosis. *Quarterly Journal of Medicine*, 21, 135–167.

McAlpine, D. M., Lumsden, C. E., & Acheson, E. G. (1972). *Multiple sclerosis: A reappraisal* (2nd ed.). Baltimore: Williams & Wilkins.

McNair, D. M., Lorr, M., & Droppleman, L. F. (1971). *Profile of Mood States*. San Diego: Education and Industrial Testing Service.

Moss, M. B., Albert, M. S., Butters, N., & Payne, M. (1986). Differential patterns of memory loss among patients with Alzheimer's disease, Huntington's disease and alcoholic Korsakoff's syndrome. *Archives of Neurology*, 43, 239–246.

Nelson, D. A., & McDowell, F. (1959). The effects of induced hyperthermia on patients with multiple sclerosis. *Journal of Neurology, Neurosurgery and Psychiatry*, 22, 113–116.

Osterrieth, P. (1946). Le test de copie d'une figure complexe. *Archives de Psychologie*, 28, 286–340.

Parsons, O. A., Stewart, K. D., & Arenberg, D. (1957). Impairment of abstracting ability in multiple sclerosis. *Journal of Nervous and Mental Disease*, 125, 221–225.

Peterson, L. R. (1966). Short-term memory. *Scientific American*, 215, 90–95.

Peyser, J. M., Edwards, K. R., Poser, J. M., & Filskov, S. B. (1980). Cognitive function in patients with multiple sclerosis. *Archives of Neurology*, 37, 577–579.

Peyser, J. M., Rao, S. M., LaRocca, N. G., & Kaplan, E. (1990). Guidelines for neuropsychological research in multiple sclerosis. *Archives of Neurology*, 47, 94–97.

Poser, C. M., Paty, D. W., Scheinberg, L., McDonald, W. I., Davis, F. A., Ebers, G. C., Johnson, K. P., Sibley, W. A., Silberberg, D. H., & Tourtellotte, W. W. (1983). New diagnostic criteria for multiple sclerosis: Guidelines for research protocols. *Annals of Neurology, 13*, 227–231.

Rao, S. M. (1986). Neuropsychology of multiple sclerosis: A critical review. *Journal of Clinical and Experimental Neuropsychology, 8*, 503–542.

Rao, S. M. (1990). Multiple sclerosis. In J. Cummings (Ed.), *Subcortical dementia* (pp. 164–180). New York: Oxford University Press.

Rao, S. M., Glatt, S., Hammeke, T. A., McQuillen, M. P., Khatri, B. O., Rhodes, A. M., & Pollard, S. (1985). Chronic progressive multiple sclerosis: Relationship between cerebral ventricular size and neuropsychological impairment. *Archives of Neurology, 42*, 678–682.

Rao, S. M., Hammeke, T. M., McQuillen, M. D., Khatri, B. O., & Lloyd, D. (1984). Memory disturbance in chronic progressive multiple sclerosis. *Archives of Neurology, 41*, 625–631.

Rao, S. M., Leo, G. J., & St. Aubin-Faubert, P. (1989). On the nature of memory disturbance in multiple sclerosis. *Journal of Clinical and Experimental Neuropsychology, 11*, 699–712.

Raven, J. C. (1958). *Standard Progressive Matrices*. London: H. K. Lewis.

Raymond, C. A. (1986). In pursuit of quarry, MS researchers draw on immunology, virology advances. *Journal of the American Medical Association, 256*, 809–816.

Raymond, P. F., Authelet, A. M., Stern, R. A., & Penny, D. (1989). *Patterns of memory function in multiple sclerosis*. Paper presented at the International Neuropsychological Society meeting, Vancouver, British Columbia.

Raymond, P. F., Stern, R. A., Authelet, A. M., & Penny, D. (1987). *A comparison of California Verbal Learning Test performance among patients with multiple sclerosis, right hemisphere vascular lesions and normal controls*. Paper presented at the International Neuropsychological Society meeting, Washington, DC.

Reitan, R. M. (1958). Validity of the Trail Making Test as an indicator of organic brain damage. *Perceptual and Motor Skills, 8*, 271–276.

Reitan, R. M., & Davison, L. A. (1974). *Clinical neuropsychology: Current status and applications*. New York: Hemisphere.

Ross, A. T., & Reitan, R. M. (1955). Intellectual and affective functions in multiple sclersosis: A quantitative study. *Archives of Neurology and Psychiatry, 73*, 663–677.

Rourke, B. P. (1989). *Nonverbal learning disabilities: The syndrome and the model*. New York: Guilford Press.

Schapira, K., Poskanzer, D. C., Newell, D. J., & Miller, H. (1966). Marriage, pregnancy and multiple sclerosis. *Brain, 89*, 419–428.

Sibley, W. A., Bamford, C. R., & Clark, K. (1985). Clinical viral infections and multiple sclerosis. *Lancet, i*, 1313–1315.

Spreen, O., & Benton, A. L. (1969). *Neurosensory Center Comprehensive Examination for Aphasia (NCCEA)*. Victoria, British Columbia: University of Victoria, Neuropsychological Laboratory.

Titcombe, A. F., & Willison, R. G. (1961). Flicker fusion in multiple sclerosis. *Journal of Neurology, Neurosurgery and Psychiatry, 24*, 260–265.

van den Burg, W., van Zomeren, A. H., Minderhoud, J. M., Prange, A. J., & Meijer, N. S. (1987). Cognitive impairment in patients with multiple sclerosis and mild physical disability. *Archives of Neurology, 44,* 494–501.

Vella, V. (1984). A review of the etiology of multiple sclerosis. *Italian Journal of Neurology Science, 5,* 347–356.

Vowels, L. M. (1979). Memory impairment in multiple sclerosis. In M. Malloy, G. V. Stanley, & K. W. Walsh (Eds.), *Brain impairment: Proceedings of the 1978 Brain Impairment Workshop* (pp. 10–22). Melbourne: University of Melbourne.

Wechsler, D. (1945). A standardized memory scale for clinical use. *Journal of Psychology, 19,* 87–95.

Wechsler, D. (1981). *Wechsler Adult Intelligence Scale—Revised.* New York: Psychological Corporation.

Weintraub, S., & Mesulam, M. M. (1988). Visual hemispatial inattention: Stimulus parameters and exploratory strategies. *Journal of Neurology, Neurosurgery and Psychiatry, 51,* 1481–1488.

16

Traumatic Brain Injury

Linda Ewing-Cobbs
Jack M. Fletcher
Harvey S. Levin

Reports in the literature have identified neuropsychological deficits in children and adolescents after severe traumatic brain injury that resemble the types of difficulties noted in children with the syndrome of Nonverbal Learning Disabilities (NLD) identified by Rourke (1989). These abnormalities include deficiencies in visual-perceptual organizational skills, psychomotor and tactile-perceptual impairment, and Performance IQ scores lower than Verbal IQ scores. Language functions tend to be less affected than visual-perceptual organizational skills (see Fletcher, 1994). In the present chapter, we review the neuroimaging, neuropathological, and epidemiological data on pediatric traumatic brain injury. Following a discussion of neuropsychological and behavioral findings, we present data from our ongoing longitudinal investigation of recovery from traumatic brain injury in children, which provide a preliminary examination of the possible presence of symptoms characteristic of the NLD syndrome.

In most of the studies reviewed, the Glasgow Coma Scale score (Teasdale & Jennett, 1974) was used to establish the severity of brain injury. This score ranges from 3 to 15 and assesses three components of consciousness: eye opening, motor response, and verbal response. Scores from 3 to 8 are regarded as reflecting a severe injury producing coma, which is defined as the absence of eye opening, inability to obey commands, and failure to utter recognizable words; scores between 9 and 12 are indicative of a brain injury of moderate severity; and scores between 13 and 15 reflect mild brain injury in patients who are generally alert, who have spontaneous eye opening, and whose verbal responses vary from confused to oriented.

NEUROIMAGING

Cerebral Computed Tomography

Early studies of the pathophysiology of closed head injury in children based on computed tomography (CT) scan findings indicated a high incidence of diffuse brain swelling, characterized by a decrease in cerebrospinal fluid spaces, compressed or obliterated mesencephalic cisterns, and small ventricles without evidence of other intracranial abnormalities (Bruce et al., 1979; Zimmerman et al., 1978). On the basis of these early studies, closed head injury in children was viewed as producing diffuse parenchymal injury in conjunction with low occurrence of focal parenchymal lesions.

In a recent report from the National Institutes of Health Traumatic Coma Data Bank, Aldrich et al. (1992) examined CT scan data prospectively collected from 111 children with severe head injury. Twenty-four percent of the sample of children had diffuse brain swelling with or without small parenchymal hemorrhages, and 17% had diffuse brain swelling without small parenchymal hemorrhages.

Neuroimaging studies report differing frequencies of occurrence of mass lesions following traumatic brain injury. CT scan results indicated focal mass lesions in 23% of 53 children studied by Bruce et al. (1979). In contrast, Berger, Pitts, Lovely, Edwards, and Bartkowski (1985) reported mass lesions in 46% of 37 children evaluated with CT scan.

Levin et al. (1992) evaluated neurobehavioral outcome during the first year following severe head injury in 103 children ages 0–15 years at injury. Bilateral diffuse swelling with midline shift of <3 mm was identified in 25% of the sample; an additional 10% had swelling with shift of >3 mm. Diffuse axonal injury, characterized by small parenchymal and/or intraventricular hemorrhages without brain swelling, shift, or mass lesions, was reported in 16%. Mass lesions, defined as a high- or mixed-density collection that was either intra- or extracerebral and 15 cc or more, were reported in 9%. Normal CT scans were seen in 9%. Levin et al. (1992) examined the relationship between the Glasgow Outcome Scale (Jennett & Bond, 1975) at 6 months after severe head injury in relation to the above-described CT scan abnormalities. Brain swelling was often associated with a poor outcome, including death, vegetative state, or severe disability. The frequency of focal brain lesions was quite low relative to the frequency of diffuse cerebral insult. Filley, Cranberg, Alexander, and Hart (1987) reported that outcome in a series of 50 consecutively admitted pediatric patients was worse in patients with diffuse brain injury plus focal lesions than in those with diffuse injury only.

Magnetic Resonance Imaging

The advent of magnetic resonance imaging (MRI) has suggested a view of the pathophysiology of closed head injury that differs from the view suggested by earlier CT studies. Levin et al. (1989) examined the occurrence of focal brain lesions visualized by MRI. Of 11 patients with severe injuries, 8 had areas of abnormal signal in the parenchyma; these 8 included 4 children with frontal lobe lesions, 3 children with primarily parietal lesions, and 1 patient with a primarily temporal lobe lesion. Nearly 50% of the severely injured patients had lesions extending to the subcortical white matter and/or deep central grey. Similarly, Mendelsohn et al. (1992) identified hemispheric lesions in 39 of 55 children and adolescents with moderate to severe closed head injury who were consecutively admitted to a pediatric trauma unit and underwent MRI at least 3 months after the injury. Abnormal signal intensity in the frontal lobes was present in 51% of the sample.

Levin et al. (1993) evaluated MRI and neurobehavioral data in 76 pediatric patients. Plotting of areas of abnormal signal on templates identified an anterocaudal gradient: Lesions occurred most frequently in the dorsolateral frontal region, the orbitofrontal region, and the frontal lobe white matter. Of the total sample, 75% had focal areas of abnormal posttraumatic signal. Forty percent of the sample, which was drawn from consecutive hospital admissions for closed head injury, had lesions restricted to or primarily in the frontal lobes. Thus, more recent MRI studies and neuropathological studies (see below) suggest that the incidence of focal lesions may be higher than previously observed. The frontal lobes are a frequent site of focal injury.

NEUROPATHOLOGY

Diffuse cerebral injury produced at the moment of impact appears to be the primary cause of brain damage following closed head injury (Adams, Mitchell, Graham, & Doyle, 1977; Strich, 1956). Strich (1956, 1970) reported pathological findings from the brains of patients with severe, diffuse closed head injuries who survived between 5 months and 1 year while remaining in a profoundly impaired or vegetative state. Strich noted subsequent white matter degeneration as the primary pathological change. In addition to generalized ventricular dilation, microscopic parenchymal lesions were visualized in the corpus callosum and the superior cerebellar peduncles. The disappearance of myelin as cerebral edema resolved was associated with the reduced bulk of the cerebral white matter. Neuronal damage was greatest in the corpus callosum, the parasagittal areas of hemispheres, the internal capsules, and the pons. Importantly, degeneration noted in the white matter was frequently asymmetrical, with tracks being damaged in one hemisphere and spared in the other.

Graham et al. (1989) completed comprehensive neuropathological studies on 87 children between 2 and 15 years of age who sustained fatal head injuries. Skull fracture was present in 72% of the cases. Large intracranial hematomas were present in 34%. Diffuse axonal injury was reported in 22%. Moreover, severe to moderately severe ischemic damage in the neocortex was identified in 61% of the cases. Brain swelling was apparent in 70%; however, there was no association of swelling with diffuse axonal injury. Cerebral contusions were present in 90% of the series. Graham et al. (1989) concluded that neuropathological findings following nonmissile head injury in children were not strikingly different from those observed in adults. Evidence of hypoxic brain damage and increased intracranial pressure was common; however, the occurrence of diffuse brain swelling appeared to be significantly higher in children. These results suggest significant involvement of cerebral white matter, but again highlight the prominent role of contusional injury to white and grey matter.

EPIDEMIOLOGY

Traumatic brain injury is a major public health concern. Annegers (1983) estimated that in the age range of 1 to 14 years in the United States, 10 per 100,000 children die from head trauma each year. This mortality rate is five times the death rate of leukemia, which is the next leading cause of death in children. Klauber, Barrett-Connor, Marshall, and Bowers (1981) reported that case–fatality ratios were highest in children under 5 years of age (17%) and in individuals 70 years of age and older.

Kraus, Fife, Cox, Ramstein, and Conroy (1986) identified all new occurrences of brain injury in 1981 in San Diego County. The major causes of pediatric brain injury included falls (35%), recreational activities (29%), and motor vehicle crashes (24%). The incidence of brain injury did not differ significantly between male and female children 1 to 4 years of age. However, significantly higher rates of injury were present for boys versus girls in the 5- to 14-year age range. Of 688 children who were admitted to a hospital, 88% had a mild brain injury, 7% had a moderate injury, and 5% had a severe injury. As Goldstein (1990) observed, head injury in children is a "silent epidemic."

DEVELOPMENTAL EFFECTS

Global Outcomes

Early reports concerning outcomes after traumatic brain injury in children indicated that mortality and morbidity rates were lower in children than in adults. However, more recent data suggest that developmental effects may be present in terms of both mortality and morbidity. Levin et al. (1992) divided their patients from the Traumatic Coma Data Bank into three age groups (0 to 4, 5 to 10, and 11 to 15 years). All patients sustained severe injuries as indicated by Glasgow Coma Scale (Teasdale & Jennett, 1974) scores of 8 or less. Analysis of the Traumatic Coma Data Bank cases (Levin et al., 1992) identified a 62% mortality rate by the end of the first year in infants and preschoolers, in comparison to the 5- to 10-year-olds, in whom the mortality rate was less than one-half that of the other children and adults. The outcomes in adolescents were similar to those identified in adults in the Traumatic Coma Data Bank. Since cases of assault or suspected child abuse were not systematically identified, it is unclear to what extent the high mortality rate in young children reflected cases of inflicted injury. Duhaime et al. (1992) inferred that nearly one-fourth of all admissions for head injury in children less than 24 months of age can be classified as inflicted.

Michaud, Rivara, Grady, and Reay (1992) evaluated outcome in 75 children and adolescents consecutively admitted to a Level I trauma center. A poor outcome was common in children less than or equal to 2 years of age; the mortality rate was 50%, and only 17% made a "good" recovery. Kriel, Krach, and Panser (1989) reported outcomes of 97 children with severe closed head injuries who were referred to a regional rehabilitation center. Children less than 6 years of age at injury had worse cognitive and motor outcomes than children ages 6 through 18 years of age at injury. Abused children had significantly worse cognitive and motor abilities than did age-matched patients who sustained accidental closed head injury. When abuse cases were excluded, no cognitive or motor differences attributable to age were present in the remaining sample.

Neuropsychological Outcomes

Neuropsychological studies have yielded data suggesting that the type of neuropsychological deficit observed following traumatic brain injury may vary with a child's developmental level at the time of injury. Similar findings have been reported in children with penetrating brain injury. In a recent study on long-term outcome from gunshot wounds to the brain in children and adolescents, Ewing-Cobbs, Thompson, Miner, and Fletcher (1994) identified differences in symptom patterns that appeared to be based on a child's developmental level at the time of injury. Intellectual and cognitive functions were significantly more impaired in children who were less than 5 years of age at the time of the gunshot wound than in older children and adolescents. Three-fourths of the younger children had IQ scores in the mentally deficient range at follow-up. Persistent deficits in school-aged children and adolescents were most prominent on measures of attention and adaptive behavior; psychometric intelligence scores recovered to the average to low-average ranges.

Studies examining intellectual function following closed head injury have generally not identified sparing of function in children. Brink, Garrett, Hale, Woo-Sam, and Nickel (1970) examined 52 patients ages 2 through 18 years at injury who were comatose for at least 1 week. The investigators identified a direct relationship between coma duration and posttraumatic IQ scores. Moreover, greater impairment was identified in children who were less than 8 years of age at the time of injury. Similarly, long-term intellectual impairment 4 to 14 years after severe closed head injury was reported by Lange-Cosack, Wider, Schlesner, Grumme, and Kubicki (1979). They reported that the late sequelae of acquired brain injury were clearly more severe in infants and young children than in school-aged children and adolescents. Abused children were included in their sample. Levin, Eisenberg, Wigg, and Kobayashi (1982) reported greater impairment of IQ scores in severely injured children than in adolescents with comparable injuries at a follow-up interval of 1 year. Several other studies of IQ recovery in school-aged children and adolescents have not reported differences attributable to age at injury (Chadwick, Rutter, Brown, Shaffer, & Traub, 1981; Klonoff, Low, & Clark, 1977; Levin & Eisenberg, 1979). Taken together, studies of mortality and morbidity following closed head injury suggest that young children are particularly vulnerable to the adverse effects of diffuse brain injury.

Rapid-Development Hypothesis

Our research group has investigated the hypothesis that skills in a rapid stage of development are more susceptible to disruption by acquired brain injury than are more overlearned and well-automatized skills. Some support for this hypothesis has been obtained in our studies of language functions following closed head injury. To illustrate, we identified greater impairment of expressive language ability during the first year after injury in infants and young children who were injured between 4 and 30 months of age than in those injured between 31 and 64 months of age (Ewing-Cobbs, Miner, Fletcher, & Levin, 1989). Our studies of language functions in school-aged children and adolescents identified greater impairment in written language in the school-aged children than in the adolescents (Ewing-Cobbs, Levin, Eisenberg, & Fletcher, 1987). We hypothesized that the type of deficit observed was related to the normal pattern of acquisition of language skills. Expressive language functions, which develop very rapidly in the early preschool years, were more disrupted by injury than were receptive language skills in children less than 31 months of age. In our school-aged sample, written language was more disrupted than other language areas. This finding is consistent with the rapid acquisition of written language skills in early primary grades.

In another study (Levin et al., 1988), we evaluated verbal learning and visual recognition memory in patients ages 6 to 8, 9 to 12, and 13 to 15 years at injury who were tested at baseline and 1 year after the injury. On a measure of visual recognition memory, severe closed head injury produced a marked deficit in all three age ranges. However, adolescents exhibited more severe and persistent impairment of verbal learning and memory than did children ages 6 to 12 years at injury. Visual recognition memory develops normally before 5 years of age; according to the rapid-development hypothesis, acquired brain injury should disrupt performance on such a measure comparably in children and adolescents. In contrast, verbal learning and memory deficiencies may be more prominent in severely injured adolescents than in school-aged children. Since semantic organization strategies develop rapidly during adolescence, cerebral injury sustained during adolescence may disrupt memory organization to a greater degree than does similar injury in school-aged children.

Thompson et al. (1994) used individual growth curve analysis to examine relationships between predictor variables reflecting injury characteristics such as CT scan findings, pupillary status, the Glasgow Coma Scale score, and the duration of impaired consciousness on a variety of motor, visual–spatial, and somatosensory outcome variables. On variables assessing visual–motor integration, psychomotor speed with the dominant hand, and speed of somatosensory processing, slower rates of change were found for severely injured younger subjects than for either older children or children sustaining milder injuries. The findings were interpreted as supporting the rapid-development hypothesis, because of the apparent increased vulnerability of rapidly emerging skills.

Investigation of the effect of developmental level at the time of injury on neuropsychological status awaits the completion of longitudinal studies that investigate the nature of changes in the acquisition of skill development by the injured brain. As findings by Goldman-Rakic (Goldman, 1974) suggest, the effect of brain injury may be manifested developmentally as a failure to acquire a skill at age-appropriate rates or levels. It will be particularly important to identify whether deficits in executive functions, which are putatively related to frontal lobe functions, show differential rates of impairment as children age. In addition, patients injured in early childhood must be followed longitudinally, to see whether their eventual symptom pattern resembles that seen in older children and adolescents.

NEUROPSYCHOLOGICAL OUTCOMES

Psychometric Intelligence

Prospective studies of intellectual recovery following closed head injury in children ages 5 to 14 years with posttraumatic amnesia persisting from 1 week to 3 months identified a reduction in Wechsler Verbal IQ and Performance IQ scores at baseline assessment, in comparison to orthopedic controls (Chadwick et al., 1981). However, by 1 year following the injury, the Performance IQ score was impaired relative to the Verbal IQ score and remained impaired through a 2-year follow-up (Chadwick, Rutter, Brown, et al., 1981). Winogron, Knights, and Bawden (1984) evaluated intellectual outcome retrospectively in 17 severely injured, 23 moderately injured, and 47 mildly injured children ranging in age from 2.5 to 17.3 years at the time of injury. The mean injury–test interval was approximately 1 year in all groups. Comparison of Wechsler Verbal IQ and Full Scale IQ scores by injury severity groups did not identify significant differences attributable to injury severity. However, the Performance IQ scores were lower in the severe group than in the mild or moderate groups; the moderate group also scored below the mild group.

Levin et al. (1982) identified a greater proportion of severely injured children with residual intellectual deficit, compared to adolescents with closed head injuries of comparable severity, at a 1-year follow-up. Although all 14 severely injured adolescents had IQ scores in at least the low-average range, one-third of the 15 severely injured children had residual intellectual deficit (defined as a Full Scale IQ score below 80). The greater proportion of children versus adolescents with residual intellectual impairment was hypothesized to be related to the more severe effects of diffuse cerebral insult on the developing brain.

Memory

Levin and Eisenberg (1979) performed an analysis of composite scores in the areas of memory, language, motor and somatosensory functioning, and visual–spatial ability; they reported that memory was the most frequently impaired neuropsychological domain. Levin et al. (1988) evaluated verbal and visual memory functions in 58 children and adolescents ages 6 to 15 years at injury, with either mild/moderate or severe closed head injury. To permit comparison across ages, scores from tests of verbal selective reminding and visual recognition memory were transformed into standard scores based on normative data. Visual recognition memory scores were lower in severely injured children than in those with mild/ moderate injuries, independent of the age at injury. However, the consistent long-term retrieval scores, reflecting retrieval of newly learned information from memory, were reduced in severely injured children relative to those with lesser injuries. At baseline, the scores from adolescents were below those obtained from children. However, at follow-up, there were no significant differences in the level of performance of children and adolescents.

Attention

Findings regarding the type and persistence of attentional disturbance following pediatric closed head injury have been inconclusive. Chadwick, Rutter, Shaffer, and Shrout (1981) identified attentional impairment in children in whom posttraumatic amnesia persisted for at least 2 weeks on the Stroop Test and on a continuous-performance test at the baseline assessment. By 4 months after the injury, these severely injured children scored lower than controls only on the continuous performance task. Group differences on measures of attention were not obtained at 1- and 2-year follow-up evaluations.

We (Kaufmann, Fletcher, Levin, Miner, & Ewing-Cobbs, 1993) evaluated the effects on attention of head injury severity and age at injury in 36 patients ages 7 to 16 years at the time of injury, using a computer-assisted, adaptive-rate continuous-performance test. In this study, the mean interstimulus interval for each of four trial blocks yielded an index of attentional efficiency. Severely injured patients scored lower than those with mild or moderate injuries at the 6-month follow-up. Young, severely injured children had the greatest impairment on the continuous-performance test. Although this study did not identify any relationships between injury severity and performance on the Wechsler Digit Span subtest, this measure of attention has generally been insensitive to the residual effects of closed head injury in adults.

Visual–Motor and Visual–Spatial Abilities

In their 1-year retrospective follow-up study of children with mild, moderate, and severe head injury, Winogron et al. (1984) identified slowing of both the dominant and nondominant hands on a finger-tapping task in the severely injured group; in addition, manual dexterity, as measured by a grooved pegboard task, was reduced only for the dominant hand in severely injured patients. In a 2¼-year prospective follow-up study, Chadwick, Rutter, Shaffer, and Shrout (1981) reported persisting deficits on a manual dexterity task requiring manipulation of pegs. The relative contributions of nonspecific motor slowing versus lateralized weakness to persistent deficits on speeded pegboard tasks remain to be studied.

Regarding tasks with visual–spatial components, Winogron et al. (1984) reported deficits on the Tactual Performance Test time-to-completion variable, and Chadwick, Rutter, Shaffer, and Shrout (1981) identified persisting difficulties on the Matching Familiar Figures Test 1 year after injury in severely injured patients. To identify further the nature of performance deficits following head injury in children, Bawden, Knights, and Winogron (1985) categorized tests from the Halstead–Reitan Neuropsychological Test Battery into those requiring high speed, moderate speed, and low to no speed. Children with severe head injuries performed significantly slower than did children with either mild or moderate head injuries on a variety of tests of motor speed, as well as on a test requiring motor speed and visual–spatial processing. When tests were divided according to the amount of speed required for performance, the severely injured patients obtained a significantly lower score on the summary measure for the highly speeded tests than on the summary measure for tests with low requirements for speed. Bawden et al. (1985) noted that the severely injured patients did not sustain a generalized deficit in motor or visual–spatial areas, since there were no severity group differences on other measures of motor strength and control and of visual–spatial abilities. The highly speeded tests included finger- and foot-tapping tests, pegboard tests, and the Coding subtest from the Wechsler Intelligence Scale for Children—Revised.

Language

We (Ewing-Cobbs et al., 1987) evaluated the nature of specific linguistic disturbance in head-injured children who exhibited no overt aphasic symptomatology. We administered the Neurosensory Center Comprehensive Examination for Aphasia (Spreen & Benton, 1969) to 23 children ages 5 to 10 years, and to 33 adolescents ages 11 to 15 years, at a median injury–test interval of 1 month. Composite scores reflecting naming, expressive language, receptive language, and written language functions were formed. Expressive language functions were more sensitive to the severity of head injury than were receptive language measures: Severely injured patients scored lower on measures of visual naming, sentence repetition, word fluency, and writing to dictation. Scores on receptive language subtests did not differ between the mild/moderate and severe injury groups. Writing to dictation was impaired in children as compared to adolescents. As previously discussed, we hypothesized that the greater impairment of written language in children as compared with adolescents was consistent with the view that rapidly emerging language skills are

more vulnerable to disruption by head injury than are more well-automatized abilities.

Jordan, Ozanne, and Murdoch (1988) evaluated language disorders
in 20 head-injured children ages 5–13 at the time of injury and in 20
normal controls. The patients were evaluated at least 12 months after
injury. Severely injured patients had Glasgow Coma Scale scores of ≤8.
However, no additional information regarding injury severity was presented that would allow for an assessment of comparability with other
samples. Patients with mild and severe injuries did not differ from each
other on any measures of specific aphasic deficits. However, patients
with severe injuries performed below controls on the overall language
quotients from tests of general language development and naming. No
significant differences were obtained on any of the Neurosensory Center
Comprehensive Examination for Aphasia subtests.

Jordan and Murdoch (1990) completed a 1-year follow-up to the
Jordan et al. (1988) assessment. Their findings were very similar, and
indicated that the severely injured children's relative impairments on
measures of general language ability and naming persisted through the
follow-up period. However, the authors noted that the scores on tests of
general language development remained in the average range. In addition, head-injured subjects' scores were lower on measures of oral fluency
and word association; this may be reflective of lexical retrieval difficulties.
Because the scores were not age-corrected, it is difficult to determine
whether the improvement that was noted on many of the measures was
related to recovery or to development.

Similar findings regarding oral fluency were reported by Chadwick,
Rutter, Shaffer, and Shrout (1981), who identified deficits in verbal fluency at baseline and on measures of object-naming latency at 1 year
in the severely injured group, in comparison to orthopedically injured
controls. In their 1-year follow-up study, Winogron et al. (1984) reported
significant severity group differences on measures of verbal fluency.

Recent research has emphasized examination of language functions
beyond the sentential level. Dennis and Barnes (1990) described discourse
deficits in head-injured children and adolescents, including problems
with interpreting ambiguous sentences and metaphors, drawing inferences, and formulating sentences from key words. Chapman et al. (1992)
evaluated narrative discourse in children and adolescents at least 1 year
after mild/moderate or severe head injury. On the basis of a story recall
task, Chapman and colleagues identified impoverished language in severely injured children; however, the complexity of language did not
differ according to injury severity. In addition, severely injured children
exhibited disruption in the story structure that was characterized by a
reduction in essential story components of setting and complicating action. More specifically, severely injured children failed to include essential

action information, did not signal a new episode, and left out more of the "gist" information than did either the children with mild/moderate head injury or the control children. The efficiency of expression, as measured by hesitational phenomena and revisions, did not differ across groups.

Executive Functions

Levin et al. (1993) investigated the relationship between deficits on measures purported to assess frontal lobe functions and MRI findings following closed head injury in 76 children ages 6 to 16 at the time of assessment, who had been injured at least 3 months previously. Patients ages 6 to 10 years were significantly impaired relative to controls on measures of concept formation and problem solving, planning, verbal fluency, design fluency, clustering on verbal memory measures, and response modulation. Moreover, severely injured children scored lower on Wechsler subtests assessing attention to visual detail, verbal abstract reasoning, and vocabulary. In contrast, deficits in the group of severely injured adolescents were apparent only on measures of concept formation/problem solving, word fluency, and design fluency. Multiple hierarchical regression analyses were used to assess whether lesion volume enhanced prediction of performance on various cognitive measures, above and beyond the variance explained by the lowest postresuscitation Glasgow Coma Scale score. The volume of left frontal lesions improved prediction of verbal fluency, problem solving, and inhibitory control. The volume of right frontal lesions enhanced the prediction of semantic clustering, verbal fluency, and inhibitory control. These findings support the relationship between the volume of frontal lobe lesion and cognitive sequelae following pediatric closed head injury.

Behavioral Changes

Early investigations of behavioral disturbance following closed head injury indicated that children with mild injuries had a higher incidence of preinjury behavioral disturbances (Brown, Chadwick, Shaffer, Rutter, & Traub, 1981). However, following the injury, severely injured children developed new psychiatric disorders at a rate that was two to three times higher than in the mildly injured children. Moreover, the likelihood of developing behavioral disturbance was significantly increased in children from homes with significant psychosocial adversity.

We (Fletcher, Ewing-Cobbs, Miner, Levin, & Eisenberg, 1990) evaluated behavioral sequelae in children and adolescents with mild ($n = 13$), moderate (n = 10), or severe (n = 22) closed head injuries; the severity ratings were based on each child's lowest Glasgow Coma Scale score and on initial CT scan findings. The Vineland Adaptive Behavior Scales (Sparrow, Balla, & Cicchetti, 1984) and the Child Behavior Checklist (Achenbach & Edelbrock, 1983) were administered as soon following the injury as possible and at 6 and 12 months after injury. Both of these measures use the parent as the informant. The baseline assessment was completed to characterize the child's behavior prior to the injury. The baseline Adaptive Behavior composite score from the Vineland did not differ at baseline for the different injury groups. However, the severely injured patients developed behavioral disturbances during the first 6 months after injury, and the decline in adaptive behavior persisted over the 12-month follow-up interval. In contrast, the Internalizing and Externalizing scores from the Child Behavior Checklist did not differ significantly across injury groups. We hypothesized that the rating scale format of the Child Behavior Checklist and the item content were less sensitive in identifying posttraumatic behavioral disturbance than was the Vineland.

RELATIONSHIP TO THE WHITE MATTER MODEL

Rourke initially described the NLD syndrome in children with developmental disorders (Rourke, 1982, 1987, 1988, 1989). He hypothesized that a variety of neurological diseases and disorders involving destruction of the cerebral white matter may produce cognitive and behavioral changes similar to those identified in patients with NLD. Closed head injury, which produces widespread damage to the cerebral white matter in addition to more focal effects produced by contusions and hemorrhage, provides a model of acquired brain injury with which to test the generalizability of the NLD syndrome.

   We (Ewing-Cobbs, Fletcher, Levin, & Boudousquie, 1993) tested the hypotheses (1) that the pattern of neuropsychological deficits in head-injured children with lower Arithmetic than Reading or Spelling scores on the Wide Range Achievement Test (WRAT; Jastak & Jastak, 1965) would be similar to that observed in individuals with the NLD syndrome; and (2) that severe closed head injury would be associated with performance similar to NLD, including relatively intact verbal abilities associated with impairment in complex psychomotor, visual-perceptual, and visual–motor abilities.

Subjects and Methods

We (Ewing-Cobbs et al., 1993) identified 75 children and adolescents between the ages of 5 and 15 years who had sustained a closed head injury and received a 1-year follow-up as part of an ongoing longitudinal study of recovery from pediatric brain injury. Exclusionary criteria included preinjury learning disability or special educational placement, psychiatric disorder, or a primary language other than English in the home.

Patients were assigned to groups with mild, moderate, or severe injuries, based on the following criteria. The patients with mild injuries ($n = 14$) were defined as those having Glasgow Coma Scale scores from 13 to 15 and no CT scan evidence of brain injury. Patients with moderate injuries ($n = 17$) had Glasgow scores from 9 through 12, or Glasgow scores from 13 to 15 and positive findings on CT scans; those with severe injuries ($n = 44$) were defined by Glasgow scores from 3 through 8, or by a duration of impaired consciousness of at least 1 day. The duration of impaired consciousness was defined as the number of days following the injury during which a patient did not respond to simple one-stage commands such as "Squeeze my hand." Table 16.1 contains neurological data by severity group.

To test the applicability of the NLD model to closed head injury, we identified patterns of achievement on the WRAT that were similar to those identified by Rourke (Rourke, 1982; Rourke & Strang, 1978). In our group with arithmetic impairment (group A), WRAT Arithmetic scores were ≤ 90 and were at least one standard deviation below either Reading or Spelling scores. The group with reading, spelling, and arithmetic impairment (group RSA) also had Arithmetic scores ≤90, as well as either Reading or Spelling scores below 90. The third group (group NI) had no impairment on the WRAT scores: Reading, Spelling, and Arithmetic scores were all >90, and the injury severity was moderate or severe. Out of 75 children, 53 met criteria for one of the three WRAT

TABLE 16.1. Neurological Information by Severity of Traumatic Brain Injury

	Severity of injury		
Variable	Mild ($n = 14$)	Moderate ($n = 17$)	Severe ($n = 44$)
Glasgow Coma Scale score (n)			
3–8	0	0	40
9–12	0	5	4
13–15	14	12	0
Duration of impaired consciousness (days)			
M	0	0.09	8.1
SD	0	0.19	7.5
Range	0	0–0.5	0.3–31.0

Note. n, number of patients. From Ewing-Cobbs, Fletcher, Levin, and Boudousquie (1993).

achievement groups. The mean age at injury was approximately 11½ years in groups A and RSA (see Table 16.2). However, patients were significantly younger in group NI, since the mean was only 8.6, F (2, 50) = 8.92, $p < .005$. The mean injury–test interval was approximately 1 year in all groups. Chi-square analysis did not identify any significant group differences in terms of gender or socioeconomic status. There were nearly twice as many males as females, and our sample was predominantly Caucasian and came from a middle-level socioeconomic background. Neither the distribution of Glasgow Coma Scale scores nor the duration of impaired consciousness differed statistically across achievement groups. The mean duration of impaired consciousness varied from 4.0 through 8.1 days. Therefore, with the exception of age, the achievement groups were comparable in terms of demographic and neurological indices.

We (Ewing-Cobbs et al., 1993) examined the type of brain injury in the three achievement groups, based on both acute CT scan and surgical

TABLE 16.2. Demographic and Neurological Information by Achievement Group

Variable	Group		
	A ($n = 17$)	RSA ($n = 9$)	NI ($n = 27$)
Age at injury (y)			
M	11.5	11.7	8.6*
SD	1.9	2.8	2.8
Injury–test interval (m)			
M	12.4	12.7	12.2
SD	1.4	1.1	0.5
Gender (n)			
Female	5	4	8
Male	12	5	19
Socioeconomic status (n)			
Low	3	1	2
Middle	14	7	24
High	0	1	1
Glasgow Coma Scale score (n)			
3–8	9	7	18
9–12	2	2	4
13–15	6	0	5
Duration of impaired consciousness (d)			
M	6.1	8.1	4.0
SD	7.7	9.0	4.9
Range	0–26.5	0.3–29.0	0–16.0

Note. d, days; m, months; y, years; n, number of subjects. From Ewing-Cobbs et al. (1993).
*$p < .005$.

reports. For group A, approximately 60% had focal right-hemisphere or bilateral pathology, while an additional 30% had primarily diffuse brain injury. Therefore, approximately 90% of group A had either focal injuries involving the right hemisphere or diffuse injuries. This is consistent with the hypothesized pathophysiological mechanisms underlying the NLD syndrome. However, these findings were based on CT scan data. More recent MRI studies highlight the role of contusional injury in the frontal lobes. As expected, 33% of group RSA had focal left-hemisphere injuries, and 44% had bilateral brain insults. Patients with no impairment on the achievement scores had fairly even representation of focal left-hemisphere, focal right-hemisphere, bilateral, and diffuse injuries.

The following tests were selected to assess a variety of neuropsychological constructs. The WRAT was used as a measure of basic academic skills. Verbal and nonverbal memory functions (Buschke, 1973; Fletcher, 1985) were assessed by means of selective reminding tasks that required storage and retrieval of new information. The consistent long-term retrieval score from each task was used as the dependent measure. Psychomotor speed was assessed with the Grooved Pegboard Test (Kløve, 1963). The Tactile Form Perception Test (Benton, Hamsher, Varney, & Spreen, 1983), which requires tactile discrimination of geometric designs made of sandpaper, was used to assess speed of tactile–spatial perception in each hand. Visual–motor integration was tested using the Beery Developmental Test of Visual–Motor Integration (Beery, 1982), which requires copying increasingly more complex geometric drawings. The Recognition Discrimination Test (Satz & Fletcher, 1979), which is a motor-free test of matching perceptually similar figures, was used to assess visual perception. Expressive and receptive language abilities were sampled with the Rapid Automatized Naming Test (Denckla & Rudel, 1974) as a measure of speed of lexical retrieval, and the Controlled Oral Word Association Test (Spreen & Benton, 1969) as a measure of oral fluency. The Peabody Picture Vocabulary Test—Revised (Dunn & Dunn, 1981) was selected as a measure of receptive vocabulary. Unless already standardized, the neuropsychological measures were transformed into z scores based on normative data for age and gender. Positive z scores always reflected better performance. To assess behavioral functioning, the Vineland Adaptive Behavior Scales (Sparrow et al., 1984) and the Child Behavior Checklist (Achenbach & Edelbrock, 1983) were used.

The data were analyzed using a multivariate approach to repeated-measures analysis of variance (ANOVA) with one between-subjects factor (achievement group) and one within-subjects factor (task). Planned comparisons among the three achievement groups were performed. To assess the effect of severity of injury on the neuropsychological variables, the analyses were repeated with injury severity as the between-subjects factor.

Academic and Neuropsychological Outcome

Table 16.3 depicts the mean WRAT scores in the three achievement groups. In group NI, mean scores on Reading, Spelling, and Arithmetic subtests were above 100 and reflected average levels of performance. In group A, mean Reading and Spelling standard scores were average, while the mean Arithmetic score was 81.3. In group RSA, all mean WRAT scores were approximately 80.

Assessment of complex psychomotor skills with the Grooved Peg-board Test identified a significant group effect, F (4, 90) = 4.31, $p <$ .003). Group NI scored in the average range with each hand, and in general performed significantly faster than did groups A and RSA (see Table 16.4). Groups A and RSA had slower left-hand performance than did group NI. The right-hand performance of group RSA was signifi-cantly slower than the other groups, which is consistent with the higher incidence of focal left hemisphere and bilateral brain injury in group RSA. Thus, group NI performed significantly faster on measures of complex psychomotor speed than did either group A or group RSA, which showed more lateralized deficiencies. The speed of tactile form perception did not differ according to either group or hand.

Significant impairment was present on both verbal and nonverbal memory measures. Analysis of verbal versus nonverbal consistent long-term retrieval scores identified a significant task effect, F (1, 42) = 7.92, $p <$ .005. Verbal selective reminding scores were lower than were nonver-bal selective reminding scores, independent of group. This pattern of

TABLE 16.3. Mean Wide Range Achievement Test (WRAT) Standard Scores by Achievement Group

	Group		
WRAT scores	A ($n = 17$)	RSA ($n = 9$)	NI ($n = 27$)
Arithmetic			
M	81.3	79.4	100.9
SD	5.6	6.8	7.9
Reading			
M	105.4	83.9	107.6
SD	7.4	5.8	10.3
Spelling			
M	97.5	80.8	104.8
SD	10.6	9.3	8.0

Note. From Ewing-Cobbs et al. (1993).

TABLE 16.4. z Scores for Neuropsychological Domains by Achievement Group

| | Group | | |
| | A | RSA | NI |
Variable	(n = 17)	(n = 9)	(n = 27)
Psychomotor speed			
Left hand			
M	−1.78	−2.13	−0.35
SD	2.35	2.12	1.33
Right hand			
M	−0.76	−2.51	0.06
SD	1.72	2.25	1.24
Tactile-perceptual speed			
Left hand			
M	−0.11	−0.21	0.22
SD	1.16	2.05	0.95
Right hand			
M	−0.21	0.35	−0.28
SD	1.21	0.63	1.72
Nonverbal memory			
M	−.02	−0.66	−0.02
SD	1.33	1.35	1.29
Verbal memory			
M	−0.99	−1.28	−0.61
SD	1.29	0.94	1.05
Composite nonverbal			
M	−0.18	−0.36	0.06
SD	0.66	0.85	0.91
Composite verbal			
M	−0.35	−0.94	0.07
SD	0.64	0.61	0.66

Note. From Ewing-Cobbs et al. (1993).

performance does not support the NLD model. Memory is one of the cognitive areas that is most vulnerable to disruption by closed head injury (Levin & Eisenberg, 1979); this specific finding may reflect the pathophysiology of closed head injury, in which focal frontal and anterior temporal lobe involvement occur frequently.

Composite scores were formed to evaluate relative performance in visual–perceptual and visual–motor as compared to verbal areas. The visual–motor score consisted of the Recognition Discrimination Test and Beery Developmental Test scores. The Rapid Automatized Naming Test, the Controlled Oral Word Association Test, and the Peabody Picture Vocabulary Test—Revised scores were included within the verbal domain. Repeated-measures ANOVA identified a significant group effect, $F(1, 49) = 3.74$, $p < .05$. Group NI had both visual–motor and verbal domain scores in the average range, and these did not differ significantly from each other. Groups A and RSA demonstrated a trend toward lower verbal than visual–motor scores. These findings did not support the predictions of the NLD model.

Behavioral Outcome

Individuals with NLD are hypothesized to have socioemotional and adaptive deficits that include poor adaptation to novelty, reduced social competence, and less emotional stability. We compared the performance of our three academic achievement groups on the Vineland Adaptive Behavior Scales Communication, Daily Living Skills, and Socialization domains (see Table 16.5). A repeated-measures ANOVA identified a trend for a significant domain $\times$ group interaction, $F(4, 84) = 2.31$, $p < .06$, and a significant group effect, $F(2, 43) = 3.32$, $p < .006$. On the Communication domain, the mean score of group RSA was significantly

TABLE 16.5. Standard Scores for Behavioral Measures by Achievement Group

	Group		
Standard scores	A ($n = 13$)	RSA ($n = 7$)	NI ($n = 26$)
Vineland Adaptive Behavior Scales[a]			
Communication			
M	84.8	71.1	89.2
SD	16.9	7.2	13.2
Daily Living Skills			
M	80.1	85.0	90.5
SD	10.5	14.6	12.2
Socialization			
M	83.2	78.9	93.7
SD	13.9	13.6	11.0
Child Behavior Checklist[b]			
Internalizing scale			
M	56.8	61.0	57.2
SD	8.9	7.9	10.2
Externalizing scale			
M	58.2	65.2	54.6
SD	6.1	8.1	10.5

Note. From Ewing-Cobbs et al. (1993).
[a] Standard score mean = 100, SD = 15.
[b] T-score mean = 50, SD = 10.

lower than were those for group A or group NI. This finding is consistent with the increased number of patients in group RSA with focal left-hemisphere or focal bilateral brain injuries. On the Daily Living Skills domain, the group A score of 80.1 was significantly below the group NI score of 90.5. The scores of both groups A and RSA fell generally in the low-average to borderline range on the Socialization domain, and were significantly lower than those of group NI. To evaluate the number of problem behaviors endorsed by parents, scores on the Vineland Maladaptive Behavior scale were compared. Since these scores are not standardized by age, analysis of covariance with age as a covariate was employed. Significantly more problem behaviors were identified in both groups A and RSA than in group NI, F $(3, 35)$ = 4.7, $p < .005$.

To evaluate the nature of behavior disorders in the three achievement groups, scores on the Internalizing and Externalizing scales of the Child Behavior Checklist were compared by means of a repeated-measures ANOVA. A significant scale × group interaction was obtained, F $(2, 39)$ = 3.79, $p < .05$. Although the group means did not differ on the Internalizing scale, group RSA had significantly higher parent ratings on the Externalizing scale than did group NI.

Severity of Injury

To determine whether the group × task interactions identified in the achievement group analysis were attributable largely to a general severity of injury factor, we completed a repeated-measures ANOVA on all the dependent measures, using injury severity as the between-subjects factor. On all cognitive and motor measures, significant group effects were obtained: Individuals with severe brain injuries performed at a lower level than did those with mild or moderate injuries. No group × task interactions were obtained, suggesting that severe closed head injury produced a global reduction in cognitive and motor abilities that did not vary across different tasks and ability domains.

Evaluation of differences in behavioral functioning among the three severity groups identified neither group nor task effects for the Internalizing and Externalizing variables from the Child Behavior Checklist or the Maladaptive Behavior scale from the Vineland. On the individual Vineland domains, scores of the severely injured group were significantly below those of the mildly injured group in all domains.

Implications for the White Matter Model

Rourke's (1989) model hypothesizes that damage to commissural fibers, association fibers interconnecting cortical regions of the same cerebral hemisphere, and/or projection fibers that project from the diencephalon to the hemispheres and from the hemispheres to the diencephalon, the brain stem, and the spinal cord would be affected by generalized white matter disease. In patients with closed head injury, there is clear neuro-pathological evidence suggesting that the primary injury is diffuse axonal injury from neuronal shear strains occurring at the time of impact (Adams et al., 1977; Strich, 1956). The generalized damage resulting from torn axonal fibers, damage to supportive glial cell structure, and degeneration of neuronal fibers that are distal to the focal area of shearing is referred to as "diffuse axonal injury." Although diffuse axonal injury effects may be widely distributed, they occur most frequently in the deep white matter areas and in the brain stem. Brain regions particularly affected by diffuse axonal injury include the corpus callosum and the parasagittal white matter, as well as dorsolateral quadrants of the midbrain. Secondary diffuse neuronal damage may occur as a result of widespread ischemia or cerebral edema. These effects typically will be additive to the more direct shear strain effects of diffuse axonal injury. Therefore, severe closed head injury is frequently associated with disruption of commis-sural, association, and projection fibers. Focal or multifocal injuries are superimposed upon this generalized damage.

However, these injuries are particularly prominent in the frontal lobes. Our group A, in which 60% of patients had focal right-hemisphere injury or primary diffuse brain injury, did not consistently show behav-ioral patterns similar to those of patients with NLD. In comparison to group NI, group A had left-hand slowing on a psychomotor task and a higher rate of maladaptive behaviors. However, scores were comparable on verbal and nonverbal memory, as well as on composite verbal and visual scores. The presence of problems in both verbal and nonverbal areas probably reflects the presence of bilateral diffuse white matter destruction plus bilateral focal damage in group A. Group RSA showed significant deficiencies on complex psychomotor, visual-perceptual, and visual–spatial tasks, and also showed significant impairment on a host of verbal tasks (including verbal learning and memory, fluency, naming, reading, and spelling). Members of this group were also more likely to have focal left-hemisphere or bilateral focal injuries. Dividing patients into groups based on their patterns of arithmetic achievement identified many cognitive and behavioral group differences that were probably related to underlying pathophysiology of brain injury.

The failure to strongly support the NLD model in this study may be related in part to the method of subject selection. Rather than select patients on the basis of patterns in achievement test scores, an alternative approach might select patients on the basis of the presence of bilateral tactile-perceptual and psychomotor deficits. Differential functioning in patients with bilateral deficiencies in these areas could be contrasted with that of comparably injured children without such deficiencies. This approach would select patients according to the variables thought to be primary and causal for the NLD syndrome, rather than dependent variables such as academic skill level (Harnadek & Rourke, 1994). An alternative strategy might involve selecting patients specifically on the basis of MRI scan evidence of diffuse axonal injury.

The problem with the latter approach is the prominent role of contusional injury superimposed on diffuse injury. Levin et al. (1993) and Levin, Mendelsohn, et al. (1994) have shown that volumetric analysis of frontal lobe lesion size accounts for significant amounts of variability beyond that accounted for by age at injury and severity of injury. These findings were especially apparent on executive function tasks hypothesized to relate specifically to prefrontal cortex. A more recent brain morphometric study showed that children with severe injuries whose MRI disclosed no areas of abnormal signal in the frontal lobe nevertheless had significant reductions in the volume of prefrontal grey matter and increased frontal lobe cerebrospinal fluid consistent with tissue loss (Levin, Fletcher, et al., in press).

Rourke (1989) proposed that neuropsychological deficits following significant closed head injury would reflect the combined effects of NLD, attentional deficits such as arousal system disturbance associated with diffuse axonal injury, and the effects of focal injury. This combination of factors was hypothesized to lead to a pattern of generalized neurobehavioral deficits (see Figure 6.1 in Rourke, 1989, p. 121). Although Rourke's (1989) model may provide a heuristic to predict the pattern of neuropsychological deficits following closed head injury, the issue of the fit of the NLD model to neuropsychological outcomes remains unsettled. To address the core issue of the fit of the model, patients with diffuse brain injuries involving the white matter without focal involvement must be studied at different ages to determine the degree of overlap of profiles with those predicted by the NLD model.

As in disorders such as Tourette syndrome (Brookshire, Butler, Ewing-Cobbs, & Fletcher, 1994), children with traumatic brain injury may have some phenotypic resemblance to children with the NLD syndrome; however, the full syndrome may not be readily apparent. In addition, current understanding of the pathophysiology of traumatic brain injury has progressed to a level of specificity beyond the descriptions of white matter disease in Rourke (1989). Even children with diffuse axonal injury show various contusional injuries that vary across cases. Many children show reductions of grey (and white) matter volume in the frontal lobes. It may be that models of outcome that address the role of the frontal lobes in executive function deficits (e.g., Pennington, 1994) may also be applicable to many children with traumatic brain injury. More generally, the considerable heterogeneity in pathophysiological mechanisms (e.g., brain swelling, focal lesions), which is complicated by developmental variables and by variations in the cause of head injury at various ages, makes a unifying interpretation of the neurobehavioral sequelae rather difficult. A multivariate approach to analyzing the injury variables will be necessary to elucidate the neurobehavioral outcomes of pediatric closed head injury, and to address the capacity of various models of brain–behavior relationships in children for explaining the variability in outcomes after such injury.

ACKNOWLEDGMENTS

Preparation of this chapter was supported in part by National Institute of Neurological Disorders and Stroke Grant No. 29462, "Accidental and Nonaccidental Pediatric Brain Injury," to Linda Ewing-Cobbs, and Grant No. 21889, "Neurobehavioral Outcome of Head Injury in Children," to Harvey S. Levin; and by National Institute of Child Health and Human Development Grant No. 27597, "Neurobehavioral Sequelae of Pediatric Head Injury," to Jack M. Fletcher. We acknowledge the assistance provided by the University Clinical Research Center at Hermann Hospital and the support of National Institutes of Health Grant No. M01-RR-02558. We are grateful to Linda Kimbrough for assistance in manuscript preparation.

REFERENCES

Achenbach, T. M., & Edelbrock, C. (1983). *Manual for the Child Behavior Checklist and Revised Behavior Profile*. Burlington: University of Vermont, Department of Psychiatry.

Adams, J. H., Mitchell, D. E., Graham, D. I., & Doyle, D. (1977). Diffuse brain damage of the immediate impact type. *Brain, 100*, 489–502.

Aldrich, E. F., Eisenberg, H. M., Saydjari, C., & Luerssen, T. G., Foulkes, M. A., Jane, J., Marshall, L. F., Marmarou, A., & Young, H. F. (1992). Diffuse brain swelling in severely head-injured children: A report from the Traumatic Coma Data Bank. *Journal of Neurosurgery, 76*, 450–454.

Annegers, J. F. (1983). The epidemiology of head trauma in children. In K. Shapiro (Ed.), *Pediatric head trauma* (pp. 1–10). Mount Kisco, NY: Futura.

Bawden, H. N., Knights, R. M., & Winogron, H. W. (1985). Speeded performance following head injury in children. *Journal of Clinical Neuropsychology, 7*, 39–54.

Beery, K. (1982). *Developmental Test of Visual–Motor Integration*. Cleveland, OH: Modern Curriculum Press.

Benton, A. L., Hamsher, K. deS., Varney, N., & Spreen, O. (1983). *Contributions to neuropsychological assessment*. New York: Oxford University Press.

Berger, M. S., Pitts, L. H., Lovely, M., Edwards, M. S. B., & Bartkowski, H. M. (1985). Outcome from severe head injury in children and adolescents. *Journal of Neurosurgery, 62*, 294–199.

Brink, J. D., Garrett, A. L., Hale, W. R., Woo-Sam, J., & Nickel, V. L. (1970). Recovery of motor and intellectual function in children sustaining severe head injuries. *Developmental Medicine and Child Neurology, 12,* 565–571.

Brookshire, B. L., Butler, I. J., Ewing-Cobbs, L., & Fletcher, J. M. (1994). Neuropsychological characteristics of children with Tourette syndrome: Evidence for a nonverbal learning disability? *Journal of Clinical and Experimental Neuropsychology, 16,* 289–302.

Brown, G., Chadwick, O., Shaffer, D., Rutter, M., & Traub, M. (1981). A prospective study of children with head injuries: III. Psychiatric sequelae. *Psychological Medicine, 11,* 63–78.

Bruce, D. A., Raphaely, R. C., Goldberg, A. I., Zimmerman, R. A., Bilaniuk, L. T., Schut, L., & Kuhl, D. E. (1979). Pathophysiology, treatment, and outcome following severe head injury in children. *Child's Brain, 2,* 174–191.

Buschke, H. (1973). Components of verbal learning in children: Analysis by selective reminding. *Journal of Experimental Child Psychology, 18,* 488–496.

Chadwick, O., Rutter, M., Brown, G., Shaffer, D., & Traub, M. (1981). A prospective study of children with head injuries: II. Cognitive sequelae. *Psychological Medicine, 11,* 49–61.

Chadwick, O., Rutter, M., Shaffer, D., & Shrout, P. E. (1981). A prospective study of children with head injuries: IV. Specific cognitive deficits. *Journal of Clinical Neuropsychology, 3,* 101–120.

Chapman, S. B., Culhane, K. A., Levin, H. S., Harward, H., Mendelsohn, D., Ewing-Cobbs, L., Fletcher, J. M., & Bruce, D. (1992). Narrative discourse after closed head injury in children and adolescents. *Brain and Language, 43,* 42–65.

Denckla, M., & Rudel, R. G. (1974). Rapid automatized naming of pictured objects, colors, letters, and numbers by normal children. *Cortex, 10,* 186–202.

Dennis, M., & Barnes, M. A. (1990). Knowing the meaning, getting the point, bridging the gap, and carrying the message: Aspects of discourse following closed head injury in childhood and adolescence. *Brain and Language, 39,* 428–446.

Duhaime, A. C., Alario, A. J., Lewander, W. J., Schut, L., Sutton, L. N., Seidl, T. S., Nudelman, S., Budenz, D., Hertle, R., Tsiaras, W., & Loporchio, S. (1992). Head injury in very young children: Mechanisms, injury types, and ophthalmologic findings in 100 hospitalized patients younger than 2 years of age. *Pediatrics, 90,* 179–185.

Dunn, L. M., & Dunn, L. M. (1981). *Peabody Picture Vocabulary Test—Revised: Manual for forms L and M.* Circle Pines, MN: American Guidance Service.

Ewing-Cobbs, L., Fletcher, J. M., Levin, H. S., & Boudousquie, A. (1993, February). Nonverbal learning disability in children and adolescents following closed head injury. In B. P. Rourke (Chair), *The "white matter" model of the nonverbal learning disability syndrome: Manifestations in neurological disease, disorder, and dysfunction.* Symposium conducted at the meeting of the International Neuropsychological Society, Galveston, TX.

Ewing-Cobbs, L., Levin, H. S., Eisenberg, H. M., & Fletcher, J. M. (1987). Language functions following closed-head injury in children and adolescents. *Journal of Clinical and Experimental Neuropsychology, 9,* 575–592.

Ewing-Cobbs, L., Miner, M. E., Fletcher, J. M., & Levin, H. S. (1989). Intellectual, motor, and language sequelae following closed head injury in infants and preschoolers. *Journal of Pediatric Psychology*, *14*, 531–547.

Ewing-Cobbs, L., Thompson, N. M., Miner, M. E., & Fletcher, J. M. (1994). Gunshot wounds to the brain in children and adolescents: Age and neurobehavioral development. *Neurosurgery*, *35*, 225–233.

Filley, C. M., Cranberg, L. D., Alexander, M. P., & Hart, E. J. (1987). Neurobehavioral outcome after closed head injury in childhood and adolescence. *Archives of Neurology*, *44*, 194–198.

Fletcher, J. M. (1985). Memory for verbal and nonverbal stimuli in learning disability subgroups: Analysis by selective reminding. *Journal of Experimental Child Psychology*, *40*, 244–259.

Fletcher, J. M. (1994). Afterword: Brain–behavior relationships in children. In S. H. Broman & J. Grafman (Eds.), *Atypical cognitive deficits in developmental disorders: Implications for brain function* (pp. 297–326). Hillsdale, NJ: Erlbaum.

Fletcher, J. M., Ewing-Cobbs, L., Miner, M. E., Levin, H. S., & Eisenberg, H. M. (1990). Behavioral changes after closed head injury in children. *Journal of Consulting and Clinical Psychology*, *58*, 93–98.

Goldman, P. S. (1974). An alternative to developmental plasticity: Heterology of CNS structures in infants and adults. In D. G. Stein, J. R. Rosen, & N. Butters (Eds.), *Plasticity and recovery of function in the central nervous system* (pp. 149–174). New York: Academic Press.

Goldstein, M. (1990). Traumatic brain injury: A silent epidemic. *Annals of Neurology*, *27*, 327.

Graham, D. I., Ford, I., Adams, J. H., Doyle, D., Lawrence, A. E., McLellan, D. R., & Ng, H. K. (1989). Fatal head injury in children. *Journal of Clinical Pathology*, *42*, 18–22.

Harnadek, M. C. S., & Rourke, B. P. (1994). Principal identifying features of the syndrome of nonverbal learning disabilities in children. *Journal of Learning Disabilities*, *27*, 144–154.

Jastak, J. F., & Jastak, S. R. (1965). *The Wide Range Achievement Test*. Wilmington, DE: Guidance Associates.

Jennett, B., & Bond, M. (1975). Assessment of outcome after severe brain damage. *Lancet*, *i*, 480–487.

Jordan, S. M., & Murdoch, B. E. (1990). Linguistic status following closed head injury in children: A follow-up study. *Brain Injury*, *4*, 147–154.

Jordon, S. M., Ozanne, A. E., & Murdoch, B. E. (1988). Long-term speech and language disorders subsequent to closed head injury in children. *Brain Injury*, *2*, 175–185.

Kaufmann, P. M., Fletcher, J. M., Levin, H. S., Miner, M. E., & Ewing-Cobbs, L. (1993). Attentional disturbance after pediatric closed head injury. *Journal of Child Neurology*, *8*, 348–353.

Klauber, M. R., Barrett-Connor, E., Marshall, L. F., & Bowers, S. A. (1981). The epidemiology of head injury: A prospective study of an entire community—San Diego County, California, 1978. *American Journal of Epidemiology*, *113*, 500–509.

Klonoff, H., Low, M. D., & Clark, C. (1977). Head injuries in children: A prospective five-year follow-up. *Journal of Neurology, Neurosurgery and Psychiatry, 40*, 1211–1219.

Kløve, H. (1963). Clinical neuropsychology. In F. M. Forster (Ed.), *The medical clinics of North America* (pp. 1069–1077). New York: Saunders.

Kraus, J. F., Fife, D., Cox, P., Ramstein, K., & Conroy, C. (1986). Incidence, severity, and external causes of pediatric brain injury. *American Journal of Diseases of Children, 140*, 687–693.

Kriel, R. L., Krach, L. E., & Panser, L. A. (1989). Closed head injury: Comparison of children younger and older than 6 years of age. *Pediatric Neurology, 5*, 296–300.

Lange-Cosack, H., Wider, B., Schlesner, H. J., Grumme, T., & Kubicki, S. (1979). Prognosis of brain injuries in young children (1 until 5 years of age). *Neuropaediatrie, 10*, 105–127.

Levin, H. S., Aldrich, E. F., Saydjari, C., Eisenberg, H. M., Foulkes, M. A., Bellefleur, M., Luerssen, T. G., Jane, J. A., Marmarou, A., Marshall, L. F., & Young, H. F. (1992). Severe head injury in children: Experience of the Traumatic Coma Data Bank. *Neurosurgery, 31*, 435–444.

Levin, H. S., Amparo, E. G., Eisenberg, H. M., Miner, M. E., High, W. M., Jr., Ewing-Cobbs, L., Fletcher, J. M., & Guinto, F. C., Jr. (1989). Magnetic resonance imaging after closed head injury in children. *Neurosurgery, 24*, 223–227.

Levin, H. S., Culhane, K. A., Mendelsohn, D., Lilly, M. A., Bruce, D., Fletcher, J. M., Chapman, S. B., Harward, H., & Eisenberg, H. M. (1993). Cognition in relation to magnetic resonance imaging in head-injured children and adolescents. *Archives of Neurology, 50*, 897–905.

Levin, H. S., & Eisenberg, H. M. (1979). Neuropsychological impairment after closed head injury in children and adolescents. *Journal of Pediatric Psychology, 4*, 389–402.

Levin, H. S., Eisenberg, H. M., Wigg, N. R., & Kobayashi, K. (1982). Memory and intellectual ability after head injury in children and adolescents. *Neurosurgery, 11*, 668– 672.

Levin, H. S., Fletcher, J. M., Kufera, J. A., Harward, H., Lilly, M. A., Mendelsohn, D., Bruce, D., & Eisenberg, H. M. (in press). Dimensions of cognition measured by the Tower of London and other cognitive tasks in head injured children and adolescents. *Deveelopmental Neuropsychology*.

Levin, H. S., High, W. M., Jr., Ewing-Cobbs, L., Fletcher, J. M., Eisenberg, H. M., Miner, M. E., & Goldstein, F. C. (1988). Memory functioning during the first year after closed head injury in children and adolescents. *Neurosurgery, 22*, 1043–1052.

Levin, H. S., Mendelsohn, D., Lilly, M. A., Fletcher, J. M., Culhane, K. A., Chapman, S. B., Harward, H., Kusnerik, L., Bruce, D., & Eisenberg, H. M. (1994). Tower of London performance in relation to magnetic resonance imaging following closed head injury in children. *Neuropsychology, 8*, 171–179.

Mendelsohn, D., Levin, H. S., Bruce, D., Lilly, M., Harward, H., Culhane, K. A., & Eisenberg, H. M. (1992). Late MRI after head injury in children: Relationship to clinical features and outcome. *Child's Nervous System, 8*, 445–452.

Michaud, L. J., Rivara, G. P., Grady, M. S., & Reay, D. T. (1992). Predictors of survival and severity of disability after severe brain injury in children. *Neurosurgery, 31*, 254–264.

Pennington, B. F. (1994). The working memory function of the prefrontal cortices: Implications for developmental and individual differences in cognition. In M. M. Haith, J. Benson, R. Roberts, & B. F. Pennington (Eds.), *Future-oriented processes in development* (pp. 243–289). Chicago: University of Chicago Press.

Rourke, B. P. (1982). Central processing deficiencies in children: Toward a developmental neuropsychological model. *Journal of Clinical Neuropsychology, 4*, 1–18.

Rourke, B. P. (1987). Syndrome of nonverbal learning disabilities: The final common pathway of white-matter disease/dysfunction? *The Clinical Neuropsychologist, 1*, 209–234.

Rourke, B. P. (1988). Syndrome of nonverbal learning disabilities: Developmental manifestations in neurological disease, disorder, and dysfunction. *The Clinical Neuropsychologist, 2*, 293–330.

Rourke, B. P. (1989). *Nonverbal learning disabilities: The syndrome and the model.* New York: Guilford Press.

Rourke, B. P., & Strang, J. D. (1978). Neuropsychological significance of variations in patterns of academic performance: Motor, psychomotor, and tactile-perceptual abilities. *Journal of Pediatric Psychology, 3*, 62–66.

Satz, P., & Fletcher, J. M. (1979). Early screening tests: Some uses and abuses. *Journal of Learning Disabilities, 12*, 56–60.

Sparrow, S. S., Balla, D. A., & Cicchetti, D. V. (1984). *Vineland Adaptive Behavior Scales.* Circle Pines, MN: American Guidance Service.

Spreen, O., & Benton, A. L. (1969). *Neurosensory Center Comprehensive Examination for Aphasia: Manual of directions.* Victoria, British Columbia: Neuropsychology Laboratory, University of Victoria.

Strich, S. J. (1956). Diffuse degeneration of the cerebral white matter in severe dementia following head injury. *Journal of Neurology, Neurosurgery and Psychiatry, 19*, 163–185.

Strich, S. J. (1970). Lesions in the cerebral hemispheres after blunt head injury. In S. Sevitt & H. B. Stoner (Eds.), *The pathology of trauma* (pp. 166–171). London: BMA House.

Teasdale, G., & Jennett, B. (1974). Assessment of coma and impaired consciousness. A practical scale. *Lancet, ii*, 81–84.

Thompson, N. M., Francis, D. J., Stuebing, K. K., Fletcher, J. M., Ewing-Cobbs, L., Miner, M. E., Levin, H. S., & Eisenberg, H. M. (1994). Motor, visual–spatial, and somatosensory skills after closed head injury in children and adolescents: A study of change. *Neuropsychology, 8*, 333–342.

Winogron, H. W., Knights, R. M., & Bawden, H. N. (1984). Neuropsychological deficits following head injury in children. *Journal of Clinical Neuropsychology, 6*, 269–286.

Zimmerman, R. A., Bilaniuk, L. T., Bruce, D., Dolinskas, C., Obrist, W., & Kuhl, D. (1978). Computed tomography of pediatric head trauma: Acute general cerebral swelling. *Radiology, 126*, 403–408.

17

Toxicant-Induced Encephalopathy

Roberta F. White
Maxine Krengel

Occupational or environmental exposure to neurotoxicants often produces a direct effect on cerebral structures or functions. These effects are toxicant-specific. Examples include hippocampal damage secondary to exposure to organic tin (Besser et al., 1987; Feldman, White, & Eriator, 1993), lesions in the white matter associated with exposure to toluene (Rosenberg, Kleinschmidt-DeMasters, et al., 1988, Rosenberg, Spitz, Filley, Davis, & Schaumberg, 1988; Filley, Heaton, & Rosenberg, 1990), and cerebellar dysfunction resulting from exposure to. methylmercury. In addition, some toxicants (e.g., chlordane) affect the production of neurotransmitters such as dopamine. Asymmetrical lesions and brain edema are also sometimes seen as effects of intoxication. Finally, neurotoxicants can affect cerebral function through other mechanisms: Anoxic encephalopathy and cerebrovascular accidents have both been described following exposure to neurotoxicants.

The mechanisms and neuropathological consequences of exposure to some neurotoxicants are known through autopsy studies of brain tissue from patients who died as a result of exposure, or through the examination of the brains of animals experimentally exposed to neurotoxicants. Both of these avenues of investigation provide fruitful information about the structural neuroanatomical consequences of intoxication in cases of extreme exposure or in the animal brain. However, these studies do not directly address the most common type of brain damage seen following exposure to neurotoxicants—that is, changes in brain function affecting cognition and behavior, but not producing death. This type of damage is often referred to in the toxicology literature as "subclinical toxicant-induced encephalopathy" because the pathological changes are generally only obvious on tests of mental function, not on a physical examination.

The existence of this form of central nervous system (CNS) damage is now well accepted and well documented in the toxicology literature, primarily because of multiple epidemiological studies of workers with well-defined exposure to specific neurotoxicants, in which clear relationships have been established between degree of exposure and outcome on psychometric tests of mentation and mood. These dose–effect relationships have been well described for environmental exposure to lead in children (Needleman et al., 1979), occupational lead exposure in adults (Baker et al., 1984, 1985), and occupational exposure to carbon disulfide (Hanninen, 1971) and organic solvents (White, Robins, Proctor, Echeverria, & Rocksay, 1994). The acceptance of the diagnosis of toxicant-induced encephalopathy as a clinical entity is demonstrated by the publication of diagnostic criteria for the syndrome by the World Health Organization (Baker & White, 1985).

Although the mechanisms of CNS action of toxicants at levels producing behavioral change in the absence of obvious clinical disease are unclear and almost certainly vary among classes of toxicants, it is intriguing that demyelination appears to be one such mechanism. This is especially so, given recent evidence from clinical neuroimaging studies that exposure to some solvents and to elemental mercury is associated with development of lesions in the white matter (Rosenberg, Kleinschmidt-DeMasters, et al., 1988; White, Moss, Proctor, & Feldman, 1993). Though these neuropathological effects are not always limited to white matter (e.g., exposure to toluene may also produce cerebellar atrophy), they represent an intriguing subtype of toxicant-induced encephalopathy that may have implications for the theoretical model of the Nonverbal Learning Disabilities (NLD) syndrome. Hence, this chapter focuses on toxicants known to have direct effects on white matter, especially toluene and elemental mercury.

FINDINGS ON MEDICAL (NEUROLOGICAL) EXAMINATION

Neurological findings in cases of toxicant-induced encephalopathy vary considerably, depending upon the severity of the exposure and resulting clinical disease. In some cases, neurological examination results are normal, with perhaps the exception of the neurologist's mental status examination. In other cases, significant neurological abnormalities may be seen. In patients exposed to toluene, cerebellar signs (gait disturbances, ataxia) may be seen. Dysarthria, nystagmus, arm incoordination, ocular flutter, and cranial nerve abnormalities have also been described in toluene abusers (Hormes, Filley, & Rosenberg, 1986). Patients with occupational exposure to elemental mercury are frequently reported to exhibit tremor (Langolf, Chaffin, Henderson, & Whittle, 1978), though behavioral changes may be prominent as well (Vroom & Greer, 1972; White, Feldman, & Travers, 1990). In addition, mercury affects the peripheral nervous system, with resultant abnormalities upon peripheral nerve examination (Vroom & Greer, 1972; White, Feldman, & Proctor, 1992).

LABORATORY STUDIES

Laboratory studies useful in the evaluation of patients exposed to solvents or mercury include measures of the toxicants or their metabolites in blood, urine, or fat. Industrial hygiene studies aimed at estimating exposure dose through assessment of occupational inhalation of toxicant vapors and other sources of exposure, or through modeling of exposure conditions, may also be quite helpful. Pharmacokinetic modeling of likely target organ absorption of specific toxicants is also at times possible and relevant.

NEUROPHYSIOLOGICAL AND NEUROIMAGING STUDIES

Several neurophysiological and neuroimaging techniques have been found to be useful in the evaluation of nervous system effects of toxicant exposure. These include nerve conduction and electromyography studies, sensory and motor evoked potentials, quantitative measures of tremor, postural balance assessment, electroencephalogram (EEG), magnetic resonance imaging (MRI), and computed tomography (CT).

Following exposure to toluene, cortical atrophy has been described on CT, with evidence of cerebellar atrophy in a subgroup of patients (Schikler, Seitz, Rice, & Strader, 1982). In addition, white matter lesions have been demonstrated on MRI studies of toluene-exposed glue sniffers (Rosenberg, Kleinschmidt-DeMasters, et al., 1988; Rosenberg, Spitz, et al., 1988). Sural nerve biopsies in glue sniffers have also revealed some demyelination, though axonal degeneration and proliferation of Schwann and mast cells were the most prominent findings.

Although there is extensive information about the neuropathological effects of exposure to *organic* mercury in humans, relatively little is known about the neuropathological effects of exposure to *elemental* mercury. On the basis of MRI studies and the results of clinical examination, one would infer the existence of damage to white matter, the cerebellum, the motor system, the visual cortex, the limbic system, and the peripheral nervous system.

EPIDEMIOLOGY

Much of the information now available on the behavioral effects of exposure to elemental mercury and toluene is based on summaries of clinical assessments of patients with well-documented intoxications. However, epidemiological investigations have also been conducted, and these have shown behavioral effects in workers with occupational exposure to toluene (Cherry, Hutchins, Pace, & Waldron, 1985) and mercury (Roels et al., 1982). Systematic studies of dose–effect relationships between exposure and behavioral measures continue to be crucial, especially if augmented by functional neuroimaging techniques.

TYPICAL TREATMENT MODALITIES

Acute intoxication from exposure to toluene or mercury is most immediately treated by withdrawal from exposure and by treatment of some acute symptoms (e.g., seizures). In the case of mercury, an elevated body burden of mercury can be lowered through the administration of chelating agents. The symptoms of chronic residual toluene or mercury encephalopathy (in which behavioral and cognitive abnormalities persist, despite normal body burdens of toxicants and cessation of exposure) are much more difficult to treat. In some cases the affective symptoms may be effectively alleviated through the use of psychopharmacological agents, but these are often ineffective. The memory and other cognitive changes (especially in executive functioning) may be quite devastating in terms of daily functioning, but difficult or impossible to alleviate with any currently known treatment modality. Simple remediative measures, such as use of memory aids and compensatory cognitive strategies, may be of some benefit. However, in our experience, these measures are usually insufficient to restore full vocational, personal, and interpersonal functioning in the patient with mild to moderate residual neuropsychological deficits in more than one functional domain.

DEVELOPMENTAL EFFECTS

The effects of exposure to the substances being highlighted in this chapter (elemental mercury and toluene) have not been systematically studied across the lifespan. However, the behavioral and neuropathological effects of other neurotoxicants (particularly methylmercury and inorganic lead) have been investigated across a wide range of developmental stages in humans. These studies suggest that developmental stage *at the time of exposure* (not at the time effects are measured or assessed) is a critical variable in the determination of the nature and severity of neuropathological and neuropsychological deficits associated with exposure. In fact, it appears that the earlier the exposure occurs, the more widespread and profound the damage will be, both pathologically and behaviorally.

This has been best described in regard to the methylmercury exposure experienced by residents of Minamata Bay in Japan, which resulted in both clinical disease and death (methylmercury is an organic form of mercury and has different toxicological properties from inorganic or elemental mercury). Neuropathological studies of tissue were conducted on patients who died as a result of exposure-induced illness. Brain tissue from children experiencing lethal intrauterine exposure to methylmercury showed severe cell loss and changes in brain cytoarchitecture; exposure in infancy produced widespread brain damage; and exposure in adulthood was associated with focal brain damage at several sites (Burbacher, Rodier, & Weiss, 1990; Choi, 1989; Marsh et al., 1980; Matsumoto, Koyo, & Takeuchi, 1965; Takeuchi, Eto, & Eto, 1979).

These neuropathological findings parallel the developmental curve of behavioral deficits associated with exposure to inorganic lead. Children exposed to lead in infancy or early childhood show widespread behavioral changes that may cover multiple or all cognitive domains (Needleman et al., 1979), even when such deficits are measured many years after the exposure (Needleman, Schell, Bellinger, Leviton, & Allred, 1988; White, Diamond, Proctor, Morey, & Hu, 1993). Adults exposed to lead show a more focal pattern of deficits limited to nonlanguage domains (Baker et al., 1985; White et al., 1990).

Although the neuropathology of these exposures clearly extends beyond white matter, the patterns of behavioral deficit closely parallel those predicted by the NLD model, with pervasive behavioral effects when pathology occurs very early and more focal deficits when pathology occurs later in development. A recent case report on two adolescents exposed to elemental mercury confirms the suggestion of widespread, diffuse effects of childhood exposure (Yeates & Mortensen, 1994), as do our own findings on a child exposed to mercury vapors at home. This child developed deficits in multiple cognitive domains when tested over several years of exposure, and continued to demonstrate these deficits in early adulthood after cessation of exposure (Diamond, White, Gerr, & Feldman, 1994).

NEUROPSYCHOLOGICAL LITERATURE

The literature on neuropsychological effects of exposure to toluene in adulthood consists mainly of descriptions of clinical examinations of patients exposed to toluene through glue sniffing or through their occupations, with limited systematic study of workers or other populations of subjects with relatively specific exposure to toluene alone. Special characteristics of the subjects evaluated in prior studies constitute a major limitation to the generalizability of results, since glue sniffers are often polysubstance abusers who may be showing the effects of exposure to neurotoxicants besides toluene (especially alcohol), and the worker subjects of some of the occupational studies have also been described as having a high rate of alcohol abuse. However, taken as a whole, the literature on behavioral effects of toluene exposure suggests that it is associated in adults with changes in attention and executive functioning, mood, motor dexterity, visual–spatial processing, and anterograde memory function. Formal language deficits and changes in basic academic skills such as reading and spelling are not generally noted. An exception to this was the study by Tsushima and Towne (1977), which described a difference in Peabody Picture Vocabulary Test scores between toluene-exposed glue sniffers and controls; however, the authors attributed this difference to pre-exposure differences between the two groups, not to an effect of toluene.

The literature on behavioral effects of exposure to elemental mercury consists of clinical assessments of workers (some of whom are identified as being diagnosed with "chronic mercurialism") and on epidemiological studies of small groups of occupationally exposed workers. This literature suggests that motor dysfunction, visual–spatial deficits, and affective/personality changes are most prominent. Memory deficits have been described, but are most often expressed as deficits in memory for visual information. (For a more complete review of literature in this area, see White et al., 1990, 1992. A comprehensive listing of studies using behavioral tests to investigate behavioral effects of specific neurotoxicants, with tables summarizing exposure types and results on specific tests, can be found in Anger, 1990.)

TYPICAL NEUROPSYCHOLOGICAL ASSESSMENT FINDINGS: FORMAL TESTING

The general pattern of neuropsychological test results seen in patients with exposure to toluene and mercury closely parallels the description provided above in the section on the neuropsychological literature. Our experience with evaluating such patients using specific neuropsychological tests is summarized below. We have also previously summarized clinical test data on a series of nine workers with mercury exposure (White et al., 1990), a case of residual mercury encephalopathy with known white matter pathology (White, Moss, et al., 1993) and patients exposed to organic solvents (White et al., 1992; White, 1995). Please note that the following summaries are all based on findings in *adult* patients.

Measures of Motor Skills

Motor deficits are most frequently seen in patients with toluene-induced encephalopathy on complex tests such as the Grooved Pegboard Test

(Tsushima & Towne, 1977) and the Wechsler Adult Intelligence Scale—Revised (WAIS-R) Digit Symbol subtest, though they can also be evident on simpler tasks such as finger tapping, particularly when the motor deficit is pronounced. It is important to note that a finding of normal finger tapping does *not* rule out a more subtle motor deficit in these patients.

Motor deficit in the form of an obvious tremor has been considered to be a *sine qua non* of mercury poisoning. However, even when the mercury-induced encephalopathy is mild or the patient does not exhibit obvious tremulousness, deficits in fine motor coordination are generally seen on tests of fine manual motor coordination, such as the Santa Ana Formboard and the WAIS-R Digit Symbol subtest.

An association between motor deficits and the occurrence of white matter lesions has been established for a variety of white matter disorders (e.g., cerebrovascular disease, multiple sclerosis). However, the contribution of cerebellar and/or basal ganglia pathology to the motor findings must be considered, especially given other clinical manifestations of exposure to these substances. It is also important to bear in mind that peripheral nervous system dysfunction can be seen following these exposures, and that numbness in the hands may contribute in some cases to the finding of a manual motor deficit on neuropsychological tasks.

Measures of Attention/Executive Functions

Vigilance on tasks such as continuous-performance tests, and deficits in simple attention on tasks such as WAIS-R Digit Span (forward) and the Trail Making Test, Part A, can be seen in patients experiencing cognitive impairment secondary to exposure to either toluene or mercury. More common, especially in cases of mild toxicant-induced encephalopathy, are impairments on tests requiring complex tracking or holding and manipulating information, such as WAIS-R Digit Span (backward); the Trail Making Test, Part B; Auditory Trails; and mental control tasks such as serial threes, WAIS-R Arithmetic, and the Paced Auditory Serial Addition Test. Deficits in attention and cognitive tracking are also common in cases of acute encephalopathy and may resolve when the patient is removed from exposure.

Tests of Memory

In the mildest form of toluene-induced encephalopathy, memory function, especially at the level of new learning and retrieval, may be disrupted because of the attentional/tracking problems experienced by the patient.

However, disorders in learning and retaining newly learned information over delays may also be affected in patients exposed to toluene. The combination of attentional and memory deficits can make tasks such as the Brown–Peterson Interference Memory Tasks, which require the patient to inhibit distractibility while retaining newly learned information, particularly problematic for these patients.

Patients with mercury-induced encephalopathy can show deficits in learning and retaining new material in both verbal and visual modalities, but they appear to be especially prone to deficits in memory for visual information. These deficits are seen for delayed recall of visual information presented in both recall and recognition formats, and do not appear to be explainable on the basis of simple visual–spatial processing impairment. We have noted these visual memory deficits on the Wechsler Memory Scale Visual Reproductions subtest (especially delayed recall), the Milner Facial Recognition Test recognition memory condition (even when performance on facial matching is normal), and the Benton Visual Recognition Test (multiple choice form of the Benton Visual Retention Test).

WAIS-R Performance Subtests

Patients with cognitive deficits attributed to toluene exposure have been reported to show significantly lower Performance IQs than to Verbal IQs (Fornazzari et al., 1983). In general, the visual–spatial/conceptual and visual–motor components of the Performance subtests appear to be problematic for these patients.

Patients with mercurialism also have problems on the WAIS-R Performance subtests for the same reasons. In a series of patients we examined, those with a more severe form of encephalopathy were particularly likely to show problems on the visual–spatial tasks, especially Block Design and Object Assembly.

Other Visual–Spatial Measures

In addition to the WAIS-R measures noted above, patients with behavioral changes secondary to mercury exposure may demonstrate deficits on a variety of visual–spatial tasks, including the matching condition of the Milner Facial Recognition Test and the Hooper Visual Organization Test, particularly if the encephalopathy is relatively severe. Performance on these tasks is especially informative in regard to visual–spatial processing, since they do not have a motor component. Drawing of the Rey–Osterrieth Complex Figure is also often affected in patients with either toluene- or mercury-induced encephalopathy, though this may be a result of deficits in planning as well as in visual–spatial processing.

Measures of Problem Solving/Cognitive Flexibility

The ability to think flexibly and to carry out reasoning tasks involving inductive and deductive reasoning may be affected following exposure to either toluene or mercury. These may be observed on tests such as the Similarities and Comprehension subtests of the WAIS-R and the Wisconsin Card Sorting Test. They may also be observed in the patient's efforts to complete tasks such as the Trail Making Test, Part B, or the Rey–Osterrieth Complex Figure.

Additional Verbal/Linguistic Measures

Tests of verbal problem solving and of word list generation may be affected following exposure to either toluene or mercury because of problems with reasoning and planning as noted above. A concrete approach to tasks may also affect the ability to construct word definitions for the WAIS-R Vocabulary subtest. In our experience, WAIS-R Information performance is rarely if ever affected in encephalopathies associated with these exposures in adults.

Formal tests of language such as naming have not been studied extensively in adults exposed to these neurotoxicants. However, our clinical experience with these patients suggests that naming, single-word reading, and the linguistic aspects of writing are unaffected in adult exposure to these substances.

Deficits in *motor* functioning can affect performance on verbal/language tests, at least qualitatively. Thus, a patient with mercury-induced encephalopathy may be dysarthric in speech production, or a patient with manual motor deficits may show impaired penmanship or letter formation in writing.

Academic Achievement

Performance on standard measures of academic knowledge is not generally affected following exposure to toluene or mercury in adulthood. These include the Wide Range Achievement Test (all subtests), the WAIS-R Information subtest, and the Peabody Picture Vocabulary Test. This situation is different in childhood exposure to mercury, which can affect performance on all such measures.

Affect/Personality

Changes in mood appear to be common following exposure to toluene, which is sometimes abused and used as a mood enhancer. Dose–effect relationships between exposure to toluene and affective outcome have been described: Low-dose exposure was associated with fatigue, and higher-dose exposure with euphoria, exhilaration, and excitement (Bor & Hurtig, 1977).

Mercury exposure has been related to flagrant changes in behavior, including the "mad hatter's syndrome"formerly seen in hat makers exposed to mercury. Prominent behavioral symptomatology associated with relatively severe mercury-induced encephalopathy may include paranoia, aggression, delusions, hallucinations, and violent behavior. Milder manifestations of mercury poisoning may include irritability, fatigue, and depression. Behavior can be violent, with homicidal or suicidal ideation and acts.

RELATIONSHIP TO THE WHITE MATTER MODEL

In our discussion of the "fit" between the predicted behavioral deficits associated with the white matter/NLD model and the deficits observed following exposure to the neurotoxicants discussed in this chapter, we first address the deficits associated with exposure during adulthood. This is followed by a brief consideration of the little knowledge we have about effects of exposure in childhood. Our discussion is organized around the central features that Rourke has defined for the NLD syndrome (Harnadek & Rourke, 1994; Rourke, 1989).

Adulthood

1. *Bilateral tactile-perceptual deficits, usually more marked on the left side of the body.* These have not been well defined in patients exposed to mercury or toluene, and would be difficult to assess accurately, given the occurrence of peripheral neuropathy in these patients. Thus, this feature of the NLD syndrome cannot be fairly addressed, given the current state of knowledge in this field.

2. *Bilateral psychomotor coordination deficiencies, often more marked on the left side of the body.* Bilateral deficits on visual–motor tasks are particularly prominent in patients with mercury-induced encephalopathy, who may show outright tremor. They are also seen in a significant portion of patients diagnosed with toluene-induced encephalopathy. The laterality of these effects is not well documented, and they appear to be most

commonly bilateral (in clinical observations). However, studies on motor function in patients exposed to neurotoxicants sometimes find greater evidence of toxicant effect on nonpreferred-hand rather than preferred-hand performance when only one hand is affected.

3. *Outstanding deficiencies in visual–spatial–organizational abilities.* Although these are not the first signs in the mildest cases of toluene-induced behavioral change, visual–spatial–organizational problems are frequently seen. They are prominent in mercury-induced encephalopathy, and extend to motor-free visual–spatial tasks involving visual organization at a purely conceptual level.

4. *Deficits in nonverbal problem solving, concept formation, and hypothesis testing.* These difficulties are seen in mild to moderate effects of exposure to either toluene or mercury, and may affect performance on numerous tests of reasoning.

5. *Very well-developed rote verbal capacities.* Patients exposed to either mercury or toluene generally demonstrate this feature of the NLD syndrome, with intact naming, reading, and spelling skills, and rote memory for information learned *prior* to exposure. However, capacity for rote learning of *new* verbal material appears to diminish significantly after exposure. Especially in mercury intoxication, the capacity for verbal learning does seem to be superior to that for learning of visual material, as would be predicted by the NLD model.

6. *Extreme difficulty in adapting to novel and otherwise complex situations.* Because of the problem-solving difficulties noted above, patients with toluene- or mercury-induced encephalopathy may have difficulty generating strategies for dealing with novel situations. This can be confounded by their affective changes and behavioral disinhibition. They may also encounter problems with complex situations, because of specific deficits in the capacity to carry out more than one procedure or mental operation simultaneously. However, if brain damage occurs during adulthood, the patient has generally overlearned many effective behavioral adjustment procedures that can be automatically invoked; this should result in less flagrant behavioral deficits than might be observed in the childhood case.

7. *Outstanding relative deficiencies in mechanical arithmetic, as compared to proficiencies in reading and spelling.* This feature of the NLD model does not fit the situation in adulthood neurotoxicant exposure, in which patients appear to retain the mechanical arithmetic knowledge that they learned in childhood. Performance of mental arithmetic on the WAIS-R Arithmetic subtest is sometimes affected, but this appears to be attributable to attentional/tracking problems rather than to dyscalculia, and there is no confirmatory evidence of mechanical arithmetic deficits on written arithmetic tests.

8. *Much verbosity of a repetitive, straightforward, rote nature.* Although some patients with toxicant-induced encephalopathies can become highly

repetitive in their recitation of the symptoms and problems that they associate with exposure, this tendency does not extend to the rest of their speech or verbal interactions. Speech is more likely to become disorganized or to diminish in verbosity than to be verbose and highly repetitive.

9. *Significant deficits in social perception, social judgment, and social interaction.* These tendencies may be seen in patients with toluene-induced encephalopathy, in that they may withdraw socially or become disinhibited. The problems appear to result from affective disturbance and loss of inhibitory controls. This differs from the childhood case, in which these behaviors appear to emanate from a more basic deficit in nonverbal processing.

In summary, the deficiencies in cognitive and behavioral processing described in the NLD model fit those associated with adulthood toxicant-induced brain damage in regard to several major features, including motor skills, visual–spatial functioning, problem solving, and life adaptation. The pattern of intact abilities (language, reading, spelling) is strikingly similar. There are differences also: the absence of mechanical arithmetic deficits, the nature of conversational output, and the degree of impairment in ability to function in complex or novel situations. Because toluene and mercury are known to affect white matter (as well as other brain structures), the role of white matter pathology in the behavioral expression appears to be prominent and to fit predictions emanating from Rourke's NLD model. The exceptions most likely reflect the fact that the damage has occurred in adulthood, allowing the patient to invoke behaviors learned in the context of intact brain function.

Childhood

Because so little is known about the effects of exposure to toluene or elemental mercury during prenatal life, infancy, and the various stages of childhood, this section is highly speculative. It is based on our experience in assessing children exposed to many types of neurotoxicants, and the very small amount of literature available on effects of elemental mercury exposure in children (which is also based entirely on clinical reports).

Especially when exposure to neurotoxicants occurs in infancy or early childhood (but sometimes even when exposure occurs in the later stages of childhood), the pattern of neuropsychological deficits is more diffuse than that seen in adults and can affect basic linguistic abilities as well as visual–spatial skills. Affected children do display significant problems in social adjustment and life adaptation, and frequently have trouble holding jobs in later life. The "learning disabilities" diagnosed for the children can cover a wide range, however, including attentional deficits, verbal processing impairments, and NLD. This occurrence of impairment in a wide variety of functional domains is consistent with Rourke's hypothesis for very early damage to white matter. It is very likely that the pattern seen in childhood exposures reflects damage to white matter (producing the kinds of changes predicted by Rourke's theory and seen in patients with known white matter pathology), plus diffuse damage to grey matter and other structures (producing widespread deficits).

VARIABILITY AND SEVERITY OF DISORDER MANIFESTATIONS

Although the common domains of functional deficit seen following exposure to such neurotoxicants as toluene and mercury are described above, there is some variability among patients in the degree of deficits and the number of domains affected. This variability can be seen even among patients who experience very similar exposures under very similar circumstances (e.g., among people in the same job category working in the same manufacturing plant). The variability in behavioral effects of exposure most likely reflects individual differences (e.g., genetic variability in sensitivity to toxicants; premorbid or familial patterns of intellectual abilities; educational history; socioeconomic status; and pre-existing medical, neurological, and psychiatric conditions), developmental variables (age and/or cognitive maturity at time of exposure), and exposure variables (duration of exposure, dosage, combinations of exposures to multiple neurotoxicants).

It is also important to understand the difference between acute manifestations of CNS dysfunction and chronic residual encephalopathy. The former occurs at the time of exposure and may remit following cessation of exposure or treatment; in some cases, no residual behavioral impairment may be evident on assessment once recovery has occurred. In the case of chronic residual encephalopathy, behavioral changes may be evident for days, months, or years in the absence of any continued exposure. Slow, gradual recovery of some functions may be seen over time, so that the expression of encephalopathic deficits may change.

DISORDERS FREQUENTLY COINCIDENT WITH OR MISDIAGNOSED AS TOXICANT-INDUCED ENCEPHALOPATHY

The most common differential diagnostic questions in evaluating patients exposed to neurotoxicants such as toluene and mercury involve differentiating between cognitive impairments caused by exposure and those representing a long-standing condition (e.g., low intellectual endowment, learning disabilities, attention deficit disorder), a psychiatric or motivational syndrome (e.g., depression, anxiety states, somatoform disorders, paranoia, personality disorders, psychosis, Ganser syndrome, malingering), other forms of "environmental disorders" (e.g., multiple-chemical sensitivity, chronic fatigue syndrome), or a neurological disease (e.g., multiple sclerosis, Parkinson disease or parkinsonism, epilepsy, Alzheimer disease, cerebrovascular dementia, cerebellar atrophy). In addition, it is important to rule out effects of exposure to other neurotoxicants (e.g., alcohol or street drugs, prescription drugs), and to discriminate (if possible) the separate effects of exposure to multiple toxicants within the same individual. These differential diagnostic considerations have been described in detail elsewhere (White et al., 1992).

REFERENCES

Anger, W. K. (1990). Worksite behavioral research: Results, sensitive methods, test batteries and the transition from laboratory data to human health. *NeuroToxicology, 11*, 629–719.

Baker, E. L., Feldman, R. G., White, R. F., Harley, J. P., Niles, C., Dinse, G., & Berkey, K.,. (1984). Occupational lead neurotoxicity—a behavioural and electrophysiologic evaluation: I. Study design and year one results. *British Journal of Industrial Medicine, 41*, 352–361.

Baker, E. L. & White, R. F. (1985). *Chronic effects of organic solvents on the central nervous system and diagnostic criteria.* Copenhagen: World Health Organization/Oslo: Nordic Council of Ministers. (Printed by the U.S. Department of Health and Human Services, Public Health Service)

Baker, E. L., White, R. F., Pothier, L. J., Berkey, C. S., Dinse, G. E., Travers, P. H., Harley, J. P., & Feldman, R. G. (1985). Occupational lead neurotoxicity: II. Improvement in behavioural effects following exposure reduction. *British Journal of Industrial Medicine, 42*, 507–516.

Besser, R., Kramer, G., Thumler, R., Bohl, J., Gutmann, L., & Hopf, H. C. (1987). Acute trimethyltin limbic cerebellar syndrome. *Neurology, 37*, 945–950.

Bor, J. W. & Hurtig, H. I. (1977). Persistent cerebellar ataxia after exposure to toluene. *Annals of Neurology, 2*, 440–442.

Burbacher, T. M., Rodier, P. M., & Weiss, B. (1990). Methylmercury developmental neurotoxicity: A comparison of effects in humans and animals. *Neuroteratology, 12*, 191–202.

Cherry, N., Hutchins, H., Pace, T., & Waldron, H. A. (1985). Neurobehavioral effects of repeated occupational exposure to toluene and paints. *British Journal of Industrial Medicine, 42*, 291–300.

Choi, B. H. (1985). The effects of methylmercury on the developing brain. *Progress in Neurobiology, 32*, 447–470.

Diamond, R., White, R. F., Gerr, F., & Feldman, R. G. (1994). *A case of developmental exposure to inorganic mercury.* Unpublished manuscript.

Feldman, R. G., White, R. F., & Eriator, I. (1993). Trimethyltin encephalopathy. *Archives of Neurology, 50,* 1320–1324.

Filley, C. M., Heaton, R. K. & Rosenberg, N. L. (1990). White matter dementia in chronic toluene abuse. *Neurology, 40,* 532–534.

Fornazzari, L., Wilkinson, D. A., Kapur, B. M., & Carlen, P. L. (1983). Cerebellar and functional impairment in toluene abusers. *Acta Neurologica Scandinavica, 67,* 319–329.

Hanninen, H. (1971). Psychological picture of manifest and latent carbon disulfide poisoning. *British Journal of Industrial Medicine, 28,* 374–381.

Harnadek, M. C. S. & Rourke, B. P. (1994). Principal identifying features of the syndrome of nonverbal learning disabilities. *Journal of Learning Disabilities, 27,* 144–154.

Hormes, J. T., Filley, C. M., & Rosenberg, N. L. (1986). Neurologic sequelae of chronic solvent vapor abuse. *Neurology, 36,* 698–702.

Langolf, G. D., Chaffin, D. B., Henderson, K., & Whittle, H. P. (1978). Evaluation of workers exposed to elemental mercury using quantitative tests of tremor and neuromuscular function. *American Industrial Hygiene Association Journal, 39,* 976–984.

Marsh, D. O., Myers, G. J., Clarkson, T. W., Amin-Zaki, L., Tikriti, S., & Majeed, M. A. (1980). Fetal methylmercury poisoning: Clinical and toxicological data on 29 cases. *Annals of Neurology, 7,* 348–353.

Matsumoto, H., Koyo, G., & Takeuchi, T. (1965). Fetal Minamata disease. *Journal of Neuropathology and Experimental Neurology, 24,* 563–574.

Needleman, H. L., Gunnoe, C., Leviton, L. A., Reed, R., Peresie, H., Maher, C., & Barett, P. (1979). Deficits in psychologic and classroom performance of children with elevated dentin levels. *New England Journal of Medicine, 300,* 689–695.

Needleman, H. L., Schell, A., Bellinger, D., Leviton, A., & Allred, E. N. (1988). The long-term effects of exposure to low doses of lead in childhood: An 11-year follow-up report. *New England Journal of Medicine, 322,* 83–88.

Roels, H., Lauwerys, R., Buchet, J. P., Bernard, A., Barthels, A., Oversteyns, M., & Gaussin, P. (1982). Comparison of renal function and psychomotor performance in workers exposed to elemental mercury. *International Archives of Occupational and Environmental Health, 50,* 77–93.

Rosenberg, N. L., Kleinschmidt-DeMasters, B. K., Davis, K. A., Dreisbach, J. N., Hormes, J. T., & Filley, C. M. (1988). Toluene abuse causes diffuse central nervous system white matter changes. *Annals of Neurology, 23,* 611–614.

Rosenberg, N. L., Spitz, M. C., Filley, C. M., Davis, K. A., & Schaumberg, H. H. (1988b). Central nervous system effects of chronic toluene abuse: Clinical, brain stem evoked response and magnetic resonance imaging studies. *Neurotoxicology and Teratology, 10,* 489–495.

Rourke, B. P. (1989). *Nonverbal learning disabilities: The syndrome and the model.* New York: Guilford Press.

Schikler, K. N., Seitz, K., Rice, J. F. & Strader, T. (1982). Solvent abuse associated cortical atrophy. *Journal of Adolescent Health Care, 9,* 37–39.

Takeuchi, Y., Eto, N., & Eto, K. (1979). Neuropathology of childhood cases of methylmercury poisoning (Minamata disease) with prolonged symptoms with particular reference to the decortication syndrome. *Neurotoxicology*, *1*, 1–20.

Tsushima, W. T. & Towne, W. S. (1977). Effects of paint sniffing on neuropsychological test performance. *Journal of Abnormal Psychology*, *86*, 402–407.

Vroom, F. G. & Greer, M. (1972). Mercury vapor intoxication. *Brain*, *95*, 305–318.

White, R. F. (1995). Clinical neuropsychological investigation of solvent neurotoxicity. In L. Chang (Ed.), *Handbook of neurotoxicology: Vol. 2. Effects and mechanisms*. San Diego: Academic Press.

White, R. F., Diamond, R. G., Proctor, S. P., Morey, C., & Hu, H. (1993). Residual cognitive deficits 50 years after lead poisoning during childhood. *British Journal of Industrial Medicine*, *50*, 613–622.

White, R. F., Feldman, R. G., & Proctor, S. P. (1992). Neurobehavioral effects of toxic exposures. In R. F. White (Ed.), *Clinical syndromes in adult neuropsychology: The practitioner's handbook* (pp. 1–51). Amsterdam: Elsevier.

White, R. F., Feldman, R. G., & Travers, P. H. (1990). Neurobehavioral effects of toxicity due to metals, solvents and insecticides. *Clinical Neuropharmacology*, *13*, 392–412.

White, R. F., Moss, M. B., Proctor, S. P., & Feldman, R. G. (1993). Magnetic resonance imaging (MRI), neurobehavioral testing, and toxic encephalopathy: Two cases. *Environmental Research*, *61*, 117–123.

White, R. F., Robins, T. G., Proctor, S. P., Echeverria, D., & Rocksay, A. (1994). Neuropsychological effects of naphtha exposure among automotive workers. *Occupational and Environmental Medicine*, *51*, 1102–1112.

Yeates, K. O. & Mortensen, M. E. (1994). Acute and chronic neuropsychological consequences of mercury poisoning in two early adolescents. *Journal of Clinical and Experimental Neuropsychology*, *16*, 209–222.

18

Conclusions and Future Directions

Katherine D. Tsatsanis
Byron P. Rourke

A major dimension of this book for readers is that a detailed summary of the current literature on several important childhood disorders is presented within one volume. Moreover, an explicit attempt is made to draw upon and integrate research findings from a variety of fields, including medical, neuropathological, neuroimaging, and neuropsychological studies. An examination of the relationships between the nature of central nervous system (CNS) dysfunction and the behavioral phenotypes of multiple neurodevelopmental disorders has thus been made possible. An important feature of using this type of information to compare clinical syndromes is the identification of general principles that should further enhance our conception of the syndromes and the brain–behavior relationships that underlie them.

At first blush, the disorders presented in this volume do not appear to have much in common: They do not share a common etiology, known genetic underpinning, or definitive pathognomonic signs or markers. Yet they are thought to be related. It is hypothesized that these disorders fall along a continuum of neurodevelopmental disease characterized by variations in the severity of expression of the Nonverbal Learning Disabilities (NLD) syndrome and its proposed relationship to white matter dysfunction. The NLD/white matter model is thus advanced as a conceptual framework with which to compare the disorders and explicate brain–behavior relationships. A perspective is presented in which pathophysiological and neuropsychological findings are integrated to account for the total expression of several childhood disorders.

The dynamic interactions of the assets and deficits in NLD, as well as the precise role of white matter dysfunction, remain to be wholly determined. That said, it remains that our aim is to further develop and refine a comprehensive theoretical model of brain–behavior relationships for these and other neurological disorders within the context of a lifespan developmental perspective. Toward this end, theoretical aspects of this model are presented below. It is hoped that these ideas may foster new avenues of research. A consideration of the disorders presented in this book and of their relationship to the NLD/white matter model provides representative illustrations of this course.

THE NLD SYNDROME AND THE WHITE MATTER MODEL

Clinical Presentation of the NLD Syndrome

The child with NLD presents with a variety of academic and socioemotional difficulties. These include difficulties in mechanical arithmetic, mathematics, reading comprehension, and science, as well as significant deficits in social perception, social judgment, and social interaction skills. This presentation is thought to be ability-based—that is, directly related to a common pattern of neuropsychological deficits and assets. Rourke (1989, 1993) has proposed asset and deficit "streams" that seek to explain the progress of these children. The NLD model can be understood in terms of a summary of assets and deficits placed within the context of a set of cause-and-effect relationships. Only the deficit stream is discussed here. For a more comprehensive treatment of this material, the reader is referred to Rourke (1989, 1993) and Rourke and Fuerst (1992). (See also Chapter 1 of this book.)

The primary neuropsychological deficits considered to be displayed by the child with NLD are impairments in tactile perception, visual perception, complex motor skills, and the ability to deal effectively with novel material. These deficits are hypothesized to eventuate in deficient tactile and visual attention, as well as restricted exploratory behavior. In turn, these secondary deficits are thought to lead to problems with memory for tactile and visual information, and to deficits in concept formation and problem solving. A set of linguistic deficiencies (e.g., repetitive, rote speech; poor psycholinguistic pragmatics; minimal speech prosody; and reliance on language for social relating, information gathering, and relief from anxiety) is also proposed to arise from these deficits. Finally, the disturbed psychosocial and emotional functioning displayed by these children is thought to be directly related to their pattern of neuropsychological deficits.

The question remains: What mechanisms are thought to underlie this developmental course? A response to this query is considered from two explanatory perspectives: cognitive development and brain maturation. Evidence is presented indicating that these two perspectives may be intimately related.

A Cognitive-Developmental Perspective

One explanation for the process by which these deficits are seen to interact lies in Piaget's emphasis on sensorimotor functioning as one of the early developmental features upon which formal operational thought is founded (Casey & Rourke, 1992). That is, the adequacy of the child's sensorimotor experience is seen to be directly related to his or her cognitive development. The external world is known to the young child principally through touch, movement, and vision. In addition, learning takes place because of a desire to know, which is outwardly manifested through motivated exploration of the environment. Manipulation of the environment through action, exploration, and experimentation yields information that is thought to lead to the formation of mental schemata. Thus, this early activity is proposed to engender the development of an understanding of cause-and-effect relationships, hypothesis testing, nonverbal concept formation, reasoning abilities, and the ability to employ symbols and representations (Casey & Rourke, 1992; Strang & Rourke, 1985).

Children with NLD are found to display tactile-perceptual, psychomotor, and visual-perceptual deficits—that is, deficits in precisely those areas that are essential to early learning. Moreover, these children demonstrate extreme difficulty in adapting to novel stimuli and are unlikely to explore their environment or seek out stimulation. In the face of a fundamental inability to organize or make sense of complex and novel stimuli, it is nevertheless easy to understand that these children can exhibit some dimensions of adequate language development. Young children receive structured auditory input and highly directed speech in their "conversations" with caregivers. In contrast, children are left to their own devices to make sense of and lend order to their visual, tactile, and (to some extent) motor world.

Moreover, certain language skills (e.g., such as verbal output, word recognition, and word decoding) are easily routinized behaviors, whereas the development of mathematical concepts and learning arising from social interaction cannot rely on routines, but requires a degree of flexibility. In addition to the formal mathematics instruction that takes place in school, children must also develop an appreciation for number *concepts*. That is, they must develop a conception of what is meant by "number," "more and less," "greater than and less than," "fraction," "conservation of quantity," and so on. Whereas number facts and procedures are taught in school, largely through a process of rote memorization, children must generally develop an understanding of the underlying mathematical concepts on their own. It is precisely at this stage that the child with NLD demonstrates difficulty in arithmetic/mathematics.

A further example of this pervasive problem can be found in the ability to interact socially. Social interaction involves the perception, evaluation, and application of nonverbal cues, all of which have been shown to be defective in children with NLD. In addition, social interaction requires the analysis of novel situations and a constantly shifting pattern of communication and give-and-take; no overlearned descriptive system can be used in coping with these. Consequently, social interaction is unlikely to be a rewarding experience for the child with NLD, and such a child may be expected to become withdrawn and socially isolated.

In this way, the manifestations of the NLD syndrome can be considered from a cognitive-developmental perspective. This approach is especially notable for its presentation of a dynamic interaction between the neuropsychological assets and deficits in the child's repertoire, as well as for the role it proposes for the child as an active agent in his or her own development. In the following section, a consideration of the relationship between NLD and CNS dysfunction is presented.

Relationship of the White Matter Model to the NLD Syndrome

Rourke (1987, 1989; see also Chapter 1) observes that children who exhibit damage to white matter or a disturbance of white matter functioning also demonstrate features of the NLD syndrome. A major theoretical principle of this model is that the more white matter that is destroyed or dysfunctional, the more likely it is that the NLD syndrome will be manifested. The role of white matter functioning has been largely neglected in past considerations of brain–behavior relationships. Therefore, prior to embarking upon further details of the relationship between the syndrome and the model, we present a consideration of the general implications of white matter functioning.

Significance of White Matter Development and Dysfunction

The significance of examining white matter tracts, particularly with respect to childhood disorders, needs to be emphasized. Few fiber tracts are completely myelinated at birth; the most rapid period of myelination occurs within the first 2 years of life (Dietrich & Bradley, 1988; Rourke, Bakker, Fisk, & Strang, 1983; see Chapters 2 and 3, this volume). Myelinogenesis is important because the functional maturity of the fiber tract appears to coincide with the termination of its myelination. Furthermore, it has been shown that postnatal growth spurts in the brain occur without a concurrent increase in neuronal proliferation; that is, cell proliferation and migration are complete at birth. Rather, the growth of dendritic processes, synaptogenesis, and myelination are said to account for these postnatal increases in brain weight (Kolb & Fantie, 1989). In addition, an important aspect of postnatal development in humans appears to be the excess production and eventual elimination of neurons, dendrites, and synapses (Huttenlocher, 1984, 1994). This suggests that a process involving the refinement of cortical connections occurs in early childhood.

Together, these findings indicate that both the development of axonal connections (white matter pathways) and the process of myelination are far from complete in the brain of the child. The integrity of white matter systems and, more specifically, the manner in which systems in the brain are connected are likely to have functional implications. This renders these late developmental events important considerations in any discussion of childhood disorders.

Whereas it may be argued that there is a clear role for white matter functioning in the expression of these childhood disorders, the exact nature of that role is not easily elucidated. The developmental immaturity of the child's brain poses a problem for prediction of his or her functional outcome, particularly with respect to white matter dysfunction. Because white matter pathway formation underlies postnatal development, it is likely to be susceptible to both intrinsic and extrinsic factors. It is probable that white matter damage or dysfunction leads to both structural and functional reorganization of the brain—that is, that alternate pathways and connections are formed to compensate for the damage (one dimension of "plasticity"). In addition, the late specification of neuronal connectivity in the brain suggests that environmental factors (e.g., an "enriched" vs. an "impoverished" environment) are more likely to exert an influence on the final "choice" of cortical targets. Third, there is the possibility that the function of a specific area in the brain may change over time: It may come to be subserved by another area (Kolb & Fantie, 1989). Thus, it is possible that this normally functional development will in fact be less adaptive in the damaged brain.

In total, these observations suggest that the resulting pattern of axonal connectivity and the changes it effects in the developing child are neither fixed nor clear. Consequently, assets and deficits may appear or disappear, as the case may be, depending upon the kinds of changes that are taking place in the "wiring" of the brain. In this context, it is worthwhile to bear in mind the second major principle in the NLD/white matter model: Which white matter is destroyed or dysfunctional, and the stage of development at which white matter is destroyed or dysfunctional, will bear upon the manifestations of the NLD syndrome.

The White Matter Model

In general, research evidence from animal and human studies (e.g., Dennis, 1976; Gravel, Sasseville, & Hawkes, 1990a, 1990b; Huttenlocher,

1984; Lassonde, Sauerwein, Chicoine, & Geoffroy, 1991; Olavarria, Serra-Oller, Yee, & VanSluyters, 1988; Ozaki & Wahlsten, 1993; Schmidt & Caparelli-Daquer, 1989) appears to point to two primary consequences of a disturbance in the normal development of white matter: (1) a reorganization or alteration in the normal path of axonal migration, and (2) a blockade of the normal process of axonal elimination. Based on these findings, it would seem that whereas the normal outlay or distribution of cell projections and terminations is found to be preserved, these two processes result in an altered pattern of connectivity in the brain. More specifically, the altered state of axonal connections is less refined and specialized. Ultimately, then, white matter dysfunction would appear to consist of an alteration in the normal circuitry of the brain that is both less evolved and less specialized. From a functional perspective, we might also hypothesize that this alteration in neuronal circuitry will bear upon specialization or lateralization of function.

In connection with this last observation, it is worthwhile to consider the role of the corpus callosum in hemisphere integration and cross-communication. If we assume that each hemisphere is prewired for specialization of some function or set of functions, then the corpus callosum is seen to enhance this functional asymmetry via its communicative and integrative role and its "regulation" of cerebral activity. By facilitating communication between the hemispheres, the corpus callosum is communicating not only what each hemisphere is doing, but also what each hemisphere need not do. It is in this sense that the development of the corpus callosum can be said to bear upon the development of cerebral lateralization. Lassonde (1986) notes that the concept of the corpus callosum as a modulator of cerebral activity predicts that "each of the two functionally different hemispheres may achieve its full potential only in the presence of the other" (p. 397).

As noted, functions that involve inter- rather than intraregional connectivity are expected to be more likely to be affected by white matter perturbations. In addition, it is predicted that white matter disturbances will have a more profound effect on higher cognitive functions (i.e., frontal systems) and right-hemispheral processing. There is evidence to suggest that the right hemisphere is characterized by relatively more white matter than grey matter, compared to the left hemisphere (Goldberg & Costa, 1981). In addition, frontal systems have been shown both to develop and to myelinate at a relatively late stage; this perhaps renders them more susceptible to white matter disease or dysfunction that occurs during these stages (Barkovich, Kjos, Jackson, & Norman, 1988; Huttenlocher, 1994; Stuss, 1992; Yakovlev & Lecours, 1967). The prediction is also based upon the supposition that both right-hemispheral processing and higher cognitive functioning are characterized by a greater degree of specification and integration—that is, by more "complex" wiring. In their capacity to deal with informational complexity, it is expected that both the right hemisphere and frontal systems display greater interregional connectivity.

In fact, the pattern of development displayed by children with NLD has been interpreted by Rourke (1982, 1987, 1989), on the basis of formulations of the Goldberg and Costa (1981) model, in terms of the roles of the left and right cerebral hemispheres in the acquisition, integration, and application of descriptive systems. The right hemisphere is seen as having a crucial role in the initial stages of the acquisition of descriptive systems, whereas the left hemisphere is well suited to deploy these codes in a routinized manner once they have been assembled. Thus, it is postulated that systems within the right hemisphere are highly efficient at processing tasks that involve novel information for which the individual has no pre-existing code. In contrast, left-hemispheral systems are thought to handle processing that takes advantage of well-routinized codes—that is, the storage and application of these overlearned descriptive systems. In light of the pattern of neuropsychological assets and deficits displayed by children with NLD, the syndrome is expected to develop under conditions that compromise the functioning of or accessibility to right-hemispheral systems.

A role for frontal systems in higher-level cognitive functioning has also been proposed. In particular, frontal systems are thought to play an integral role in executive control of novel responses (i.e., in directing, planning, and organizing lower-level systems toward a selected goal), as well as a metacognitive role involving awareness of oneself and one's relation to the environment (Stuss, 1992). Results of studies using quantified electroencephalographic (qEEG) measures of intracortical connections offer support for the first role. In particular, postnatal cerebral maturation has been found to be characterized by the establishment of reciprocal connections between regions of the frontal lobes and posterior, central, and temporal cortical regions (Case, 1992; Thatcher, 1994). Moreover, the finding of an anterior–posterior gradient of development in the formation of these connections has been interpreted to suggest a mechanism of integration by frontal systems of elemental sensorimotor units to form higher-level abstractions and systems of abstraction (Thatcher, 1994).

It is further interesting to note that these qEEG studies revealed a left–right hemisphere pole of development, evidenced by predominantly left-hemisphere growth spurts followed by predominantly right-hemisphere growth spurts (Thatcher, 1994). Cycles in the left hemisphere consisted of a developmental sequence involving a progressive lengthening of intracortical connections between posterior sensory areas and frontal regions. Cycles in the right hemisphere, however, consisted of a sequential consolidation of long-distance frontal connections to shorter-distance posterior sensory connections (Thatcher, 1994). These results were interpreted to suggest a process of functional integration of differentiated subsystems in the left hemisphere, and a process of functional differentiation of previously integrated systems and formation of specialized subsystems in the right hemisphere (Thatcher, 1994). Although the models involve different levels of functioning, these results are thought to be consistent with Goldberg and Costa's (1981) formulation of left- and right-hemispheral roles. In both cases, the left hemisphere predominates in the utilization and integration of systems that are fully formed, whereas the right hemisphere is involved in the assembly of new systems.

In the previous discussion, the manifestation of the NLD syndrome has been presented within the context of Piaget's formulation of cognitive maturation. It is interesting to note that postnatal spurts in brain growth coincide with Piaget's main stages of intellectual development (Kolb & Fantie, 1989). Moreover, as was suggested earlier, this increase in weight is accounted for by growth of dendritic processes, synaptogenesis, and myelination, as compared to an increase in neuronal proliferation. In a similar vein, the results of the qEEG studies are especially notable because they indicate that brain maturation progresses in a discontinuous manner, and, moreover, that the stages in brain maturation are consistent with Piagetian theory (Case, 1992; Hudspeth & Pribram, 1990, 1992; Thatcher, 1994). Intracortical connections have been found to demonstrate growth spurts and plateaus overlapping with the stages of cognitive development described by Piaget.

It would make sense that the sort of change that takes place in development is structured to deal effectively with and adapt to environmental complexity. A fundamental aspect of this process would appear to consist of a dynamic interplay between integration and differentiation (in Piagetian terms, assimilation and accommodation) of single units to yield functionally more specialized or higher-order systems. This mechanism is also thought to engender a dichotomy between the processing of highly predictable, expected, or routine events and the processing of events that are novel or unexpected. As the discussion above illustrates, this process is represented at several levels of brain development and cognitive maturation. (This distinction has also been made at the level of neural processes. For examples, see Berry, Bradley, & Borges, 1978, and Greenough, 1986.)

Summary of Relations between the NLD Syndrome and the White Matter Model

In sum, the pattern of neuropsychological assets and deficits, academic performance, and socioemotional functioning exhibited by the child with NLD may be seen to arise from primary deficits in the following: visual perception, tactile perception, complex motor skills, and adaptation to novel stimuli. Important outcomes of these primary deficits include deficient concept formation, reasoning abilities, and the ability to employ symbols and representation. The manifestation of this pattern of neuropsychological assets and deficits may be understood in terms of complementary brain maturation explanations, in addition to a cognitive-developmental perspective.

When the performance of children with NLD (or any other group of children with some form of abnormality) is compared to that of their normally achieving peers, it is often assumed that the perceptual capacities of the groups are comparable—that is, that any observed discrepancy between them arises from differences or deficits in central processing as opposed to disparate input. Our discussion of white matter dysfunction should make it abundantly clear that this assumption should be questioned. In other words, an altered pattern of axonal connections in the brain can be reasonably expected to affect the way in which information is received.

An example of this notion is provided by Dennis's (1976) research on acallosal subjects. Dennis tested acallosal subjects on a series of finger localization tasks and found that they showed difficulty in accurately perceiving the distribution or interrelationship of fingers on either hand. She concluded that their perception of stimulus topography was impaired, and proposed that this deficit reflected a limitation of ipsilateral sensory pathways (as opposed to constituting a central processing defect, for example). Whereas contralateral projections permit the coding of stimulus topography, ipsilateral sensory pathways do not supply this information.

Furthermore, the ability to shift abruptly and simultaneously from one activity to another would seem to be an important mark of a well-functioning brain. It has been hypothesized that the fundamental effect of white matter dysfunction is an altered pattern of axonal connectivity that is both less evolved and less specialized. An ongoing process of refinement of axonal and synaptic connections in the formation of white matter pathways is thus expected to bear upon the brain's ability to process new information and respond to changes in functional demands.

In connection with this last expectation, white matter perturbations were predicted to have a more profound effect on right-hemispheral systems, and hence on higher-order cognitive processing. Distinct roles for the hemispheres have been proposed, in which the left hemisphere is generally responsible for integrating well-formed descriptive systems, whereas the right hemisphere is thought to be responsible for assembling those descriptive systems. In this way, one outcome of white matter dysfunction may be reflected in the inability of the child with NLD to form schemata of his or her world—that is, to form descriptive systems that entail both coding and representing novel experiences (right-hemispheral functioning), and to apply those systems effectively and efficiently (left-hemispheral functioning). Interhemispheric communication via the corpus callosum is expected to permit more precise definition of these cerebral hemispheral functions.

A role has further been postulated for the frontal lobes in integrating lower-level (e.g., sensorimotor) systems to form higher levels of abstraction. There is also evidence to suggest that the frontal lobes develop from two independent but parallel systems (Thatcher, 1994). The functions thought to be subserved by these systems also reflect a dynamic interplay of assimilation and accommodation. It is interesting to note that the mediofrontal regions, which are thought to be involved in anticipatory or predictive behaviors, are connected through the corpus callosum, whereas the laterofrontal regions are not.

Finally, evidence has been presented to indicate that stages of cognitive maturation and brain maturation coincide. In particular, growth spurts in brain weight and intracortical connections have been found to overlap with Piaget's proposed stages of cognitive maturation.

The discussion to this point illustrates that the manifestation of the NLD syndrome can be viewed in terms of the complex and complementary interaction of cognitive, brain maturational, and experiential factors. In the following section, the neurodevelopmental disorders included in this book are discussed in relation to some of these elements. Specifically, it is proposed that the behavioral phenotypes of these disorders correspond to the developmental presentation of the NLD syndrome. In addition, a role for white matter perturbations in the expression of the NLD syndrome in these disorders is advanced.

A SPECTRUM/HIERARCHY OF NEUROLOGICAL DISEASE, DISORDER, AND DYSFUNCTION

A spectrum of neurodevelopmental disorders characterized by variations in the severity of expression of the NLD syndrome has been hypothesized. In this connection, we have attempted to present the forms of neurological disease, disorder, and dysfunction contained in this book in terms of a hierarchy (see Table 18.1 for a summary of this). This endeavor is also reflected in the order of the book's table of contents—beginning with those diseases and forms of dysfunction in which the NLD syndrome is manifested most clearly, and moving to those in which the phenotypic manifestations of the NLD syndrome are less well defined and/or obscured by other types of neuropsychological dysfunction.

A fuller description of the features of this hierarchy is presented in the following list. It is structured in a manner that assumes the reader will refer to Table 18.1.

1. The levels within this hierarchy denote decreasing phenotypic similarity to the various neuropsychological assets and deficits that constitute the manifestations of the NLD syndrome. The levels are as follows:

TABLE 18.1. Nonverbal Learning Disabilities: Overview of Manifestations in Neurological Disease, Disorder, and Dysfunction

Level 1

Callosal agenesis (uncomplicated)
Asperger syndrome
Velocardiofacial syndrome
Williams syndrome
de Lange syndrome
Hydrocephalus (early, shunted)
Congenital hypothyroidism

Level 2

Sotos syndrome
Prophylactic treatment for acute lymphocytic leukemia (long-term survivors)
Metachromatic leukodystrophy (early in disease progression)
Turner syndrome
Fetal alcohol syndrome (high-functioning)

Level 3

Multiple sclerosis (early to middle stages)
Traumatic brain injury (diffuse white matter perturbations)
Toxicant-induced encephalopathies (affecting white matter)
Autism (high-functioning)

Suggestive

Fragile-X syndrome (high-functioning)
Leukodystrophies other than metachromatic (early in disease progression)
Haemophilus influenzae meningitis
Neurofibromatosis (early to middle stages of disease progression)
Early-treated phenylketonuria
Intracranial hemorrhage (early)
Congential adrenal hyperplasia
Prader–Willi syndrome
Insulin-dependent diabetes mellitus (very early onset)

Difficult to classify

Cerebral palsy of perinatal origin

Similar, but basically different

Tourette syndrome

Level 1: *Virtually all* of the NLD assets and deficits are manifested.

Level 2: A *considerable majority* of the NLD assets and deficits are evident.

Level 3: *Many* of the NLD assets and deficits are manifested by a *significant subset* of children with these disorders.

2. Prophylactic treatment, of course, is not a form of neurological disease. It is included at Level 2 because children who are long-term survivors of acute lymphocytic leukemia (ALL) and who have received very high doses of whole-brain cranial irradiation and some other types of therapies frequently exhibit a considerable majority of the NLD assets and deficits.

3. The category labeled "Suggestive" contains a number of diseases for which the literature is highly suggestive of patterns of NLD assets and deficits in a significant subset of children so afflicted. These diseases will be examined from the perspective of the NLD/white matter model in the future.

4. Many children with cerebral palsy of perinatal origin exhibit a considerable majority of the NLD assets and deficits. However, because of the wide variety of etiologies and manifestations considered under this rubric, the classification by level of NLD manifestations is rendered problematic.

5. Tourette syndrome is one example of a neurological disorder wherein several of the NLD manifestations are evident. However, there are also many basic differences, which suggest strongly that Tourette syndrome should not be considered within the group of neurological disorders that can be characterized in terms of the NLD spectrum (Brookshire, Butler, Ewing-Cobbs, & Fletcher, 1994).

6. It is very probable that this hierarchy will change somewhat as more becomes known about the neuropsychological manifestations of the diseases in question.

7. It is likely that other forms of neurological disease, disorder, and dysfunction will be added to this hierarchy.

8. It would appear highly probable that advances in neuroimaging of white matter functioning, neuropathological findings regarding white matter perturbations, and other advances in the specification of the developmental and functional neuroanatomy of myelination will throw considerable light upon the underpinnings of this NLD hierarchy.

EVIDENCE FROM THE HIERARCHY REGARDING THE NLD SYNDROME PHENOTYPE AND THE WHITE MATTER MODEL

The NLD Syndrome Phenotype

Ideally, we would have liked to examine this proposed hierarchy by rating the disorders in this book according to the extent to which they display the pattern of neuropsychological assets and deficits manifested in NLD. However, a systematic investigation of the hypothesis was rendered difficult by differences in the depth and quality of the neuropsychological studies representing each disorder. In particular, there was a relative paucity of studies examining tactile-perceptual abilities; in addition, few studies undertook a comprehensive investigation of speech and language skills. Thus, it is difficult to comment precisely on the extent to which the phenotypes of these neurological disorders are congruent with that of the NLD syndrome.

In general, a pattern of deficits in visual–spatial, complex psychomotor, and concept-formation skills in the face of relatively well-preserved verbal skills was found to characterize virtually all of the disorders. Poor mechanical arithmetic performance relative to reading and spelling performance was also demonstrated in the majority of cases. In addition, it was found that rote material was dealt with more effectively than was novel information. Many of the children described in this book showed a need for regularity, routine, and structure in their cognitive and social activities. As well, a pattern of hyperactivity in early childhood followed by shy, withdrawn, or immature behavior in later years was commonly observed.

The White Matter Model

Disturbances in white matter functioning were also in evidence. The disorders may be classified into three general groups on the basis of the type of white matter perturbations manifested: disorders involving abnormal white matter development, degeneration of myelin, and damage to white matter.

Abnormal White Matter Development

Callosal agenesis clearly signifies the abnormal development of a major set of white matter pathways. This primary disturbance probably has profound effects on the organization of cortical connections in general. Callosal agenesis is also an associated feature of hydrocephalus. There is evidence to suggest that hydrocephalus affects other white matter pathways as well, and may result in the long term in disruption of the process of myelination in the brain.

Several disorders (e.g., velocardiofacial [VCF] syndrome, de Lange syndrome [DLS], Sotos syndrome [SS], and fetal alcohol syndrome [FAS]) are characterized by prenatal defects in neuronal proliferation and migration. These disturbances are expected to lead to both a structural and a functional reorganization in the brain: Alternate pathways and connections may be formed in response to these primary defects. The development and organization of axonal connections depend upon the number and location of cortical neurons. Furthermore, dendritic arborization and synaptic development are related to early cell migration (Menkes, 1990). In either case, an influence on CNS development and maturation, affecting both grey and white matter, is probable. Although the evidence for Williams syndrome (WS) is less clear, its phenotypical similarity to these other disorders would suggest a comparable course of development.

In addition to a primary disturbance in cell migration and pathway formation, the aforementioned disorders also share important physical features. These include the following: characteristic craniofacial anomalies, growth deficiency, malformation of organs (especially heart, kidneys, and gastrointestinal organs), and endocrine dysfunction. Secondary effects of poor organ and endocrine development, affecting nutrition, oxygen requirements, and hormone production and secretion, are also expected to have a deleterious effect on CNS maturation and white matter development.

A similar hypothesis has been proposed for Turner syndrome (TS). The lack of an X chromosome in females with TS is expected to have an effect on neuronal migration and patterns of connectivity in the developing brain. In addition, abnormal levels of hormones, particularly during adolescence, may have a late-occurring effect on brain maturation. Thyroid deficiency is also thought to affect the pattern of synaptic connections and axonal projections in the child with congenital hypothyroidism (CH). The idea that CH has an overall negative effect on cell proliferation, neuronal differentiation, gliogenesis, myelinogenesis, and synaptogenesis has gained wide acceptance.

White Matter Degeneration

Demyelination is evidenced in metachromatic leukodystrophy (MLD), the prophylactic treatment of ALL, and multiple sclerosis (MS). Degeneration of white matter is also associated with exposure to some toxicants, such as toluene and elemental mercury.

Damage to White Matter

The destruction of white matter characterizes the remaining disorder. Widespread damage to white matter is a major consequence of traumatic brain injury (TBI); in addition to focal lesions, TBI has been shown to produce diffuse axonal injury.

An Exception

Asperger syndrome (AS) represents the only disorder discussed in this book for which a white matter association has not been clearly established.

Research on this disorder has only recently begun in earnest. It is expected that, given its phenotypical similarity to the other disorders described herein, investigations of the neuropathological underpinnings of AS will reveal evidence of white matter perturbations.

Deficit—Timing Interactions

Clearly, white matter dysfunction encompasses a broad range of conditions. It includes TBI, in which a segment of white matter is damaged at one point in time; demyelinating diseases, in which white matter is progressively destroyed; and various disorders (e.g., CH) in which the *development* of white matter is affected. Although all of the conditions described in this book, with the exception of AS, can be seen to affect white matter in some way, it is important that a distinction be made among the events that have led up to it. Specifically, fundamental differences in the timing, extent, and nature of the insult to white matter in these various conditions should have a bearing upon their neuropsychological presentation and, within the present context, upon the extent to which their phenotypes resemble that of the NLD syndrome.

The timing of specific ontogenetic processes—neuronal proliferation and differentiation; the multiplication of glial cells and their differentiation; the establishment of synaptic connections; and myelination—is likely to differ in various regions of the brain. Moreover, the timing, sequence, or coordination of these events may be interdependent, such that events in one region of the brain depend upon the development and sequence of events in another. Thus, the consequences of an insult will not similarly affect all regions of the brain. The effects of the insult will depend on the stage and rate of development of the respective areas of the brain, as well as on the ways in which these disparate regions interact. The nearer to the beginning of cell differentiation and reproduction that the insult occurs, the more severe and widespread the consequences of the insult may be expected to be.

Types of Studies

Both within- and across-group studies lend themselves well to investigations of the effects of timing on brain—behavior relationships. A substantial degree of phenotypic variability has been seen to characterize each of the disorders described in this book. And, among these children, some were observed to exhibit the NLD syndrome to a greater extent than others. Comparisons of these subgroups permit an examination of the effects of the three critical variables mentioned above (type, extent, and timing of disturbances) on white matter functioning and on behavioral expression of the disorder. Disorders such as MLD, TBI, and the treatment of ALL, in which the insult to white matter occurs at different stages in development, lend themselves especially well to this type of study. Deficit—timing interactions may be further elucidated by within-group studies of children with CH, TS, and FAS. In these cases, the influence of a lack of thyroid hormone, lack of estrogen, and maternal alcohol use, respectively, during critical periods of development may be examined, to reveal when different neuropsychological functions and their underlying substrates are most profoundly affected. Disorders occurring in adulthood, such as MS and toxicant-induced encephalopathy, are especially interesting for what they reveal about the effects of disruptions to white matter on well-established behavioral patterns. These disorders are suggestive of the susceptibility of different sites in the brain and of different neuropsychological functions to late-occurring white matter perturbations. Also, a comparison of different toxicant-induced encephalopathies at different ages would be expected to shed considerable light on this general issue.

Across-group investigations permit an even wider range of studies. Although each of the disorders in this book exhibited the NLD syndrome to a degree, there are areas of divergence that may be attributed to differences in timing. Early developments in morphogenic disorders—such as VCF, DLS, and SS as well as FAS—are expected to have widespread effects on white matter formation, and these may also engender more generalized effects on grey matter structures. Hormonal influences in disorders such as CH and TS are likely to exert their effects during a critical window of development, and may have their greatest effect on the development of right-hemispheral systems. Later-occurring disturbances in MLD and the prophylactic treatment of ALL are proposed to have a more profound long-term impact on functions normally thought to be subserved by frontal systems. This is also expected to be true of TBI, in which the frontal lobes appear to be especially susceptible to injury. In each case, the importance of longitudinal studies to track the long-term effects of these disorders on brain maturation and organization cannot be overemphasized.

Within- and across-group studies are also interesting for what they can reveal about brain–behavior relationships in general. This kind of research permits reciprocal predictions between profiles of neuropsychological abilities and deficits, and what might be dysfunctional in the brain. In this way, research hypotheses may be guided by an exploration of the events that correspond between CNS dysfunction and the neuropsychological profiles obtained in various neurodevelopmental disorders. A review of the chapters in this book reveals shared deficits among several disorders for which there may also be a common brain correlate. These are outlined below:

1. Superficially well-developed verbal skills were evident in children with hydrocephalus, WS, AS, TS, and FAS. Research on children with WS has implicated a role for vermal areas VI and VII of the cerebellum in language development (see Chapter 6). It would be well to examine this area in children with AS, TS, FAS, and hydrocephalus. In addition, an investigation of corpus callosum involvement in language functioning is suggested.

2. General deficits in attention—a feature not congruent with the NLD syndrome—have been found to characterize children treated for ALL and children with FAS. The neocerebellum has been implicated in the voluntary coordination of selective, accurate, and rapid shifts of attention, on the basis of research with autistic children (Courchesne et al., 1994). This role for the cerebellum could be further examined in children with FAS and in long-term survivors of ALL. In MLD, the cerebellum is largely spared, and attention deficits of this nature would not be expected.

3. A notable similarity in the physical and behavioral phenotype of FAS and suspected genetic disorders such as the VCF syndrome, WS, and DLS warrants exploration. A common mechanism may be responsible for the interference with normal gene expression.

4. On a free-recall task, requiring hierarchical processing of visual information, children with FAS were found to show deficits in recall and reproduction of local but not global features. The reverse pattern was found in children with WS. An examination of differences in CNS dysfunction in these two groups of children may lead to a brain correlate for this observed difference.

5. A consistent association between the integrity of white matter pathways and various aspects of visual-perceptual functioning has been found. Further research is needed to elucidate the specific dimensions of this relationship.

6. Whereas impaired arithmetic performance was found to be a consistent feature of childhood neurodevelopmental disorders, in the adult-onset disorders (such as MS and toxicant-induced encephalopathy), deficits in mechanical arithmetic skills were not observed. Presumably, this type of discrepancy is indicative of the differential effect of the timing of an insult to white matter on the development of descriptive systems versus access to or the application of pre-existing systems.

7. Finally, two important aspects of the NLD syndrome are social adjustment and emotional behavior, which are integral dimensions of development. Many of the children described in this book showed impaired social competence and mild emotional disturbance. Although these developments can be understood from an exclusively psychosocial perspective, it would also be interesting to explore the role of cortico-limbic connections. These connections may represent the integration of

higher-order systems with regions typically thought to be involved in the expression of emotions.

FUTURE DIRECTIONS

Although each of the chapters in this book provides an expansive synthesis of the research literature, the depth and quality of research both within and across disorders were quite discrepant. This restricted a systematic integration of the findings. A review of the chapters points to a greater need for the following:

1. Comprehensive neuropsychological investigations.
2. Neuroimaging and neuropathological studies.
3. Sophisticated integration of neuropsychological and neurological findings.
4. Large-scale cross-sectional and longitudinal investigations.
5. Multicenter studies.

Discrepancies in the depth and quality of the research make it difficult to draw many firm conclusions, but it does seem abundantly clear that it is no longer acceptable to think of brain–behavior relationships solely in terms of grey matter structures or a limited notion of neuronal functioning. CNS functioning is dependent upon several events that extend beyond the structure of the neuron itself. These include neuronal proliferation and migration, cell differentiation, axon and dendrite growth, axon guidance and target recognition, and synaptic formation. In addition to an unfolding sequence of genetically determined events, internal and external factors may have an impact upon the development of the brain. Events that may be involved with the modification of cortical connections—such as nerve cell death, the formation and elimination of excess axonal connections and synapses, and trophic factors such as hormones and neurotransmitters—cannot be neglected. In addition, it is important to consider a role for environmental events, such as learning experiences, in refining cortical connections.

The mechanisms underlying these events are not well understood, and there is even less appreciation of their functional role. However, they clearly merit our attention. In this book, we have tried to draw attention to the importance of white matter functioning and its relationship to the presentation of the NLD syndrome. Several neurodevelopmental disorders that are thought to manifest the NLD syndrome to varying degrees and to exhibit white matter disturbance have been presented. Other disorders, not mentioned in this book, are also thought to share aspects of the NLD phenotype. It is suspected that neuronal structures, cortical connections, and neurotransmitter functioning form a basic triad, the dynamic interplay of which underlies most neurodevelopmental and neuropsychiatric disorders. The degree of involvement of any one of these elements is likely to affect the classification of the disorder. Thus, although Tourette syndrome is an example of a disorder that shares several features of the NLD syndrome, it is not thought to fall within this continuum. It may be the case that this syndrome is characterized by a degree of white matter disturbance (and thus shares some aspects of the basic NLD phenotype), but that neurotransmitter functioning plays a bigger role in its expression, particularly with respect to the regulation of behavior.

The time is ripe in neuropsychology for a perspective that seeks to do more than draw simple correspondences between brain and behavior functioning in the developing child. A progressive role is one in which our knowledge of cognitive and behavioral maturation is integrated with our knowledge of brain maturation, and presented within a framework that acknowledges the importance of experiential factors and the child's position as an active agent in his or her development. We feel that the contents of this book constitute an important step in this direction.

REFERENCES

Barkovich, A. J., Kjos, B. O., Jackson, D. E., Jr., & Norman, D. (1988). Normal maturation of the neonatal and infant brain: MR imaging at 1.5T. *Radiology, 166,* 173–180.

Berry, M., Bradley, P., & Borges, S. (1978). Environmental and genetic determinants of connectivity in the central nervous system: An approach through dendrite field analysis. In M. A. Corner, R. E. Baker, N. E. van de Poll, D. F. Swaas, & H. B. M. Uylings (Eds.), *Progress in brain research: Vol. 48. Maturation of the nervous system* (pp. 133–146). New York: Elsevier.

Brookshire, B. L., Butler, I. J., Ewing-Cobbs, L., & Fletcher, J. M. (1994). Neuropsychological characteristics of children with Tourette syndrome: Evidence for a nonverbal learning disability? *Journal of Clinical and Experimental Neuropsychology, 16,* 289–302.

Case, R. (1992). The role of the frontal lobes in the regulation of cognitive development. *Brain and Cognition, 20,* 51–73.

Casey, J. E., & Rourke, B. P. (1992). Disorders of somatosensory perception in children. In I. Rapin & S. J. Segalowitz (Eds.), *Handbook of neuropsychology: Vol. 6. Child neuropsychology* (pp. 477–494). New York: Elsevier.

Courchesne, E., Lincoln, A. J., Townsend, J. P., James, H. E., Akshoomoff, N. A., Saitoh, O., Yeung-Courchesne, R., Egaas, B., Press, G. A., Haas, R. H., Murakami, J. W., & Schreibman, L. (1994). A new finding: Impairment in shifting attention in autistic and cerebellar patients. In S. Broman & J. Grafman (Eds.), *Atypical cognitive deficits in developmental disorders: Implications for brain function* (pp. 101–137). Hillsdale, NJ: Erlbaum.

Dennis, M. (1976). Impaired sensory and motor differentiation with corpus callosum agenesis: A lack of callosal inhibition during ontogeny? *Neuropsychologia, 14*, 455–469.

Dietrich, R. B., & Bradley, W. G. (1988). Normal and abnormal white matter maturation. *Seminars in Ultrasound, CT, and MR, 9*(3), 192–200.

Goldberg, E., & Costa, L. D. (1981). Hemisphere differences in the acquisition and use of descriptive systems. *Brain and Language, 14*, 144–173.

Gravel, C., Sasseville, R., & Hawkes, R. (1990a). Maturation of the corpus callosum of the rat: I. Influence of thyroid hormones on the topography of callosal projections. *Journal of Comparative Neurology, 291*, 128–146.

Gravel, C., Sasseville, R., & Hawkes, R. (1990b). Maturation of the corpus callosum of the rat: II. Influence of thyroid hormones on the number and maturation of axons. *Journal of Comparative Neurology, 291*, 147–161.

Greenough, W. T. (1986). What's special about development? Thoughts on the bases of experience-sensitive synaptic plasticity. In W. T. Greenough & J. M. Juraska (Eds.), *Developmental neuropsychobiology* (pp. 387–407). Orlando, FL: Academic Press.

Hudspeth, W. J., & Pribram, K. H. (1990). Stages of brain and cognitive maturation. *Journal of Educational Psychology, 82*(4), 881–884.

Hudspeth, W. J., & Pribram, K. H. (1992). Psychological indices of cerebral maturation. *International Journal of Psychophysiology, 12*, 19–29.

Huttenlocher, P. R. (1984). Synapse elimination and plasticity in developing human cerebral cortex. *American Journal of Mental Deficiency, 88*(5), 488–496.

Huttenlocher, P. R. (1994). Synaptogenesis in human cerebral cortex. In G. Dawson & K. W. Fischer (Eds.), *Human behavior and the developing brain* (pp. 137–152). New York: Guilford Press.

Kolb, B., & Fantie, B. (1989) Development of the child's brain and behavior. In C. Reynolds & E. Fletcher-Janzen (Eds.). *Handbook of clinical child neuropsychology.* New York: Plenum Press.

Lassonde, M. L. (1986). The facilitatory influence of the corpus callosum on intrahemispheric processing. In F. Lepore, M. Ptito, & H. H. Jasper (Eds.), *Two hemispheres—one brain: Functions of the corpus callosum* (pp. 385–401). New York: Alan R. Liss.

Lassonde, M. L., Sauerwein, H., Chicoine, A.-J., & Geoffroy, G. (1991). Absence of disconnexion syndrome in callosal agenesis and early callosotomy: Brain reorganization or lack of structural specificity during ontogeny? *Neuropsychologia, 29*(6), 481–495.

Menkes, J. H. (1990). *Textbook of child neurology* (4th ed.). Philadelphia: Lea & Febiger.

Olavarria, J., Serra-Oller, M. M., Yee, K. T., & VanSluyters, R. C. (1988). Topography of interhemispheric connections in the neocortex of mice with congenital deficiencies of the callosal commissure. *Journal of Comparative Neurology, 270*, 575–590.

Ozaki, H. S., & Wahlsten, D. (1993). Cortical axon trajectories and growth cone morphologies in fetuses of acallosal mouse strains. *Journal of Comparative Neurology, 336*, 595–604.

Rourke, B. P. (1982). Central processing deficiencies in children: Toward a developmental neuropsychological model. *Journal of Clinical Neuropsychology, 4*(1), 1–18.

Rourke, B. P. (1987). Syndrome of nonverbal learning disabilities: The final common pathway of white-matter disease/dysfunction. *The Clinical Neuropsychologist, 1*(3), 209–234.

Rourke, B. P. (1989). *Nonverbal learning disabilities: The syndrome and the model.* New York: Guilford Press.

Rourke, B. P. (1993). Arithmetic disabilities, specific and otherwise: A neuropsychological perspective. *Journal of Learning Disabilities, 25,* 1–25.

Rourke, B. P., Bakker, D. J., Fisk, J. L., & Strang, J. D. (1983). *Child neuropsychology: An introduction to theory, research, and clinical practice.* New York: Guilford Press.

Rourke, B. P., & Fuerst, D. R. (1992). Psychosocial dimensions of learning disability subtypes: Neuropsychological studies in the Windsor Laboratory. *School Psychology Review, 21,* 360–373.

Schmidt, S. L., & Caparelli-Daquer, E. M. (1989). The effects of total and partial callosal agenesis on the development of morphological brain asymmetries in the BALB/cCF mouse. *Experimental Neurology, 104,* 172–180.

Strang, J. D., & Rourke, B. P. (1985). Adaptive behavior of children who exhibit specific arithmetic disabilities and associated neuropsychological abilities and deficits. In B. P. Rourke (Ed.), *Neuropsychology of learning disabilities: Essentials of subtype analysis* (pp. 302–328). New York: Guilford Press.

Stuss, D. T. (1992). Biological and psychological development of executive functions. *Brain and Cognition, 20,* 8–23.

Thatcher, R. W. (1994). Cyclic cortical reorganization: Origins of human cognitive development. In G. Dawson & K. W. Fischer (Eds.), *Human behavior and the developing brain* (pp. 232–266). New York: Guilford Press.

Yakovlev, P. I., & Lecours, A. R. (1967). The myelogenetic cycles of regional maturation of the brain. In A. Minkowski (Ed.), *Regional development of the brain in early life* (pp. 3–69). Philadelphia: F. A. Davis.

Treatment Program for the Child with NLD

Byron P. Rourke

Outlined in this appendix are some common features of an integrated and carefully orchestrated program of intervention that my colleagues and I have found to be helpful for children and adolescents who exhibit the NLD syndrome. Much of this material is adapted from Strang and Rourke (1985) and Rourke (1989). The program involves the child's principal caregivers (parents, teachers, therapists) at every step of the way. For example, one of the first steps in a remediation/habilitation program is to provide the parents with appropriate information concerning the nature and significance of their child's neuropsychological assets and deficits. Often the child's parents require fairly constant counseling and support in order to gear their expectations and their parenting methods and techniques to fit the child's most salient developmental needs.

A note regarding the NLD syndrome in relation to the treatment program is in order here. In view of the particular pattern of neuropsychological strengths and deficits exhibited by children with NLD—their difficulties in benefiting from nonverbal experiences, their unusual reliance on language as a primary tool for adaptation, the confusion of their parents and other caretakers concerning the nature or significance of their condition, and the inappropriate expectations of such children by all concerned—many of the initial phases of the treatment program are focused on the perceptions of the parents and other caretakers. Although not all children who exhibit the NLD syndrome have identical developmental histories or behave exactly as outlined in the body of this work, the behavioral outcomes for such children are remarkably similar. At the same time, it is clear that the ability of a child's primary caretakers to understand his or her deficits early in life, and to generate appropriate expectations for such a child, is an important factor in determining the degree to which the child will exhibit maladaptive or atypical behavior in later childhood. Thoughtful guidance from the child's parents and specialized forms of treatment outside of the home situation are also important determinants of general prognosis. Finally, the *degree* of neuropsychological impairment would appear to be an important consideration. Children whose abilities are outstandingly impaired and who exhibit the full constellation of neuropsychological deficits characteristic of the NLD syndrome would appear to be the ones most at risk for maladaptive consequences.

Remediation and habilitation for the child with NLD are crucial but difficult. Part of this difficulty relates to the impression that persists in the minds of many involved in the educational process and others: that a child who reads and spells well could not possibly have any outstanding educational needs. This being the case, such children are seldom involved in educational programs that are appropriate for their special learning needs. This is particularly unfortunate, because if treatment is not instituted fairly early and on all fronts (including academic) in such a child's life, the prognosis tends to be quite bleak. With these remarks as background, the following general principles of intervention are offered. These principles are framed as suggestions to the child's principal caregivers. Our ordinary practice is to present these to the principal caretakers and, in the process, to make modifications as necessary to accommodate specific individual, family, community, and other factors that are operative in the particular case.

1. Observe the child's behavior closely, especially in novel or complex situations.

During this first potentially informative exercise, caregivers should focus on what the child *does* and disregard what the child *says*. This should help the parent, therapist, and/or teacher to develop a better appreciation of the child's potentially outstanding adaptive deficits and to shape their own cognitive "set" for interventions with the child. One of the most frequent criticisms of remedial intervention programs with this particular type of child is that remedial authorities are unaware of the extent and significance of the child's deficits. Through direct observation under these conditions, it should become apparent that the child is very much in need of a systematic, well-orchestrated program of intervention.

Examples: A therapist can arrange for parents to observe their child at play with other children; can videotape such interactions or solitary behavior in the classroom; and can explain the results of standardized rating scales of social behavior and other relevant dimensions—for example, the Nonverbal Learning Disabilities Scales (Rourke, 1993) and the Vineland Adaptive Behavior Scale (Sparrow, Balla, & Cicchetti, 1984)—that are completed by persons who are very familiar with the child.

2. Adopt a realistic attitude.

Once it has been established that the child's behavior is nonadaptive, particularly in new or otherwise complex situations, a caregiver must then be realistic in assessing the import and impact of the child's neuropsychological assets (e.g., "automatic" language skills, rote memory) and deficits (e.g., visual–spatial–organizational skills). In the classroom, for instance, it should be readily apparent that the child's well-developed word recognition and spelling abilities are not sufficient for him or her to benefit from many forms of formal and informal instruction, especially for those subjects requiring visual–spatial–organizational and/or nonverbal problem-solving skills. This being the case, there are really only two educational alternatives: to adopt special procedures for the presentation of material of the latter variety, or to avoid such material altogether. Some suggestions for "special procedures" follow.

3. Teach the child in a systematic, "step-by-step" fashion.

Whenever possible, a parts-to-whole verbal teaching approach should be used. As a rule of thumb, the therapist or teacher should take note that if it is possible to talk about an idea, concept, or procedure in a straightforward fashion, then the child should be able to grasp at least some aspects of the material. On the other hand, if it is not possible to put into words an adequate description of the material to be learned (e.g., as in explaining time concepts), it will probably be quite difficult for the child with NLD to benefit from the instruction.

   It should also be kept in mind that the child will learn best when each of the verbal "steps" is presented in the correct sequence, because of his or her inadequate problem-solving skills and associated organizational difficulties with novel (even linguistically novel) material. A secondary benefit of this teaching approach is that the child is provided with a set of verbal rules that can be written out and then reapplied whenever it is appropriate to do so. This is particularly important for the teaching of mechanical arithmetic operations and procedures.

   The principal impediment to engaging in this rather slow and painstaking approach to teaching the child with NLD is the caregiver's (faulty) impression that the child is much more adept and adaptable than is actually the case. This increases the probability that the caregiver will start the program at a level that is too sophisticated for the child, and will proceed at too fast a clip for the child's information-processing capacities. The child with NLD, on the other hand, tends to respond quite appreciatively and appropriately to an approach that is slow, repetitive, and highly redundant.

4. Encourage the child to describe in detail important events that are transpiring in his or her life.

The fourth remedial recommendation applies not only to teaching sessions with the child, but also to any situation in which the child does not seem to appreciate fully the significance of his or her behavior or the behavior of others. For example, when there is an incident on the playground in which the child has encountered interpersonal difficulty, the teacher or therapist should ask the child to explain in detail the events that transpired and his or her perceptions of the cause of the incident and its effects. The caregiver should encourage the child to focus on the relevant aspects of the situation and point out the irrelevancies that are brought up. Through discussion, the child should be helped to become aware of discrepancies between his or her perceptions (regarding the situation in question) and the perceptions of others. In teaching situations, one useful technique is to encourage the child to "reteach" the teacher or therapist (or, in some situations, to teach other children) the procedure or concept that he or she has been taught. This will help to increase the probability that the child has understood the necessary information, that it has been analyzed and integrated, and that it will be applied in future situations.

5. Teach the child appropriate strategies for dealing with particularly troublesome situations that occur on a frequent, everyday basis.

In many cases, children with NLD do not generate appropriate problem-solving strategies independently because they are unaware of the actual requirements of the situation. At other times, the childen may be unable to generate appropriate strategies because this particular type of endeavor requires basic neuropsychological competencies that the childen have not developed. For both of these reasons, such children need to be taught appropriate strategies for handling the requirements of frequently occurring troublesome situations. The teacher or therapist will find that the step-by-step requirements for teaching this type of child are quite similar to those that would be employed effectively for much younger children. Once again, it should be emphasized that the most frequent error made by adult caretakers in such situations is to overestimate the capacities of children with NLD to learn and to apply adaptive problem-solving solutions and techniques for coping.

6. Encourage the generalization of learned strategies and concepts.

Although the majority of "normal" children see how one particular strategy or procedure may apply to a number of different situations, and/or how certain concepts may apply to a wide range of topics, the child with NLD usually exhibits difficulties with this form of generalization. For example, it is common to find that although the child with NLD has been trained assiduously in visual attention and visual tracking skills in the laboratory or therapeutic setting, he or she fails to employ the skills effectively in everyday life (e.g., when it would be propitious to examine some aspects of a person's physical characteristics in order to enhance recognition of that person in the future). It is abundantly clear not only that the child with NLD needs to be taught specific skills in a step-by-step fashion, but also that transitional or generalization skills need to be addressed in an identical manner.

Related to these difficulties is a very persistent and pervasive deficit in the judgment of cause-and-effect relationships. For example, the child with NLD may not discern, even after hundreds of experiences with a particular event, that there is nascent within it a reasonable and easily inferrable causal linkage. For example, the child may not discern that there is a causal connection between flipping a light switch and the illumination or extinguishing of a light. Most often, the child has to be shown quite explicitly that (say) the up position on the light switch signals "on," and the down position "off." The vast majority of persons unfamiliar with NLD fail to see that such relationships have to be brought quite explicitly to the child's attention, because children with NLD do not make the same sort of inferences regarding cause and effect that are arrived at spontaneously and without difficulty by children not so afflicted.

7. Teach the child to refine and use appropriately his or her verbal (expressive) skills.

As has been pointed out previously, it is quite probable that the child with NLD will come to use verbal (expressive) skills much more frequently and for much different reasons than do most children. For example, such a child may repeatedly ask questions as a primary way of gathering information about a new or otherwise complex situation. This may be quite inappropriate for many situations (e.g., those of a social nature), in which nonverbal behaviors are much more important for feedback and direction.

The content of the child's verbal responses may also be problematic. A common observation is that the child with NLD may begin to make a reply by directly addressing the question asked, but then may gradually drift off into a completely different topic. At the very least, the tangential nature of such utterances has the effect of alienating the listener. Specific training should be undertaken that is directed at "what to say," "how to say," and "when to say" aspects of language as these questions apply to the child's problem areas. However, as with other aspects of remediation mentioned above, there is the problem of generalization of learning in this sort of training exercise. The child with NLD tends not to be flexible and adaptive in the application of learned habits, even when these are in his or her areas of "strength" (i.e., verbal skills).

For these and other reasons, it is usually necessary to spend considerable time and effort to train the child to stop, look, listen, and weigh alternatives, even in what may appear to the casual observer to be mundane, straightforward situations. Failure to anticipate the consequences of their actions often leads children with NLD to rush into situations where they are very likely to suffer physical and/or psychological harm. Their usual tendency is to avoid such situations after repeated failure and pain. The caregiver's role is to help a child to deal effectively with such situations, rather than to encourage the child's understandable tendency to avoid them altogether.

8. Teach the child to make better use of his or her visual—spatial—organizational skills.

It should be borne in mind that children tend to "lead with their strong suit" in situations that are in any way problematic for them. For example, if a child exhibits an outstanding area of disability (e.g., visual—spatial skills) in combination with relatively intact abilities (e.g., verbal receptive and expressive skills), he or she tends to use the better-developed (verbal) skills whenever it is possible, although inappropriate, to do so. This encourages a situation in which the poorly developed skills (e.g., visual—spatial skills) are not challenged or "exercised"; hence, optimal development may not be realized. The tendency to "play the strong suit" also encourages the child with NLD to develop a very wide variety of ways to use language-related skills, many of which are clearly maladaptive.

To increase the likelihood that the child's visual modality and associated perceptive and analytic abilities will be developed and used optimally, a younger child of this type could be taught to name visual details in pictures as a way of encouraging him or her to pay attention to these details. In conjunction with this exercise, the child could be asked to talk about the relationship between various details in a picture (e.g., intersecting lines) as a way of drawing attention to the complexity, importance, and significance of visual features of stimulus presentation.

When the child is older, remedial suggestions and exercises should be more "functional" or practical in nature, but at the same time should address directly the child's outstanding areas of difficulty. For example, most social situations require the child to decipher or decode the nonverbal behaviors of others in order to interpret them properly. It is clear that the child with NLD is quite deficient in abilities that are crucial for the development of nonverbal social-analytic skills. Therefore, a caregiver might create "artificial" social situations that require the child to rely only on his or her visual receptive and other nonverbal skills for interpretation. This could be done with pictures, films, or even contrived "real-life" situations for which there is no verbal feedback available. After an exercise of this type, the caregiver should discuss the child's perception of the social situation and of his or her most appropriate role in the situation. At the same time, the caregiver might provide the child with strategies for deciphering the most salient nonverbal dimensions inherent in these contrived social situations.

9. Teach the child to interpret visual information when there is "competing" auditory information.

Training the child to focus on visual stimuli when auditory stimuli are available is usually more complex than the suggested remedial interventions already mentioned. This recommendation is particularly important in attempting to teach the child to deal more effectively with novel social situations. In these situations, it is important not only to interpret others' nonverbal behavior correctly, but also to interpret what is being said in conjunction with these nonverbal cues. In most cases, this type of training should be undertaken only when there has been adequate work and progress in the previously mentioned areas.

Example: A caregiver can have the child observe videotaped interactions that contain varying degrees of complexity in terms of physical and psychological cause-and-effect relationships. The child should be encourage to examine all of the information available before generating a "solution" to the problem and/or anticipating the next step in the action sequence. In this genre of activities, as in so many others, it is necessary to adopt ways and means to quell the child's rather predominant tendency to proceed without due concern for all (or even most) of the elements necessary to comprehend and deal effectively with complex or novel situations.

10. Teach appropriate nonverbal behavior.

Many children with NLD do not appear to have adequately developed nonverbal behavior. For example, such children often present with a somewhat "vacant look" or other inappropriate facial expressions. This is especially true of those individuals who are found to exhibit marked neuropsychological deficits. A child with NLD may smile in situations in which such behavior is quite inappropriate (e.g., when he or she is experiencing failure with a task). It is important to attempt to teach more appropriate nonverbal behavior, keeping in mind the concepts introduced in association with the refinements of the child's verbal expressive skills. In this connection, teaching the child "what to do" and "how and when to do it" should be the focus of concern. For example, some children may not know how or when to convey their feelings in a nonverbal manner. The use of informative pictures, imitative "drills," work with a mirror, and other techniques and concrete aids can prove to be invaluable in this type of training. This sort of intervention may also serve to make the child more aware of the significance of the nonverbal behavior of others.

Example: The caregiver can encourage the development of mime by having the child confine his or her own communication to nonverbal means for certain periods during the day, and by encouraging the child to interpret the mimed communication of others on videotape or in real-time interactions. Although the child with NLD will find this to be very difficult to countenance initially, staying with a regimen that involves regular periods of nonverbal communication (both sending and receiving) can be very effective in achieving worthwhile adaptive goals.

11. Facilitate structured peer interactions.

It is not always possible to promote social training in unstructured social situations, because these are largely beyond the reach of the remedial therapist or teacher. For instance, when the child is on the playground, it is not often possible to regulate his or her play in any way (at least to the extent that it promotes positive social growth for the socially impaired youngster). However, intramural activities of one sort or another, clubs, and formal community groups can provide a forum for social training if they are exploited in a proper manner. Unfortunately, because many children of this type tend to be somewhat socially withdrawn, they may not be encouraged to join their peers in social activities of any kind, because their parents and other caregivers may see a need to protect the children from such encounters.

This raises the thorny issue of "overprotection." Although sensitive caregivers are often accused of this, it is clear that they may be the only ones who have an appreciation for a child's vulnerability and lack of appropriate skill development. Balancing the need for protection with the need for expanded horizons and encounters with physical and social reality is never easy. Understanding that this is a difficult realm within which to exercise prudence (i.e., to dare wisely) is the first—and very necessary—step to engaging in the complex series of judgments and activities that constitute effective intervention for children with NLD.

12. Promote, encourage, and monitor "systematic" explorative activities.

One of the most potentially harmful tacks that a well-meaning therapist can take with a child with NLD is to leave the child to his or her own devices in activities that lack sufficient (or any) structure (e.g., ambient play situations with other children). On the other hand, it is quite worthwhile to design specific activities through which the child is encouraged to explore his or her environment. For example, exploratory activity may be encouraged within the structure of a gross motor program. In this setting, the child could be provided with the opportunity to explore various types of apparatus and the exercises that would suit each apparatus. In this situation, it is important that such children do not feel that they are competing with their peers. In addition, following the lesson, a child should be required to give the instructor some verbal feedback and perhaps accompanying demonstrations regarding the activities that have transpired.

13. Teach the child how to use age-appropriate aids to reach a specific goal.

One potential "aid" for an older child with NLD is a hand calculator, which can be used to provide the child with a way of checking the accuracy of his or her mechanical arithmetic work. After the child has completed a question independently, he or she can be allowed to redo the same question with a hand calculator. This gives the child a means for checking the accuracy of the answer (as long as the hand calculator is used correctly). If it is found that the solution is incorrect, the child should then be encouraged to rework the question with pen and paper. At the high school level, hand calculators should probably be used whenever possible, so that the adolescent or young adult will develop at least a functional grasp of common mathematical operations and their applications in everyday life situations.

Another aid that can be used, especially for the younger child of this type, is a digital watch. We have found that many such children have difficulty in reading the hands of a traditional clock face, and that this imposes further limitations on their already impoverished appreciation of time concepts. A digital watch is more easily read and can serve as a concrete tool for the teaching of elementary time concepts.

In all of this, there is no substitute for creative approaches to the provision of therapeutic "aids." This is especially the case for the exploitation of the vast potential of computers as prosthetic/therapeutic devices. Programs that allow for appropriate and helpful corrective feedback for difficult academic subjects; those that take the child in a step-by-step fashion through any number of quasi-social and problem-solving situations; those that present material in a systematic, sequenced fashion that draws the child's attention to the process of problem-solving development—all of these and many more dimensions of the creative use of computer software are potentially of considerable benefit for the child and adolescent with NLD.

14. Help the child to gain insight into situations that are easy for him or her and those that are potentially troublesome.

It is important for older children and adolescents with NLD to gain a reasonably realistic view of their capabilities. This is certainly more easily said than done. In this regard, a therapist's expectations always need to be in concert with a child's abilities, since gains in this area may prove to be marginal at best. For instance, a child's practical insight may be limited to "I am good at spelling and have problems with math." However, if the child is provided with consistent and appropriate feedback from concerned and informed adults regarding his or her performances in various kinds of situations, fairly sophisticated insights may develop. This is especially important with respect to perceiving the need to use prelearned strategies in appropriate situations. Furthermore, it is important for children with NLD to learn that they do have some cognitive strengths and that these strengths can be used to advantage in specific situations.

15. Work with all of the child's caregivers to help them with insight and direction regarding the child's most salient development needs.

All of the recommendations that have been made above can be incorporated by all caregivers into their interactions with a child with NLD. We have found that well-motivated caregivers who have an intuitive or learned appreciation of such a child's adaptive strengths and weaknesses most often create a milieu at home or elsewhere in which the child prospers and in which adaptive deficits are minimized. Unfortunately, this ideal caregiver–child relationship is not often found; in consequence, it is often necessary for the concerned professional to assume a major responsibility for guiding the child's principal caregivers. In some cases, it may be advisable and/or necessary to employ highly structured "parenting" programs (e.g., Directive Parental Counseling; Holland, 1983) to assist various caregivers in the habilitational process.

16. Other recommendations.

Among the other specific educational recommendations for a child with NLD are the following:

a. Teach and emphasize reading comprehension skills as soon as the child has gained a functional appreciation of sound–symbol correspondence.

b. Institute regular drills early in the child's educational career to facilitate development of his or her handwriting skills.

c. Before any copying task, teach the child to read the material to be copied carefully.

d. Teach the child (verbal) strategies that will help him or her to organize written work.

e. Teach mechanical arithmetic in a systematic, verbal, step-by-step fashion, as outlined in some detail elsewhere (see above and Strang & Rourke, 1985).

f. Involve the child as much as possible in skill-level-appropriate physical education experiences. With respect to this point, it should be borne in mind that motor learning of all sorts is difficult but necessary for the child with NLD.

Indeed, since such children learn to decode words and spell at superior levels without any appreciable teaching or other assistance, it would be well to substitute various types of "physical" activities during times when word decoding and spelling are being "taught" to classmates.

17. Be cognizant of the therapist's/remedial specialist's role in preparing the child with NLD for adult life.

Special educators, in particular, should assume a major role in preparing the child with NLD for adult life. Unlike most educational programs, in which the primary goal is to help the child to master a particular curriculum, the program required by children with NLD is one that focuses primarily on the development of life skills. A child's mastery of the standard academic curriculum is insignificant if he or she is not prepared to meet the social and other adaptive demands of independent living. Indeed, we have found through longitudinal follow-up that some children with NLD as adults have developed rather seriously debilitating forms of psychopathology. Thus, it is clear that remedial/habilitational interventions with such children should always be consonant with their short- and long-term remedial needs and with their remedial capacities.

A final note

For further information regarding principles of intervention and their applications for the child and adolescent with NLD, the interested reader may wish to consult the following: Cermak and Murray (1992); Foss (1991); Rourke (1985, 1989, 1991); Rourke, Bakker, Fisk, and Strang (1983); Rourke and Del Dotto (1994); Rourke, Fisk, and Strang (1986); Rourke and Fuerst (1991).

REFERENCES

Cermak, S. A., & Murray, E. (1992). Nonverbal learning disabilities in the adult framed in the model of human occupation. In N. Katz (Ed.), *Cognitive rehabilitation models for intervention in occupational therapy* (pp. 258–291). Boston: Andover Medical.

Foss, J. M. (1991). Nonverbal learning disabilities and remedial interventions. *Annals of Dyslexia, 41*, 128–140.

Holland, C. J. (1983). *Directive Parental Counseling: The counselor's guide*. Bloomfield Hills, MI: Midwest Professional Publishing.

Rourke, B. P. (Ed.). (1985). *Neuropsychology of learning disabilities: Essentials of subtype analysis*. New York: Guilford Press.

Rourke, B. P. (1989). *Nonverbal learning disabilities: The syndrome and the model*. New York: Guilford Press.

Rourke, B. P. (Ed.). (1991). *Neuropsychological validation of learning disability subtypes*. New York: Guilford Press.

Rourke, B. P. (1993). *Nonverbal Learning Disabilities Scale*. Unpublished manuscript, University of Windsor, Ontario.

Rourke, B. P., Bakker, D. J., Fisk, J. L., & Strang, J. D. (1983). *Child neuropsychology: An introduction to theory, research, and clinical practice*. New York: Guilford Press.

Rourke, B. P., & Del Dotto, J. E. (1994). *Learning disabilities: A neuropsychological perspective*. Thousand Oaks, CA: Sage.

Rourke, B. P., Fisk, J. L., & Strang, J. D. (1986). *Neuropsychological assessment of children: A treatment-oriented approach*. New York: Guilford Press.

Rourke, B.P., & Fuerst, D. R. (1991). *Learning disabilities and psychosocial functioning: A neuropsychological perspective*. New York: Guilford Press.

Sparrow, S. S., Balla, D. A., & Cicchetti, D. V. (1984). *The Vineland Adaptive Behavior Scales: A revision of the Vineland Social Maturity Scale by Edgar A. Doll*. Circle Pines, MN: American Guidance Service.

Strang, J. D., & Rourke, B. P. (1985). Adaptive behavior of children who exhibit specific arithmetic disabilities and associated neuropsychological abilities and deficits. In B. P. Rourke (Ed.), *Neuropsychology of learning disabilities: Essentials of subtype analysis* (pp. 302–328). New York: Guilford Press.

Index